Atlas of Neuroradiology

Atlas of Neuroradiology

STEVEN J. WILLING, M.D.
Associate Professor of Radiology
University of Alabama at Birmingham
Birmingham, Alabama

W.B. SAUNDERS COMPANY
A Division of Harcourt Brace & Company
PHILADELPHIA LONDON TORONTO
MONTREAL SYDNEY TOKYO

W.B. SAUNDERS COMPANY
A Division of Harcourt Brace & Company

The Curtis Center
Independence Square West
Philadelphia, Pennsylvania 19106

Library of Congress Cataloging-in-Publication Data

Willing, Steven J.
Atlas of neuroradiology / Steven J. Willing. — 1st ed.

p. cm.

ISBN 0–7216–4219–5

1. Nervous system—Radiography—Atlases. I. Title
[DNLM: 1. Brain Diseases—radiography—atlases. 2. Spinal Diseases—radiography—atlases. 3. Head—radiography—atlases. WL 17 W733a 1995]

RC349.R3W54 1995 616.8'04757—dc20

DNLM/DLC 95-4087

ATLAS OF NEURORADIOLOGY ISBN 0–7216–4219–5

Printed in the United States of America

Last digit is the print number: 9 8 7 6 5 4 3 2 1

Preface

Textbooks come in many forms. Some are comprehensive and scholarly, and used mostly for reference. Others are written to teach, offering a thorough treatment of their chosen subject and assuming little knowledge on the part of the reader. This book is written to be used—as an easy "viewbox" reference in the day-to-day practice of neuroradiology, with attention to differential diagnosis. It assumes that the reader is already acquainted with the necessary understanding of anatomy and examination techniques. This book is also designed for radiology residents, who are preparing for oral boards, and for neurologists, otolaryngologists, and neurosurgeons, who are in training or practice.

My intent has also been to present the neuroimaging features of the most significant and common disease states with an approach to differential diagnosis. To this end, the emphasis is on illustration rather than explanation. Those of us who are visually oriented find a picture is superior to a thousand words—it takes less time to assimilate. Although some clinical information is presented, it is purposefully concise.

There are many subjects that beg to be included here but are beyond the purpose and scope of this volume. The user will not find herein any systematic discussion of normal anatomy or examination technique or extensive bibliographies. Many less common conditions have been omitted entirely, as I have chosen to concentrate on those most frequently encountered. Fractures (craniofacial, spinal) have been excluded for the most part, because there is seldom doubt in their differential diagnosis. Fractures are basically skeletal, not neurologic or otolaryngologic, conditions.

I have endeavored to include all imaging modalities essential to the practice of neurodiagnosis, including MRI, CT, myelography, angiography, and sonography. In the era of MRI, the role of CT and myelography has diminished. In certain cases, their inclusion herein may seem anachronistic; however, both techniques remain in wide use and indeed offer their own unique anatomic perspective, at times complementing the corresponding MRI findings.

Completing each chapter is a list of recommended readings that amplify the material presented. I have tried to select articles that represent the largest series, the most recent series, or the most comprehensive discussion. My deliberate intent has been to focus on current radiologic journals, so that the references may be easily accessible to most practicing radiologists.

I hope you will find this book useful in your daily practice.

STEVEN J. WILLING, M.D.

Acknowledgments

Heartfelt thanks are extended to all those who assisted in the preparation of this volume. The cases illustrated herein were accumulated from many sources. Special thanks to Dr. Stuart Royal of the Children's Hospital of Birmingham and Dr. Betty Brooks of the Mulberry Diagnostic Imaging Center for allowing me free access to their teaching collections. Over a dozen colleagues contributed individual cases for this volume. Particular thanks go to Drs. Taher El Gammal, Alan Lovell, Loretta Shearer, and Pamela Van Tassel for their many contributions.

Virtually all of the photography herein is the product of our department photographer, Mr. Tony Zagar, whose hard work and patience eased this project to its completion.

Deep appreciation is extended to all of my colleagues in Neurology, Neurosurgery, and Otolaryngology at the University of Alabama at Birmingham, who skillfully and compassionately cared for most of the patients illustrated herein and who honor us with their referrals for neuroimaging.

Contents

CHAPTER **ONE**

General Manifestations of Intracranial Diseases

TABLE 1–1 | Types of Cerebral Edema

Type	Causes	Location	Differential	Pathology
Interstitial	Hydrocephalus	Periventricular white matter	Ischemic leukoencephalopathy Periventricular leukomalacia	Escape of CSF through ependyma into extracellular space
Vasogenic	Tumor Inflammation Acute demyelination Infarction	White matter tracts	Gliosis Ischemic encephalopathy	Defective blood-brain barrier with increase in extracellular water
Cytotoxic	Anoxia Toxins	Gray and/or white matter	Tumor	Failure of sodium pump with intracellular edema but normal extracellular space

Edema

Edema is a condition of increased tissue water. The essential imaging findings consist of (1) mass effect and (2) diminished attenuation on computed tomography (CT) or hyperintensity on T2-weighted magnetic resonance imaging (MRI). There are three forms of edema: vasogenic, cytotoxic, and interstitial, which are summarized in Table 1–1.

Vasogenic Edema

Vasogenic edema is the accumulation of water in the extracellular compartment of the brain, usually resulting from disruption of the blood-brain barrier. The usual causes are neoplasms, especially metastatic, and inflammation. Its characteristic appearance is the presence of diminished attenuation on CT (hyperintensity on T2-weighted MRI), which conforms to white matter tracts and accentuates the gray-white junction. Low attenuation limited to the white matter, however, is not specific (Table 1–2). Vasogenic edema causes mass effect, whereas other common causes of white matter attenuation or signal abnormality (atrophy, gliosis, demyelination) result in parenchymal loss (negative mass effect). Intravenous contrast helps in many instances, as the pathologic processes underlying vasogenic edema (tumor, abscess) frequently enhance with contrast, whereas most other causes of diminished attenuation do not. Most radiologically apparent edema is vasogenic in nature, including that resulting from cerebral infarction.

Cytotoxic Edema

Cytotoxic edema is the presence of increased intracellular water due to a toxic or anoxic insult leading to failure of the sodium-ATPase pump. The usual cause is acute ischemic infarction. In the first few hours of cerebral infarction cytotoxic edema produces mild effacement of sulci with subtle or indetectable signal alterations on MRI. Established infarction, containing both cytotoxic and vasogenic edema, appears as homogeneous low attenuation on CT and hyperintensity on T2-weighted MRI affecting both gray and white matter, usually in a recognizable vascular distribution. Diffusion-weighted MRI is a promising technique for the diagnosis of pure cytotoxic edema. With this technique, normal diffusion causes signal loss, whereas areas of diminished diffusion associated with cytotoxic edema appear hyperintense.

TABLE 1–2 | Pathologic Correlates of White Matter Hypodensity (CT)/Hyperintensity (T2-Weighted MRI)

Normal
Immature brain
Edema
Inflammation (abscess, encephalitis) Primary neoplasm Metastases Acute ischemia Diffuse axonal injury
Gliosis/Encephalomalacia
Surgery Trauma Chronic ischemia
Atrophy
Enlarged perivascular spaces Chronic ischemia
Abnormal Myelin
Multiple sclerosis Other demyelinating diseases Aging related demyelination Dysmyelinating diseases
Replacement
Astrocytoma Hamartoma

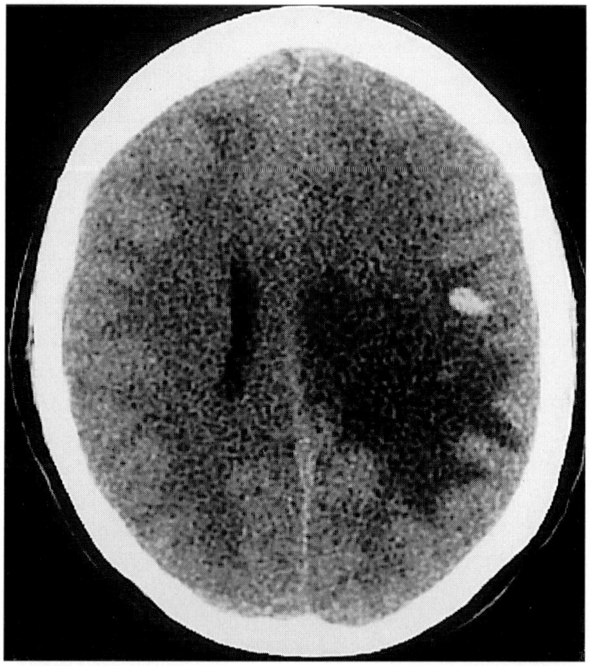

Figure 1–1. Vasogenic edema. CT shows enhancing metastasis at the gray-white junction on the left. Marked vasogenic edema is confined to the white matter and accentuates the gray-white junction.

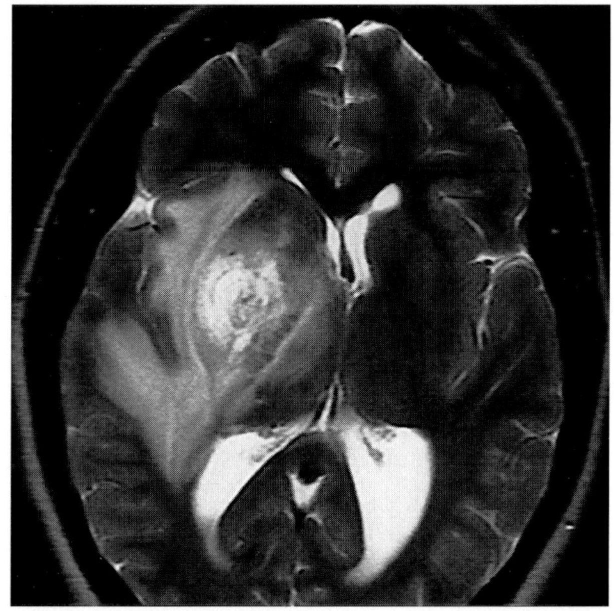

Figure 1–2. Vasogenic edema due to mass in lentiform nuclei. Marked vasogenic edema is present in right internal and external capsules and temporal lobe white matter. There is sparing of insular gray matter.

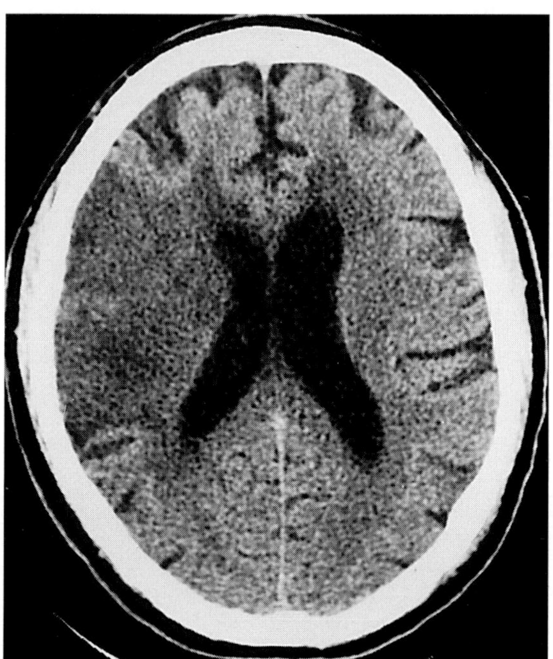

Figure 1–3. Cytotoxic edema (acute right middle cerebral infarction). There is diminished attenuation of gray and white matter of the right frontal lobe with loss of the gray-white junction. Most of the observed hypodensity is due to the vasogenic component of edema.

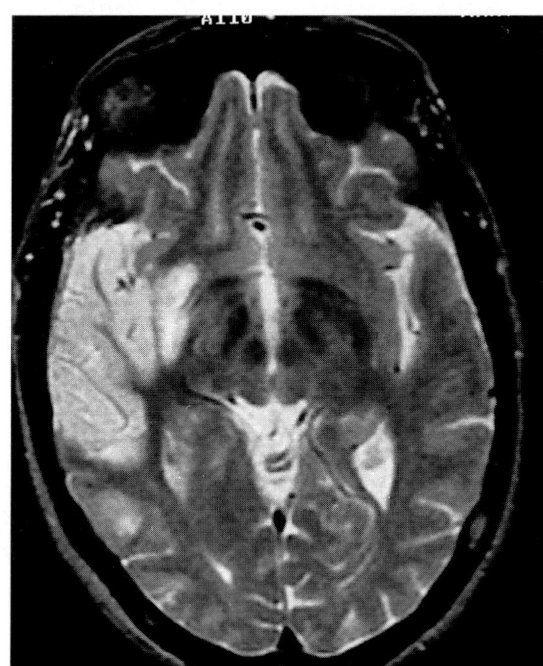

Figure 1–4. Cytotoxic edema (acute right middle cerebral infarction). There is marked hyperintensity of the right basal ganglia, insular cortex, and anterior temporal lobe affecting both gray and white matter. Most of the observed hyperintensity is due to the vasogenic component of edema.

Infarction Versus Tumor

The diagnosis is often evident from the clinical presentation, since infarction usually occurs with the abrupt onset of a neurologic deficit, whereas symptoms of tumor are more gradual in onset. Anatomic conformity to a classic vascular distribution supports the diagnosis of infarction. The finding of gray matter involvement helps to distinguish infarction from vasogenic edema of other causes, as does the use of intravenous contrast. The differentiation of infarction from neoplasm still may remain problematic, particularly if the tumor does not enhance or the infarct is subacute and does enhance. In unresolved cases, it may be helpful to repeat the examination in 4 to 6 weeks. By that time, mass effect due to infarction should be diminished or resolved, whereas that due to untreated tumor will be static or increased.

Interstitial Edema

Interstitial edema is the presence of increased water in the periventricular white matter due to hydrocephalus. It appears as a rim of low attenuation or hyperintensity surrounding the lateral ventricles, whose walls may become indistinct. Ependymal tears due to extreme stretching of the ventricular walls with subsequent leakage of cerebrospinal fluid (CSF) are regarded as the underlying mechanism.

It sometimes can be difficult to distinguish hydrocephalus with interstitial edema from ischemic leukoencephalopathy, atrophy, and ventricular dilatation ex vacuo. The diagnosis of hydrocephalus should not rest solely on the finding of enlarged ventricles with periventricular hyperintensity. Additional findings should be present to make the diagnosis of hydrocephalus, which is addressed later in this chapter. (See also Ischemic Leukoencephalopathy, Chapter 5.)

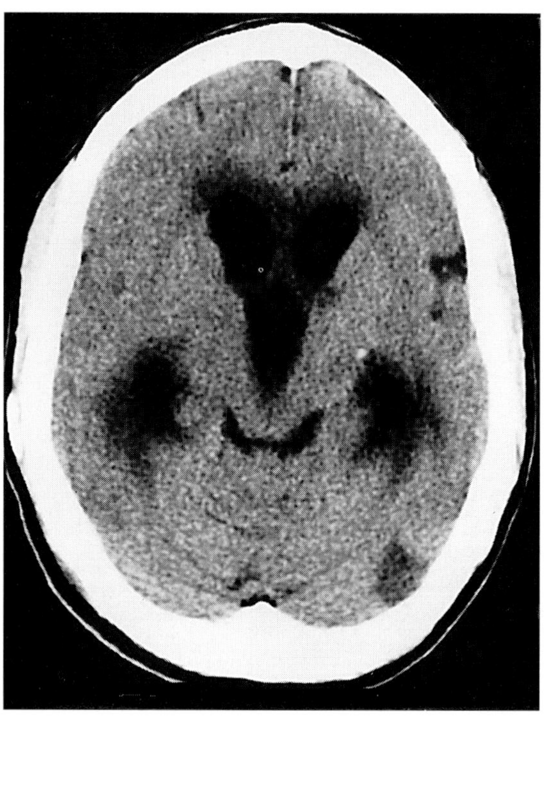

Figure 1–5. Interstitial edema. Axial CT shows hydrocephalus with bilateral, diffuse, and symmetric periventricular low attenuation and blurring of the ventricular margins.

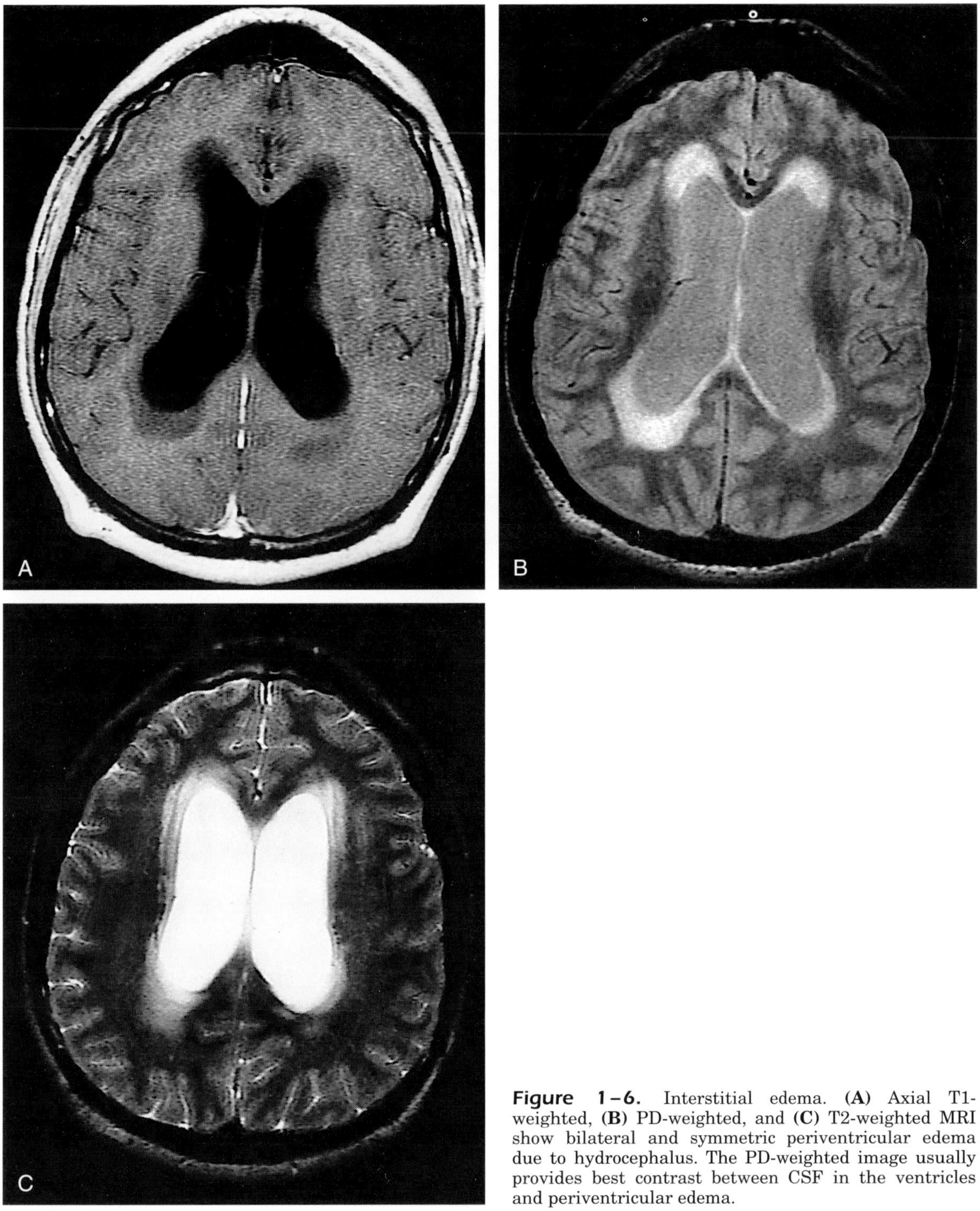

Figure 1–6. Interstitial edema. **(A)** Axial T1-weighted, **(B)** PD-weighted, and **(C)** T2-weighted MRI show bilateral and symmetric periventricular edema due to hydrocephalus. The PD-weighted image usually provides best contrast between CSF in the ventricles and periventricular edema.

Mass Localization

Before an accurate differential diagnosis can be given for an intracranial mass, it must first be correctly determined whether the mass is intraaxial (within the brain or ventricles) or extraaxial (arising outside the brain). The ability to localize a mass within the brain is less critical to the diagnosis but essential to treatment.

Extraaxial Versus Intraaxial

The useful criteria for differentiating extraaxial from intraaxial mass lesions are listed in Table 1–3. The following two criteria are unreliable in making this determination:

1. Vasogenic edema of adjacent white matter. Although usually associated with intraaxial pathology, vasogenic edema is common with meningiomas and may be encountered with other extraaxial masses.
2. Direct contiguity and broad interface with brain surface, meninges, or inner table. Although usually regarded as evidence of an extraaxial mass, this finding is common with superficial glioblastomas and a characteristic feature of primary cerebral lymphoma.

Text continued on page 12

TABLE 1–3 | Extraaxial Versus Intraaxial Mass Lesions

Extraaxial	Intraaxial
Bony changes: Hyperostosis (CT) Erosion Remodeling Enlargement of a foramen Interruption of inner table signal void (MRI) Thickened bone with increased or decreased signal intensity (T1-weighted MRI)	Bony changes extremely rare
Displacement of pial vessels away from inner table, falx, or tentorium	Vessels displaced toward or flattened against inner table, falx, or tentorium
Invasion of a dural sinus	Sinus invasion extremely rare
White matter buckling	Infiltration and replacement of gray and white matter
Widening of subarachnoid space adjacent to tumor	Subarachnoid space effaced
Dural tail sign (thickening and enhancement of adjacent meninges with smooth tapering away from tumor)	Dural tail rare but occasionally occurs with superficial malignant lesions (glioblastoma and metastases)
Tumor on both sides of falx in absence of commissural involvement	May cross midline via corpus callosum, especially glioblastoma and lymphoma
Hypointense rim at interface of brain with tumor due to CSF (T1-weighted MRI)	Indistinct interface of tumor with brain
Very thin rim of enhancement at tumor-brain interface due to enhancing meninges (seen with nonenhancing lesions such as dermoids and epidermoids)	If ring enhancing, enhancing wall tends to be thick
Tumor on both sides of the tentorium in absence of brainstem involvement	Cerebral and cerebellar hemispheric tumors do not cross the tentorium Brainstem and pineal region tumors may bridge the tentorial incisura

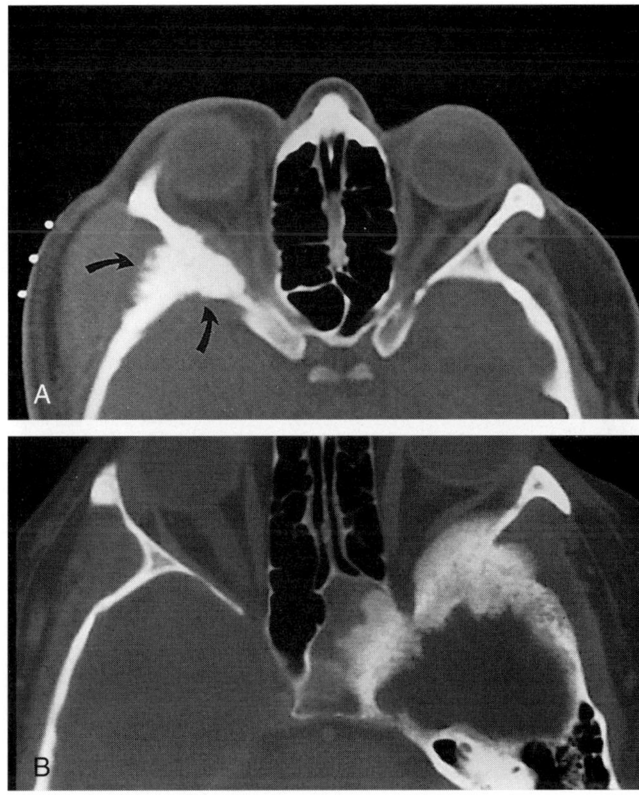

Figure 1–7. Hyperostosis of sphenoid wing. **(A)** CT shows thickening and sclerosis of right greater sphenoid wing (arrows) due to extracranial meningioma in the right temporal fossa **(B)**. There is dense hyperostosis of the left sphenoid wing due to meningioma.

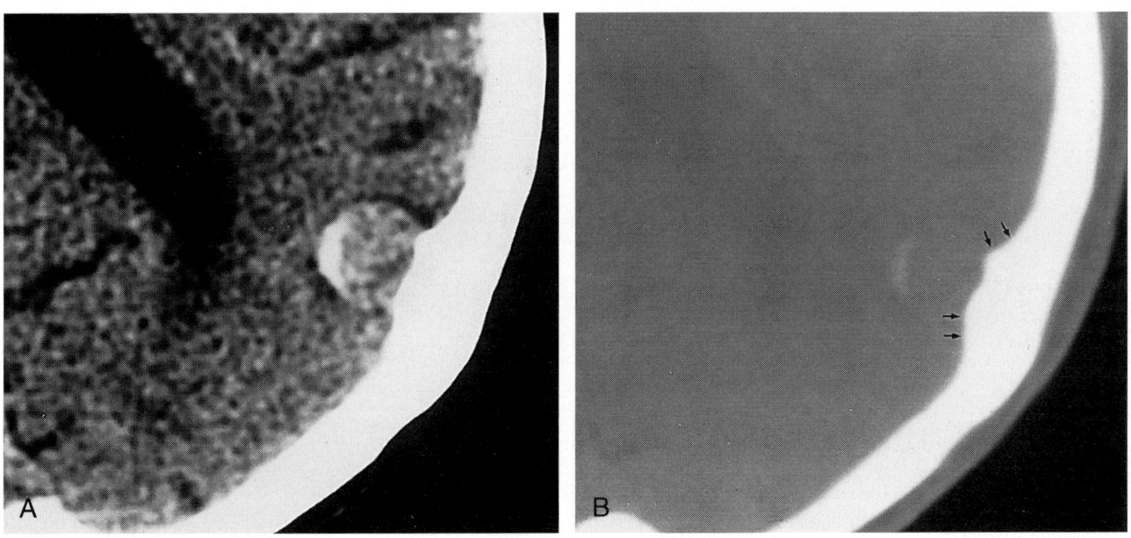

Figure 1–8. Hyperostosis. **(A)** CT soft tissue window and **(B)** bone window show focal thickening of the calvarium (arrows) associated with a small partly calcified meningioma.

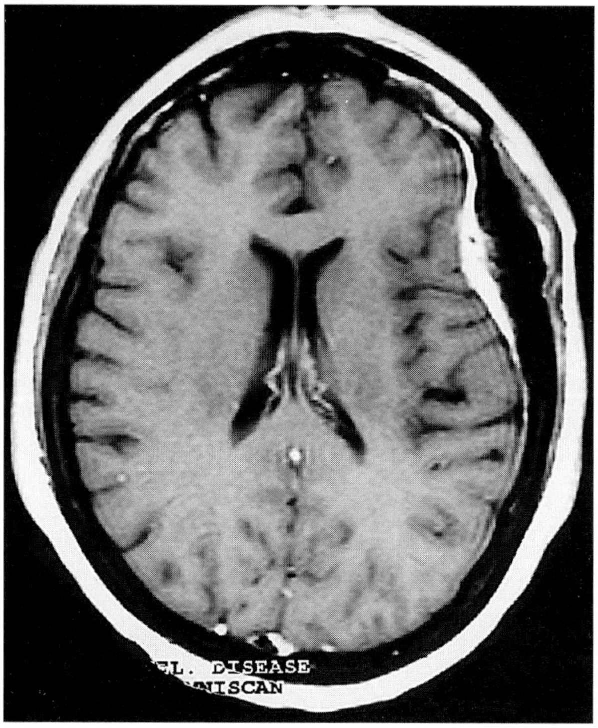

Figure 1–9. Hyperostosis. Contrast-enhanced MRI shows thickening of the skull overlying an en plaque meningioma of the left frontal region. The thickened bone is markedly hypointense and does not enhance, reflecting dense sclerosis and absence of marrow formation.

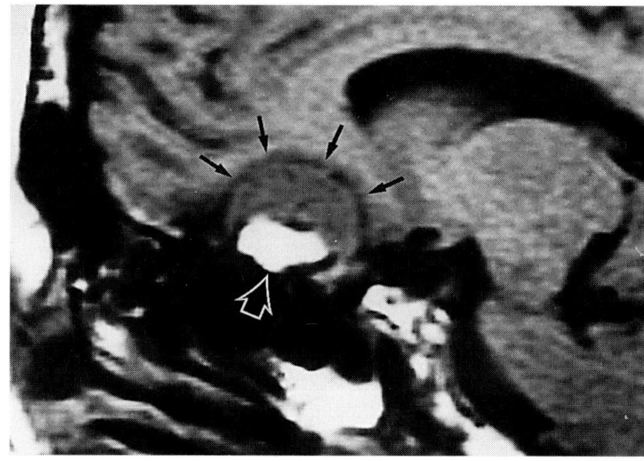

Figure 1–10. Hyperostosis. Sagittal T1-weighted MRI shows a meningioma of the tuberculum sella. The fatty marrow (open arrow) within the hyperostotic bone is markedly hyperintense. The tumor is demarcated above by a thin hypointense rim of CSF (small arrows).

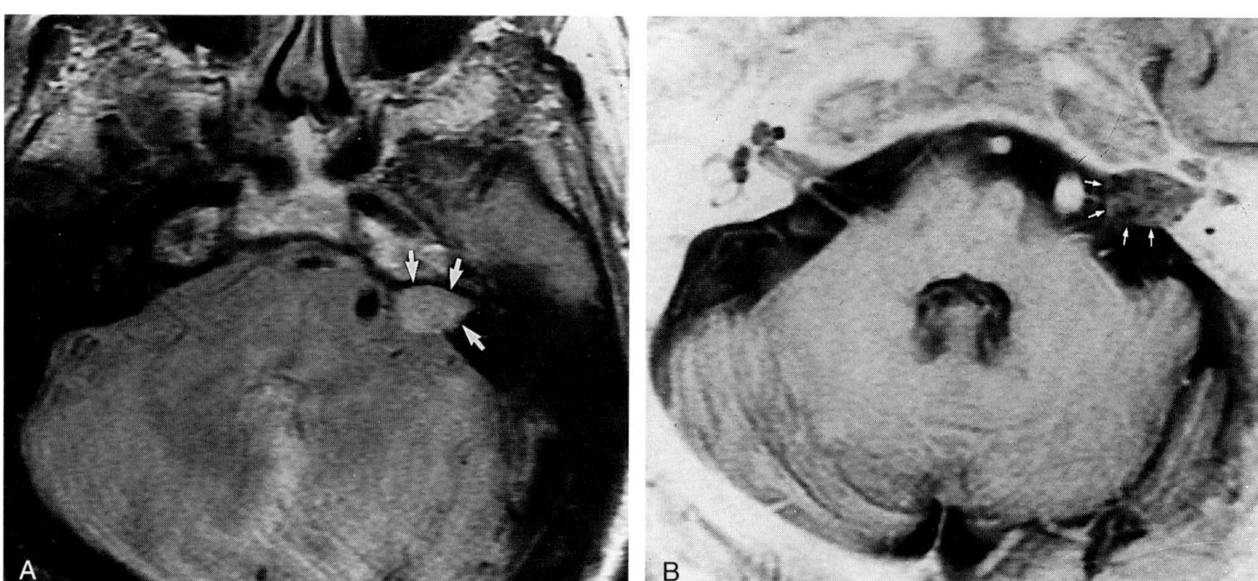

Figure 1–11. Foraminal enlargement (acoustic neuroma). **(A)** Axial PD-weighted MRI shows enlargement of the left internal auditory canal (arrows) and a hyperintense mass. **(B)** MR cisternogram shows capping of the tumor (arrows) by CSF in the cerebellopontine angle cistern.

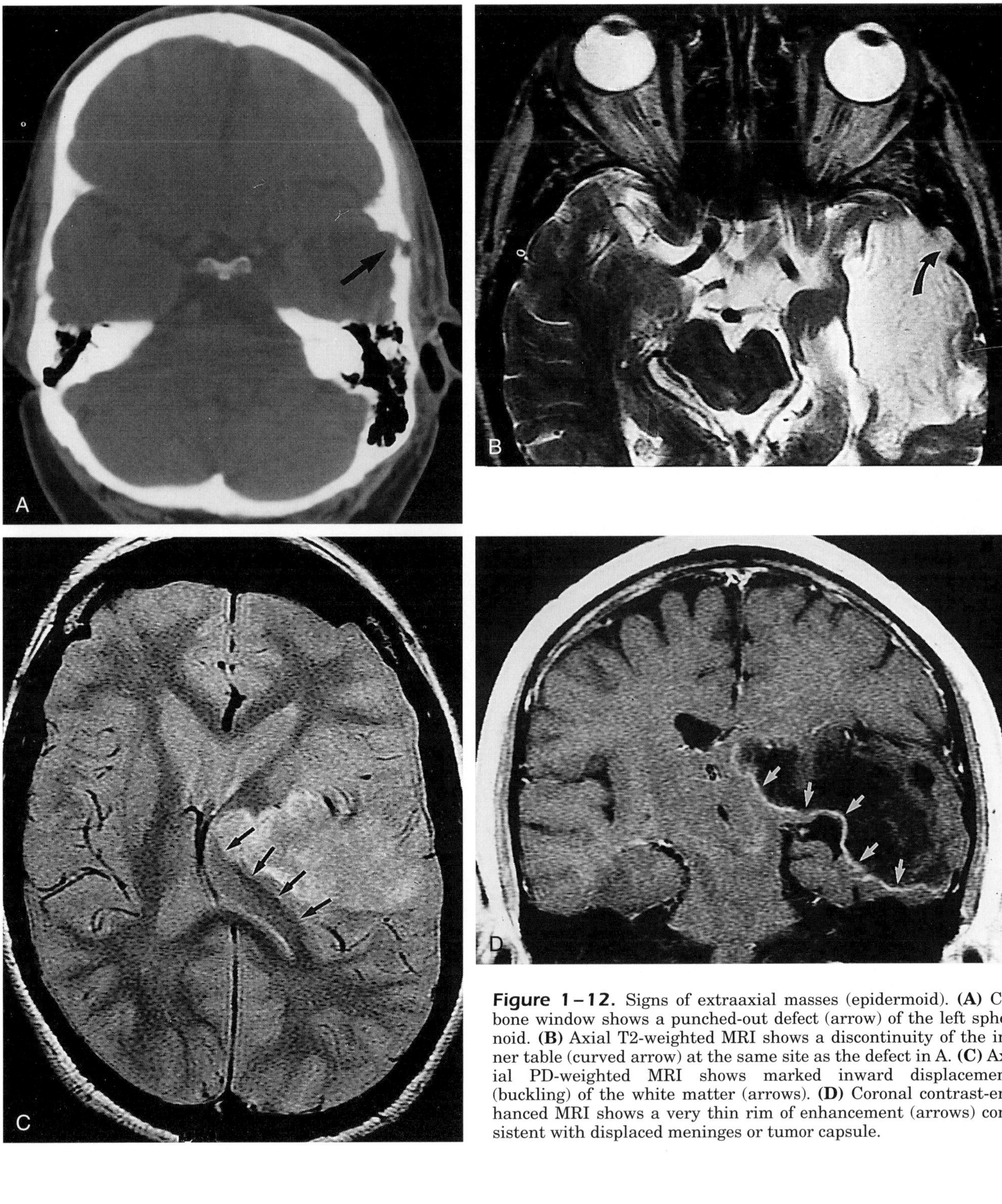

Figure 1–12. Signs of extraaxial masses (epidermoid). **(A)** CT bone window shows a punched-out defect (arrow) of the left sphenoid. **(B)** Axial T2-weighted MRI shows a discontinuity of the inner table (curved arrow) at the same site as the defect in A. **(C)** Axial PD-weighted MRI shows marked inward displacement (buckling) of the white matter (arrows). **(D)** Coronal contrast-enhanced MRI shows a very thin rim of enhancement (arrows) consistent with displaced meninges or tumor capsule.

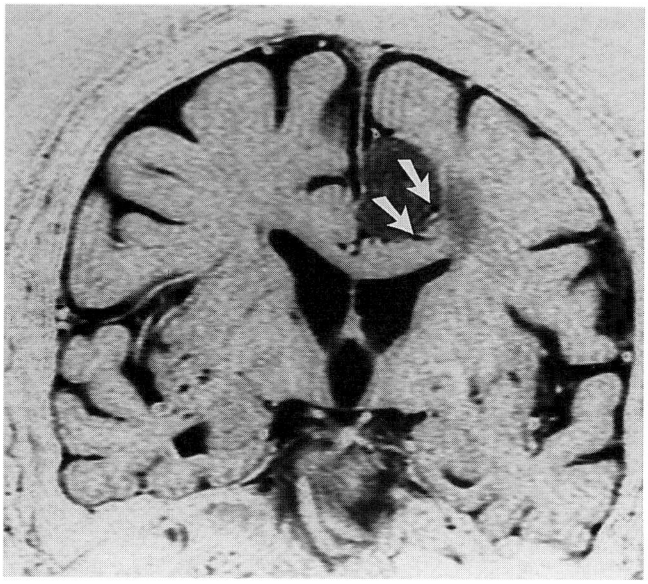

Figure 1–13. Displaced pial vessels. Coronal MR cisternogram shows pial vessels (arrows) displaced by falcine meningioma.

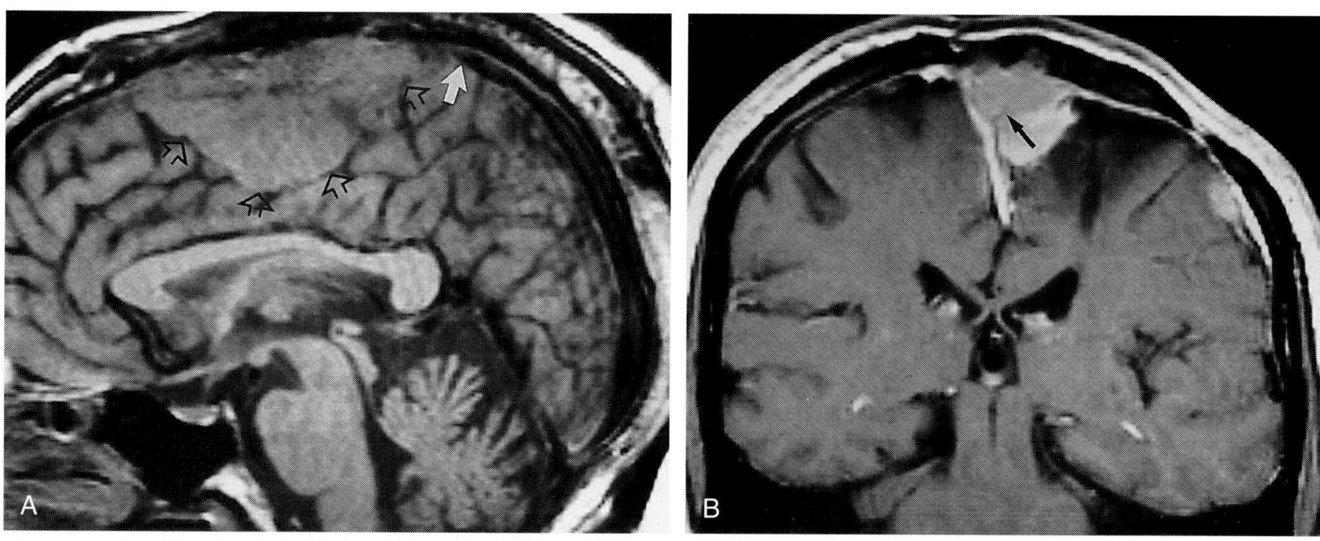

Figure 1–14. Invasion of the sagittal sinus. **(A)** There is occlusion of the superior sagittal sinus due to a parasagittal meningioma (open arrows). Note the discontinuity of the normal sinus flow void, which resumes (arrow) posterior to the mass. **(B)** Coronal contrast-enhanced MR shows replacement of the sagittal sinus by tumor (arrow).

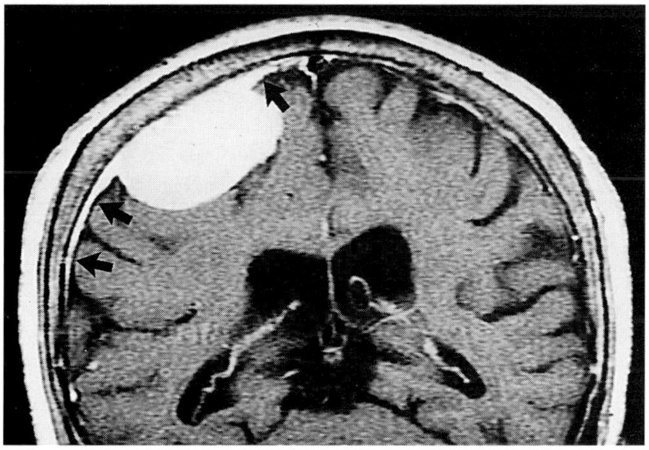

Figure 1–15. Dural tail sign. Arrows show tapered thickening of enhanced meninges adjoining a convexity meningioma.

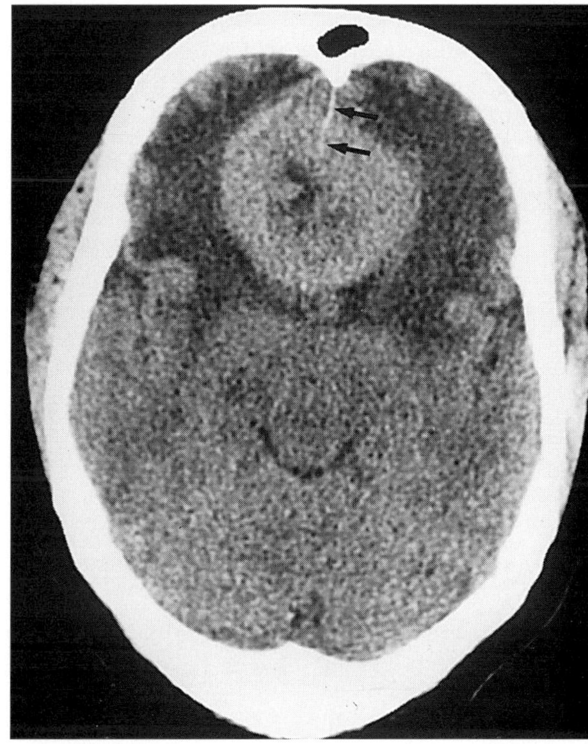

Figure 1–16. Tumor on both sides of falx. A large falcine meningioma spans both anterior fossae, causing edema in both frontal lobes. Arrows indicate the anterior falx.

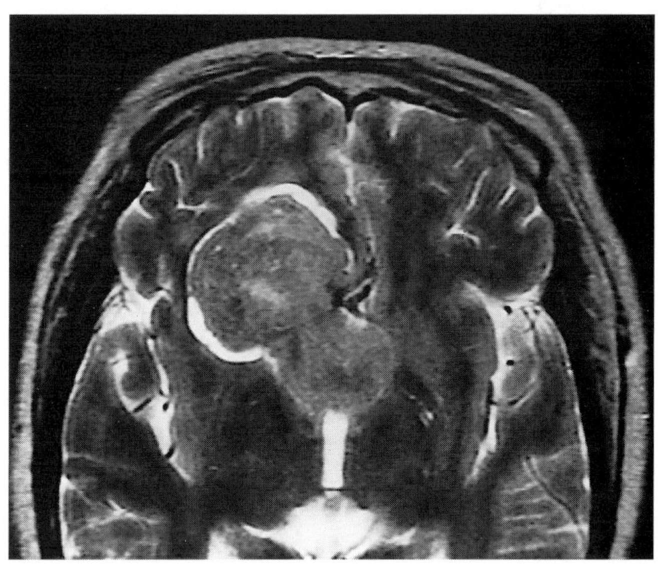

Figure 1–17. CSF rim sign. Axial T2-weighted MRI shows a hyperintense rim of CSF surrounding a large pituitary adenoma.

Lobar Localization

Precise localization of cortical pathology is most readily accomplished with sagittal and coronal MRI. Many lobar boundaries are distinctly marked by sulci or fissures. Some lack distinct surface landmarks, however, such as the boundaries between occipital and temporal lobes, the lateral boundary between occipital and parietal lobes, and the posterior boundary between parietal and temporal lobes.

On a lateral view of the cerebral hemispheres, the boundaries between lobes are marked by the following structures:

Lobe	Boundaries
Frontal	Sylvian fissure
	Central sulcus
Parietal	Sylvian fissure
	Central sulcus
	Angular gyrus
	(capping superior temporal sulcus)
Temporal	Sylvian fissure

On a median view of the cerebral hemispheres, the boundaries between lobes are marked by the following structures:

Lobe	Boundaries
Frontal	Cingulate sulcus
	Central sulcus
Parietal	Parieto-occipital fissure
	Central sulcus
Occipital	Parieto-occipital fissure
Temporal	No distinctive landmark

Identification of the Central Sulcus

On a midline sagittal MRI, the central sulcus is the first sulcus anterior to the ascending marginal ramus of the cingulate sulcus. From that point, it can be traced laterally on sequential sections. A method described by Iwasaki et al enables identification of the central sulcus from axial sections (CT or MRI), using the medullary pattern of hemispheric white matter. On a lateral parasagittal image through the sylvian fissure, the central sulcus is the second fissure posterior to the anterior ascending ramus (precentral sulcus is the first), as described by Ebeling et al.

The identification of primary motor cortex is critical in the surgical approach of nearby mass lesions. Unfortunately, all imaging-based methods are subject to errors caused by interobserver variation and distortion by mass lesions. Functional methods, such as magnetoencephalography (MEG), may provide the most accurate localization of specific areas.

Herniations

An intracranial mass of sufficient size will result in displacement of contiguous cerebral structures into adjoining anatomic compartments. This causes pressure effects on the adjacent brain and vascular structures, which may result in cerebral injury, hemorrhage, or infarction. Most cases are due to intracranial hemorrhages, especially post-traumatic, and neoplasms. The imaging features of the various forms of herniation are listed next. Not all findings must be present to establish a diagnosis. Certain findings, such as secondary infarctions, occur only in advanced cases.

Subfalcine Herniation

- Herniation of cingulate gyrus beneath free edge of falx cerebri
- Compression of ipsilateral lateral ventricle
- Enlargement of contralateral lateral ventricle (due to obstruction of foramen of Monro)
- Anterior cerebral territory infarctions (due to compression of callosomarginal artery against falx)

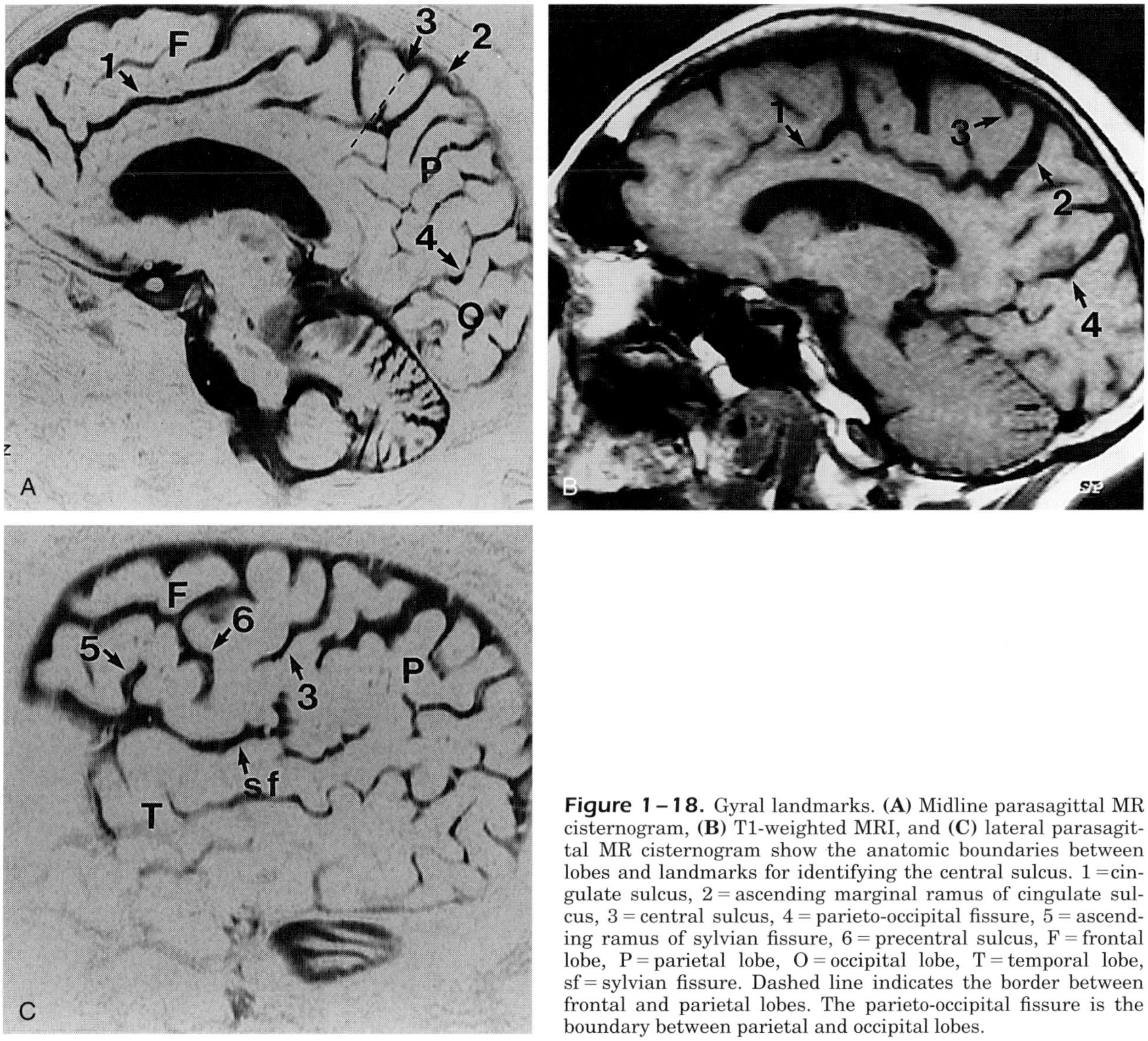

Figure 1–18. Gyral landmarks. **(A)** Midline parasagittal MR cisternogram, **(B)** T1-weighted MRI, and **(C)** lateral parasagittal MR cisternogram show the anatomic boundaries between lobes and landmarks for identifying the central sulcus. 1 = cingulate sulcus, 2 = ascending marginal ramus of cingulate sulcus, 3 = central sulcus, 4 = parieto-occipital fissure, 5 = ascending ramus of sylvian fissure, 6 = precentral sulcus, F = frontal lobe, P = parietal lobe, O = occipital lobe, T = temporal lobe, sf = sylvian fissure. Dashed line indicates the border between frontal and parietal lobes. The parieto-occipital fissure is the boundary between parietal and occipital lobes.

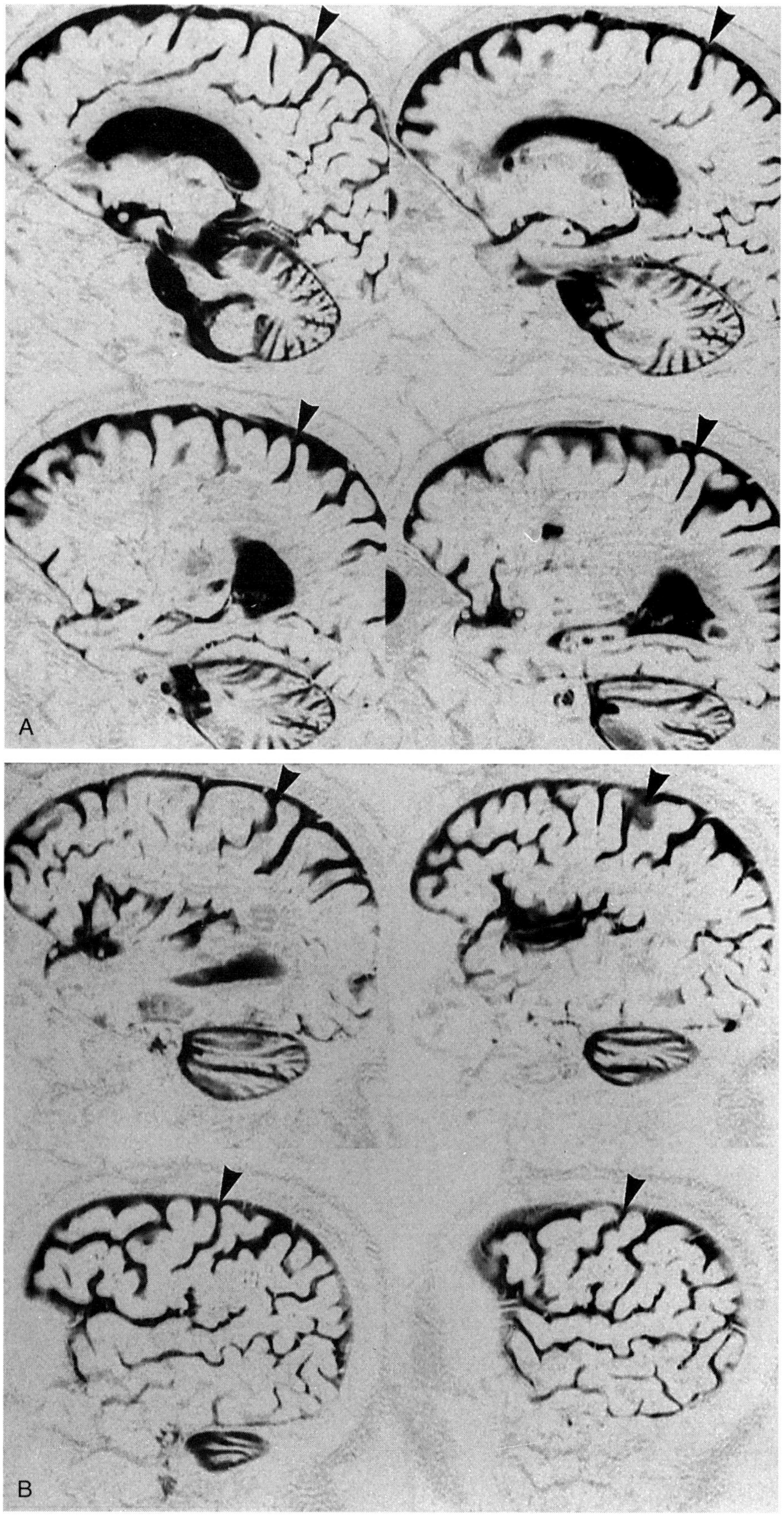

Figure 1–19. Localization of central sulcus. **(A,B)** Sagittal MRI cisternogram shows the position of the central sulcus (arrowheads), which may be localized by midline or lateral landmarks and traced back.

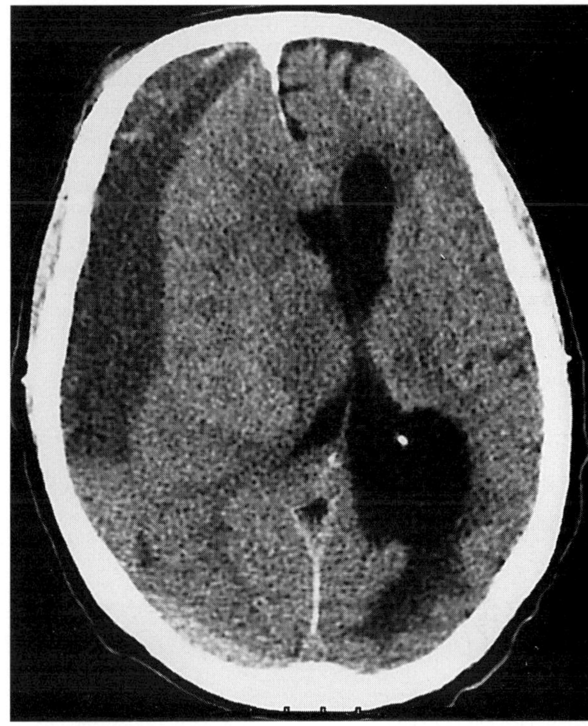

Figure 1–20. Subfalcine herniation. Axial CT shows contralateral displacement of the right lateral ventricle due to a large subdural hematoma.

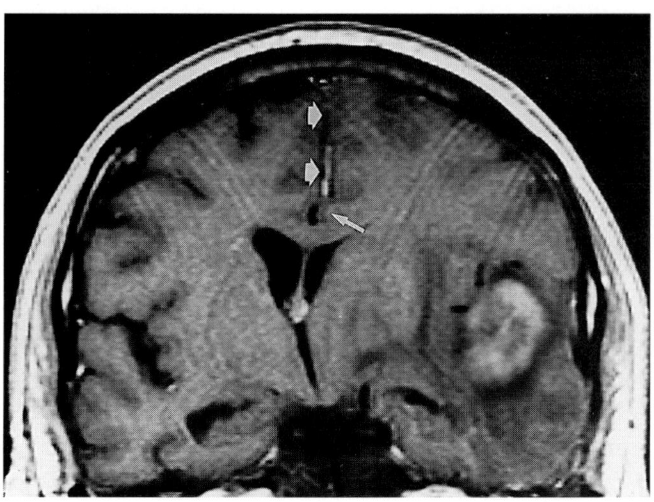

Figure 1–21. Subfalcine herniation (temporal lobe astrocytoma). Coronal contrast-enhanced MRI shows herniation of the left cingulate gyrus (long arrow) beneath the falx (short arrows).

Descending Transtentorial Herniation

- Herniation of uncus and parahippocampal gyrus across free edge of tentorium into posterior fossa
- Rotation or displacement of brainstem
- Enlargement of ipsilateral cerebellopontine angle cistern
- Flattening of ipsilateral suprasellar cistern (early)
- Obliteration of suprasellar, parasellar, and interpeduncular cisterns (late)
- Total effacement of subarachnoid spaces
- Anteroposterior elongation of midbrain
- Inferomedial displacement of posterior cerebral artery (PCA)
- PCA infarcts due to compression against edge of tentorium
- Brainstem hemorrhage (Duret's hemorrhages due to stretching of perforating arteries and usually occurring in midline pons and midbrain)
- Kernohan's notch (injury of contralateral cerebral peduncle due to compression against edge of tentorium)
- Contralateral hydrocephalus

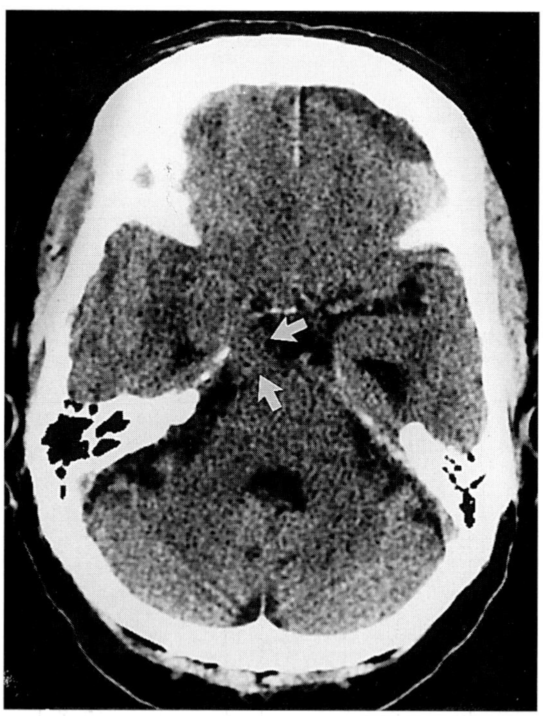

Figure 1–22. Transtentorial herniation (subdural hematoma). The herniated uncus (arrows) is seen in cross section on CT at the level of the suprasellar cistern.

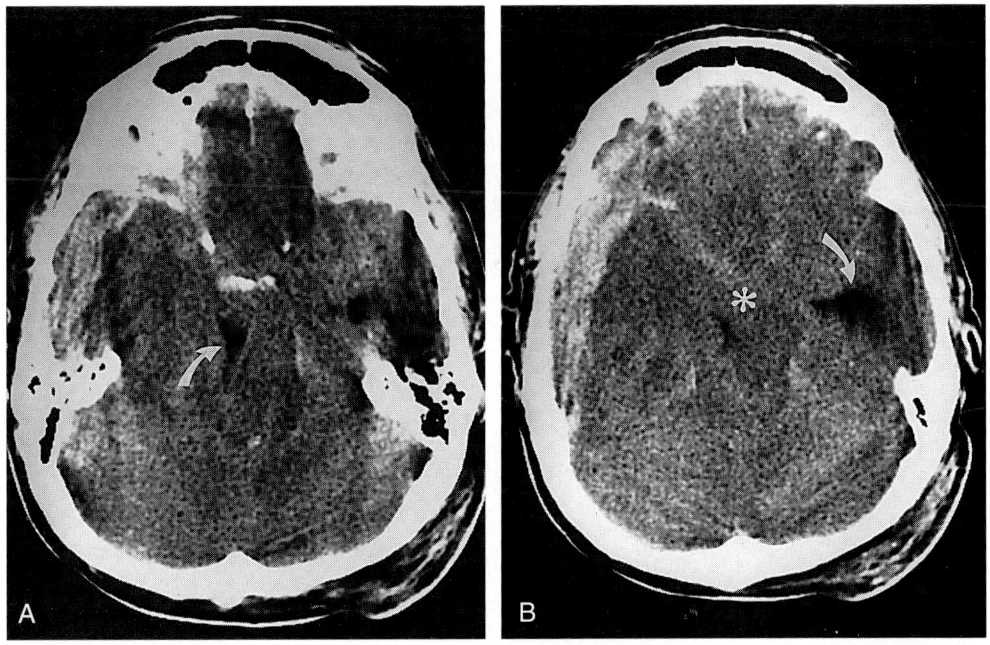

Figure 1–23. Transtentorial herniation (right subdural hematoma). **(A)** CT shows enlargement of the ipsilateral ambient cistern (arrow) due to contralateral brainstem displacement. **(B)** Scan at higher level shows obliteration of the suprasellar cistern (asterisk) and quadri-geminal cistern and dilatation of the contralateral temporal horn (arrow).

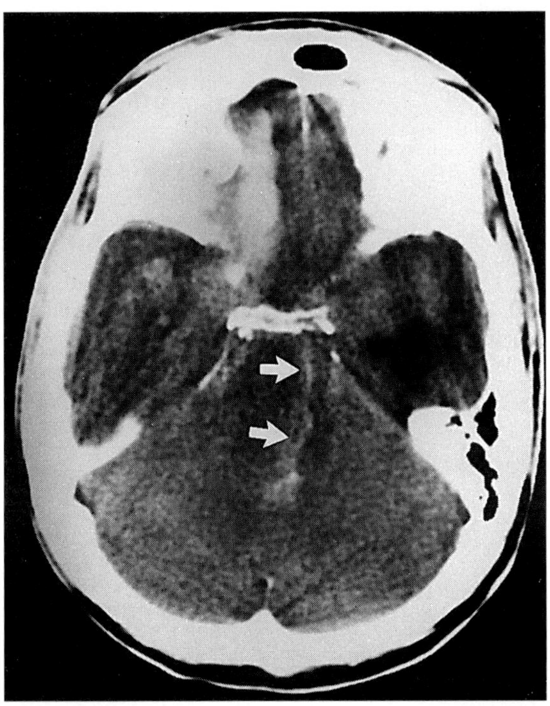

Figure 1–24. Transtentorial herniation (right subdural hematoma). CT shows hemorrhage in the pons (arrows). This probably represents Duret's hemorrhages, although similar hemorrhages may result from tentorial impingement (Kernohan's notch).

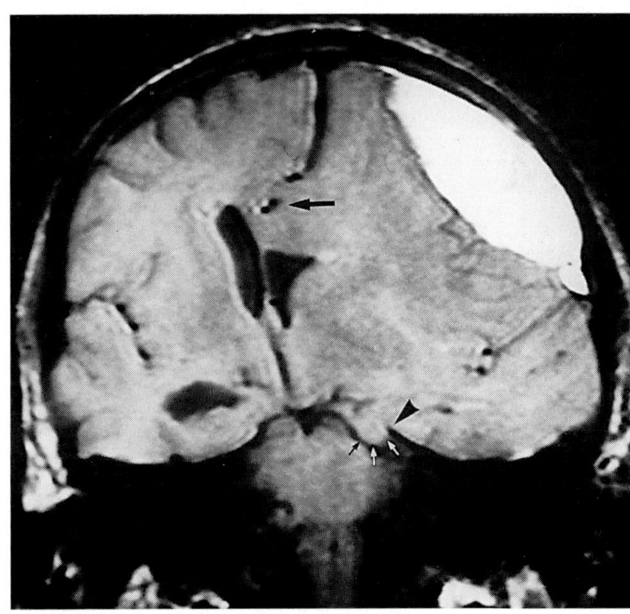

Figure 1–25. Transtentorial herniation (subacute subdural hematoma). Coronal T1-weighted MRI allows direct visualization of the herniated uncus (small arrows). Arrowhead marks the free edge of the tentorium. Note the marked contralateral displacement of anterior cerebral arteries (long arrow) due to subfalcine herniation.

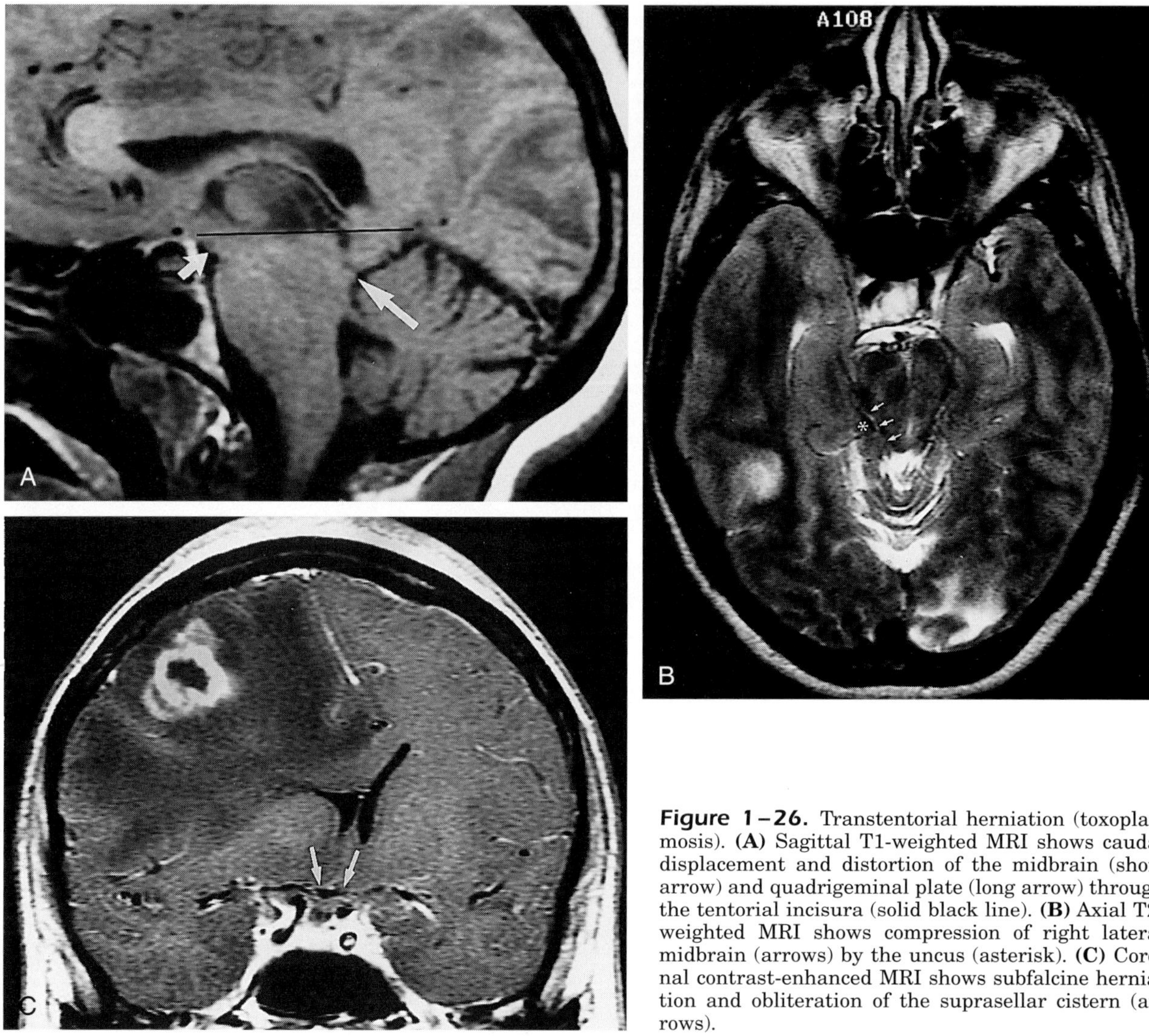

Figure 1–26. Transtentorial herniation (toxoplasmosis). **(A)** Sagittal T1-weighted MRI shows caudal displacement and distortion of the midbrain (short arrow) and quadrigeminal plate (long arrow) through the tentorial incisura (solid black line). **(B)** Axial T2-weighted MRI shows compression of right lateral midbrain (arrows) by the uncus (asterisk). **(C)** Coronal contrast-enhanced MRI shows subfalcine herniation and obliteration of the suprasellar cistern (arrows).

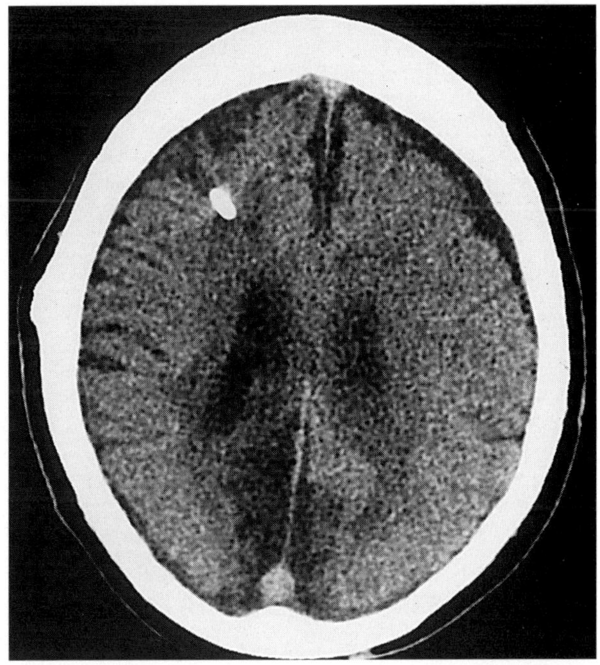

Figure 1–27. Transtentorial herniation. Axial CT shows bilateral chronic PCA infarcts due to previous episode of herniation (head trauma with diffuse axonal injury and edema).

Ascending Transtentorial Herniation

- Upward herniation of vermis and cerebellar hemispheres through tentorial incisura
- Distortion or effacement of quadrigeminal and superior cerebellar cisterns
- Hydrocephalus due to compression of aqueduct
- Posterior flattening of third ventricle
- Anterior displacement of brainstem
- Obliteration of pontine cisterns

Tonsillar Herniation

- Herniation of cerebellar tonsils through foramen magnum (normal tonsils should not extend more than 3 mm below foramen magnum)
- Obliteration of cisterna magna
- Anterior displacement of medulla
- Effacement of subarachnoid space anterior to tonsils
- Hemorrhage or infarction of tonsils (infrequent)

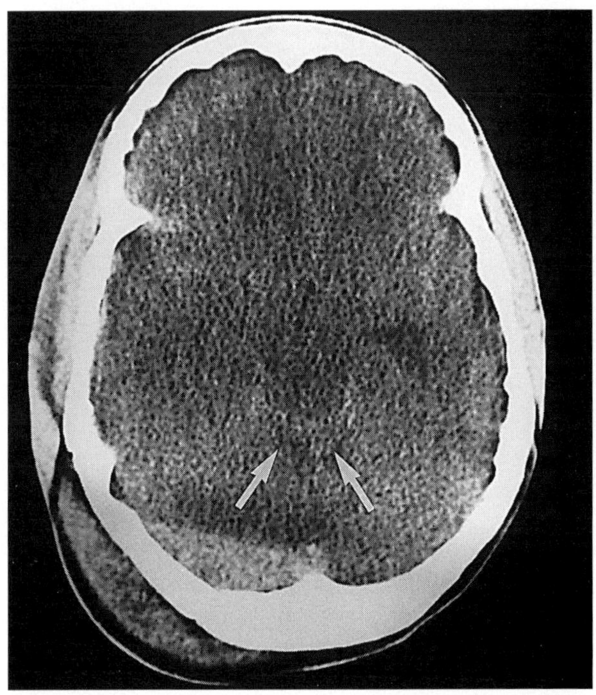

Figure 1–28. Ascending transtentorial herniation (posterior fossa epidural hematoma). CT shows obliteration of the superior cerebellar cistern (arrows) and dilatation of the left temporal horn.

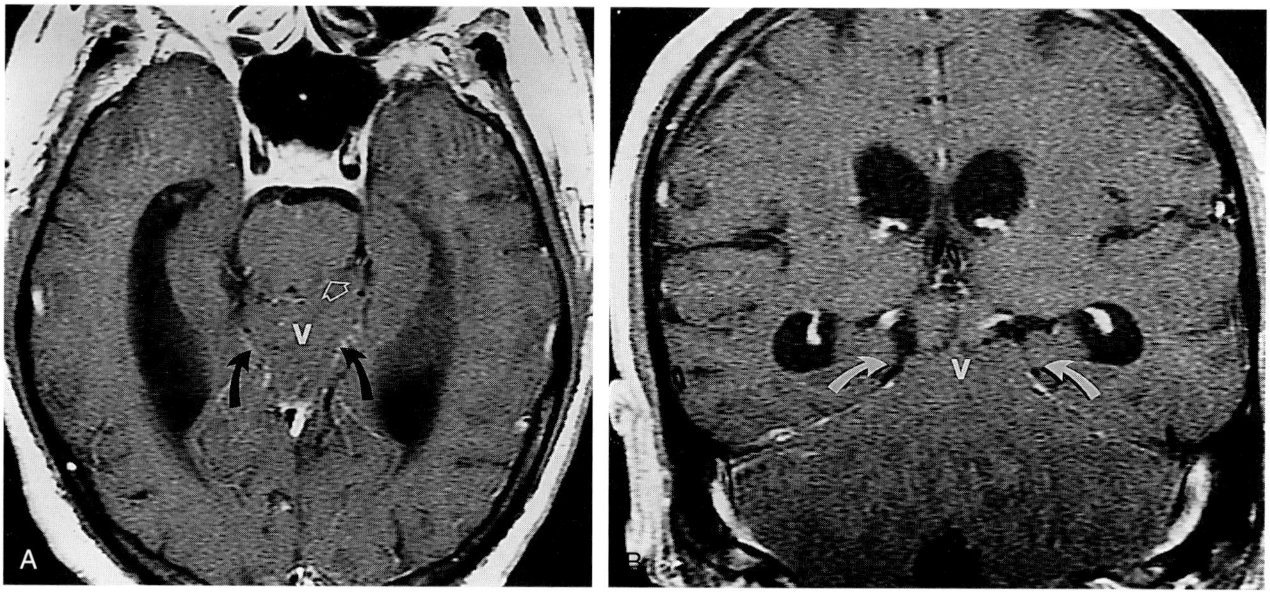

Figure 1–29. Ascending transtentorial herniation (cerebellar metastasis). **(A)** Axial and **(B)** coronal contrast-enhanced MRI show upward herniation of the cerebellar vermis (V) through the tentorial incisura (arrows). Hydrocephalus is present. The herniating vermis displaces and compresses the brainstem (open arrow).

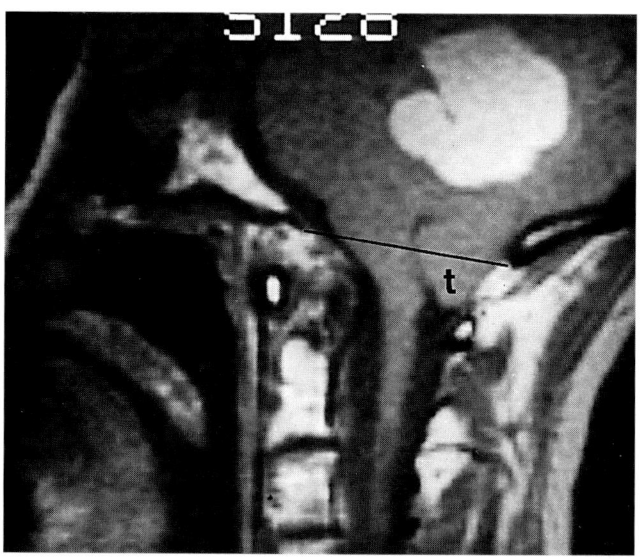

Figure 1–30. Tonsillar herniation (cerebellar metastasis). Sagittal T1-weighted MRI shows a hyperintense cerebellar mass, causing herniation of the tonsils (t) through the foramen magnum (solid line). There is obliteration of the cisterna magna and premedullary cisterns.

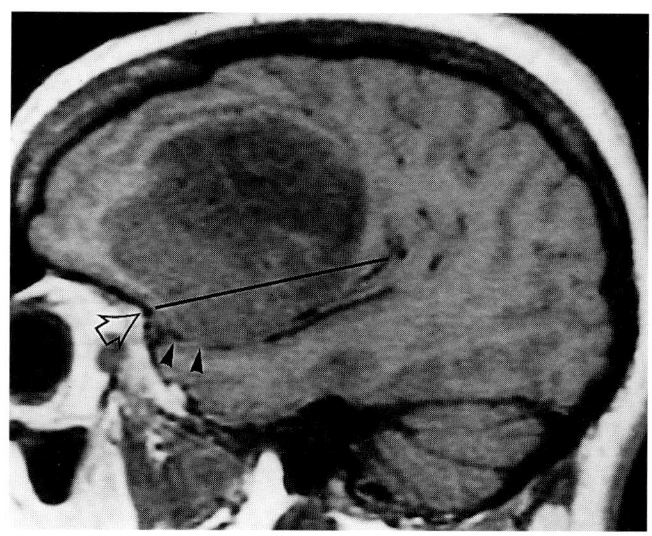

Figure 1–31. Transalar (transsphenoidal) herniation (anaplastic astrocytoma). Sagittal T1-weighted MRI shows downward herniation of the frontal lobe (arrowheads) behind the sphenoid ridge (open arrow). Solid line indicates normal position of sylvian fissure.

Transsphenoidal Herniation

- Descending: posterior herniation of frontal lobe over greater wing of sphenoid
- Ascending: anterior herniation of temporal lobe across sphenoid ridge

Fungus Cerebri

- Herniation of cerebral cortex through traumatic or postoperative skull defect
- Infarction of herniated tissue due to vascular compression

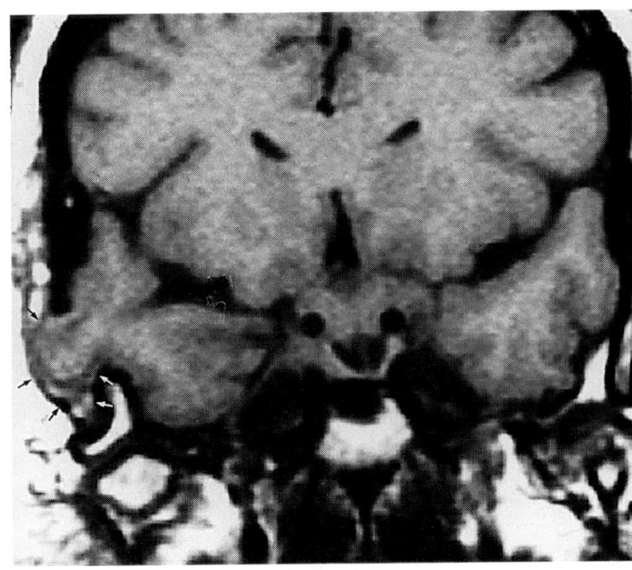

Figure 1–32. Fungus cerebri (pituitary adenoma). Coronal T1-weighted MRI shows herniation of middle temporal gyrus (arrowheads) through a craniotomy defect. No mass effect is present.

Hydrocephalus

Diagnosis

The sine qua non of hydrocephalus is dilatation of the ventricular system; however, the majority of patients with enlarged ventricles have atrophy and not hydrocephalus. The following imaging findings may be present in hydrocephalus and help to distinguish hydrocephalus from atrophy:

1. Ventricular dilatation without, or disproportionately greater than, sulcal enlargement
2. Effacement of cortical sulci
3. Periventricular interstitial edema
4. Dilatation of temporal horns (one of the most sensitive and specific indicators)
5. Rounded third ventricle (walls parallel and straight in atrophy)
6. Ballooning of anterior recesses of third ventricle
7. Mammillopontine distance of less than 10 mm
8. Thinning (less than 6 mm) and elevation of corpus callosum
9. Depression of posterior fornix
10. Narrowing of ventricular angle (remains normal in atrophy)
11. Widening of frontal horn radius (usually smaller in atrophy)
12. Ventricular diverticula, especially through choroid fissure or from posterior third ventricle (rare)

The most problematic cases are those with severe deep atrophy or, at the other extreme, minimally enlarged ventricles. In such circumstances, one cannot always be absolute about the diagnosis or its exclusion.

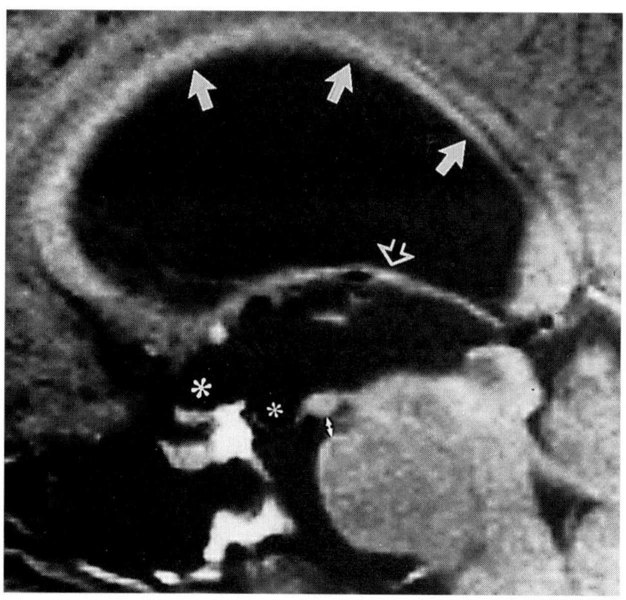

Figure 1–33. Hydrocephalus. Sagittal midline MRI shows thinning and elevation of the corpus callosum (solid arrows), depression of the fornix (open arrow), ballooning of the supraoptic (large asterisk) and infundibular (small asterisk) recesses of the third ventricle, and narrowing of the mammillopontine distance (small double arrow).

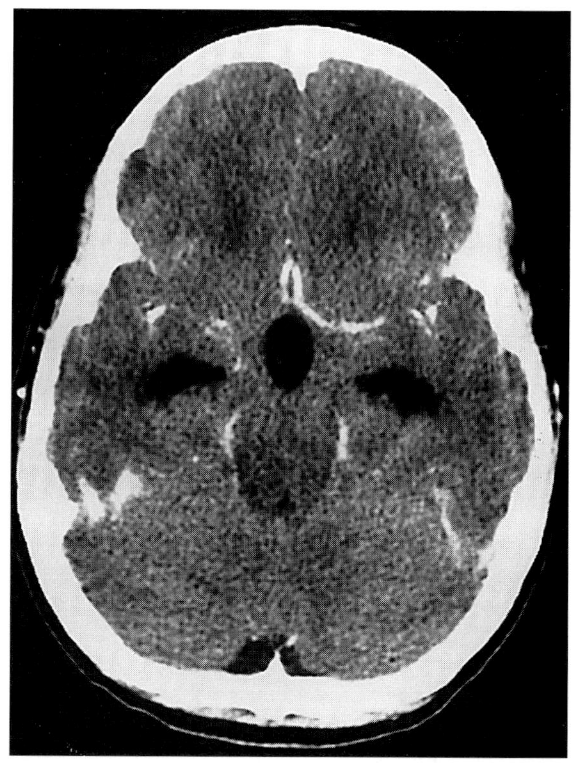

Figure 1–34. Hydrocephalus. Axial CT with contrast shows a dilated third ventricle with convex lateral walls and bilateral temporal horn dilatation.

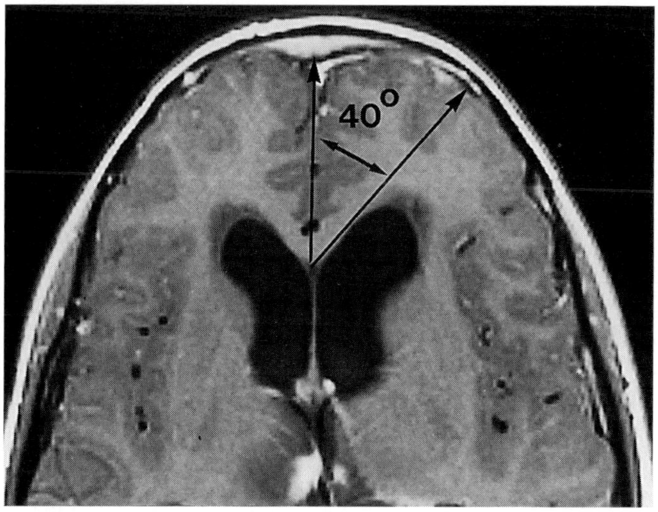

Figure 1-35. Hydrocephalus (ventricular angle). The method of measuring the ventricular angle is illustrated, giving a result of 40°. The angle tends to be smaller in hydrocephalus and larger in atrophy.

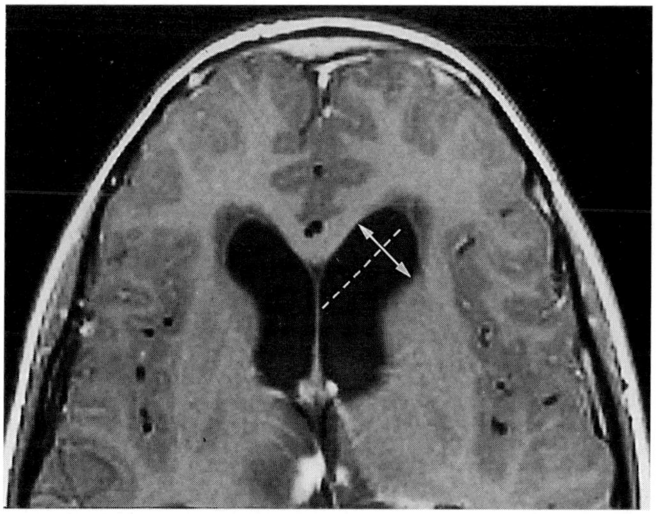

Figure 1-36. Hydrocephalus. The frontal horn radius represents one half the maximum diameter of the frontal horn perpendicular to the long axis (dashed line) of the frontal horn. This measurement tends to be larger in hydrocephalus and smaller in atrophy.

Noncommunicating Hydrocephalus

Synonym: Intraventricular obstructive hydrocephalus (IVOH).

Noncommunicating hydrocephalus results from an impedance of CSF outflow from the ventricles. It may occur at the foramen of Monro (e.g., colloid cyst, subfalcine herniation), third ventricle, aqueduct (e.g., aqueductal stenosis, pineal tumors, transtentorial herniation), fourth ventricle (usually tumors), or fourth ventricular outlet foramina (e.g., Dandy-Walker malformation).

Communicating Hydrocephalus

Synonym: Extraventricular obstructive hydrocephalus (EVOH).

Communicating hydrocephalus describes an impairment of CSF clearance distal to the fourth ventricular outlet. It usually results from disease of the subarachnoid space, such as subarachnoid hemorrhage, meningitis, or leptomeningeal metastases. Impaired CSF resorption by the arachnoid villi is the postulated mechanism. In contrast to obstructive hydrocephalus, the sulci may remain quite prominent in this condition. An idiopathic and self-limited form, designated external hydrocephalus, is seen in infants who manifest enlarging head circumference with enlarged frontal or frontoparietal subarachnoid spaces.

Normal Pressure Hydrocephalus

Normal pressure hydrocephalus (NPH) is a condition of the elderly manifested by ventricular dilatation in association with the clinical triad of ataxia, dementia, and incontinence. There is no obstruction to CSF flow in a classic sense. The pathologic basis is poorly understood, but diminished compliance of the ventricular walls has been implicated.

The differentiation of NPH from atrophy is a classic diagnostic dilemma. Factors in favor of NPH include temporal horn enlargement, rounding of the anterior third ventricle, and, most important, ventricular dilatation disproportionately greater than the degree of sulcal enlargement. NPH is discussed further in Chapter 5.

Injuries

Atrophy

Atrophy is one of the most frequent abnormalities encountered with neuroimaging. The most common form is associated with aging but unrelated to primary central nervous system (CNS) disease. Age-related atrophy begins to manifest around age 50 years and then increases steadily in both prevalence and severity into later decades. It is highly individual in nature, with the brains of many people over 70 years of age still well within the size range of those of younger adults. The cerebral white matter is primarily affected. Atrophy occurs secondarily with a broad spectrum of diseases, particularly ischemic and degenerative disorders. Reversible loss of brain volume has been observed in some conditions, which may lead to a false-positive diagnosis of atrophy (Table 1–4).

Superficial (cortical) atrophy describes the presence of enlarged cortical fissures and sulci with or without enlarged ventricles. In cases related to normal aging, the parasagittal frontal, parietal, and temporal lobes are most affected.

Deep atrophy connotes atrophic enlargement of the third and lateral ventricles. One of the earliest changes related to aging is enlargement of the third ventricle due to regression of the median nuclei of the thalami. Widening of the third ventricle may begin around age 50. Progressive enlargement of the lateral ventricles is a result of white matter loss and begins during the seventh decade. The dubious expression *hydrocephalus ex vacuo* is sometimes used to describe deep atrophy.

A particularly common finding in the elderly is atrophic enlargement of the perivascular or Virchow-Robin spaces, a condition also referred to as état criblé. This results in the common MRI finding of isolated hyperintensities in the lower third of the lentiform nuclei, tiny punctate hyperintensities in the gray matter, and fine linear hyperintensities in the white matter of the cerebral convexities. A few dilated perivascular spaces in the inferior basal ganglia are a common normal finding in younger individuals.

TABLE 1–4 Causes of Reversible Cerebral Volume Loss

Chronic alcoholism
Anorexia nervosa
Cushing disease
Corticosteroid therapy
Chemotherapy

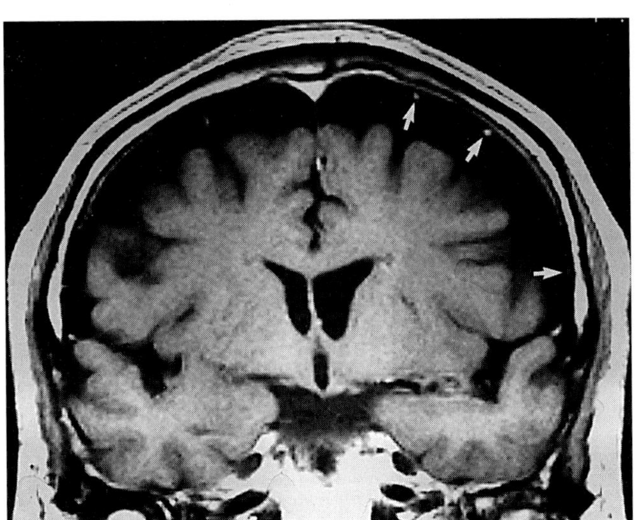

Figure 1–37. Cortical atrophy. Coronal T1-weighted MRI shows volume loss of the frontal lobes and marked enlargement of the subarachnoid space. The close apposition of cortical veins (arrows) to the inner table enables confident exclusion of subdural effusion.

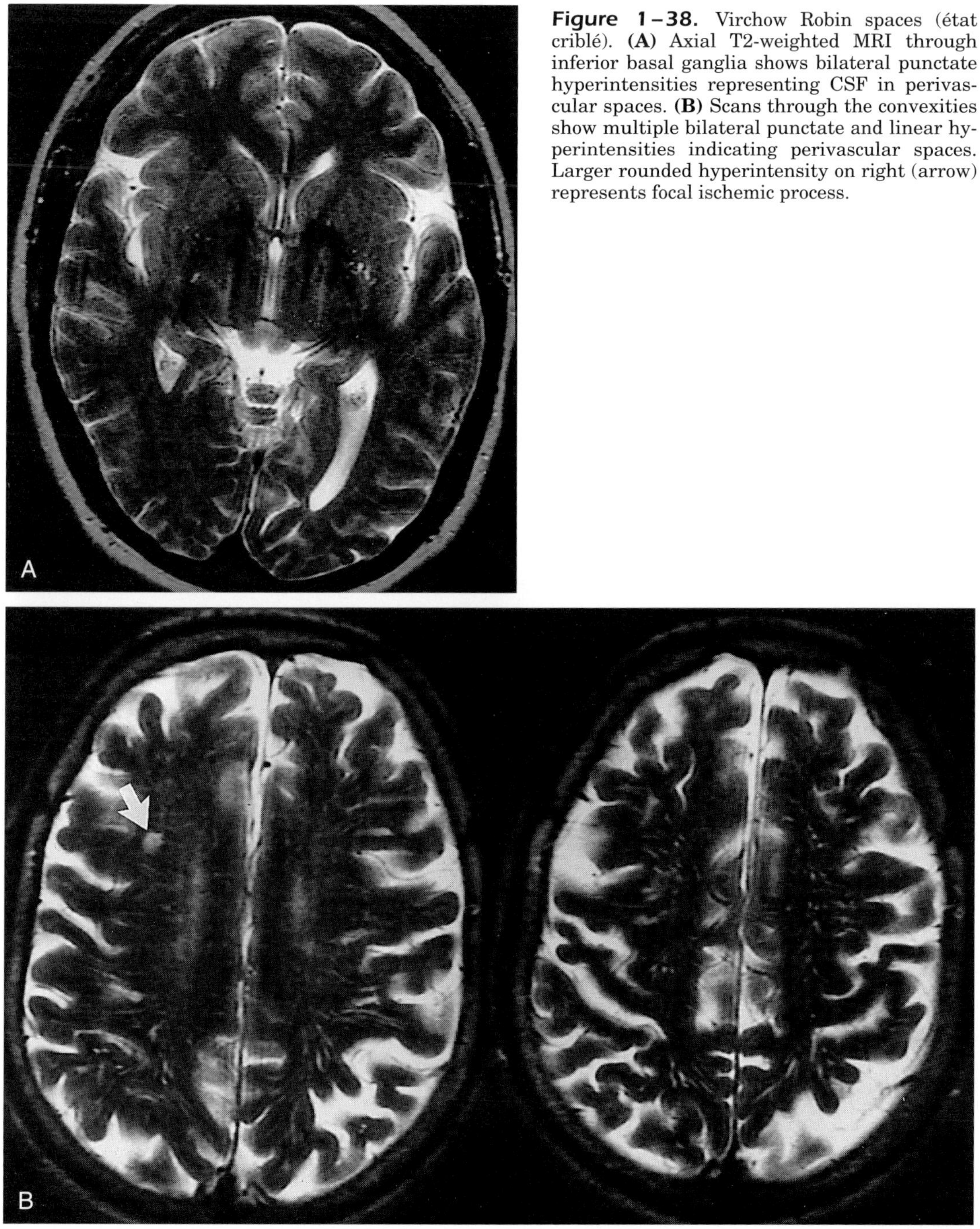

Figure 1–38. Virchow Robin spaces (état criblé). **(A)** Axial T2-weighted MRI through inferior basal ganglia shows bilateral punctate hyperintensities representing CSF in perivascular spaces. **(B)** Scans through the convexities show multiple bilateral punctate and linear hyperintensities indicating perivascular spaces. Larger rounded hyperintensity on right (arrow) represents focal ischemic process.

Focal glial and neuronal loss within the white matter may allow accumulation of water in the enlarged extracellular spaces, resulting in diminished attenuation of the white matter on CT and hyperintensities on T2-weighted MRI associated with ventricular enlargement. Common causes for this secondary form of deep atrophy include ischemic leukoencephalopathy, periventricular leukomalacia, radiation therapy, and HIV encephalitis.

A potential pitfall lies in the finding of unifocal or multifocal low attenuation foci in the brain (hyperintensities on T2-weighted MRI). Although in the majority of cases, especially among the elderly, these result from ischemia, a host of other entities may produce this appearance, including old trauma, acute and chronic demyelination, metastases, and inflammatory diseases. One should be wary when white matter abnormalities coexist with any suggestion of mass effect (or even the absence of expected atrophy) or when they appear to follow white matter tracts; both are possible indicators of vasogenic edema. In the presence of these findings, intravenous contrast should be considered.

Cerebellar atrophy, especially as an isolated occurrence, is less often seen with normal aging and more likely to be related to a specific disorder. Signs of cerebellar atrophy include enlargement of the sulci, fourth ventricle, and cerebellopontine angle cisterns. The cisterna magna is too highly variable in normal size to be useful as an indicator of atrophy.

Numerous linear and volumetric measurement techniques have been used to quantify cerebral and cerebellar atrophy, but these are almost never used clinically. Most neuroradiologists rely on a subjective impression of the cross-sectional images, and this appears to be adequate in most situations.

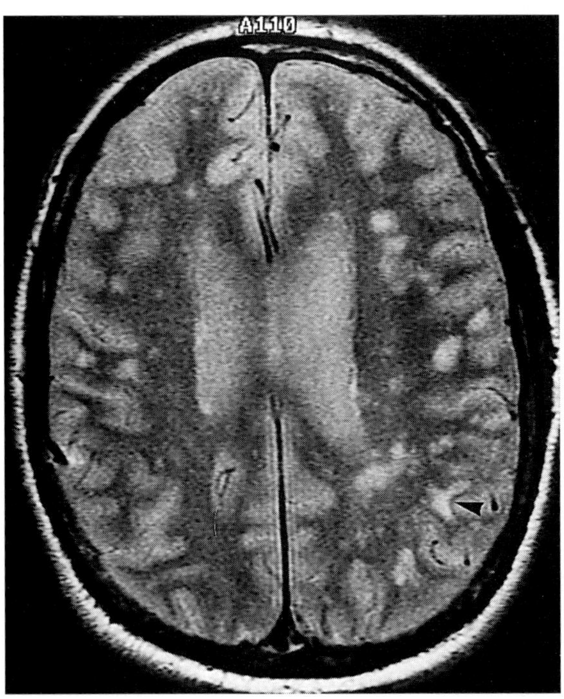

Figure 1–39. Deep white matter atrophy (chronic ischemic leukoencephalopathy). Axial PD-weighted MRI shows multiple subcortical white matter hyperintensities representing atrophy and gliosis. Note the sparing of subcortical U fibers (arrowhead), which are better vascularized.

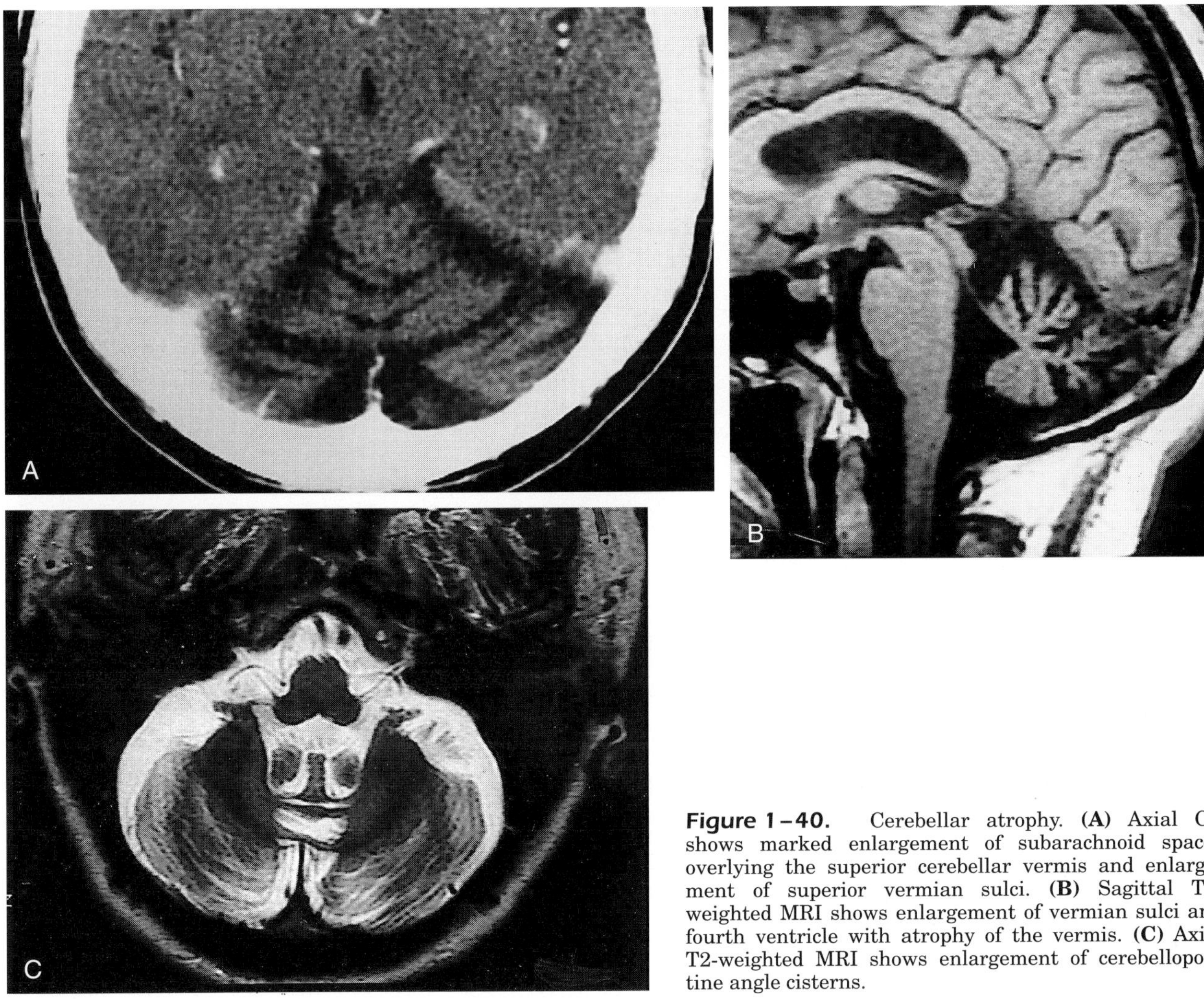

Figure 1-40. Cerebellar atrophy. **(A)** Axial CT shows marked enlargement of subarachnoid spaces overlying the superior cerebellar vermis and enlargement of superior vermian sulci. **(B)** Sagittal T1-weighted MRI shows enlargement of vermian sulci and fourth ventricle with atrophy of the vermis. **(C)** Axial T2-weighted MRI shows enlargement of cerebellopontine angle cisterns.

Encephalomalacia

Encephalomalacia is the presence of cystic or microcystic parenchymal cavities containing CSF that result from a cerebral injury causing necrosis of both neuronal and glial elements. Gross atrophy is almost invariably present. The most common cause is cerebral infarction. Other causes include trauma, hemorrhage, or fulminant infections (especially intrauterine or neonatal). Encephalomalacia must be differentiated from gliosis, which usually coexists at the periphery of encephalomalacia and often exists in isolation. On T1-weighted MRI, encephalomalacia should be nearly isointense with CSF, although volume averaging with residual glial tissue may result in slightly higher signal intensities. Gliosis, although hypointense, should continue to manifest a higher signal intensity than CSF.

Gliosis

Synonyms: Astrocytosis, astrogliosis.

Almost any injury to the brain results in hypertrophy and proliferation of glial elements (gliosis) at the site of neural damage. Surgery and trauma are common causes. Gliosis usually develops at the periphery of infarcts, and in less severe cases glial tissue may survive throughout the infarcted territory while the more vulnerable neurons do not. Such an infarct results in gliosis without encephalomalacia.

Because myelin is hydrophobic, replacement of myelin by glial tissue results in a relatively increased water content and therefore diminished attenuation on CT and hyperintensity on T2-weighted MRI.

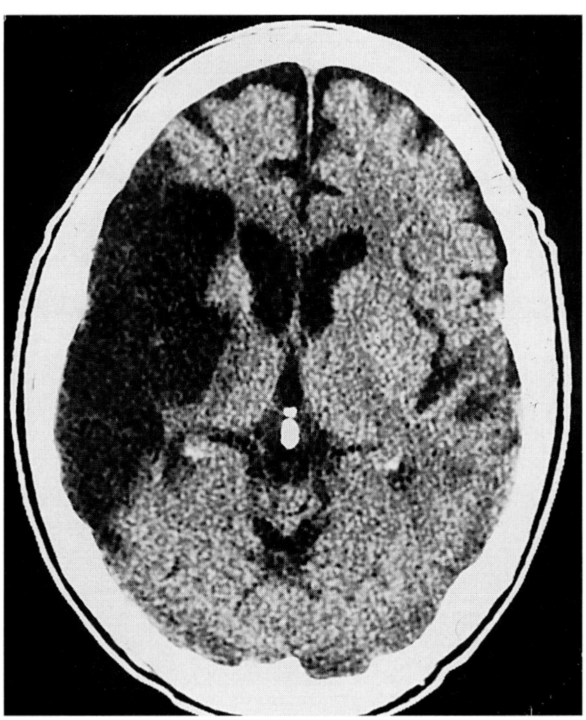

Figure 1-41. Encephalomalacia (old right MCA infarct). An extensive portion of the right MCA territory is isodense with CSF.

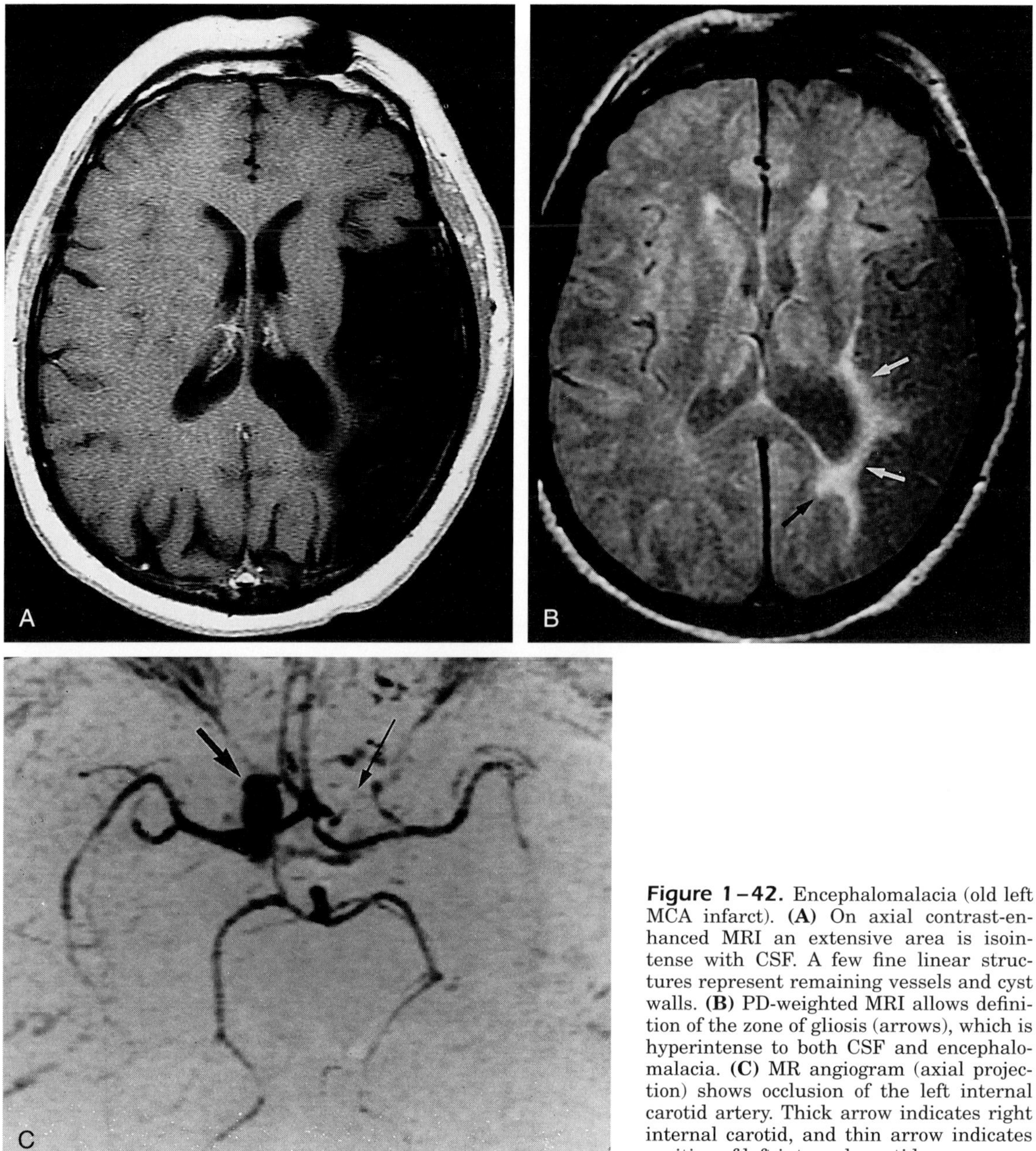

Figure 1–42. Encephalomalacia (old left MCA infarct). **(A)** On axial contrast-enhanced MRI an extensive area is isointense with CSF. A few fine linear structures represent remaining vessels and cyst walls. **(B)** PD-weighted MRI allows definition of the zone of gliosis (arrows), which is hyperintense to both CSF and encephalomalacia. **(C)** MR angiogram (axial projection) shows occlusion of the left internal carotid artery. Thick arrow indicates right internal carotid, and thin arrow indicates position of left internal carotid.

Porencephaly

Porencephaly is the presence of a CSF-filled cavity in the brain parenchyma without ependymal or arachnoid lining. It may or may not communicate with the ventricles or subarachnoid space. Common causes include severe hemorrhagic events (especially neonatal) and surgical resection. Some cases are congenital, arising from an in utero ischemic event or other injury. Porencephaly must be distinguished from other cystic mass lesions (see Chapter 4) and ventricular diverticula secondary to hydrocephalus or agenesis of the corpus callosum. Mass effect is rarely seen with porencephaly.

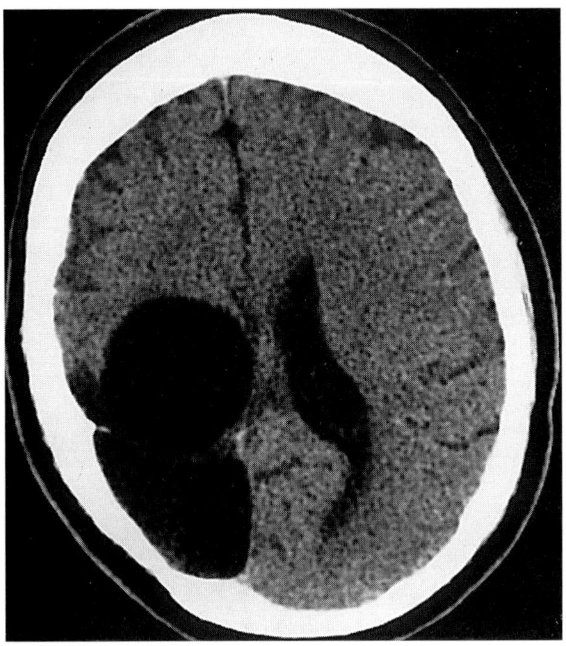

Figure 1–43. Porencephaly (partial hemispherectomy for Sturge-Weber syndrome). Axial CT shows a large cyst isointense with CSF and continuous with the lateral ventricle. The right hemicranium is hypoplastic. (Surgery was performed in childhood.)

Hemorrhage

Computed Tomography

Because of the limited sensitivity of MRI for both acute parenchymal (<12 hours old) and subarachnoid hemorrhage, CT remains the imaging procedure of choice for the detection of acute intracranial hemorrhage.

Acute Hemorrhage (1 Hour to 3 Days)

Acute clot manifests itself on CT as a hyperdense mass with well-defined borders ranging from 50 to 100 Hounsfield units (HU). Parenchymal hematoma will exhibit a low attenuation rim of varying size due to edema. Various circumstances, however, may contribute to a lower attenuation even to the point of isodensity with brain. These circumstances include low hematocrit, hyperacute hematoma composed of unclotted whole blood, or dilution (hemorrhage into cystic- or CSF-containing spaces).

Subacute Hemorrhage (4 Days to 3 Weeks)

As the hematoma resorbs, the margins become fuzzy and the attenuation of the clot progressively decreases, eventually becoming isodense with brain. Diminution of the mass effect takes place more slowly. During this period, ring enhancement develops at the original margins of the hematoma and may persist for months.

Chronic Hemorrhage (>3 Weeks)

Chronic hematoma is characterized by hypodensity with respect to brain. It will eventually disappear completely, leave a small area of low attenuation, or leave a porencephalic cavity isodense with CSF. Both mass effect and enhancement disappear during this stage, taking somewhat longer the larger the original hematoma.

Text continued on page 38

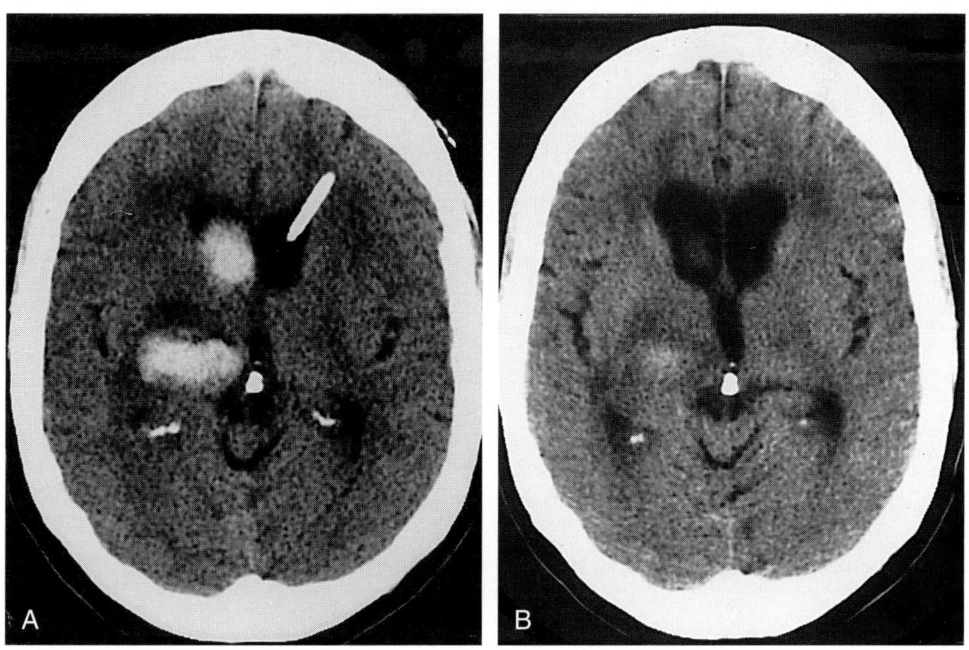

Figure 1–44. Evolution of ICH. **(A)** CT shows acute right thalamic and intraventricular hemorrhage. **(B)** After 13 days the intraventricular clot is nearly gone. The thalamic hemorrhage has become largely isodense with a small central area remaining slightly hyperdense. Mild mass effect is still present.

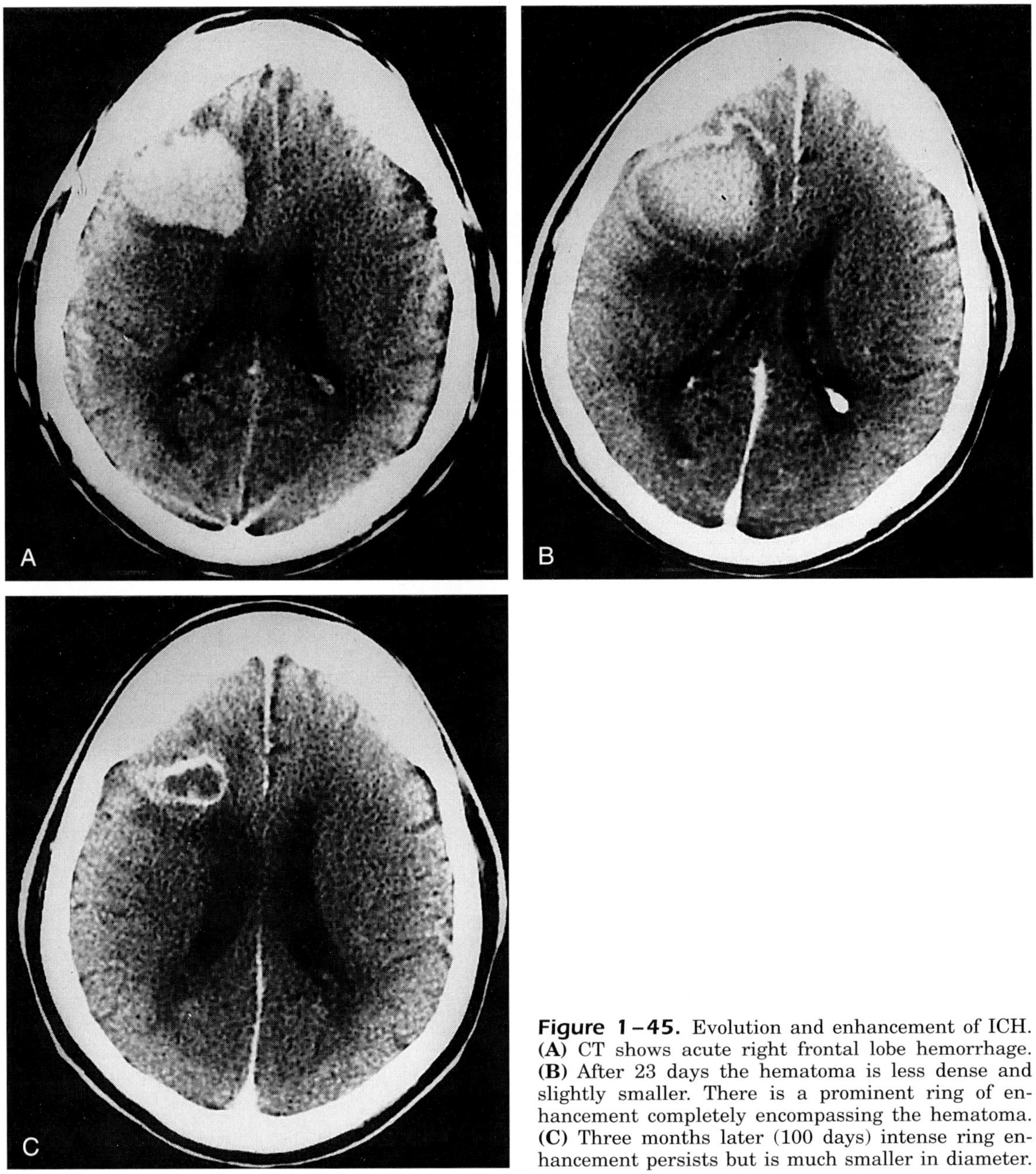

Figure 1–45. Evolution and enhancement of ICH. **(A)** CT shows acute right frontal lobe hemorrhage. **(B)** After 23 days the hematoma is less dense and slightly smaller. There is a prominent ring of enhancement completely encompassing the hematoma. **(C)** Three months later (100 days) intense ring enhancement persists but is much smaller in diameter.

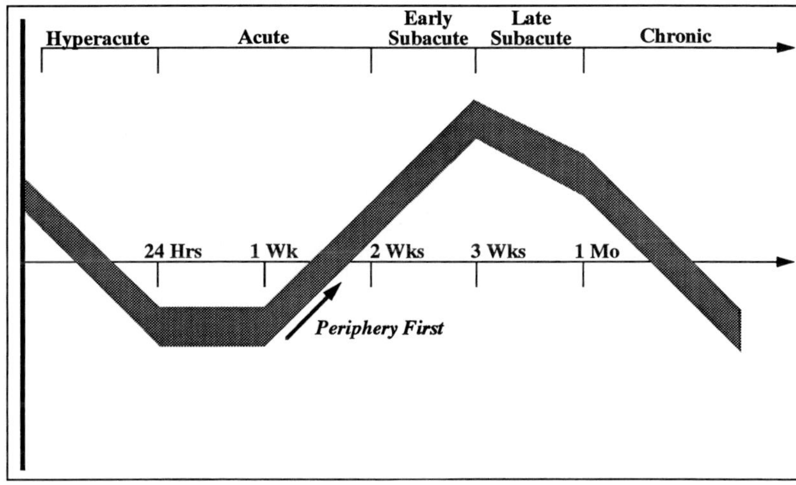

Figure 1–46. Signal intensity of ICH, T1-MRI plotted against time.

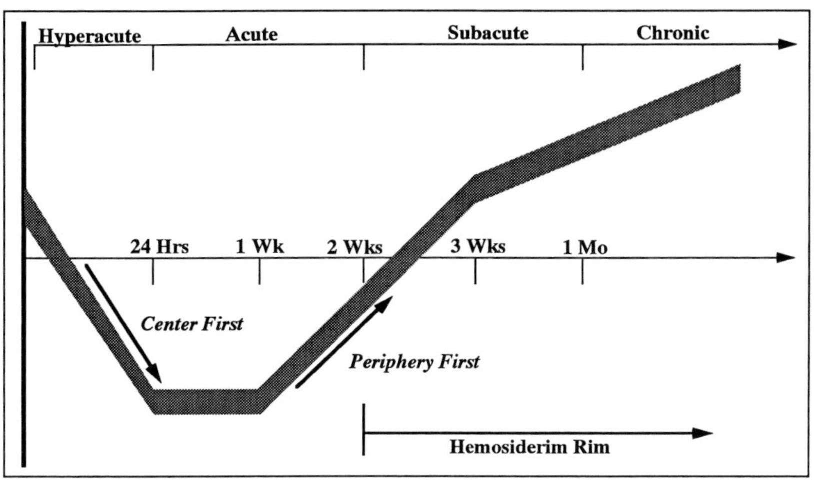

Figure 1–47. Signal intensity of ICH, T2-MRI plotted against time.

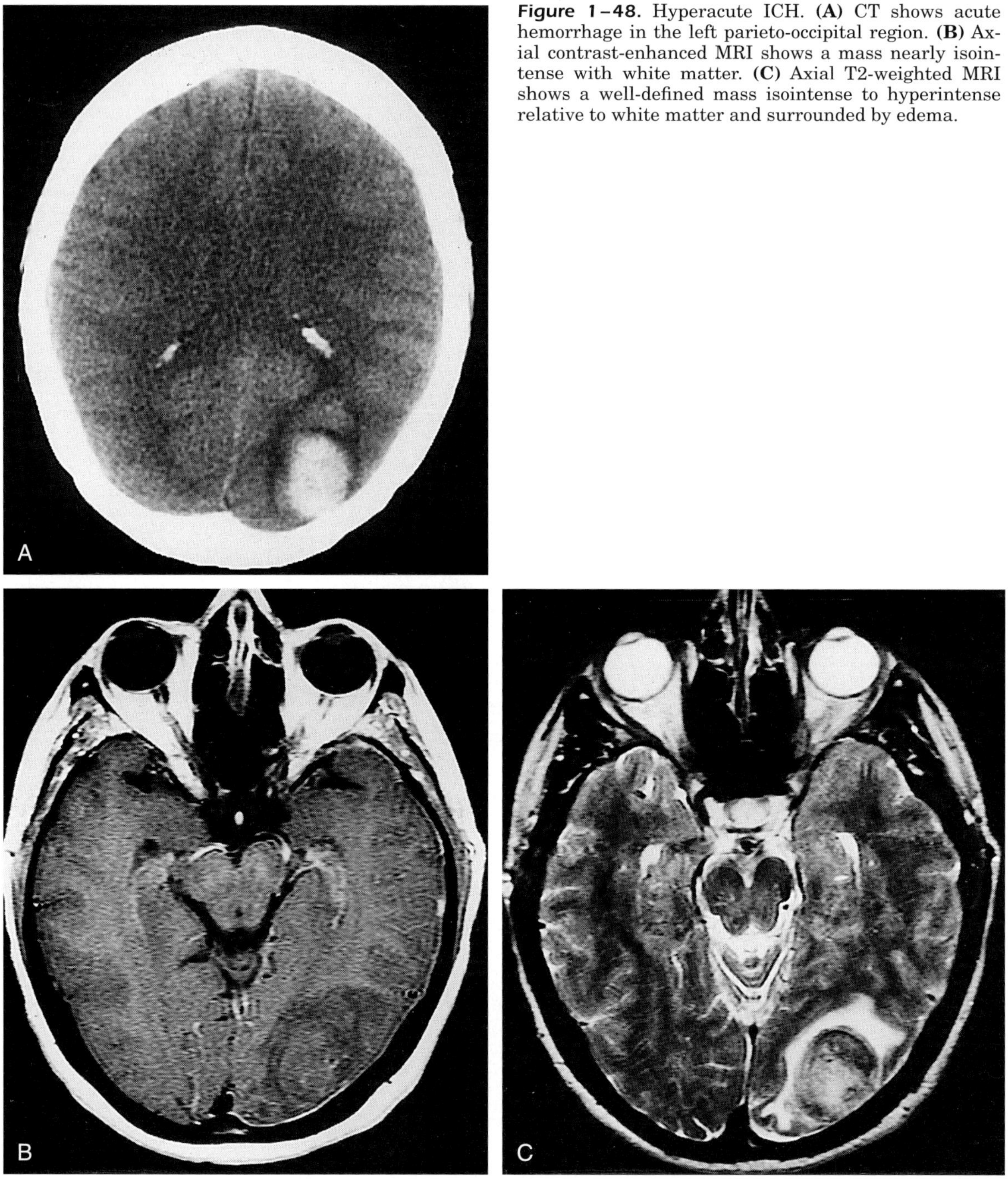

Figure 1–48. Hyperacute ICH. **(A)** CT shows acute hemorrhage in the left parieto-occipital region. **(B)** Axial contrast-enhanced MRI shows a mass nearly isointense with white matter. **(C)** Axial T2-weighted MRI shows a well-defined mass isointense to hyperintense relative to white matter and surrounded by edema.

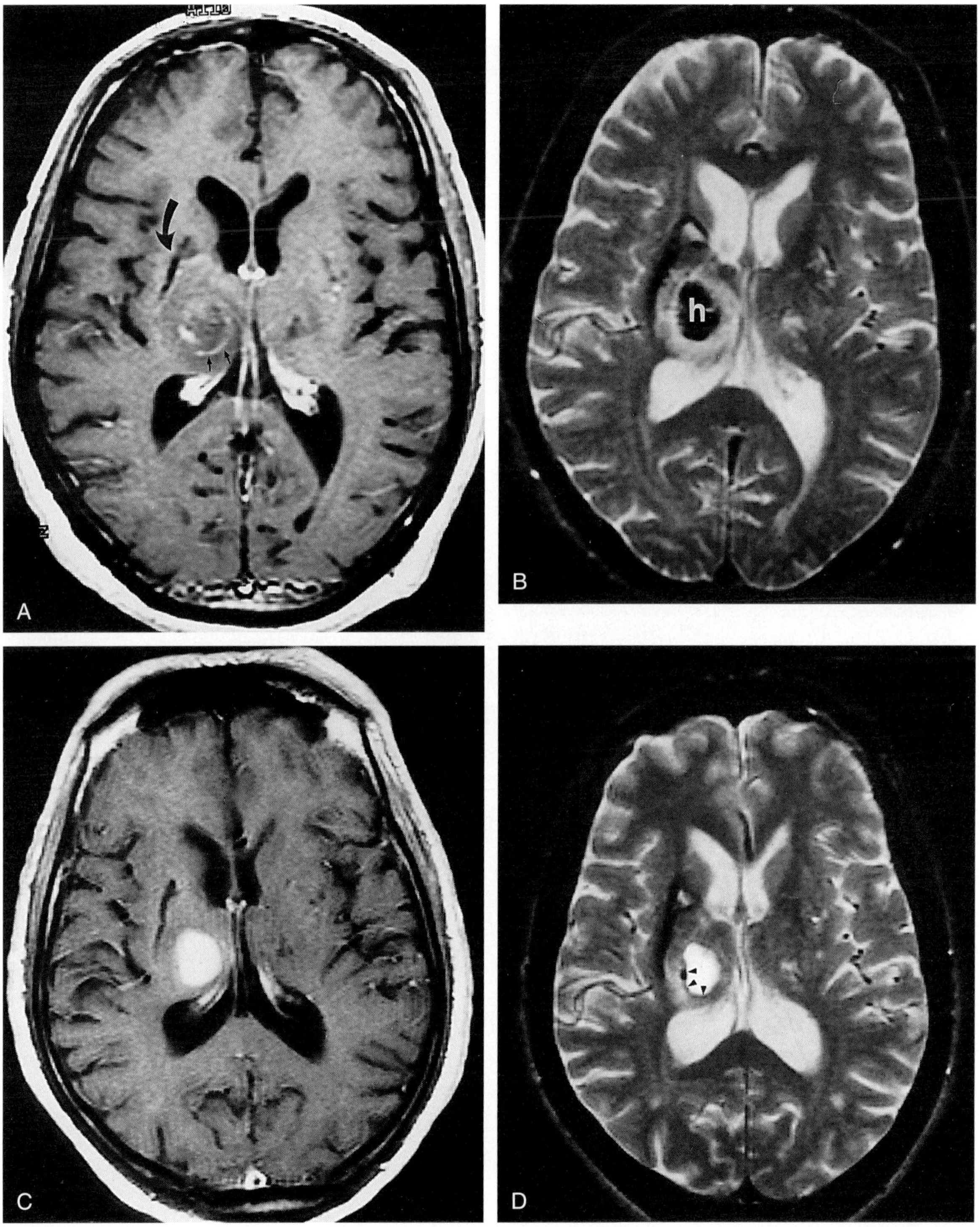

Figure 1–49. Acute and subacute ICH. **(A)** T1-weighted, contrast-enhanced MRI 36 hours after onset of right thalamic hemorrhage shows mixed hypointensity and hyperintensity in the center of the hematoma with a hypointense rim of edema. There is faint ring enhancement. Note also residual of old hemorrhage (curved arrow) in the right putamen. **(B)** T2-weighted MRI at 36 hours shows marked central hypointensity (h = hematoma) with a hyperintense rim of edema. **(C)** T1-weighted MRI with contrast 14 days later shows the hematoma is homogeneously hyperintense. **(D)** T2-weighted MRI after 14 days shows the hematoma is homogeneously hyperintense with a thin hypointense hemosiderin rim (arrowheads). (Reprinted with permission from Willing, SJ. Magnetic Resonance Imaging of Intracerebral Hemorrhage. *Contemporary Diagnostic Radiology* 17(4):1–6, 1994.)

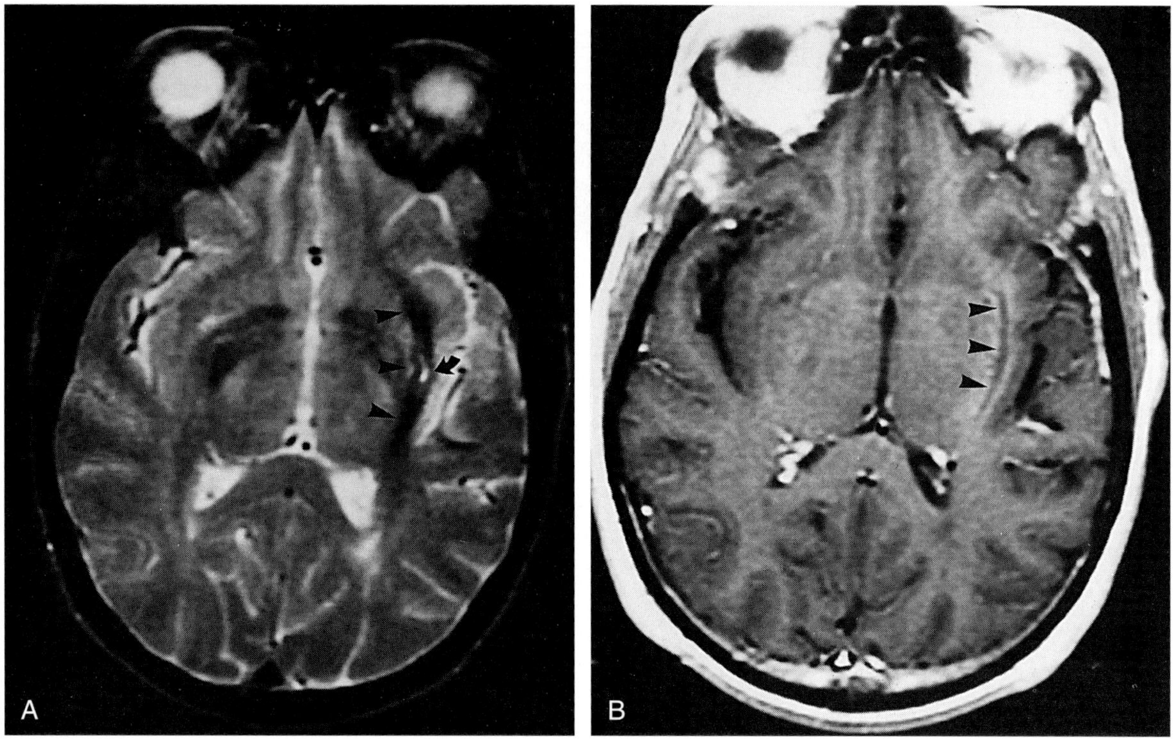

Figure 1–50. Chronic ICH. **(A)** Axial T2-weighted MRI shows hypointensity of the left putamen and external capsule due to hemosiderin (arrowheads) with a small hyperintense residual cavity (curved arrow). **(B)** T1-weighted scan shows a hypointense cleft (arrowheads) corresponding to the hemosiderin accumulation in A. (Reprinted with permission from Willing,SJ. Magnetic Resonance Imaging of Intracerebral Hemorrhage. *Contemporary Diagnostic Radiology* 17(4):1–6, 1994.)

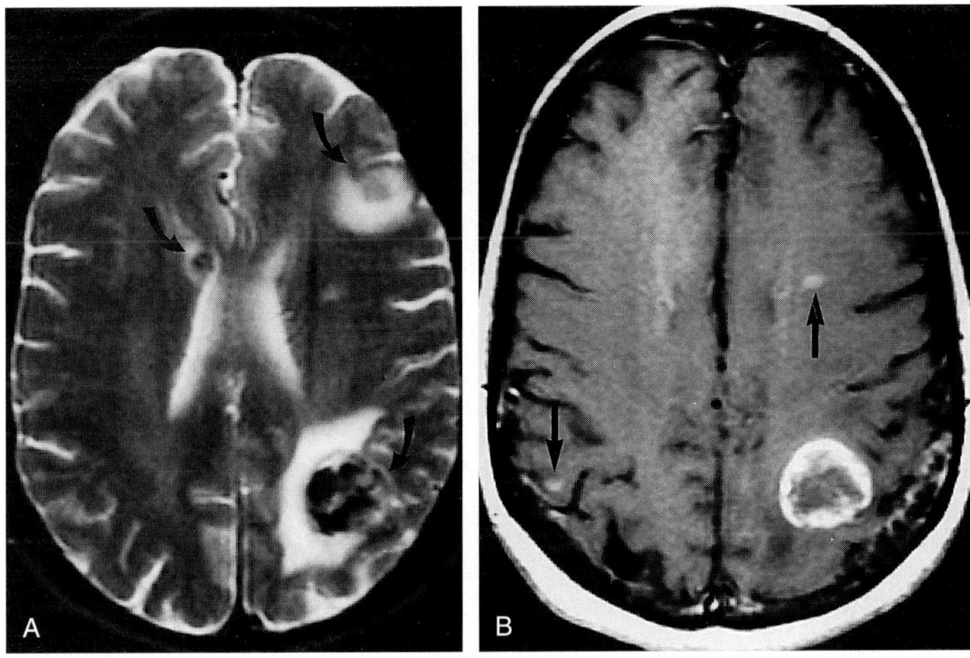

Figure 1–51. Hemorrhagic lung metastases. **(A)** T2-weighted MRI shows metastases (arrows) in the left frontal lobe, left parietal lobe, and right caudate head. The left parietal lesion is heterogeneous with areas of marked hypointensity representing acute hemorrhage. **(B)** Contrast-enhanced, T1-weighted sequence shows a hyperintense rim due to both methemoglobin and enhancement. Other enhancing lesions are present (arrows). The finding of multiple lesions points to the diagnosis of metastases.

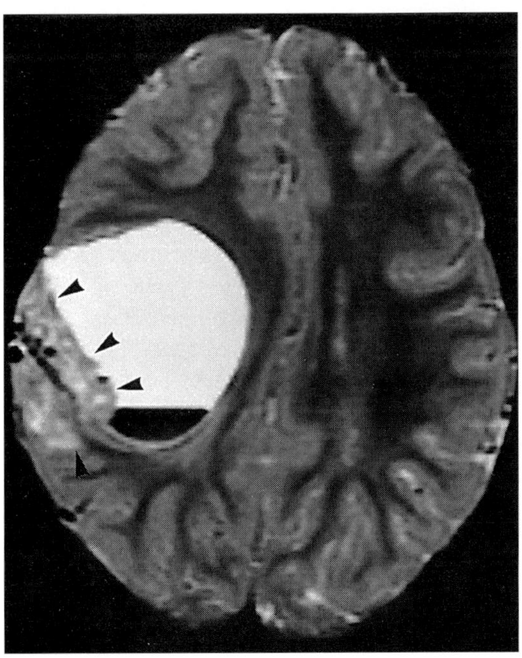

Figure 1–52. Hemorrhagic peripheral neuroectodermal tumor. Axial T2-weighted MRI shows a fluid-fluid level within a large cavity. The hypointense dependent portion represents acute hemorrhage. Although small fluid levels may be transiently encountered in spontaneous hematoma, such a finding generally indicates hemorrhage into a preexisting cavity. Note the irregular and heterogeneous mass on the lateral aspect of the cavity (arrowheads). (Courtesy of Alan Lovell, MD, Birmingham, AL.)

Magnetic Resonance Imaging

Intracerebral Hematoma

The MRI appearance of intracerebral hematoma is a function of many factors, including time, drugs, and systemic or local metabolic states. From a practical standpoint, the important considerations are the scanning technique being employed and the age of the hematoma.

T2-Weighted Images. Hyperacute hemorrhage (<12 hours old) is composed of plasma and intact oxygenated red blood cells. The high water content and absence of paramagnetic effects result in hyperintensity on T2-weighted images. Almost immediately after the hemorrhagic event, several concurrent processes begin. Local aggregation of clotting factors and platelets entraps the extravasated red blood cells, tending to squeeze out serum with its high water content. Hence, there is a local redistribution of water resulting in edema at the periphery of the clot and dehydration within. Soon after, the oxyhemoglobin of extravasated red blood cells releases its molecular oxygen (desaturates) to become deoxyhemoglobin. This effect begins and is first apparent in the more hypoxic center of the hematoma.

Unlike oxyhemoglobin, deoxyhemoglobin is paramagnetic, meaning that it becomes magnetized in the presence of a magnetic field (such as the static field of an MRI scanner). This local strengthening of the magnetic field around each individual red blood cell results in local peaks and valleys of the magnetic field at the cellular level. Mobile water protons diffusing through this locally inhomogeneous field rapidly become dephased, and this dephasing cannot be refocused by the 180° pulse of a spin echo sequence. Because dephasing results in accelerated signal loss with long echo times (TEs), the acute clot (>12 hours, up to 7 days) appears dark on T2-weighted images. This effect is referred to as T2 proton relaxation enhancement. Peripheral edema, of course, is moderately hyperintense relative to adjacent brain.

In the subacute stage (1 week to 1 month), deoxyhemoglobin is oxidized to methemoglobin. Methemoglobin is also paramagnetic. As long as it remains intracellular, it also results in local magnetic field inhomogeneity and T2 shortening. However, the red blood cells soon lyse, releasing methemoglobin into the extracellular fluid compartment. The released methemoglobin diffuses more or less evenly throughout the extracellular fluid. With the paramagnetic agent now homogeneously distributed, the local magnetic field once again becomes homogeneous, and proton dephasing can again be refocused by the 180° pulse. The hematoma begins to increase in signal intensity on T2-weighted images because of both the loss of proton relaxation enhancement and the overlap of hyperintensity resulting from T1 shortening (discussed subsequently).

At the periphery of the hematoma, methemoglobin breaks down to hemosiderin, which is phagocytized by macrophages. Hemosiderin is also paramagnetic, and its heterogeneous accumulation within the intracellular compartment of macrophages results in T2 shortening, as with intracellular deoxyhemoglobin. The resulting hemosiderin rim seen on T2-weighted images begins to form at about 2 weeks.

In the chronic stage (beyond 1 month), resorption of the central clot may lead to a complete resolution, a residual small cleft, or following extensive parenchymal destruction a porencephalic cavity that fills with CSF. The high water content within the cavity leads to a permanent area of hyperintensity. The hypointense hemosiderin rim persists indefinitely.

T1-Weighted Images. Hyperacute hematoma may exhibit mild hyperintensity on T1-weighted images due to the high proton density and the overlap of T2 effects. Acute hematoma may be isointense to hypointense relative to adjacent brain probably due to the predominance of rapid T2-related signal loss. Although deoxyhemoglobin is paramagnetic, the iron is deeply embedded within the globin protein and inaccessible to free water. For significant T1 shortening, the hydrogen proton of free water must approach within 3 angstroms of the unpaired iron electrons. Edema surrounding the hematoma is mildly hypointense, as with edema of other etiologies.

The first event specifically altering T1 relaxation occurs in the subacute stage when deoxyhemoglobin is oxidized to methemoglobin. The resulting change in molecular configuration allows the hydrogen proton to approach within 3 angstroms of the unpaired electrons of the ferric ion. This facilitates an event called proton-electron dipole-dipole interaction, which markedly enhances T1 relaxation in a manner similar to gadolinium. Serial T1-weighted images in this stage show increasing hyperintensity of the hematoma beginning at the periphery.

The T1-shortening effect of methemoglobin occurs whether it is intracellular or extracellular and persists until the methemoglobin is degraded to hemosiderin, which is also paramagnetic but hydrophobic and therefore inaccessible to the hydrogen proton of water.

In the chronic stage, the hematoma gradually diminishes in signal intensity, approaching isointensity with CSF as all blood products are resorbed. The clot center may completely resolve or leave behind a small cleft or fluid-filled cavity of variable size. The hemosiderin rim cannot usually be detected on T1-weighted images.

Subdural Hematoma

The MRI appearance of subdural hematoma versus time is similar to the pattern for parenchymal hematoma. There are, however, a few differences. The propensity of chronic subdural hematomas to rebleed may result in a layering phenomena and an appearance of blood in varying stages of breakdown. Hemosiderin is infrequent in chronic subdural hematomas unless rebleeding has occurred. Finally, methemoglobin may be cleared more rapidly, so that chronic subdural hematomas approach isointensity with CSF much earlier than parenchymal hematomas.

Summary: MRI of Intracerebral Hemorrhage

Field strength above 0.15 Tesla (T) and spin echo sequences reveal the following:

1. Hyperacute hemorrhage (<24 hours) resembles proteinaceous fluid (bright on T1-weighted imaging/brighter on T2-weighted imaging).
2. Acute clot turns dark in 24 to 48 hours (very dark on T2-weighted imaging) beginning centrally.
3. Clot in evolution turns progressively brighter on both T1- and T2-weighted imaging beginning peripherally.
4. Mature hematoma (approximately 2 weeks) is very bright.
5. Dark peripheral rim (hemosiderin ring) forms in about 2 weeks and lasts indefinitely.
6. Old chronic hematoma (>1 month) approaches CSF signal patterns as blood products are resorbed, leaving a CSF-filled cavity.
7. Appearance may vary somewhat depending on field strength of the magnet.
8. The rules do not always apply.

Differential Diagnosis

The imaging findings of hemorrhage are virtually pathognomonic. The challenge is usually not to diagnose the hemorrhage itself but if possible to ascertain the etiology of the hemorrhage. The differential diagnosis of spontaneous intracerebral hemorrhage is addressed in Chapter 7. The issue to be considered here is differentiation of primary hemorrhage from tumoral hemorrhage. Much attention has been focused on this issue, and several helpful MRI findings have been identified, which are summarized in Table 1–5.

TABLE 1–5 | Primary Hemorrhage Versus Hemorrhagic Tumor: MRI Appearance

Primary Hemorrhage	Tumoral Hemorrhage
Fairly regular temporal evolution	Delayed temporal evolution
Hyperintensity of subacute clot begins peripherally	Hyperintensity of subacute clot may begin centrally
More consistently homogeneous	Often heterogeneous, reflecting hemorrhage in various stages of evolution
Only clot and edema present	Mass accompanying hematoma
Usually complete hemosiderin ring beginning at 2 weeks	Hemosiderin ring beginning later and frequently discontinuous
Edema proportionate to size of hematoma	Edema often greater
Absence of layering effects	Blood-fluid levels due to hemorrhage into cyst
Faint, fuzzy ring enhancement in subacute stage and thick, intense ring enhancement in chronic stage	Lumpy, irregular, and locally intense enhancement unrelated to age of hemorrhage

RECOMMENDED READINGS

Edema

Cowley,AR. Influence of Fiber Tracts on the CT Appearance of Cerebral Edema: Anatomic-Pathologic Correlation. *AJNR* 4:915–925, 1983.

Sevick,RJ, Kanda,F, Mintorovitch,J, et al. Cytotoxic Brain Edema: Assessment with Diffusion-weighted MR Imaging. *Radiology* 185:687–690, 1992.

Turski,PA, Perman,WH, Hald,JK, Houston,LW, Strother,CM, Sackett,JF. Clinical and Experimental Vasogenic Edema: In Vivo Sodium MR Imaging. *Radiology* 160:821–825, 1986.

Mass Localization

Curnes,JT. MR Imaging of Peripheral Intracranial Neoplasms: Extraaxial vs. Intraaxial Masses. *J Comput Assist Tomogr* 11:932–937, 1987.

Ebeling,U, Steinmetz,H, Huang,Y, Kahn,T. Topography and Iden-tification of the Inferior Precentral Sulcus in MR Imaging. *AJR* 153:1051–1056, 1989. *AJNR* 10:937–942, 1989.

Goldsher,D, Litt,AW, Pinto,RS, Bannon,KR, and Kricheff,II. Dural "Tail" Associated with Meningiomas on Gd-DTPA-enhanced MR Images: Characteristics, Differential Diagnostic Value, and Possible Implications for Treatment. *Radiology* 176:447–450, 1990.

Iwasaki,S, Nakagawa,H, Fukusumi,A, et al. Identification of Pre- and Postcentral Gyri on CT and MR Images on the Basis of the Medullary Pattern of Cerebral White Matter. *Radiology* 179:207–213, 1991.

Sobel,DF, Gallen,CC, Schwartz,BJ, et al. Locating the Central Sulcus: Comparison of MR Anatomic and Magnetoencephalographic Functional Methods. *AJNR* 14:915–925, 1993.

Steinmetz,H, Huang,Y. Two-Dimensional Mapping of Brain Surface Anatomy. AJNR 12:997–1000, 1991.

Tiede,U, Bomans,M, Höhne,KH, et al. A Computerized Three-Dimensional Atlas of the Human Skull and Brain. *AJNR* 14:551–559, 1993.

Wilms,G, Lammens,M, Marchal,G, et al. Prominent Dural Enhancement Adjacent to Nonmeningiomatous Malignant Lesions on Contrast-Enhanced MR Images. *AJNR* 12:761–764, 1991.

Herniations

Ishikawa,M, Kikuchi,H, Fujisawa,I, Yonekawa,Y. Tonsillar Herniation on Magnetic Resonance Imaging. *Neurosurgery* 22:77–81, 1988.

Osborn,AG. Diagnosis of Descending Transtentorial Herniation by Cranial Computed Tomography. *Radiology* 123:93–96, 1977.

Osborn,AG, Heaston,DK, Wing,SD. Diagnosis of Ascending Transtentorial Herniation by Cranial Computed Tomography. *AJR* 130:755–760, 1978.

Osborn,AG. Secondary Effects of Intracranial Trauma. *Neuroimaging Clin North Am* 1:461–474, 1991.

Hydrocephalus

El Gammal,T, Allen,MB, Brooks,BS, Mark,EK. MR Evaluation of Hydrocephalus. *AJNR* 8:591–597, 1987. *AJR 149:* 807–813, 1987.

Fitz,CR, Harwood-Nash,DC. Computed Tomography of Hydrocephalus. *Comput Tomogr* 2:91–108, 1978.

Maytal,J, Alvarez,LA, Elkin,CM, Shinner,S. External Hydrocephalus: Radiologic Spectrum and Differentiation from Cerebral Atrophy. *AJR* 148:1223–1230, 1987.

Injuries

Allen,JH, Martin,JT, McLain,LW. Computed Tomography in Cerebellar Atrophic Processes. *Radiology* 130:379–382, 1979.

Braffman,BH, Zimmerman,RA, Trojanowski,JQ, et al. Brain MR: Pathologic Correlation with Gross and Histopathology. 1. Lacunar Infarction and Virchow-Robin Spaces. *AJR* 151:551–558, 1988.

Braffman,BH, Zimmerman,RA, Trojanowski,JQ, et al. Brain MR: Pathologic Correlation with Gross and Histopathology. 2. Hyperintense White-Matter Foci in the Elderly. *AJR* 559–566, 1988.

Drayer,BP. Imaging of the Aging Brain. Part I. Normal Findings. *Radiology* 166:785–796, 1988.

Drayer,BP. Imaging of the Aging Brain. Part II. Pathologic Conditions. *Radiology* 166:797–806, 1988.

Golomb,J, Kluger,A, Gianutsos,J, et al. Nonspecific Leukocephalopathy Associated with Aging. *Neuroimaging Clin North Am* 5:33–44, 1995.

Kolawole,TM, Patel,PJ, Mahdi,AH. Porencephaly: Computed Tomography (CT) Scan Findings. *Comput Radiol* 11:53–58, 1987.

LeMay,M. Radiologic Changes of the Aging Brain and Skull. *AJR* 143:383–389, 1984.

Hemorrhage

Atlas,SW, Grossman,RI, Gomori,JM et al. Hemorrhagic Intracranial Malignant Neoplasms: Spin-Echo MR Imaging. *Radiology* 164:71–77, 1987.

Chaney,RK, Taber,KH, Orrison,WW, Hayman,LA. Magnetic Resonance Imaging of Intracerebral Hemorrhage at Different Field Strengths: A Review of Reported Intraparenchymal Signal Intensities. *Neuroimaging Clin North Am* 2:25–52, 1992.

Cohen,WA, Hayman,LA. Computed Tomography of Intracranial Hemorrhage. *Neuroimaging Clin North Am* 2:75–87, 1992.

Destian,S, Sze,G, Krol,G, Zimmerman,RD, Deck,MDF. MR Imaging of Hemorrhagic Intracranial Neoplasms. *AJNR* 9:1115–1122, 1988.

Fobben,ES, Grossman,RI, Atlas,SW, et al. MR Characteristics of Subdural Hematomas and Hygromas at 1.5 T. *AJR* 153: 589–595, 1989.

Gentry,LR, Godersky,JC, Thompson,B, and Dunn,VD. Prospective Comparative Study of Intermediate-Field MR and CT in the Evaluation of Closed Head Trauma. *AJNR* 9:91–100, 1988.

Gomori,JM, Grossman,RI. Mechanisms Responsible for the MR Appearance and Evolution of Intracranial Hemorrhage. *Radiographics* 8:427–440, 1988.

Pfleger,MJ, Hardee,EP, Contant,CF, Hayman,LA. Sensitivity and Specificity of Fluid-Blood Levels for Coagulopathy in Acute Intracerebral Hematomas. *AJNR* 15:217–224, 1994.

Taber,KH, Ford,JJ, Hayman,LA. Magnetic Resonance Imaging Appearance of Hemorrhage: Sources of Image Contrast. *Neuroimaging Clin North Am* 2:61–74, 1992.

CHAPTER TWO

Congenital Brain Anomalies

A logical system of classification forms a cognitive foundation for the understanding and diagnosis of congenital brain anomalies. This chapter is organized using a modification of the classification system proposed by van der Knapp and Valk.

The imaging diagnosis of congenital CNS disorders differs from that of other disease categories in that intravenous contrast is almost never indicated in the absence of neoplasia (thus excepting the phakomatoses). The diagnosis relies mostly on anatomic alterations, whereas attenuation (CT) or signal abnormalities (MRI) are less useful. Hence the imaging findings for the conditions described herein are presented by anatomy rather than by imaging modality.

The application of MRI to congenital disorders over the past 10 years has yielded an unprecedented clarity of anatomic depiction and facilitated improved understanding of the embryologic basis for many malformations. There are instances, such as migrational disturbances or malformations of the craniocervical junction, where MRI is indispensable. Nonetheless, it is still possible to make a correct diagnosis with CT or even ultrasound in many cases.

Differential Diagnosis

The diagnosis of congenital malformations can be very straightforward sometimes and extremely difficult other times. Anomalies such as dysgenesis of the corpus callosum occur both individually and as a component of more complex malformations. Sometimes more than one complex anomaly may be present, as in the association of holoprosencephaly with the Dandy-Walker malformation. Most anomalies occur along a continuum of severity, and precise subclassification of conditions like holoprosencephaly and the Dandy-Walker complex can be a hairsplitting and probably inconsequential exercise. Lastly, despite our improved understanding and the wonder of MRI, not every malformation can be easily labeled.

A simplified algorithm with which to evaluate an unknown case is given in Figure 2–1; however, no representation is made that this will include *all* possibilities. Table 2–1 indicates the extent to which the major malformations overlap in their findings. Tables 2–2 through 2–4 are provided as further aids in the differential diagnosis.

TABLE 2–1 Anomalies Associated with Individual Disorders

	Extracranial Cyst	Posterior Fossa Cyst	Tonsillar Herniation	Gross Cortical Defects	Absent Septum Pellucidum	Tumors	Hydrocephalus	Defect of Corpus Callosum	Dysplastic Brain
Encephalocele	+	•		•	•		•	•	•
Meningocele	+	•		•	•		•	•	
Chiari III	+		+		•		+	•	•
Dandy-Walker malformation		+					•	•	•
Dandy-Walker variants		+					•	•	•
Chiari I			+				•		
Chiari II			+		•		+	•	•
Holoprosencephaly				•	•			•	
Hydranencephaly				+	•			•	
Porencephaly				+			•		
Schizencephaly				•	•			•	+
Septo-optic dysplasia					+			•	
Neurofibromatosis						•	•		•
Tuberous sclerosis						+	•		+
Lipoma						+		•	•
Aqueductal stenosis							+		
Lissencephaly							•	•	+
Dysgenesis of corpus callosum								+	
Heterotopia								•	+
Focal cortical dysplasia									+
Hemimegalencephaly									+
Sturge-Weber syndrome									+

\+ = Always or nearly always present
• = May be present

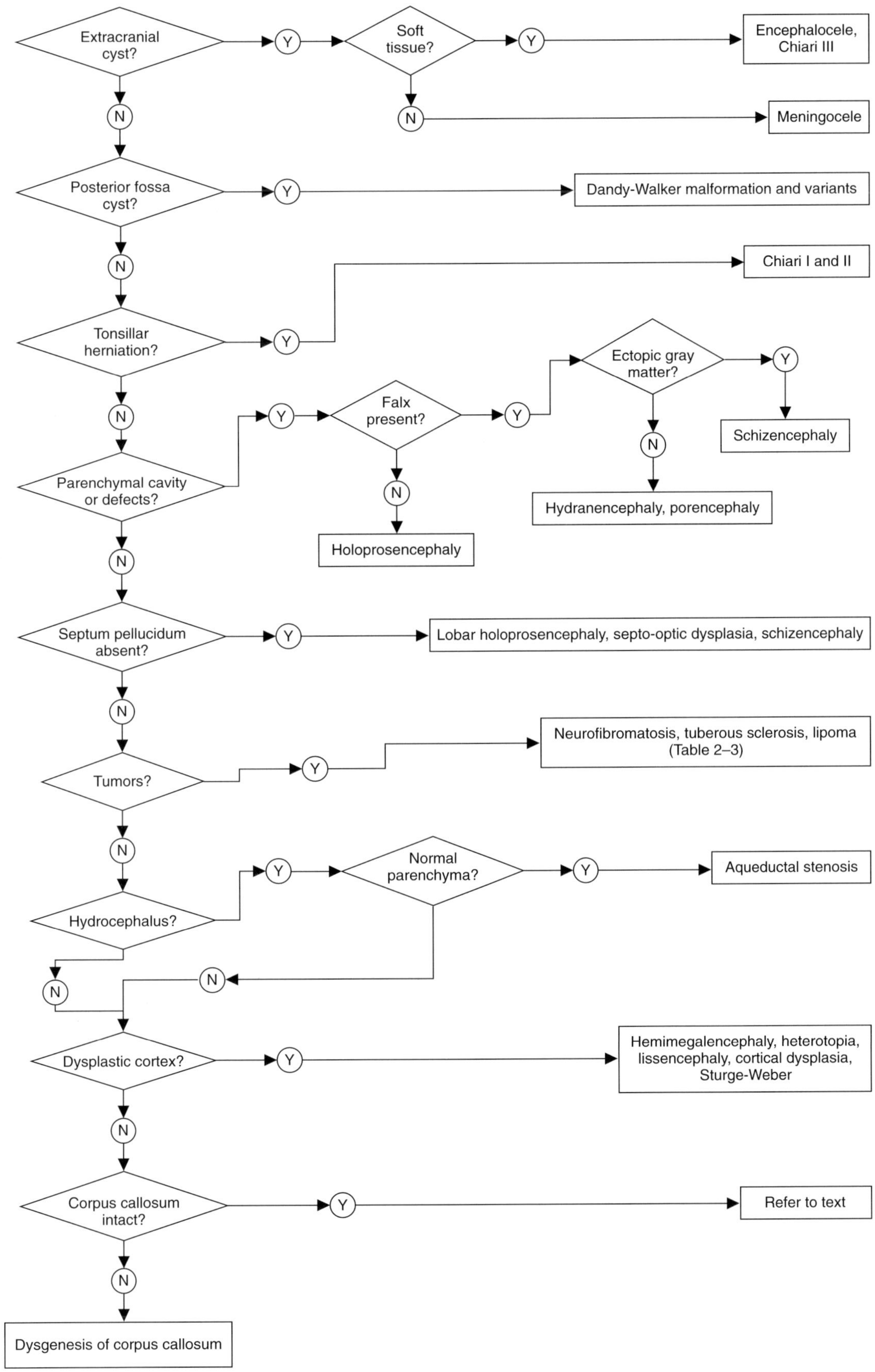

Figure 2–1. Algorithmic approach to differential diagnosis.

TABLE 2-2 | Differential Diagnosis of Partial or Complete Cortical Defects

Condition	Features
Holoprosencephaly	Partial or complete absence of cerebral hemispheres, absent falx cerebri
Hydranencephaly	Partial or complete absence of cerebral hemispheres, distinguished from holoprosencephaly by presence of intact falx cerebri
Schizencephaly	Unilateral or bilateral hemispheric cleft with continuous wall of gray matter from surface to lateral ventricle
Porencephaly	Cerebral cavity not lined by gray matter; may otherwise resemble schizencephaly
Meningoencephalocele	Extracerebral herniation of CSF or brain tissue always present

Disorders of Dorsal Induction (Neural Tube Defects)

Chiari I

The Chiari I malformation is a congenital hindbrain deformity in which there is downward displacement of the cerebellar tonsils with a normally positioned fourth ventricle. There is no increased incidence of myelomeningocele. Patients usually present during adulthood with symptoms of brainstem compression or syringohydromyelia. Many cases are incidentally detected on MRI performed

TABLE 2-3 | Congenital Malformations Associated with Neoplasia

Condition	Neoplasms	Distinguishing Features
Neurofibromatosis I	Extracranial plexiform neurofibromas Optic gliomas Brainstem gliomas Hypothalamic gliomas Arachnoid cysts Spinal cord gliomas Vascular malformations	Diagnosis based on clinical criteria, including ophthalmic, cutaneous, and osseous findings Café au lait spots, axillary freckling, and cutaneous neurofibromas Hypoplasia of sphenoid wing common Over 10 times more common than NF-2
Neurofibromatosis II	Cranial nerve schwannomas Ependymomas Meningiomas Spinal cord ependymomas	Definitive diagnosis based on bilateral acoustic schwannomas
Sturge-Weber syndrome	Leptomeningeal vascular malformation	Intense localized meningeal enhancement with atrophy and calcification of underlying cortex Port-wine stain
Lipoma	Benign lipoma	Not a true neoplasm Absence of mass effect
Tuberous sclerosis	Subependymal hamartomas Gyral hamartomas (tubers) Giant cell astrocytomas	Calcified subependymal hamartomas are diagnostic Giant cell astrocytomas usually at foramen of Monro, often cause hydrocephalus Numerous systemic findings
Hemimegalencephaly	Hemispheric hypertrophy	Not a true neoplasm Diffusely enlarged hemisphere with increased white matter

TABLE 2–4 **Differential Diagnosis of Dysplastic Brain**

Condition	Pathology	Features
Chiari II	Stenogyria	Abnormally small gyri
Lissencephaly	Agyria	Shallow or absent sulci
Schizencephaly	Transcortical cleft	Open or closed cleft
	Ectopic gray matter	Continuous seam of gray matter from pia to ependyma
Hemimegalencephaly	Hypertrophy	Enlarged hemisphere with increased white matter
Heterotopia	Ectopic gray matter	Gray matter rests deep within hemispheric white matter or lining the lateral ventricles
Focal cortical dysplasia	Pachygyria Polymicrogyria	Thickened gyri, accessory sulci due to gyral infolding
Sturge-Weber syndrome	Hypoplasia or atrophy	Atrophy and calcification develop beneath leptomeningeal vascular malformation
Tuberous sclerosis	Cortical hamartomas	Enlarged gyri with altered signal on MRI, calcifications
Neurofibromatosis	Hamartomas (?)	Nonspecific hyperintensities in basal ganglia, brainstem, and cerebellum
Lipoma	Hypoplasia	Hypoplasia of structures immediately contiguous to fatty mass

for unrelated indications. Symptoms are rare with herniations less than 5 mm but are present in 70% with herniations of 5 to 10 mm and in virtually all with herniations exceeding 12 mm.

Primary Abnormalities

- Herniation of cerebellar tonsils below the foramen magnum (>3 mm) which may be unilateral or asymmetric
- Fourth ventricle in normal position (but inferior recess may be elongated)

Ancillary Findings

- Syringohydromyelia in 30–50% of cases with peak frequency at cervical levels 4 through 6
- Ventral angulation of brainstem at foramen magnum (cervicomedullary kinking)
- Hydrocephalus in up to 44%
- Mamillopontine distance normal or reduced
- Craniospinal anomalies (atlanto-occipital assimilation, platybasia, basilar invagination)
- Pointed tonsillar tip rather than usual rounded appearance
- Effacement of cisterna magna

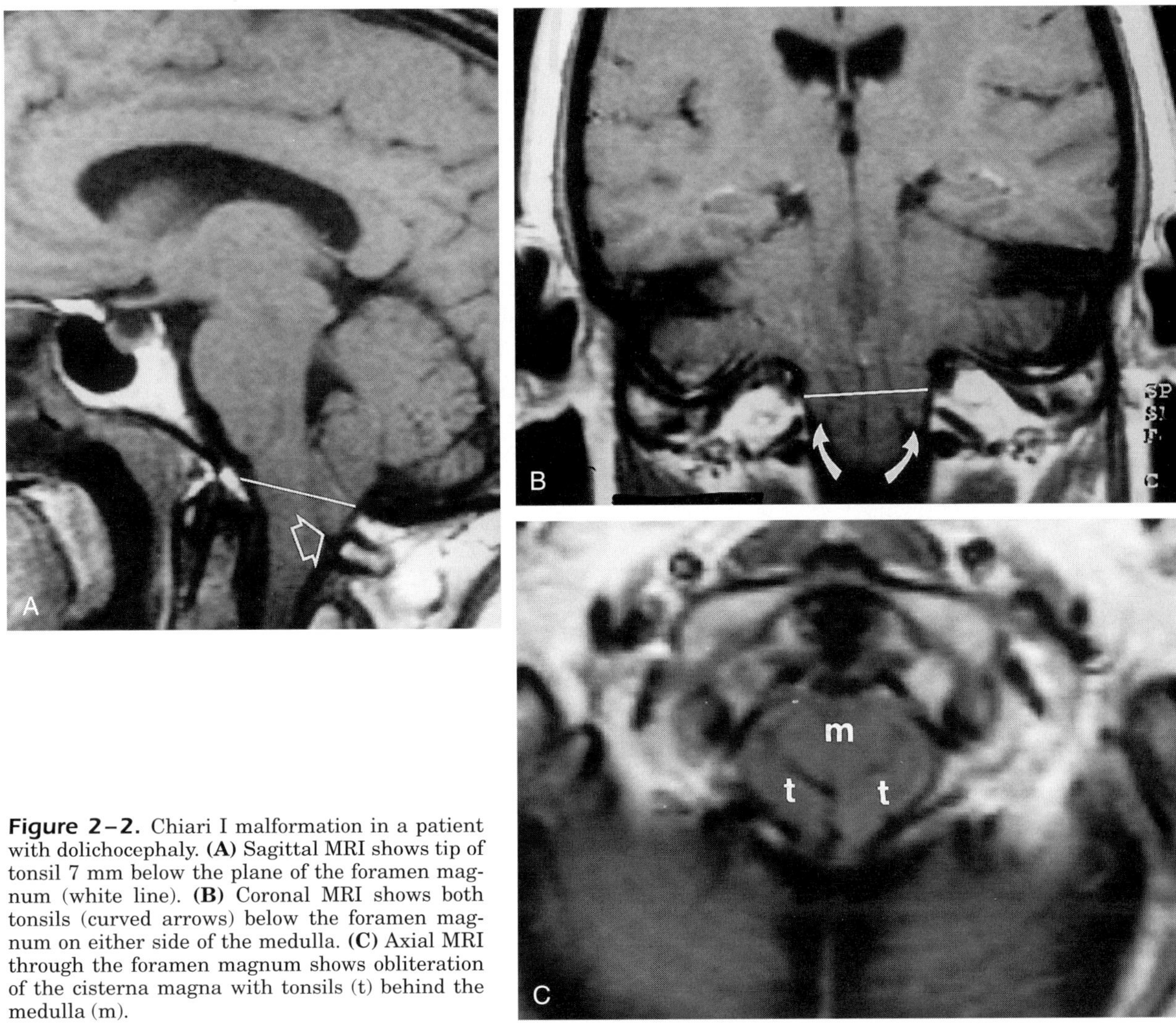

Figure 2–2. Chiari I malformation in a patient with dolichocephaly. **(A)** Sagittal MRI shows tip of tonsil 7 mm below the plane of the foramen magnum (white line). **(B)** Coronal MRI shows both tonsils (curved arrows) below the foramen magnum on either side of the medulla. **(C)** Axial MRI through the foramen magnum shows obliteration of the cisterna magna with tonsils (t) behind the medulla (m).

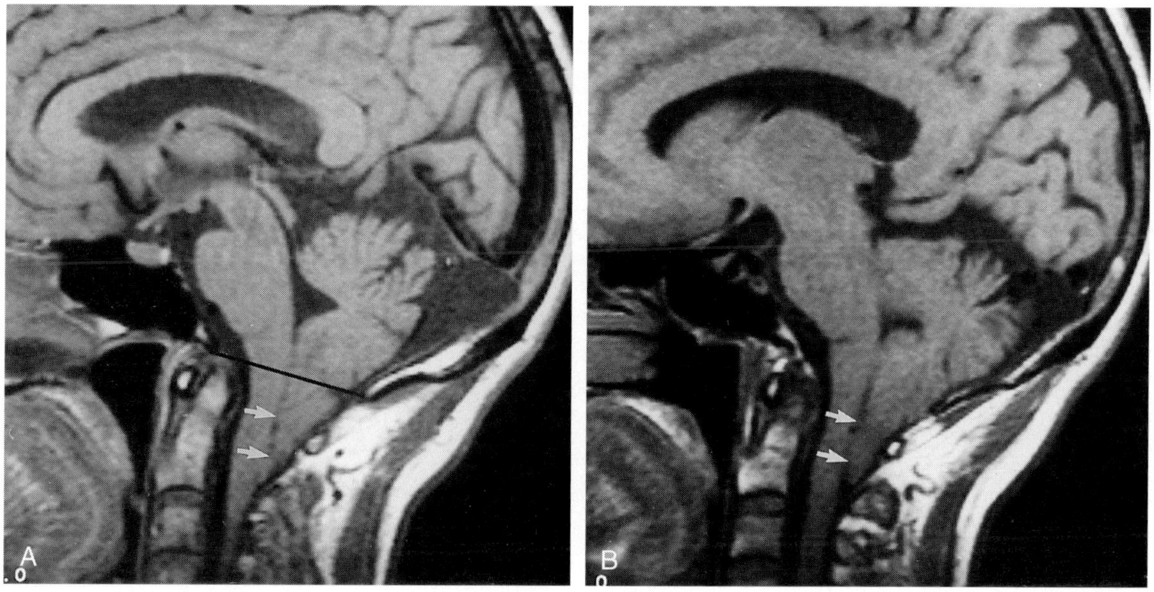

Figure 2–3. Chiari I. **(A)** Right and **(B)** left cerebellar tonsils (arrows) extend 30 mm below the foramen magnum (black line in **A**). Note the pointed appearance of the tonsillar tips.

Chiari II

Synonym: Arnold-Chiari II.

The Chiari II malformation is a complex and variable congenital hindbrain deformity almost invariably associated with a myelomeningocele. The incidence of myelomeningocele (and thus the Chiari II) varies by location, ranging from 3 in 10,000 births in Japan to 125 in 10,000 in Wales. It has been proposed that the neural tube defect is the primary abnormality and that the cranial abnormalities arise secondary to an in utero CSF leak and inadequate ventricular distension. About 20% of patients develop symptoms of brainstem, cranial nerve, and spinal cord compression, usually in infancy.

A Chiari II malformation with a cervico-occipital encephalocele (see following section) is considered a Chiari III malformation. The Chiari IV malformation is severe cerebellar hypoplasia or agenesis with hypoplasia of the pons and medulla.

Primary Abnormalities

- Caudal displacement of fourth ventricle, brainstem, cerebellar tonsils, and vermis through foramen magnum
- Meningomyelocele and obstructive hydrocephalus almost always present
- Small posterior fossa
- Dysplastic tentorium with wide incisura and low insertion

Ancillary Findings

Skull

- Lückenschädel skull (disappears after age 6 months)
- Petrous bone scalloping in 70–90%
- Concave scalloping of the clivus in up to 80%
- Concave scalloping of dens

Cerebral Hemispheres

- Polymicrogyria (or stenogyria, an area of very small but histologically normal gyri)
- Fenestration or partial absence of falx with gyral interdigitation across midline in 20–80%
- Dysgenesis of the corpus callosum

Lateral Ventricles

- Hydrocephalus in up to 90%
- Inferior pointing of the frontal horns of the lateral ventricles
- Absence of the septum pellucidum in 40%
- Colpocephaly (nonhydrocephalic enlargement of the trigones and occipital horns)

Third Ventricle

- Enlargement of the massa intermedia in 80–90%
- Enlargement of suprapineal recess
- Pseudodiverticula of anterior (lamina terminalis) and inferior (hypothalamus) walls

Brainstem

- Increased mamillopontine distance (maximum normal is 12 mm) from stretching of midbrain
- Caudal displacement of pons and medulla
- Flattening of ventral pons
- Nonvisualization of the cerebral aqueduct in up to 70%
- Wide prepontine cistern
- Tectal beaking from fusion and deformity of the quadrigeminal plate

Cerebellum/Posterior Fossa

- "Towering cerebellum" or pseudomass from upward herniation of cerebellum through incisura
- Downward herniation of cerebrum through incisura and flattening of superior cerebellum
- Vertically oriented straight sinus
- Cerebellum hypoplastic and poorly differentiated with craniocaudal elongation
- Poor visualization of folia
- Cerebellum wrapped around brainstem, causing "triple peak" appearance on axial sections
- Obliteration of cisterna magna and cerebellopontine angle cisterns
- Fourth ventricle thin, elongated, and possibly obliterated
- Ballooning of the fourth ventricle in about 5%

Spine

- Foramen magnum enlarged in 75%
- Constriction of spinal canal at C1 by fibrous band
- Cervicomedullary kink (herniation of medulla posterior to spinal cord) in up to 70%
- Syringohydromyelia
- Caudal displacement of cervical cord

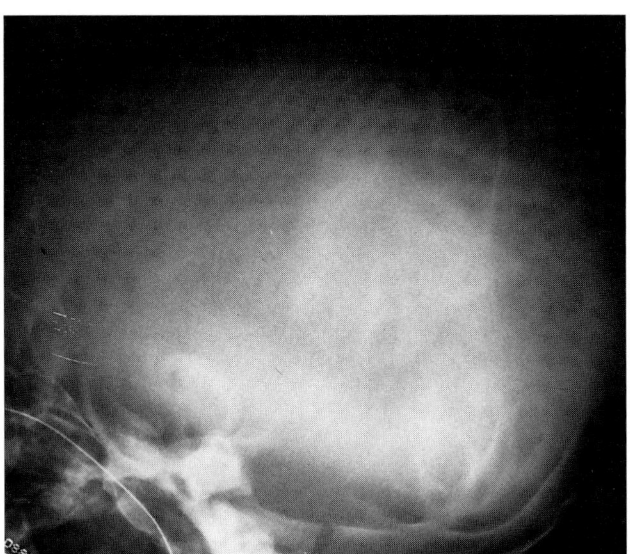

Figure 2–4. Arnold Chiari II. Skull radiograph shows the trabecular appearance of lückenschädel skull.

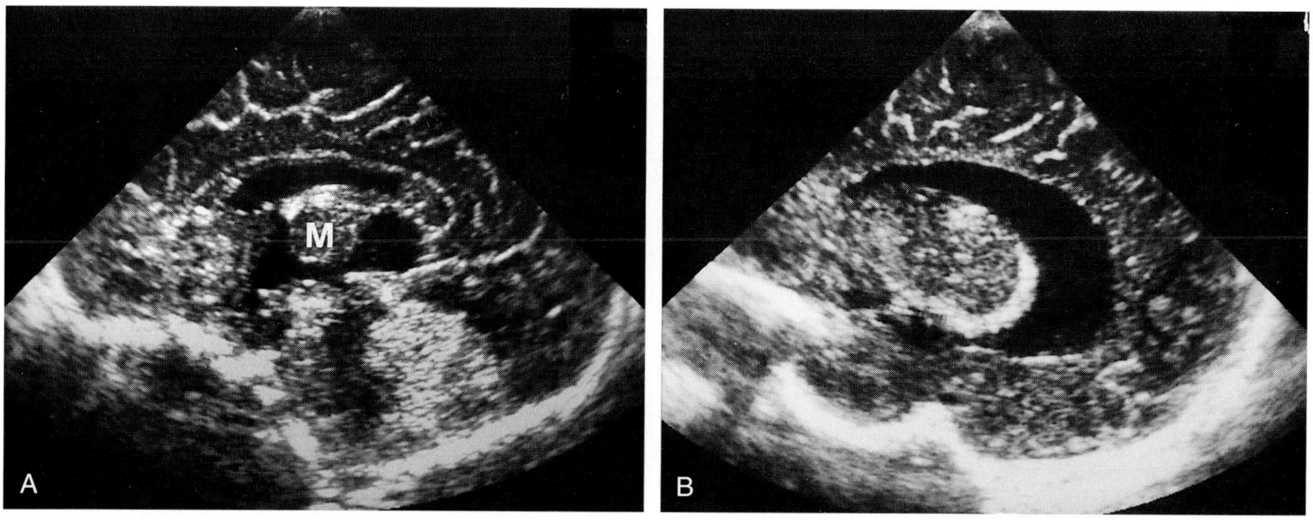

Figure 2–5. Arnold Chiari II. **(A)** Midline sagittal sonogram shows enlargement of the massa intermedia (M). **(B)** Parasagittal sonogram through lateral ventricle shows mild ventricular enlargement and colpocephaly.

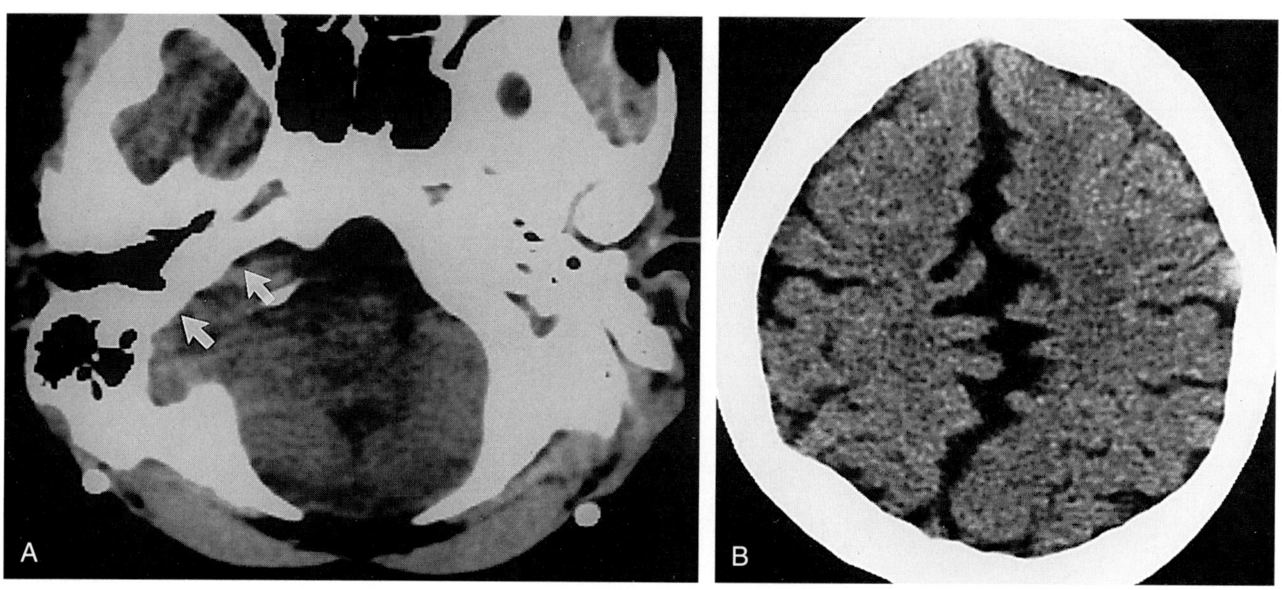

Figure 2–6. Arnold Chiari II. **(A)** CT of skull base shows enlargement of the foramen magnum and scalloping (arrows) of the right petrous bone. **(B)** Scan through vertex shows partial absence of the falx with a mild degree of gyral interdigitation.

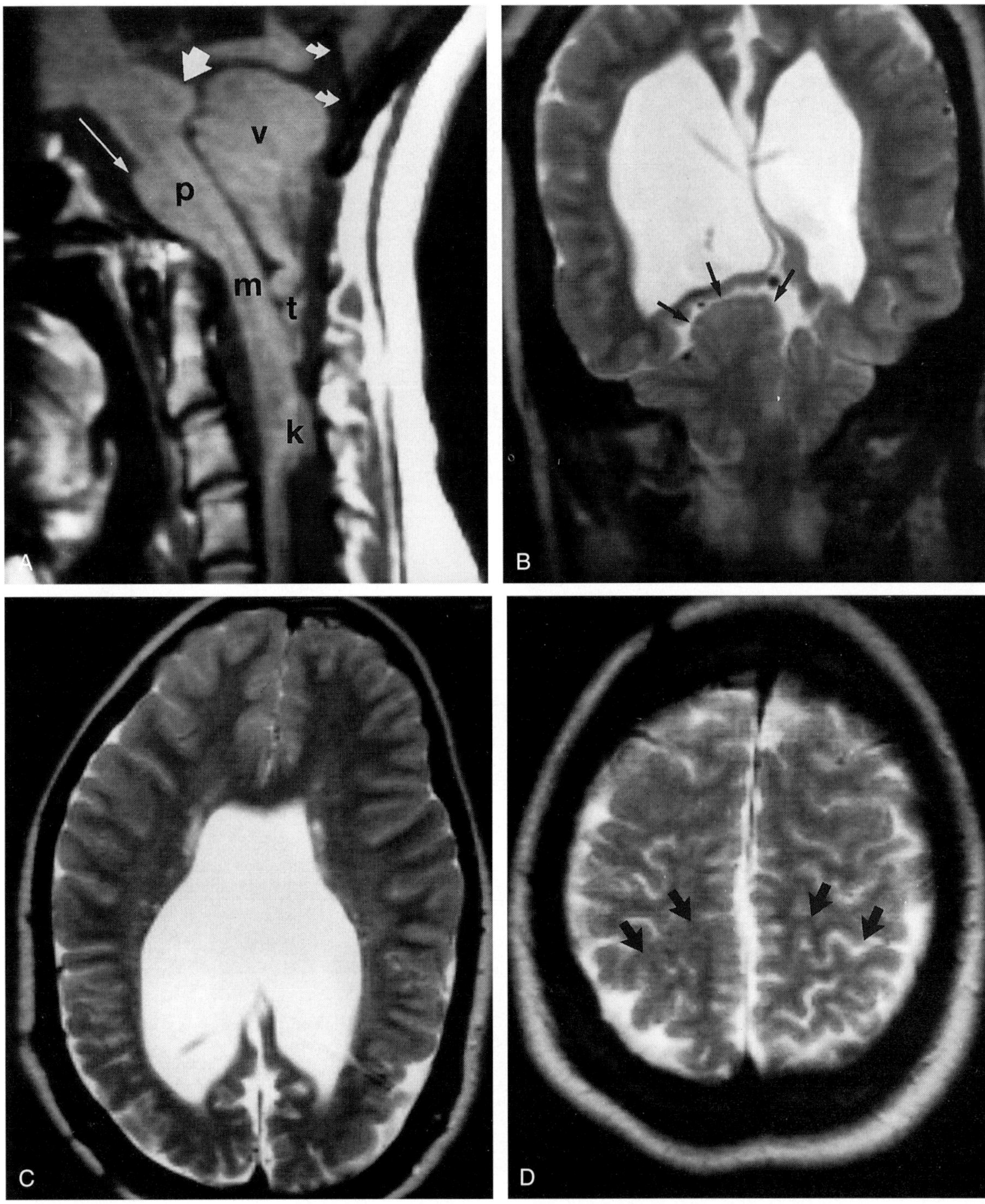

Figure 2–7. Arnold Chiari II. **(A)** Sagittal MRI illustrates the primary abnormalities of the Chiari II malformation with caudal displacement of the tonsils (t), vermis (v), medulla (m), and fourth ventricle through an enlarged foramen magnum. A cervicomedullary kink (k) is present behind C3. The vermis is small and dysplastic, lacking normal folia. Caudal displacement of the pons (p) has resulted in an increased mammillopontine distance (long thin arrow). Tectal beaking is present (thick arrow). The fourth ventricle is thin and elongated. Curved arrows indicate the vertical course of the straight sinus. **(B)** Coronal T2-weighted MRI shows a dysplastic tentorium with wide incisura and small posterior fossa with towering cerebellum (arrows). **(C)** Axial scan through lateral ventricles shows absence of the septum pellucidum, hydrocephalus, and colpocephaly. **(D)** Axial MRI through vertex shows areas of abnormally small gyri (stenogyria) posteriorly (arrows).

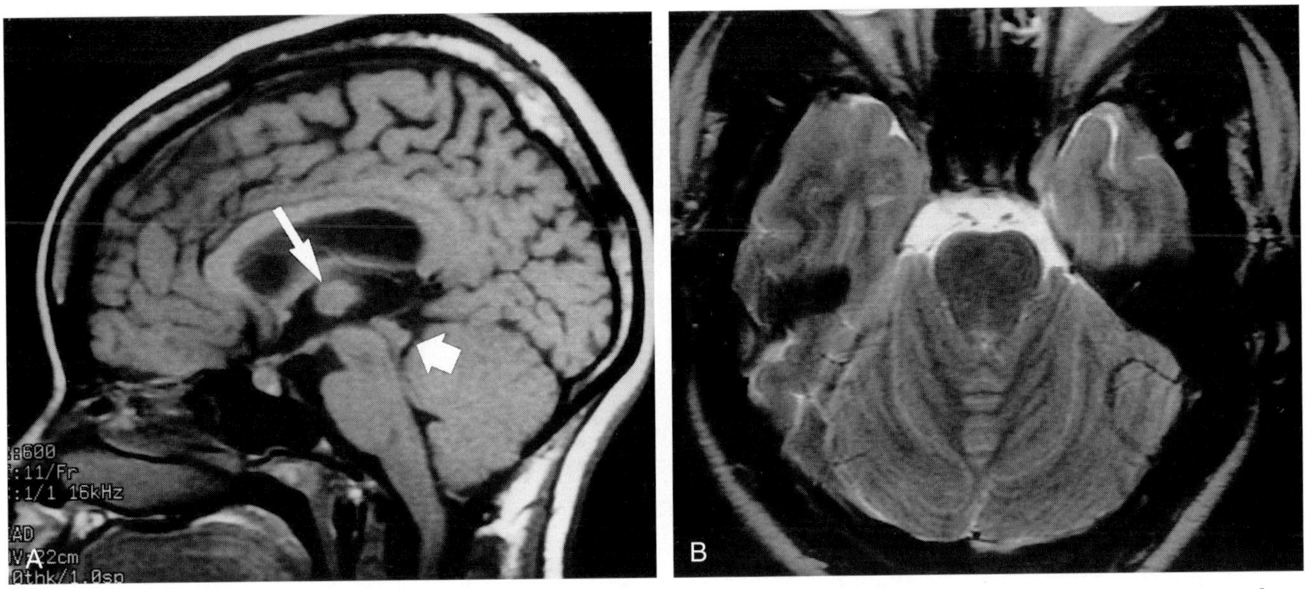

Figure 2–8. Arnold Chiari II. **(A)** Sagittal MRI in a milder case shows enlargement of the massa intermedia (long arrow) and tectal beaking (short arrow). **(B)** On axial section the cerebellum is wrapped around both sides of the brainstem resulting in the triple peak appearance.

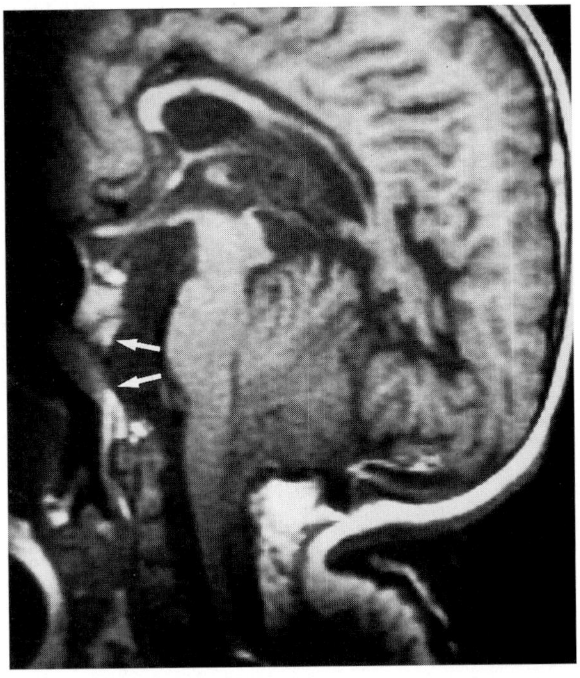

Figure 2–9. Arnold Chiari II. Sagittal MRI illustrates a wide prepontine cistern, scalloping of the clivus (arrows), and callosal dysgenesis. (Courtesy of Dr. Loretta Shearer, Louisville, KY.)

Encephalocele

Encephaloceles are congenital herniations of brain and meninges through a skull defect and result from incomplete closure of the neural tube. They are one tenth as common as myelomeningoceles with an incidence of 1 to 3 per 10,000 births. Most occur in the occipital region, and the diagnosis is clinically evident at birth. The prognosis is related to the size of the herniation and the amount of brain tissue within the sac. Simple meningoceles portend a favorable outcome, whereas cases with significant brain herniations have a poor prognosis.

Primary Abnormalities

- Midline skull defect with hernia sac containing CSF (meningocele) or brain and CSF (meningoencephalocele)
- Location:

Occipital	70%
Parietal	10%
Frontal	9%
Nasal	9%

Ancillary Findings

- Microcephaly
- Islands of disorganized tissue lining the walls of the sac
- Hydrocephalus
- Defects of posterior arches of upper cervical vertebra (seen with low occipital encephaloceles)
- Absence of anterior commissure, septum pellucidum, and fornix in 80%
- Partial or complete agenesis of corpus callosum
- Absence or severe hypoplasia of cerebellar hemispheres
- Dandy-Walker cysts

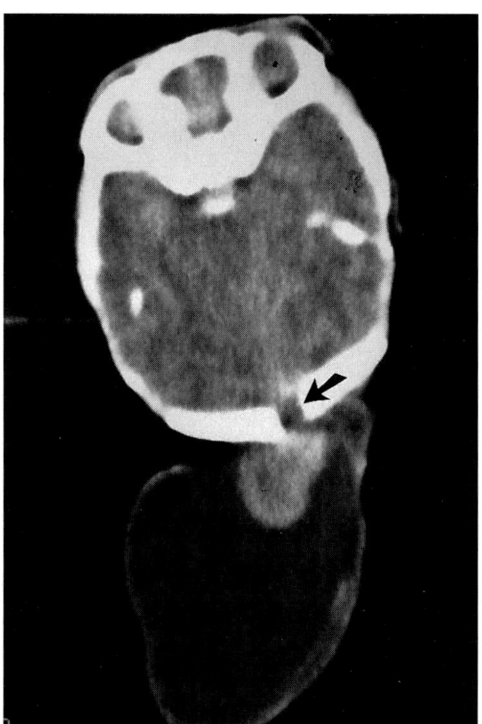

Figure 2–10. Meningoencephalocele. Axial CT shows a large occipital meningoencephalocele containing brain and CSF. Note the midline skull defect (arrow).

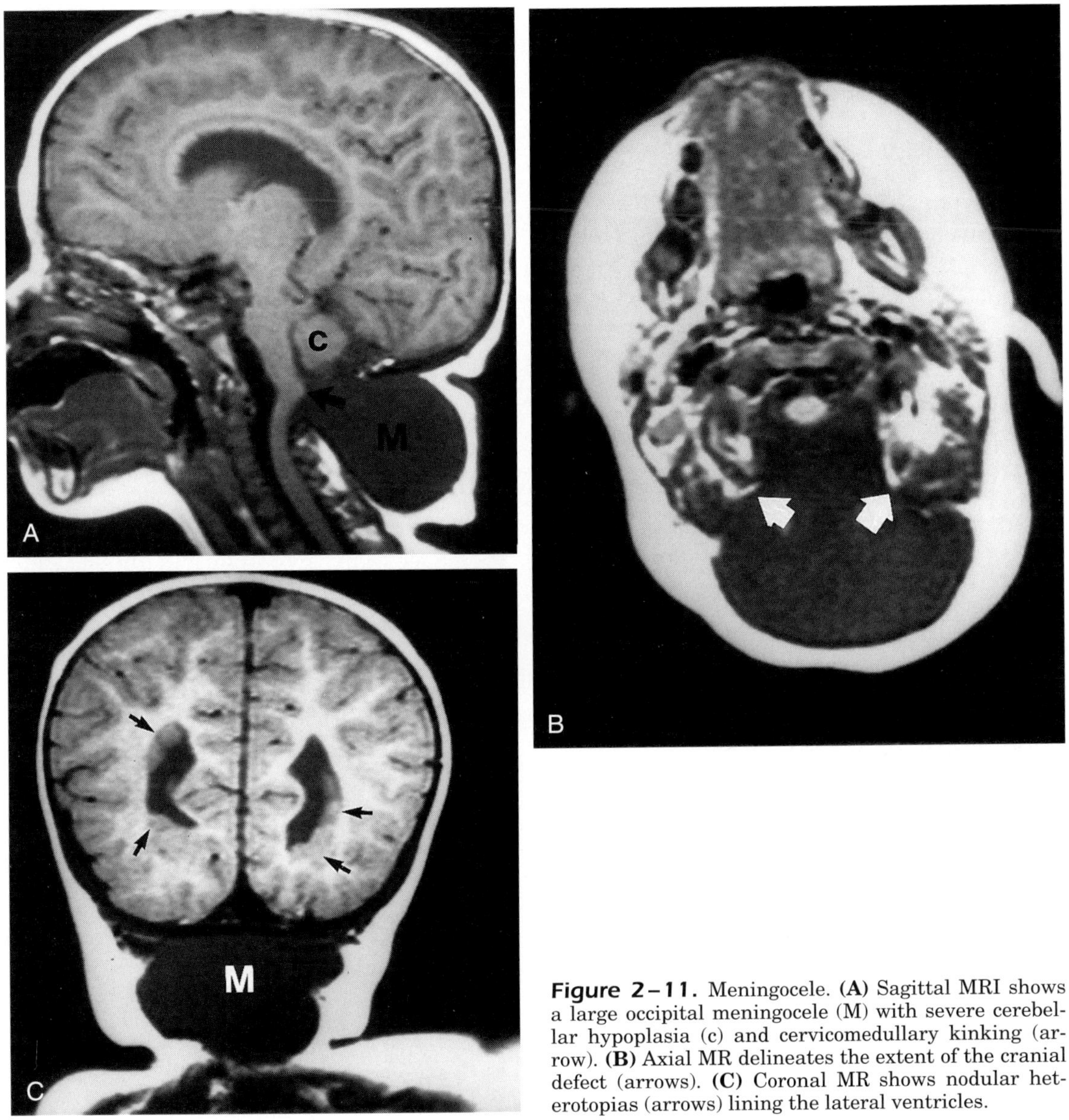

Figure 2–11. Meningocele. **(A)** Sagittal MRI shows a large occipital meningocele (M) with severe cerebellar hypoplasia (c) and cervicomedullary kinking (arrow). **(B)** Axial MR delineates the extent of the cranial defect (arrows). **(C)** Coronal MR shows nodular heterotopias (arrows) lining the lateral ventricles.

Disorders of Ventral Induction (Hemispheric Organization)

Holoprosencephaly

Holoprosencephaly is a condition in which there is failure or incomplete diverticulation of the primitive forebrain. The result may range from persistence of a single midline cerebrum and monoventricle (alobar), to partial hemispheric development (semilobar), to nearly complete diverticulation with only partial fusion of the frontal lobes (lobar holoprosencephaly). The incidence is approximately 1 in 10,000 live births. Most are isolated in nature, but the condition is associated with trisomy 13 and a long list of less common conditions.

Alobar Holoprosencephaly

Primary Abnormalities

- Single holoventricle (oval, round, or horseshoe shaped) with no differentiation of the ventricular system
- Absence of third ventricle, sylvian fissure, opercular cortex, falx, interhemispheric fissure, corpus callosum, and tentorium
- Absence of internal cerebral veins, superior and inferior sagittal sinuses, straight sinuses, and vein of Galen
- Fusion of thalami and basal ganglia in the midline

Ancillary Findings

- Microcephaly
- Trigonocephaly (triangular shaped head)
- Dorsal sac or cyst may compress the monoventricle anteriorly
- Pancake of cerebral cortex anteriorly (the holoprosencephalon) with pachygyria
- Azygous (single) anterior cerebral artery

Facial Anomalies

- Cyclopia (single midline orbit)
- Cebocephaly (hypotelorism and single nostril)
- Ethmocephaly (midline proboscis between orbits)
- Cleft lip or palate

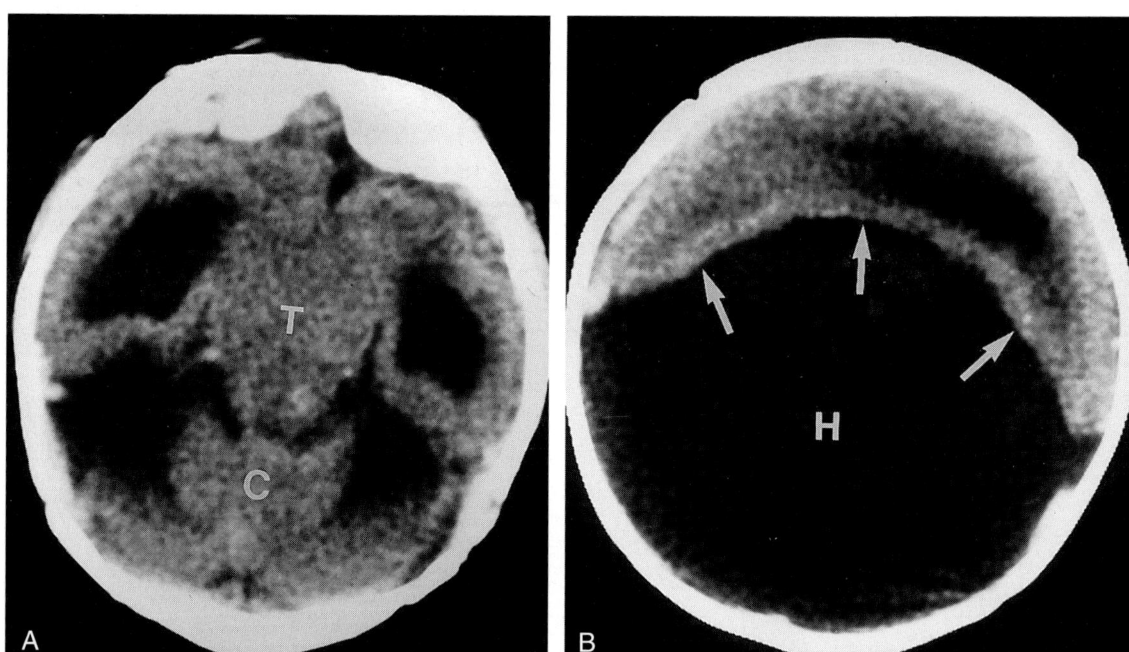

Figure 2–12. Alobar holoprosencephaly. **(A)** Lower CT section shows the midline mass of fused thalami (T). More posteriorly is the superior cerebellum (C). **(B)** Higher section shows the large holoventricle (H), absence of the falx, and anterior pancake of the cerebral cortex (arrows).

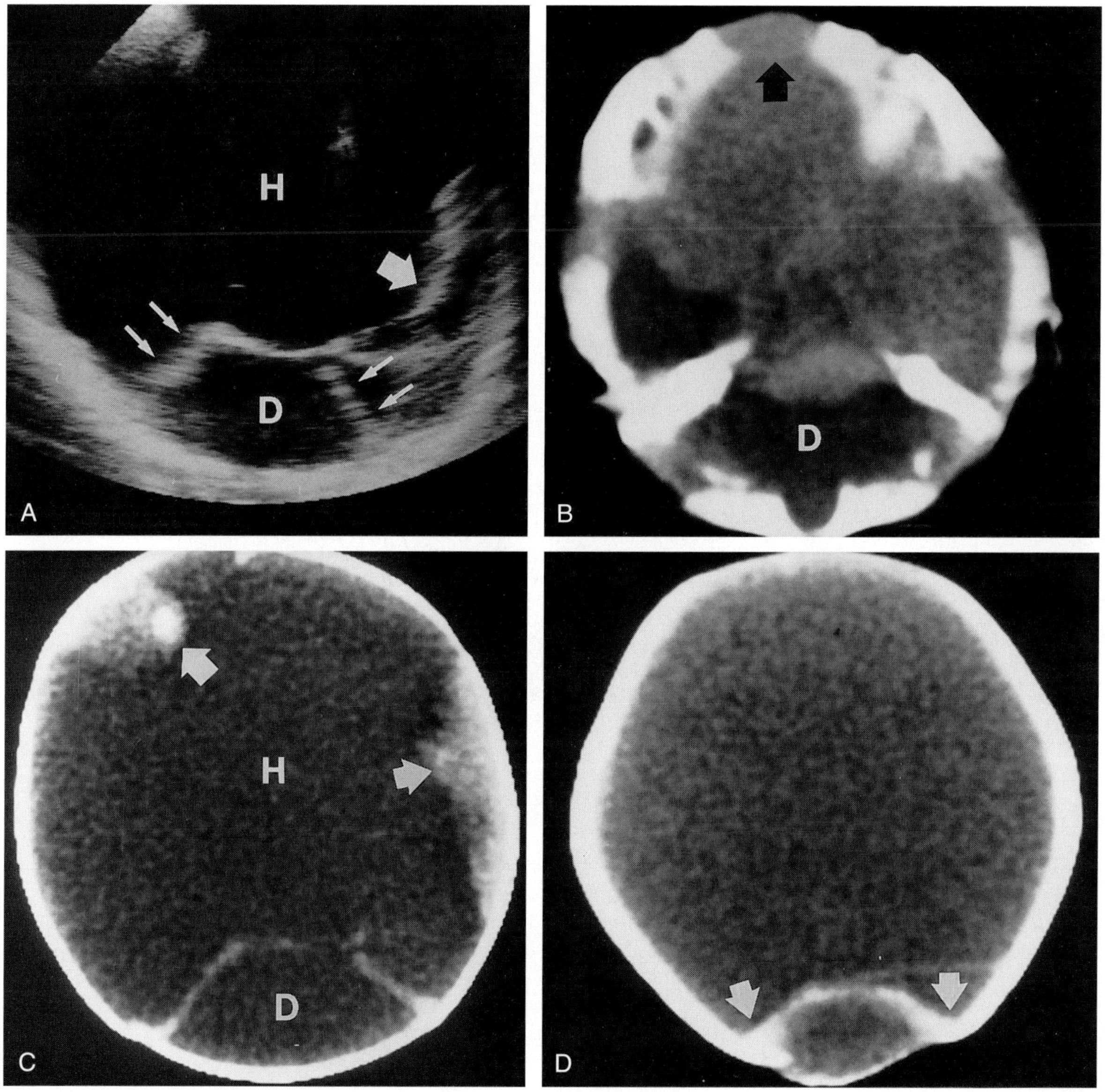

Figure 2–13. Alobar holoprosencephaly and Dandy-Walker cyst. **(A)** Coronal sonogram shows absence of the falx, large holoventricle (H), flattened cortex (large arrow), and Dandy-Walker cyst (D). Small arrows indicate the tentorium. **(B)** CT through posterior fossa shows Dandy-Walker cyst (D). Flattened featureless cortex occupies the anterior cranial vault. There is a large anterior frontal bone defect (arrow). **(C)** Higher section shows the Dandy-Walker cyst bounded by the tentorium, a large cerebral holoventricle (H), and the superior limit of the cortical pancake (arrows). **(D)** Scan near the vertex shows abnormally high tentorial attachment (arrows) and absence of the falx. The last feature distinguishes this case from hydranencephaly.

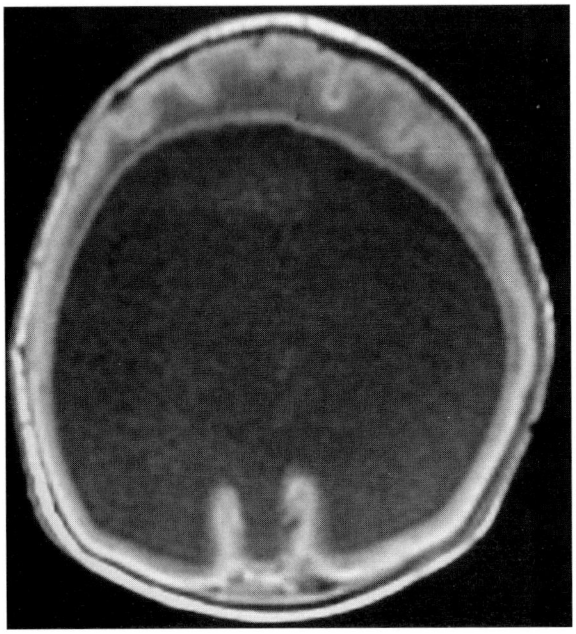

Figure 2–14. Alobar holoprosencephaly. Axial MRI shows the large holoventricle, ventral pancake of cerebral cortex, and absence of the falx. (Courtesy of Dr. Frank Raila, Jackson, MS.)

Semilobar Holoprosencephaly

Primary Abnormalities

- Cerebral monoventricle with some formation of occipital and/or temporal horns

Ancillary Findings

- Partial development of third ventricle, posterior interhemispheric fissure, falx, dural sinuses, deep veins, and corpus callosum
- Partial cleavage of thalami by rudimentary third ventricle
- Holoprosencephalon may be thicker and cover more of the monoventricle
- Dorsal cyst smaller than in alobar form

Lobar Holoprosencephaly

Primary Abnormalities

- Partial fusion of the frontal lobes with a shallow anterior interhemispheric fissure

Ancillary Findings

- Hypoplastic falx and shallow interhemispheric fissure anteriorly
- Absence of the septum pellucidum with squared off frontal horns
- Otherwise normal formation of the cerebral hemispheres

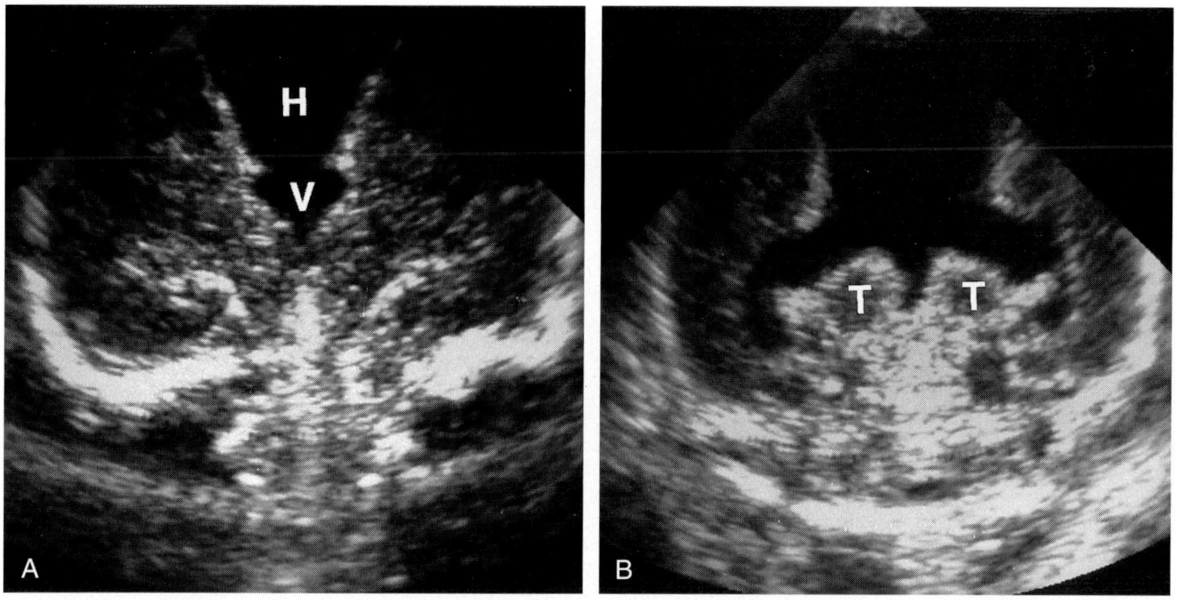

Figure 2–15. Semilobar holoprosencephaly. **(A)** Coronal sonogram shows a midline holoventricle (H), greater parenchymal development, and partial formation of the third ventricle (V). **(B)** More posterior section shows almost complete separation of the thalami (T). The falx is absent.

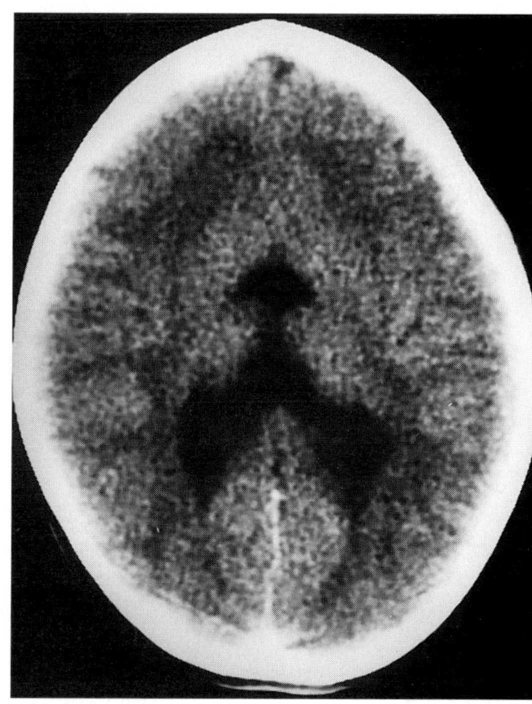

Figure 2–16. Semilobar holoprosencephaly. CT shows midline fusion of the lateral ventricles and partial development of the falx. The septum pellucidum is absent.

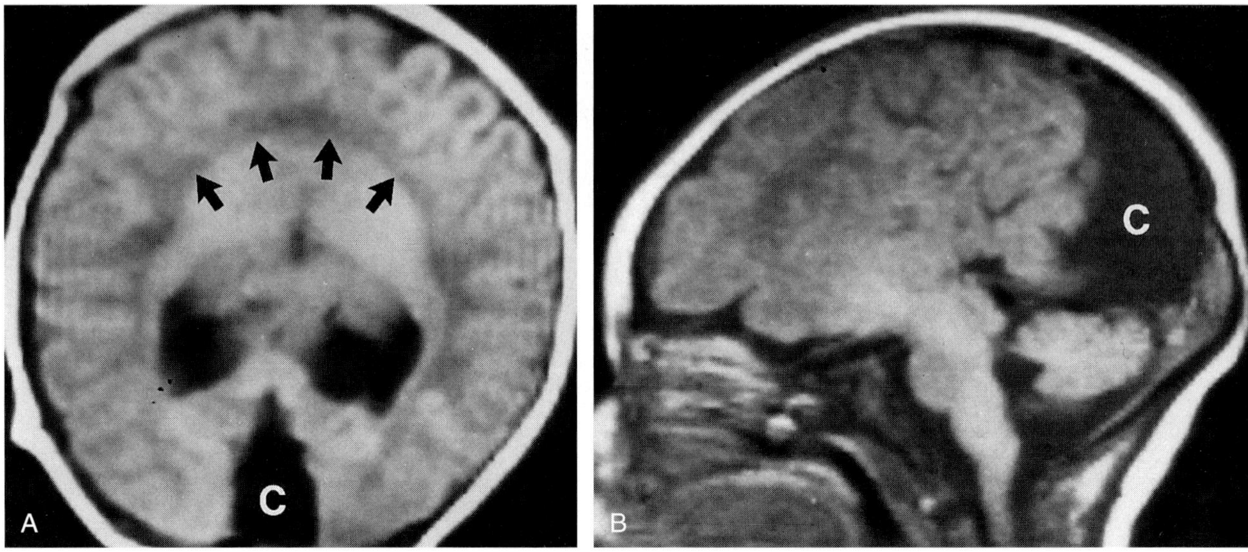

Figure 2–17. Lobar holoprosencephaly. **(A)** Axial and **(B)** sagittal MRI show complete development of third and lateral ventricles. The corpus callosum is dysplastic. The key finding is the continuous anterior rind of cortex (arrows) with absence of the anterior falx and interhemispheric fissure. A dorsal cyst is present (C).

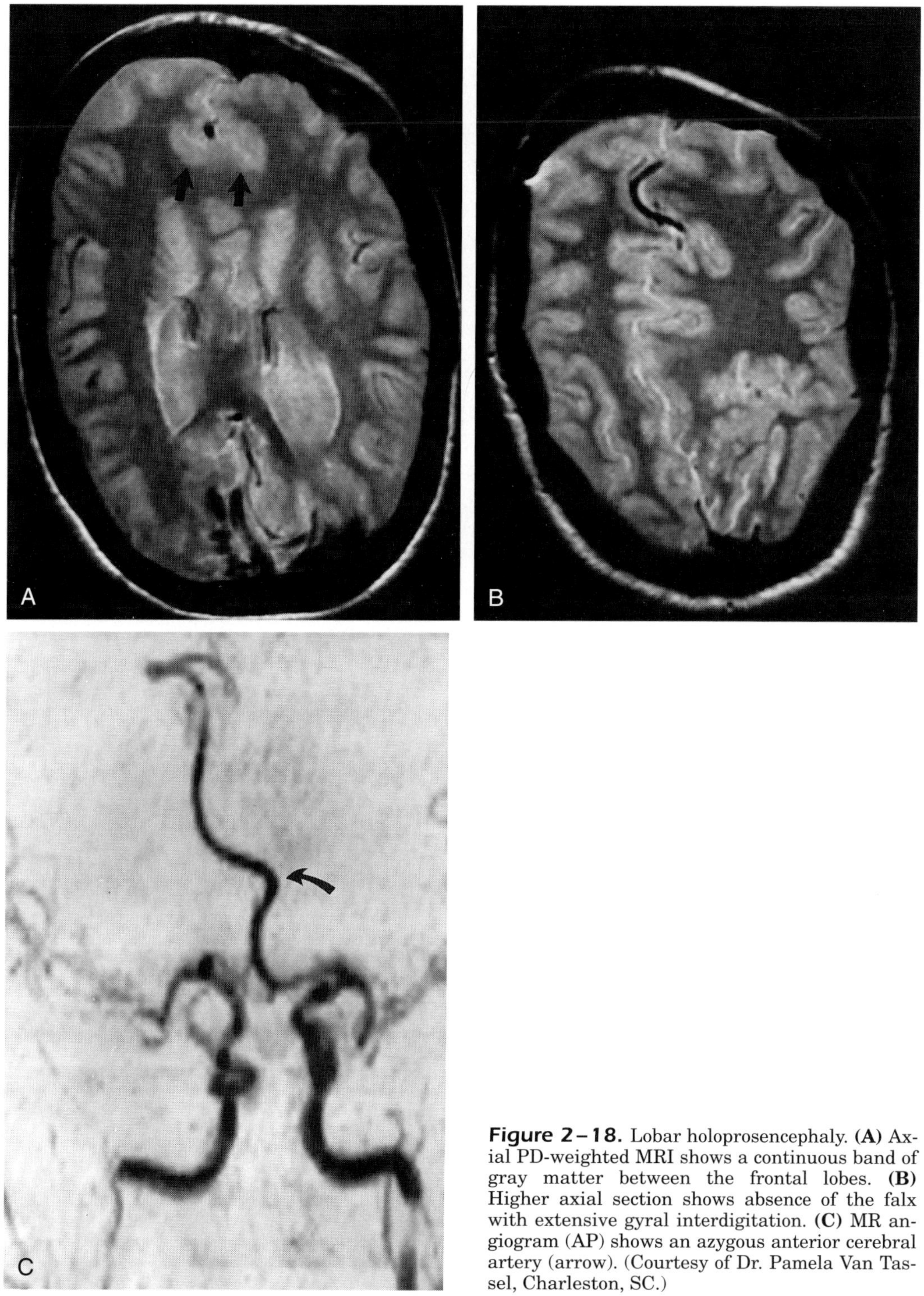

Figure 2–18. Lobar holoprosencephaly. **(A)** Axial PD-weighted MRI shows a continuous band of gray matter between the frontal lobes. **(B)** Higher axial section shows absence of the falx with extensive gyral interdigitation. **(C)** MR angiogram (AP) shows an azygous anterior cerebral artery (arrow). (Courtesy of Dr. Pamela Van Tassel, Charleston, SC.)

Septo-optic Dysplasia

Septo-optic dysplasia (de Morsier syndrome) consists of absence of the septum pellucidum with hypoplasia of the optic nerves or chiasm. The etiology is not known, although it may be a mild form of holoprosencephaly (incomplete diverticulation of the prosencephalon). Affected patients present with congenital blindness and often develop symptoms of hypopituitarism. Imaging is less sensitive than clinical examination for the optic nerve deficiency; thus, absence of the septum pellucidum may be the only imaging finding. Absence of the septum pellucidum by itself, however, does not establish the diagnosis. Up to 50% of patients diagnosed clinically also have schizencephaly. This latter group exhibits varying degrees of septal hypoplasia and may represent a distinct clinical entity.

Primary Abnormalities

- Absent (or incomplete) septum pellucidum
- Optic nerve hypoplasia

Ancillary Findings

- Dilated frontal horns with inferior pointing
- Small optic nerves and chiasm
- Enlarged suprasellar cistern
- Dilatation of anterior recesses of third ventricle
- Lower than normal fornix
- Small pituitary, hypoplastic, or absent infundibulum
- Colpocephaly
- Diffuse white matter hypoplasia
- Hypoplasia of corpus callosum

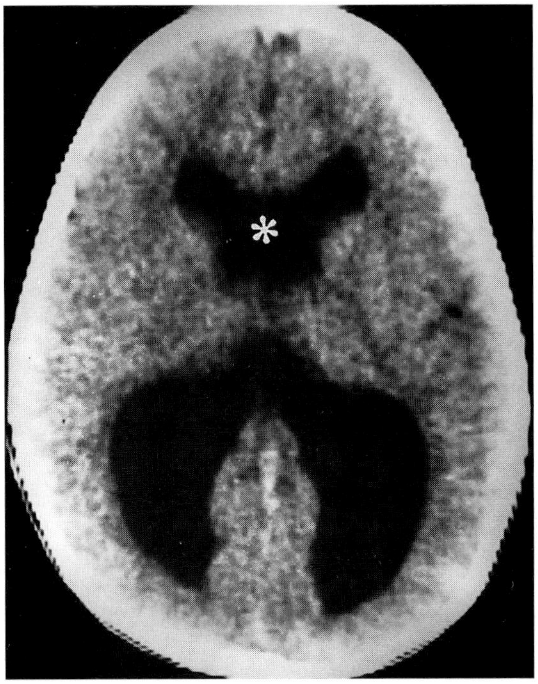

Figure 2–19. Septo-optic dysplasia. CT shows absence of the septum pellucidum (asterisk), dilated frontal horns, and colpocephaly.

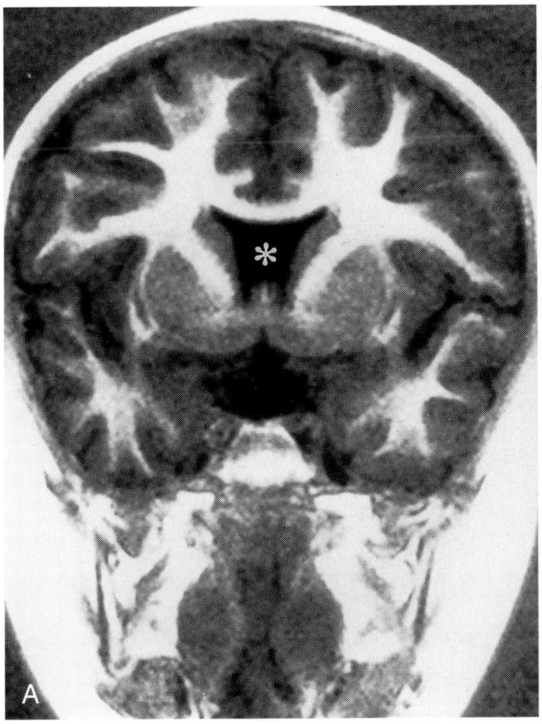

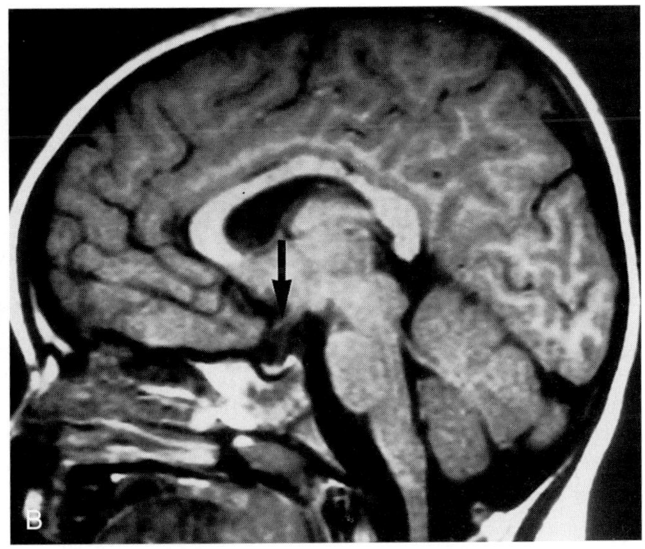

Figure 2–20. Septo-optic dysplasia. **(A)** Coronal MRI (IR sequence) shows absence of the septum pellucidum (asterisk). The optic chiasm is poorly visualized. **(B)** Sagittal view shows a severely hypoplastic optic chiasm (arrow) and a small pituitary gland.

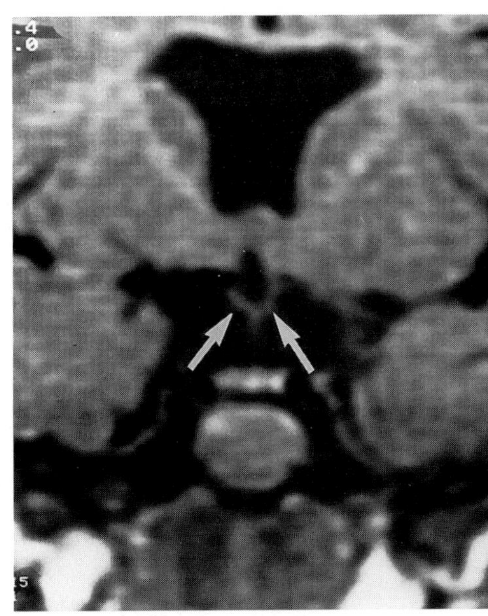

Figure 2–21. Septo-optic dysplasia. Coronal MRI shows absence of the septum pellucidum and severe hypoplasia of optic chiasm (arrows).

Dandy-Walker Malformation

Dandy-Walker malformation (DWM) represents the most severe form in a spectrum of cystic posterior fossa malformations anchored at the other end by megacisterna magna. DWM occurs with an incidence of about 0.3 per 10,000 births. It is believed to result from an in utero obstruction of the fourth ventricle by a fetal membrane, although the membrane may proceed to lyse (forming a patent foramen of Magendie) by birth. Over 80% of patients present with progressive hydrocephalus, usually after birth but before 3 months of age.

Primary Abnormalities

- Cystic dilatation of fourth ventricle communicating with posterior fossa cyst
- Absence or hypoplasia of vermis
- Enlarged posterior fossa

Ancillary Findings

Skull and Dura

- Macrocephaly
- Dolichocephaly
- Scalloping of petrous pyramids
- Elevated tentorial insertion with vertically oriented incisura
- Elevation of torcular
- Falx cerebelli usually absent

Cerebellum and Brainstem

- Residual superior vermis displaced upward by the retrocerebellar cyst
- Anterior and lateral displacement of cerebellar hemispheres
- Hypoplastic cerebellar hemispheres
- Brainstem small and hypoplastic or compressed

Ventricles

- Hydrocephalus

Dandy-Walker Cyst

- Massively dilated fourth ventricle displaces cerebellar hemispheres anteriorly and vermis superiorly
- Cyst may herniate through foramen magnum

Associated Anomalies

- Dysgenesis of corpus callosum
- Migrational anomalies
- Holoprosencephaly

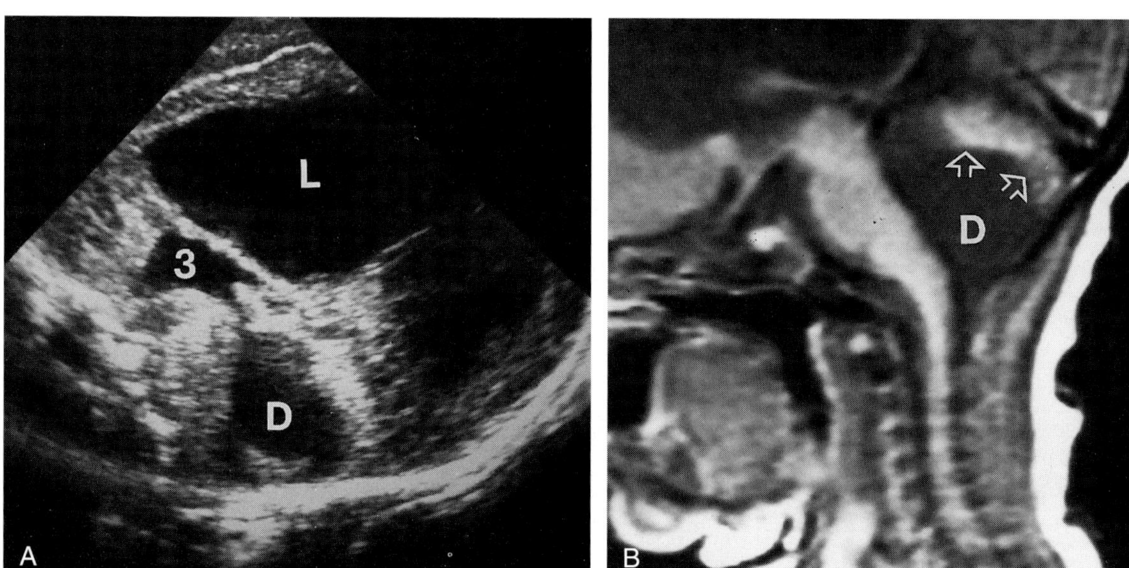

Figure 2–22. Dandy-Walker malformation. **(A)** Sagittal sonogram shows severe hydrocephalus and a posterior fossa cyst. L = lateral ventricles, 3 = third ventricle, D = Dandy-Walker cyst. **(B)** Sagittal MRI shows the cyst (D) and upward displacement of the residual cerebellar vermis (arrows).

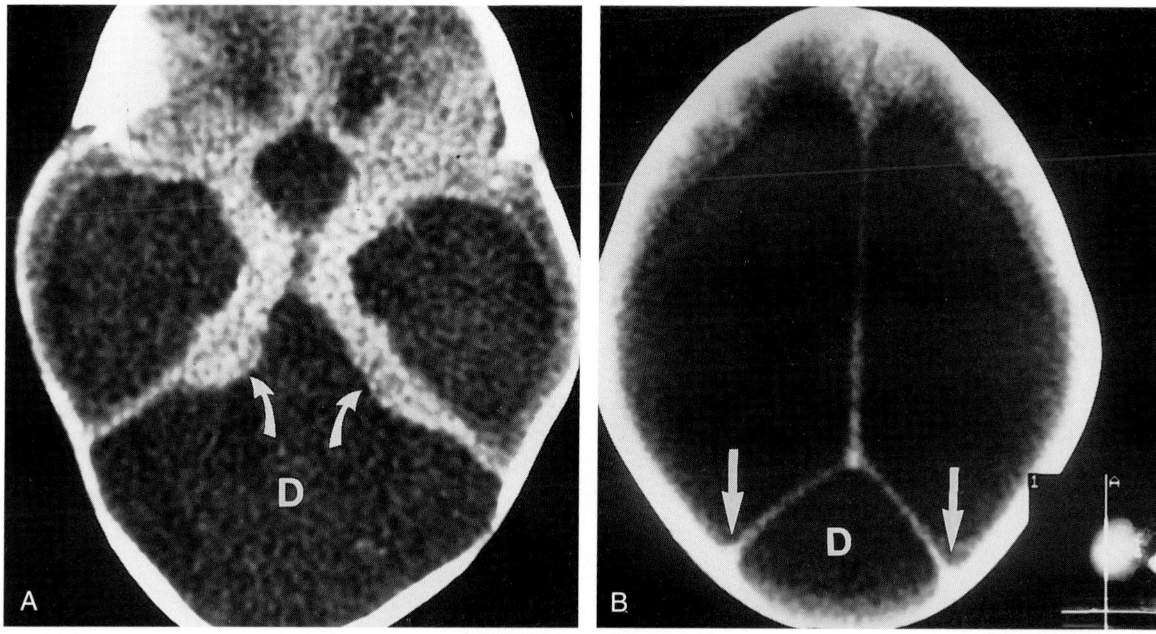

Figure 2–23. Dandy-Walker malformation. **(A)** CT shows Dandy-Walker cyst (D), anterolateral displacement of hypoplastic cerebellar hemispheres (arrows), and massive hydrocephalus. The posterior fossa is dramatically enlarged, and the falx cerebelli is absent. **(B)** On higher section there is severe hydrocephalus and marked elevation of the tentorial insertion (arrows). A thin rim of cortex allows differentiation from hydranencephaly, and the intact falx excludes holoprosencephaly. (Courtesy of Dr. Loretta Shearer, Louisville, KY.)

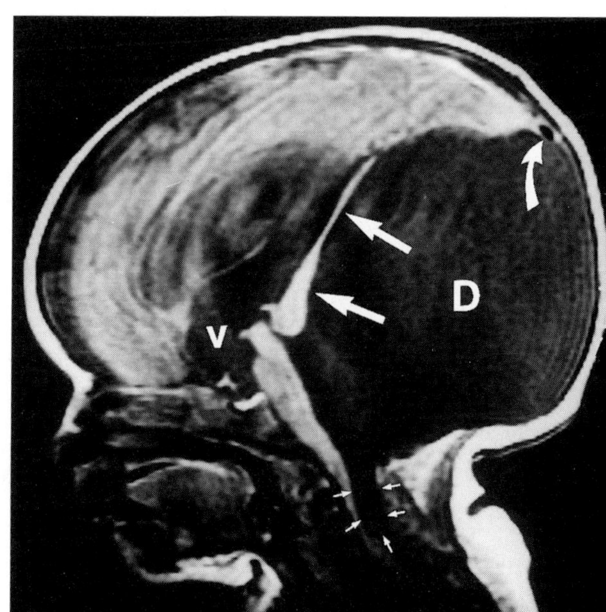

Figure 2–24. Dandy-Walker malformation. Sagittal MRI shows massive expansion of the posterior fossa by Dandy-Walker cyst (D) resulting in macrocephaly. The torcular is elevated (curved arrow) along with the tentorial insertion. The brainstem is compressed, the hypoplastic vermis (straight arrows) is markedly elevated, and the third ventricle (v) is markedly distended. Note compression of the cervical cord due to herniation of cyst (small arrows) through the foramen magnum. (Courtesy of Dr. Alan Lovell, Birmingham, AL.)

Dandy-Walker Variant

The Dandy-Walker variant differs from DWM by the presence of a normal-size posterior fossa and better-formed fourth ventricle. It is twice as common as DWM, composing one third of cystic posterior fossa malformations. Affected children may present with hydrocephalus or developmental delay.

Primary Abnormalities

- Hypoplasia of the vermis with dilatation of the fourth ventricle
- Normal-size or mildly enlarged posterior fossa

Ancillary Findings

- Hydrocephalus sometimes present
- Falx cerebelli may be present
- Hypoplastic cerebellar hemispheres
- Better-formed fourth ventricle and less cerebellar hypoplasia and deformity than in the classic DWM

Associated Anomalies

- Agenesis of corpus callosum
- Migrational anomalies

Megacisterna magna is a retrocerebellar arachnoid cyst with expansion of the posterior fossa. The fourth ventricle and vermis are normally developed. It is about four times as common as DWM, composing 54% of cystic posterior fossa malformations. The patients present with hydrocephalus or developmental delay. The delay is due to associated supratentorial anomalies.

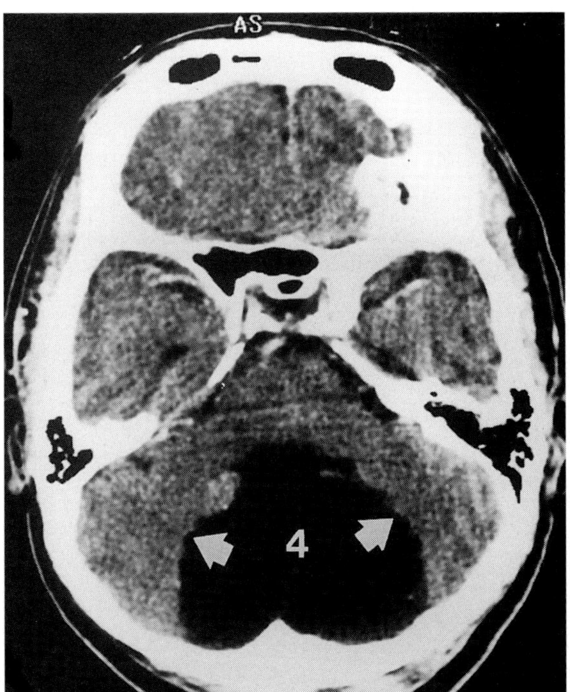

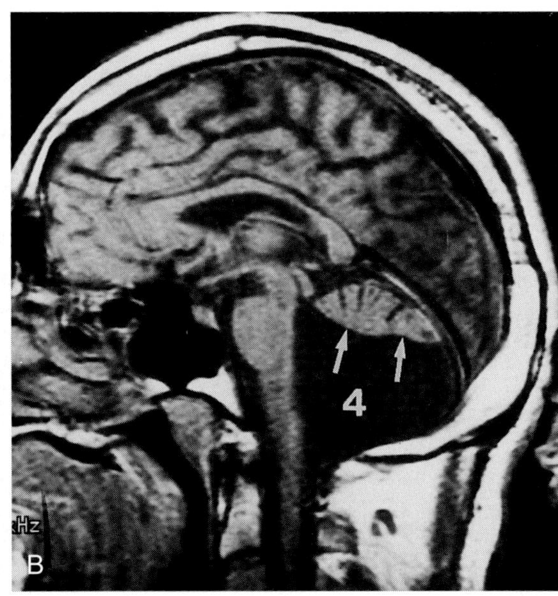

Figure 2–25. Dandy-Walker variant. **(A)** Axial CT shows an enlarged fourth ventricle (4) and lateral displacement of the cerebellar hemispheres (arrows). The posterior fossa is moderately enlarged, and the falx cerebelli is absent. **(B)** Sagittal MRI shows the enlarged fourth ventricle, elevation of a well-formed superior vermis (arrows), and agenesis of the inferior vermis. There was no hydrocephalus.

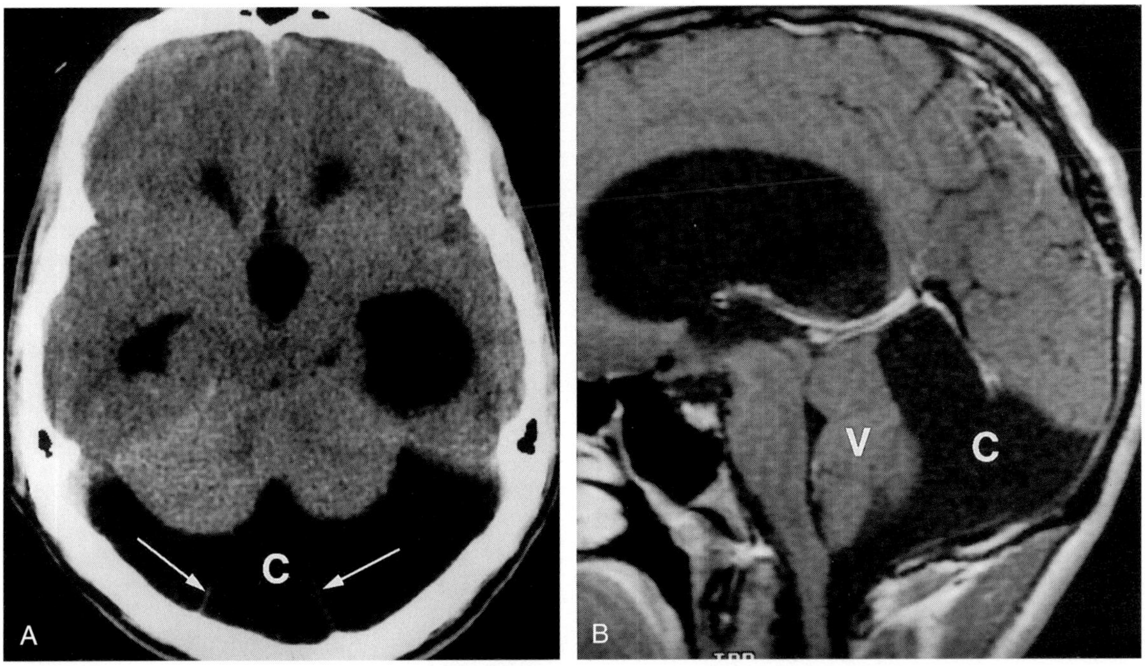

Figure 2–26. Megacisterna magna (retrocerebellar arachnoid cyst). **(A)** Axial CT shows a large posterior fossa cyst (C), severe hydrocephalus, and anterior displacement of the cerebellum. Arrows indicate leaves of a bifid falx cerebelli. **(B)** Sagittal MRI shows the arachnoid cyst (C) and ventral compression of a fully formed vermis (V), fourth ventricle, and brainstem.

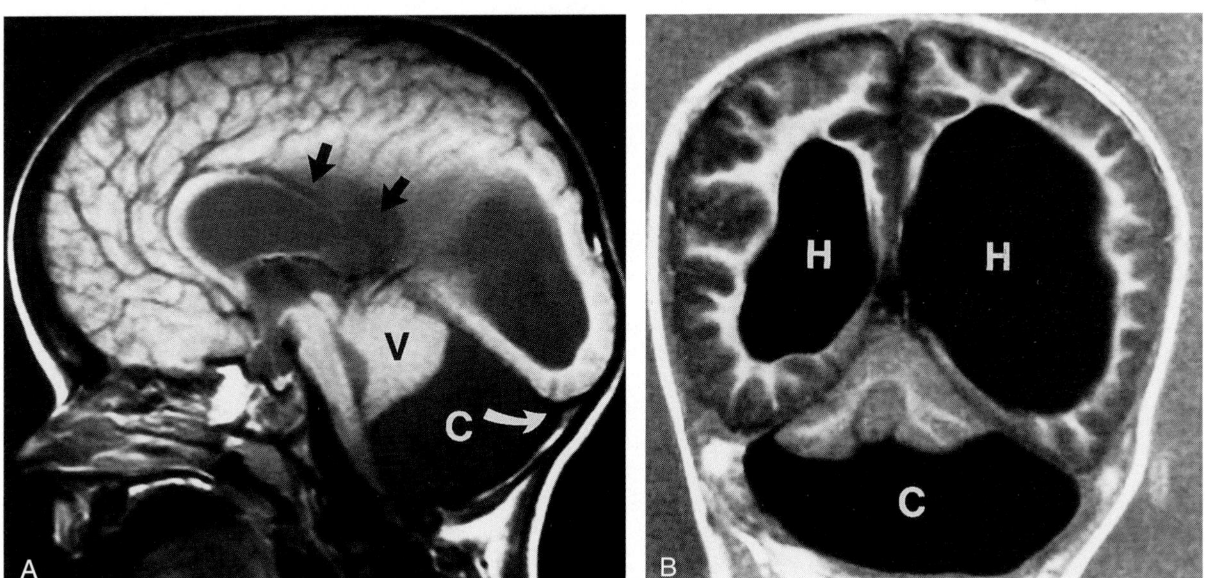

Figure 2–27. Megacisterna magna. **(A)** Sagittal and **(B)** coronal MRI show an arachnoid cyst (C) with elevation of a dysplastic vermis lacking normal folia. Note severe hydrocephalus (H), normal tentorial insertion (curved arrow), and dysgenesis of the corpus callosum (straight arrows).

Disorders of Neuronal Proliferation, Differentiation, and Histogenesis

Sturge-Weber Syndrome

The Sturge-Weber syndrome (encephalotrigeminal angiomatosis) consists of a facial vascular capillary angioma (port wine stain) and an ipsilateral leptomeningeal angiomatosis of the occipital lobe. Most cases are sporadic in origin. The meningeal angioma is associated with impaired venous drainage. The resultant parenchymal venous stasis leads to atrophy, gliosis, demyelination, and cortical calcification, manifesting clinically with homonymous hemianopsia, seizures, and hemiparesis.

Primary Abnormalities

- Leptomeningeal vascular malformation (LVM) in the subarachnoid space overlying the occipital and posterior temporoparietal regions but sometimes more extensive
- Most often unilateral, although bilateral involvement not rare
- Best demonstrated by contrast-enhanced MRI

A similar imaging appearance is seen in meningioangiomatosis. This condition is usually more focal and is associated with neurofibromatosis.

Ancillary Findings (All Ipsilateral to LVM)

- Dilated, tortuous deep hemispheric and medullary veins
- Buphthalmos (congenital glaucoma with enlarged globe)
- Enlarged choroid plexus due to angiomatous change
- Progressive atrophy of cortex underlying the LVM and possibly entire hemisphere
- Cerebral cortical calcifications underlying the LVM begin to appear on CT by 1 year of age
- Hyperintensity of involved gyri and subjacent white matter on T2-weighted MRI

Skull

- Calvarial thickening
- Increased pneumatization of paranasal sinuses
- Elevation of the petrous ridge and lesser wing of the sphenoid
- Ipsilateral shift of falx
- Above findings sometimes referred to as Dyke-Davidoff-Masson syndrome

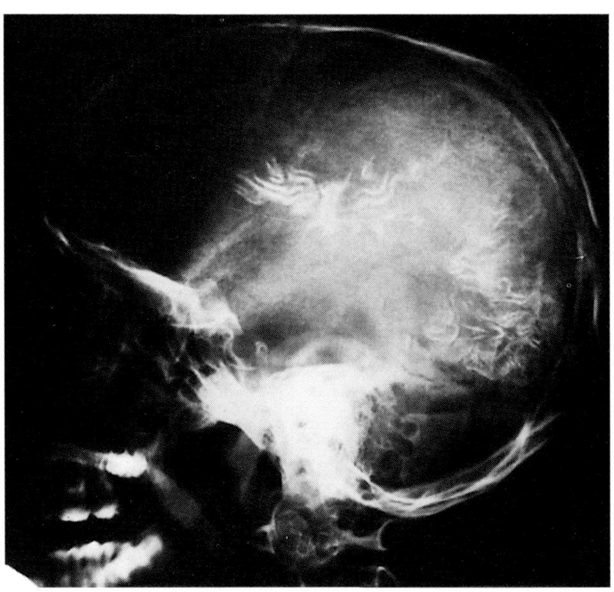

Figure 2–28. Sturge-Weber. Lateral skull radiograph shows extensive occipital and parietal cortical calcification. The calcification of apposing gyri separated by intervening sulci produces the parallel lines or tram track calcifications.

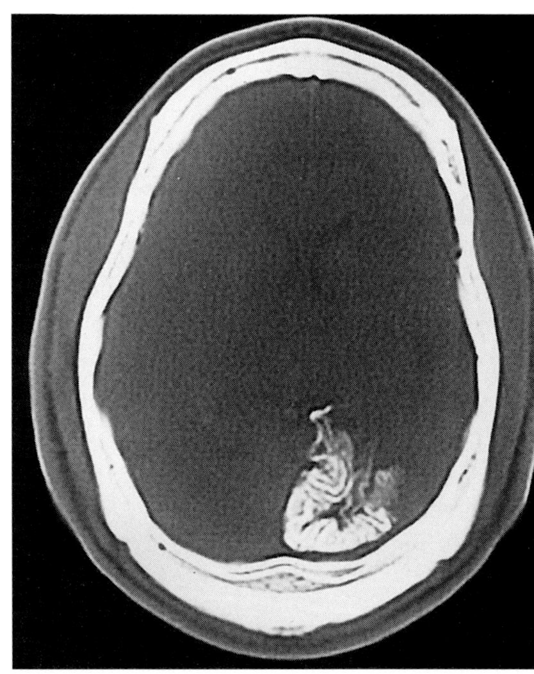

Figure 2–29. Sturge-Weber. Axial CT (bone window) shows heavy gyral calcification of the left occipital lobe. There is only minimal hemispheric asymmetry.

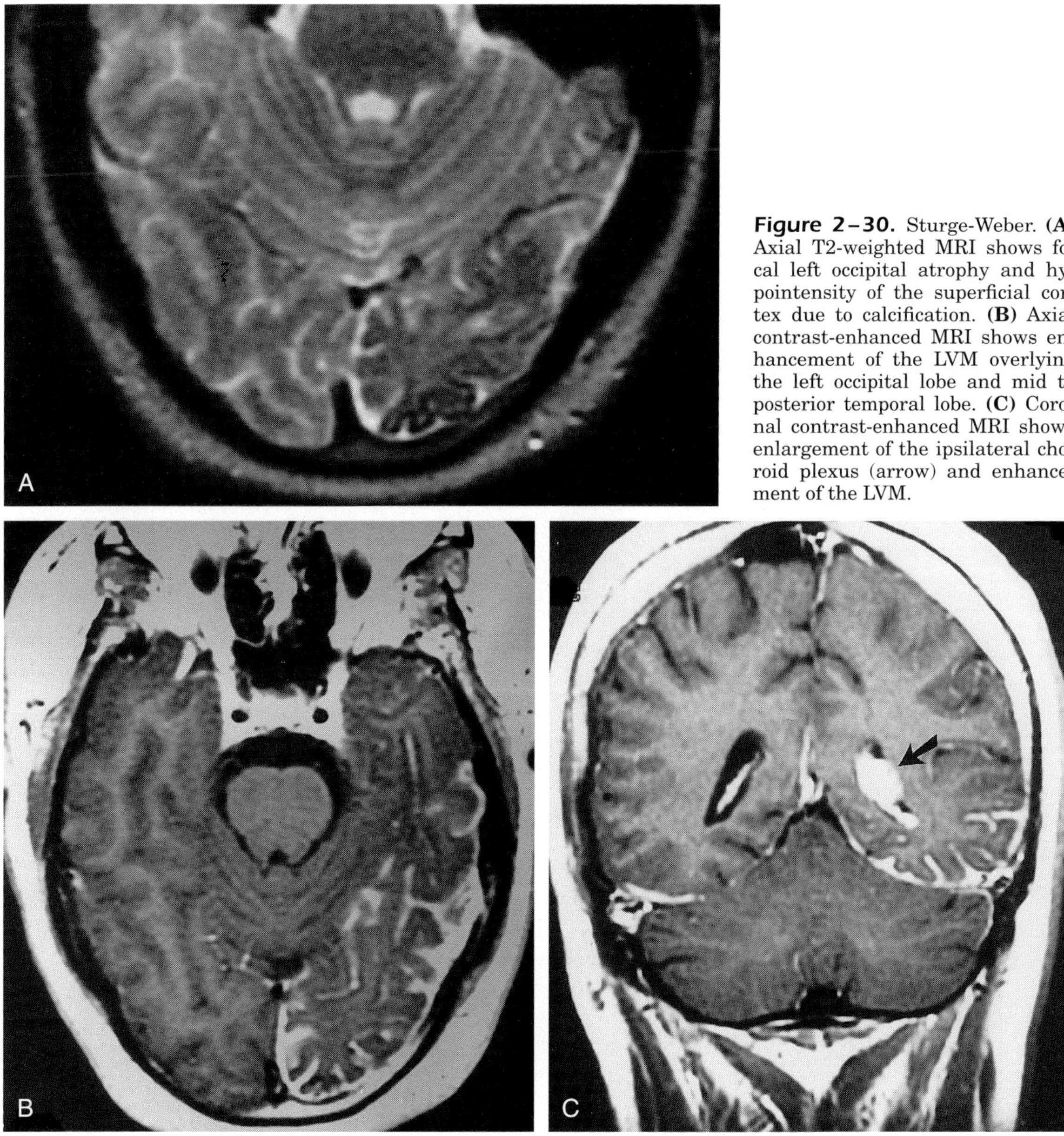

Figure 2–30. Sturge-Weber. **(A)** Axial T2-weighted MRI shows focal left occipital atrophy and hypointensity of the superficial cortex due to calcification. **(B)** Axial contrast-enhanced MRI shows enhancement of the LVM overlying the left occipital lobe and mid to posterior temporal lobe. **(C)** Coronal contrast-enhanced MRI shows enlargement of the ipsilateral choroid plexus (arrow) and enhancement of the LVM.

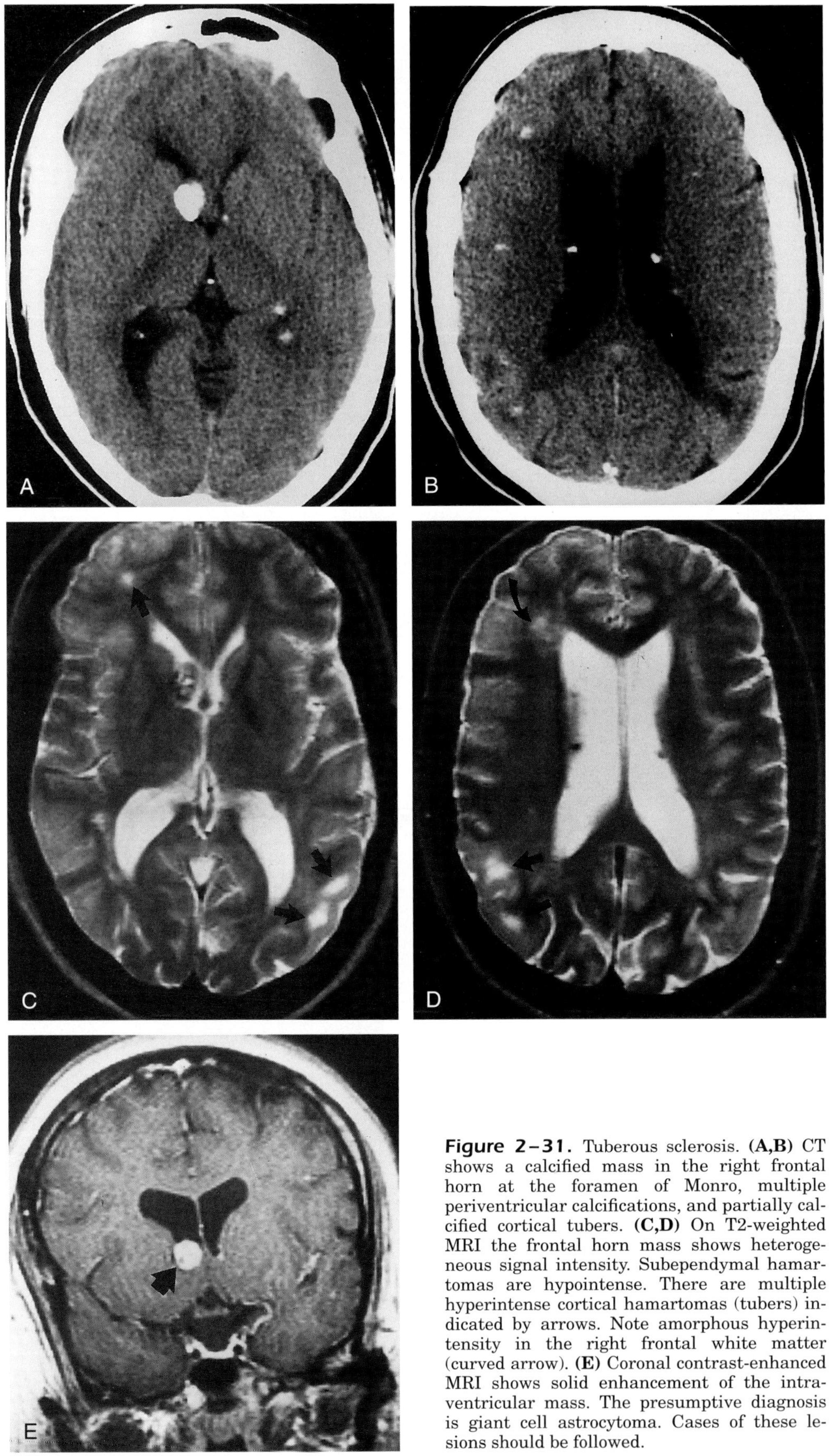

Figure 2–31. Tuberous sclerosis. **(A,B)** CT shows a calcified mass in the right frontal horn at the foramen of Monro, multiple periventricular calcifications, and partially calcified cortical tubers. **(C,D)** On T2-weighted MRI the frontal horn mass shows heterogeneous signal intensity. Subependymal hamartomas are hypointense. There are multiple hyperintense cortical hamartomas (tubers) indicated by arrows. Note amorphous hyperintensity in the right frontal white matter (curved arrow). **(E)** Coronal contrast-enhanced MRI shows solid enhancement of the intraventricular mass. The presumptive diagnosis is giant cell astrocytoma. Cases of these lesions should be followed.

Tuberous Sclerosis

Tuberous sclerosis (TS) (Bourneville's disease) is a common phakomatosis that has been tentatively linked to chromosome 9. Most cases arise from spontaneous mutations, and the overall prevalence is 1 in 20,000 persons. It derives its name from the tough gliotic cortical hamartomas present in the first reported cases. TS is a multisystemic disorder, and the cerebral abnormalities listed here need not be present to make a diagnosis.

Primary CNS Abnormalities

Subependymal Nodules

- Small periventricular hamartomas
- Typically calcified
- Occur along lateral borders of the lateral ventricles, especially caudothalamic groove

Cortical Tubers

- Multiple hamartomas of the gyri
- Most common in the frontal lobes
- Hypointense on T1-weighted and hyperintense on T2-weighted MRI
- May cause gyral expansion
- May involve gray matter, white matter, or both
- May show calcification on CT

Ancillary Findings

- White matter abnormalities
  - Hyperintense on T2-weighted MRI
  - Linear, curvilinear, wedge shaped, or amorphous
  - No mass effect
- Hydrocephalus
- Cortical heterotopias
- Infarcts
- Ventricular dilatation (nonhydrocephalic)
- Retinal hamartomas

Giant Cell Astrocytomas

- Occur in about 10% of patients with TS
- Enhancing and often calcified mass almost always occurring in the lateral ventricle near the foramen of Monro
- Heterogeneously hypointense on T1-weighted and hyperintense on T2-weighted images
- May exhibit signal voids from enlarged vessels
- Hydrocephalus typical (obstruction of one or both lateral ventricles)
- Edema absent

Systemic Findings

- Multiple facial angiofibromas (adenoma sebaceum)
- Periungual or subungual fibroma
- Renal angiomyolipomas
- Cardiac rhabdomyoma
- Pulmonary lymphangiomyomatosis

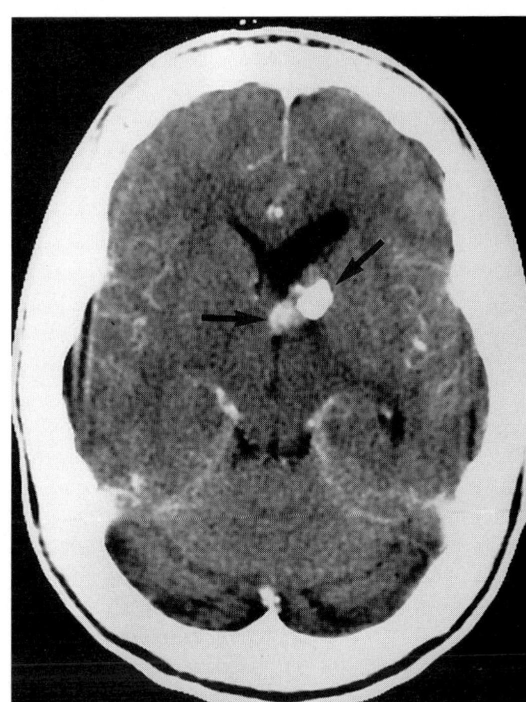

Figure 2–32. Giant cell astrocytoma. Axial contrast-enhanced CT shows an enhancing and a calcified mass (arrows) at the left foramen of Monro with enlargement of the left lateral ventricle.

Neurofibromatosis

There are as many as eight clinical subtypes of neurofibromatosis (NF); however, types 1 and 2 account for 99% of the total. NF-1 is an autosomal dominant disorder linked to chromosome 17, with a prevalence of about 1 in 4,000. NF-2 has been linked to chromosome 22 and is also autosomal dominant, with a lower prevalence of 1 in 50,000. Diagnostic imaging serves as an adjunct to physical examination in making the diagnosis, especially in identifying cranial and spinal neoplasia and skeletal deformities.

Neurofibromatosis Type 1

Primary Abnormalities

Two of the following must be present:

- Six or more café au lait spots
- Two or more neurofibromas
- One or more plexiform neurofibromas
- Axillary or inguinal freckling
- Optic glioma
- Two or more iris hamartomas
- One or more distinctive bone lesions
- A first-degree relative with NF-1

Ancillary Findings

Brain

- Multifocal hyperintensities on T2-weighted MRI in basal ganglia, centrum semiovale, internal capsule, brainstem, and cerebellum in up to 80%
- Juvenile pilocytic astrocytomas of the optic pathways in up to 30%
- Brainstem gliomas
- Pilocytic astrocytomas of the hypothalamus
- Arachnoid cysts
- Cranial nerve schwannomas

Extracranial

- Hypoplasia of sphenoid wing
- Plexiform neurofibroma
- Buphthalmos (enlarged globe)

Spine (See Chapter 11)

- Spinal cord gliomas
- Lateral meningoceles
- Spinal neurofibromas
- Vertebral scalloping
- Kyphoscoliosis

Vascular

- Vascular malformations
- Moyamoya disease
- Pseudoaneurysms and dissections of carotid or vertebral arteries

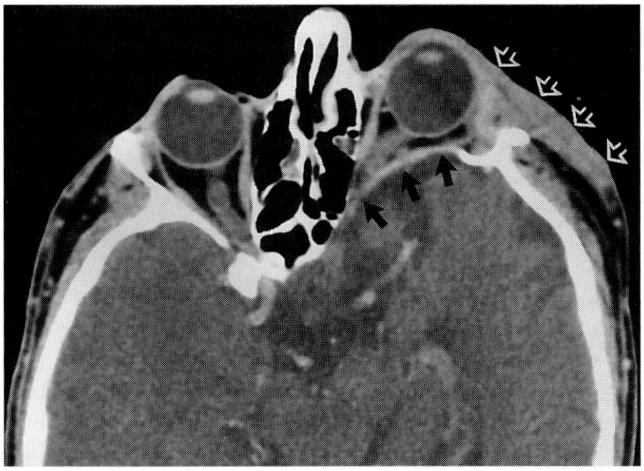

Figure 2–33. Neurofibromatosis I. Axial contrast-enhanced CT shows anterior expansion of the left middle fossa secondary to sphenoid wing hypoplasia (arrows) producing proptosis, relative enlargement of the left optic globe (buphthalmos), and plexiform neurofibroma of the left face (open arrows).

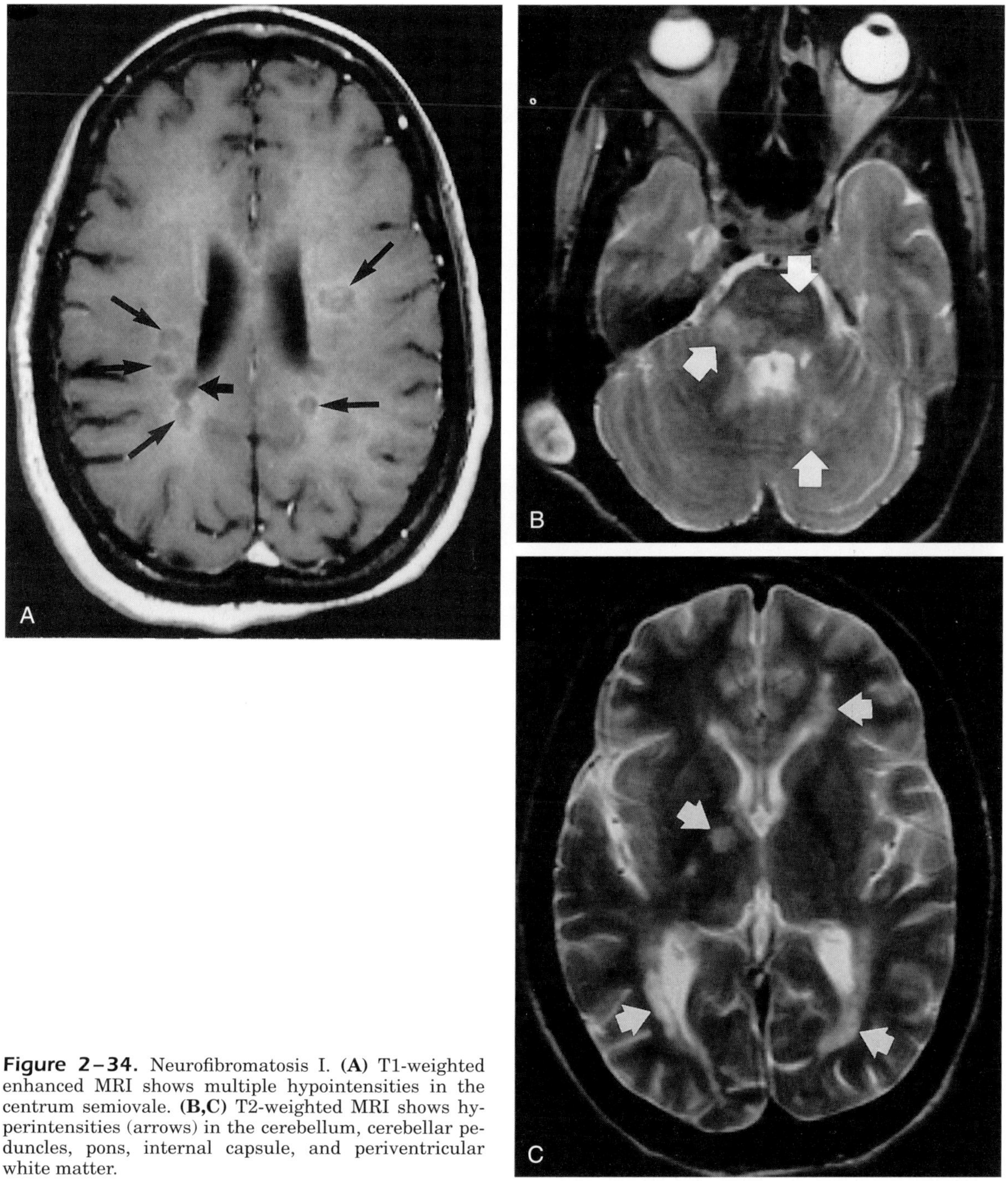

Figure 2–34. Neurofibromatosis I. **(A)** T1-weighted enhanced MRI shows multiple hypointensities in the centrum semiovale. **(B,C)** T2-weighted MRI shows hyperintensities (arrows) in the cerebellum, cerebellar peduncles, pons, internal capsule, and periventricular white matter.

Neurofibromatosis Type 2

Primary Abnormalities

- Bilateral schwannomas of the eighth cranial nerve

Ancillary Findings

- Schwannomas of other cranial nerves, especially fifth and seventh
- Ependymomas of brain and spinal cord
- Solitary or multiple meningiomas

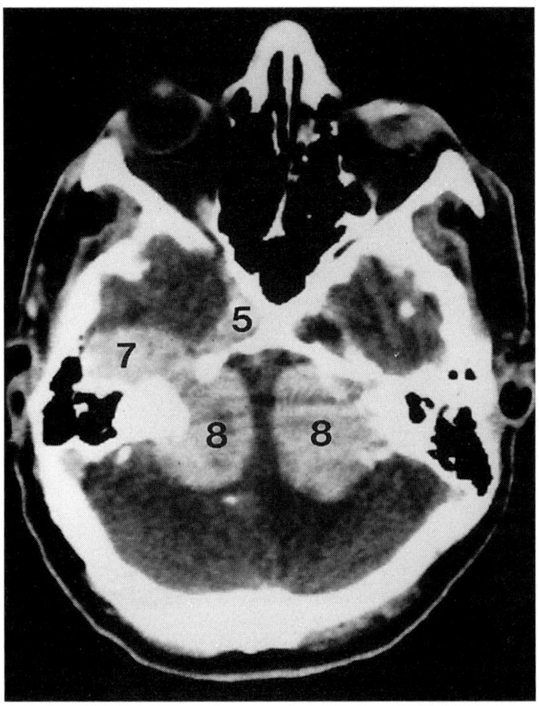

Figure 2–35. Neurofibromatosis II. CT shows enhancing schwannomas of both the acoustic nerves (8), the right facial nerve (7), and the right trigeminal nerve (5).

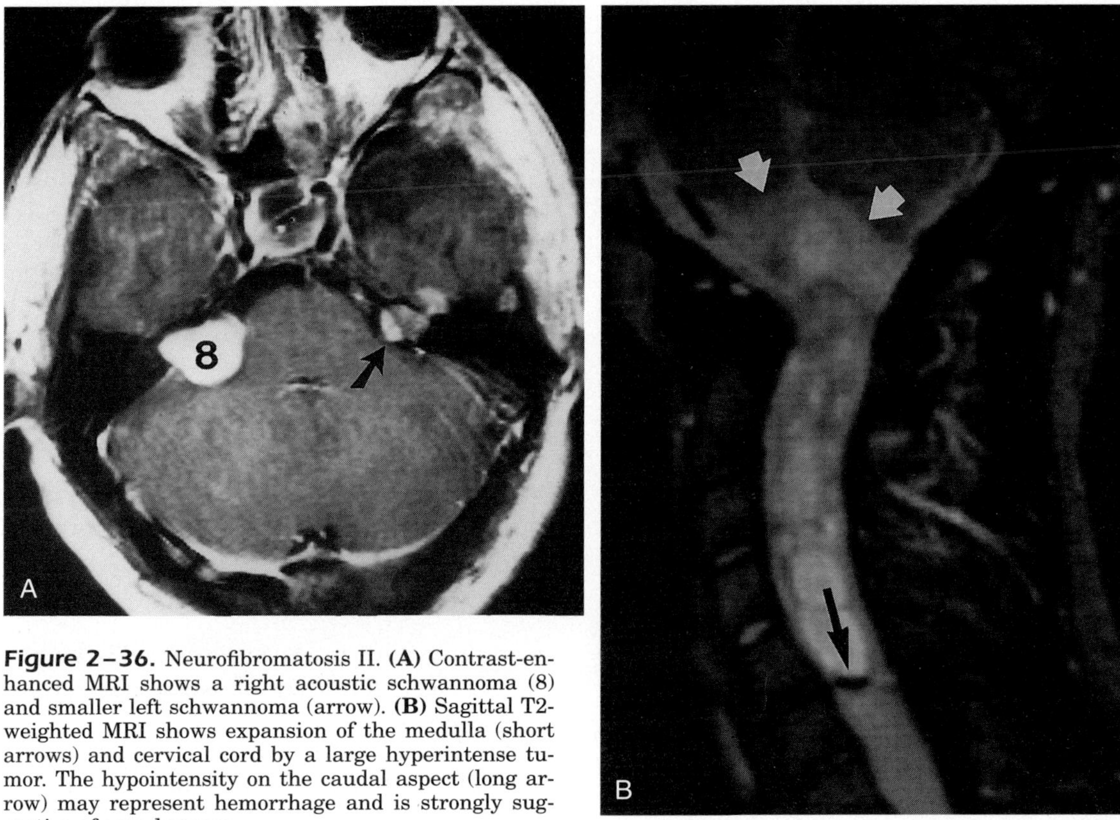

Figure 2–36. Neurofibromatosis II. **(A)** Contrast-enhanced MRI shows a right acoustic schwannoma (8) and smaller left schwannoma (arrow). **(B)** Sagittal T2-weighted MRI shows expansion of the medulla (short arrows) and cervical cord by a large hyperintense tumor. The hypointensity on the caudal aspect (long arrow) may represent hemorrhage and is strongly suggestive of ependymoma.

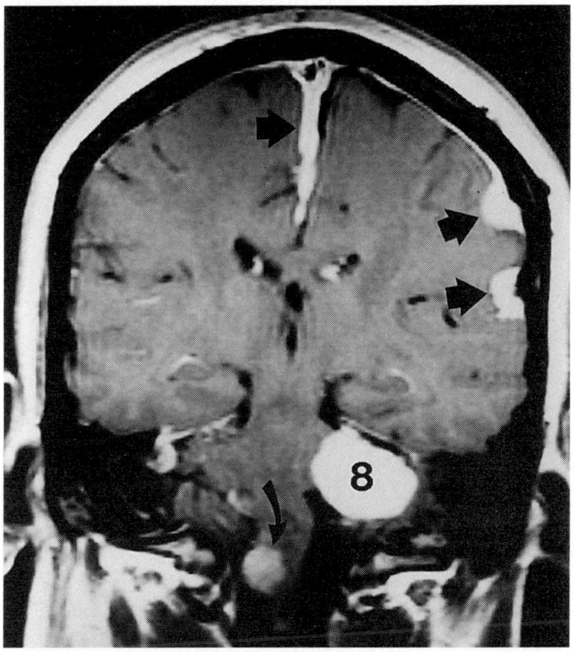

Figure 2–37. Neurofibromatosis II. Contrast-enhanced MRI shows multiple meningiomas (thick arrows), a large left acoustic schwannoma (8), and a right hypoglossal schwannoma (curved arrow).

Aqueductal Stenosis

Aqueductal stenosis is a leading cause of intraventricular obstructive (noncommunicating) hydrocephalus in children and young adults. It may occur as a sporadic congenital malformation, in association with other congenital disorders, or as an acquired disorder. Pathologically the aqueduct may be stenotic, forked into multiple small channels, obstructed by a thin glial septum, or occluded by an acquired mass of fibrillary gliosis. Most patients present before 25 years of age with signs and symptoms of hydrocephalus.

Primary Abnormalities

- Hydrocephalus with enlarged third and lateral ventricles and normal fourth ventricle
- Narrowing of the aqueduct of Sylvius—with a proximal obstruction the aqueduct appears diffusely small and with distal stenoses (more common) there is dilatation of the aqueduct proximal to the stenosis

Ancillary Findings

- Tectum is intrinsically normal but may be secondarily deformed from compression by a dilated suprapineal recess or enlarged temporal lobes or may be thinned by a dilated aqueduct.
- Specialized MRI techniques may be employed to assess presence of flow through the aqueduct.

Associated Anomalies

- Chiari I malformation
- Chiari II malformation
- Neurofibromatosis

Hemimegalencephaly

This is a rare congenital condition consisting of unilateral hypertrophy and dysplasia of a cerebral hemisphere. The embryogenesis is unknown, although some type of insult during the second trimester has been postulated. Affected patients present in infancy with seizures, hemiparesis, or enlarged head circumference. Intellectual impairment is always present but variable in severity.

Primary Abnormalities

- Hypertrophy of cerebral hemisphere with lateral ventricular dilatation
- Cortical dysplasia with cortical thickening and abnormal gyral pattern (shallow sulci and thick gyri)

Ancillary Findings

- Midline shift toward unaffected side
- Increased quantity of white matter on the affected side
- Diminished attenuation (CT) or hyperintensity (T2-weighted MRI) in white matter on affected side due to gliosis
- Nodular gray matter heterotopias
- Cortical dysplasia ranging from agyria to polymicrogyria with normal white matter
- Degree of hypertrophy inversely related to severity of cortical dysplasia

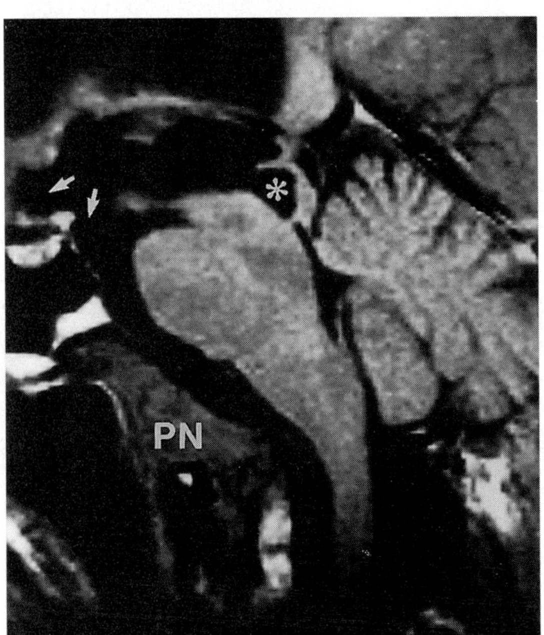

Figure 2–38. Aqueductal stenosis. Sagittal MRI shows marked ballooning of the aqueduct (asterisk) with distal occlusion. Hydrocephalus is present with ballooning of the anterior recesses of the third ventricle. There is marked reduction of the mammillopontine distance. The fourth ventricle is of normal size. This patient had NF-1. Note plexiform neurofibroma (PN) of the clivus and C1.

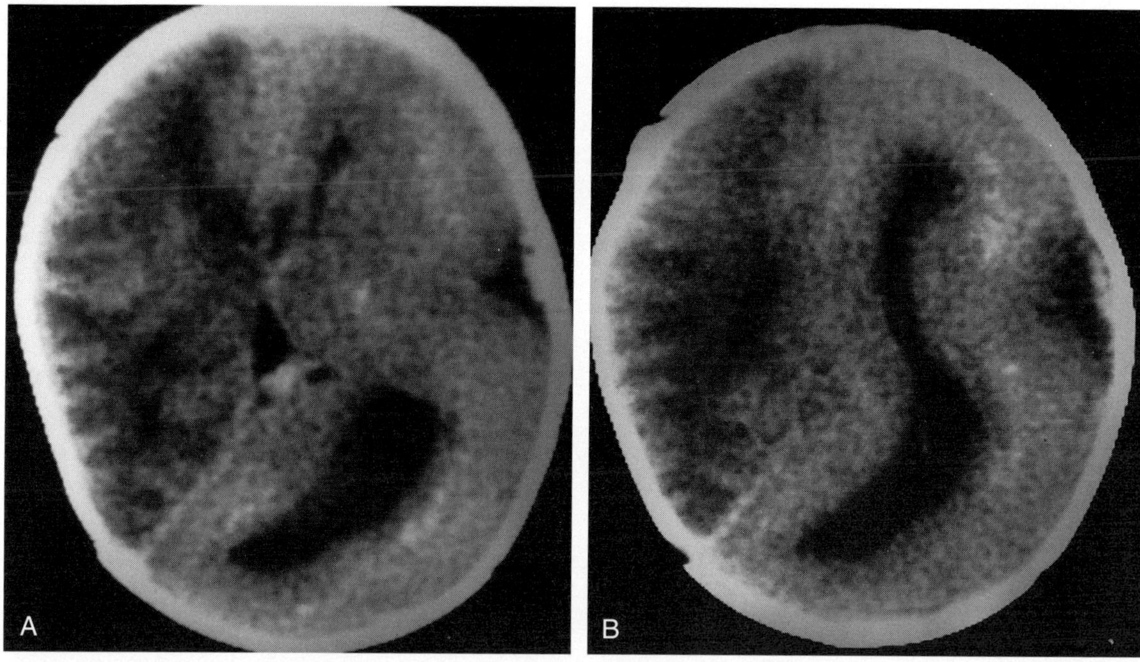

Figure 2–39. Hemimegalencephaly. **(A,B)** Axial CT shows marked hypertrophy of the left hemisphere, enlargement of the left lateral ventricle, and cortical dysplasia with a shallow sylvian fissure and absence of normal gyral development.

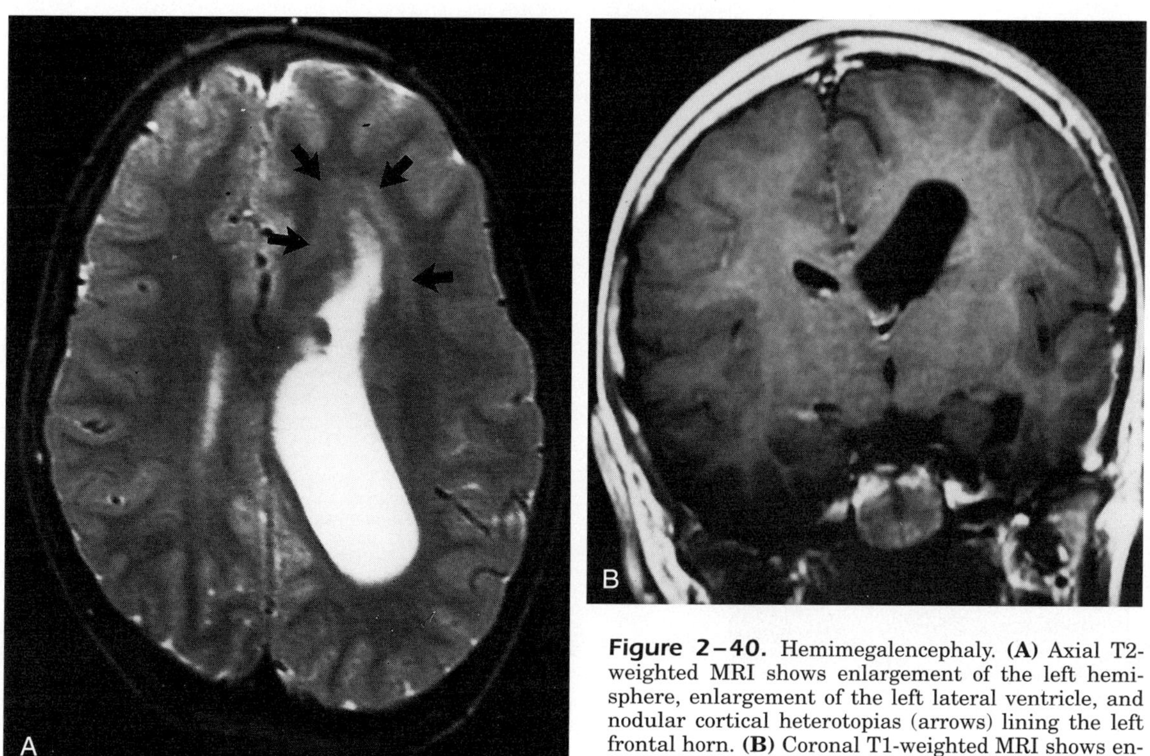

Figure 2–40. Hemimegalencephaly. **(A)** Axial T2-weighted MRI shows enlargement of the left hemisphere, enlargement of the left lateral ventricle, and nodular cortical heterotopias (arrows) lining the left frontal horn. **(B)** Coronal T1-weighted MRI shows enlargement of the left hemisphere and lateral ventricle with an increased quantity of white matter.

Neuronal Migration Disturbances

Lissencephaly

Lissencephaly is the most severe of the migrational disorders, which result from faulty migration of neurons from the germinal matrix to their proper cortical destination. Lissencephaly usually occurs in isolation but also occurs in a variety of congenital syndromes. Affected patients present in infancy with hypotonia, microcephaly, and intractable seizures.

Primary Abnormalities

- Agyria (complete absence of gyri) or agyria with areas of pachygyria
- Flat, smooth brain surface due to near complete absence of gyri
- Hourglass configuration of the brain on axial section due to smooth brain surface and shallow sylvian fissures (opercula fail to develop)
- Abnormally thickened gray matter with relative paucity of white matter

Ancillary Findings

- Linear gray-white junction with absence of normal digitations
- Microcephaly
- Decrease in size of brainstem
- Gray matter heterotopias
- Hydrocephalus
- Colpocephaly
- Hypoplasia or dysplasia of corpus callosum

Associated Anomalies

- Numerous genetic syndromes
- Dandy-Walker cyst

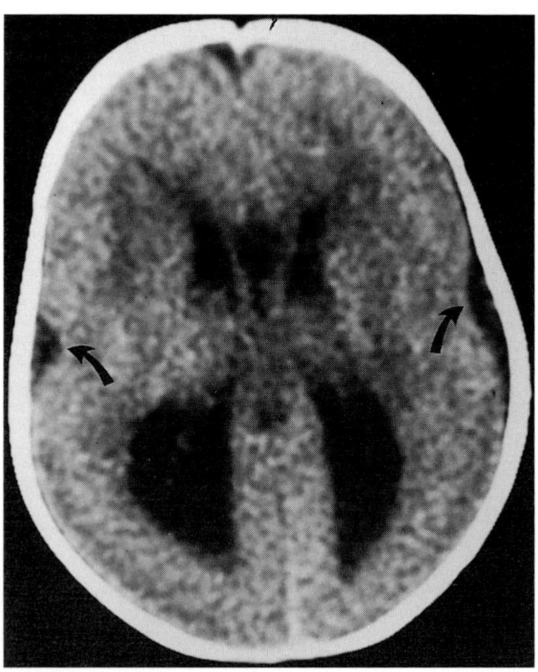

Figure 2–41. Lissencephaly. Axial CT shows extremely shallow sylvian fissures (arrows), absence of sulci, and colpocephaly.

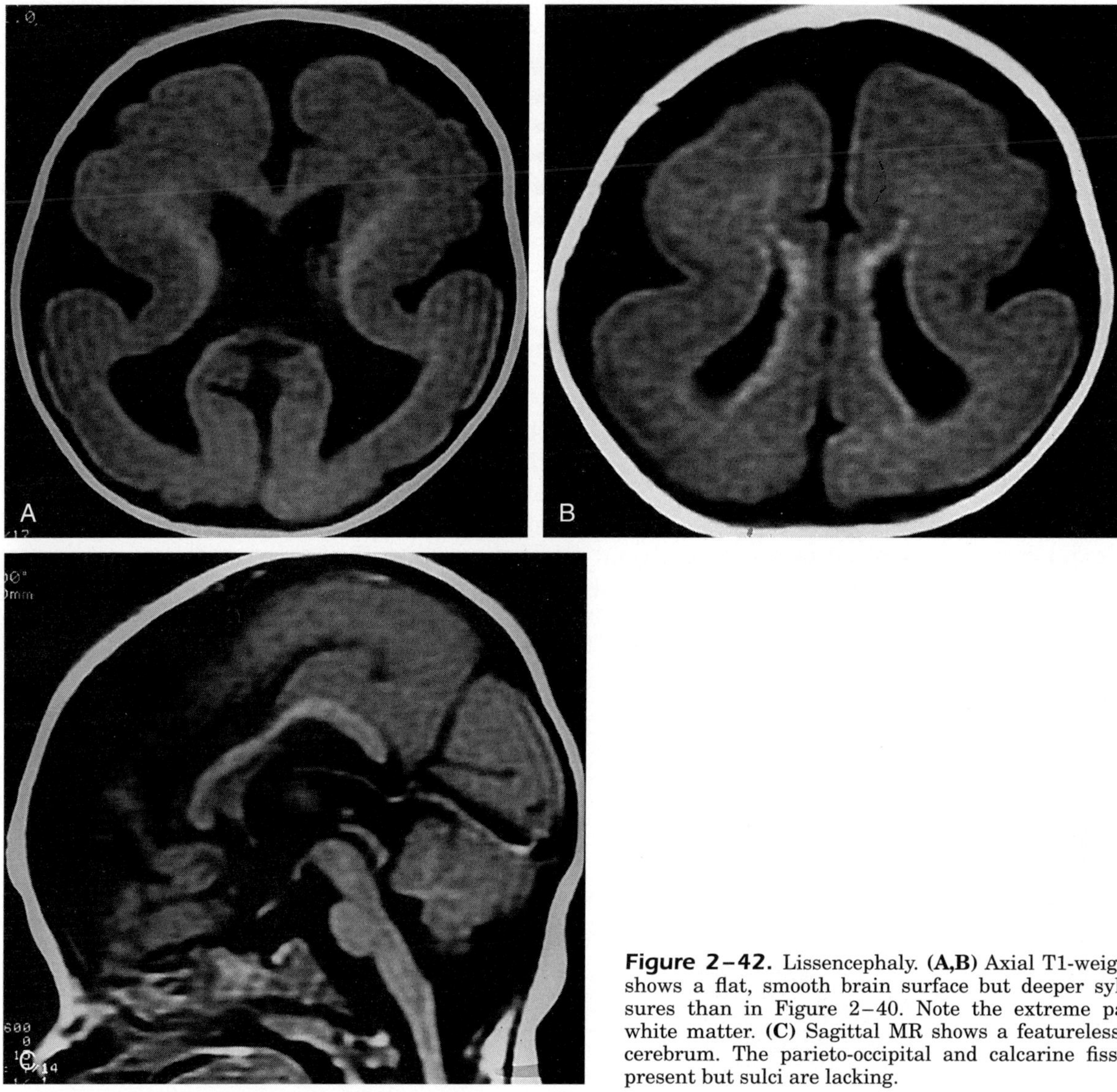

Figure 2–42. Lissencephaly. **(A,B)** Axial T1-weighted MR shows a flat, smooth brain surface but deeper sylvian fissures than in Figure 2–40. Note the extreme paucity of white matter. **(C)** Sagittal MR shows a featureless midline cerebrum. The parieto-occipital and calcarine fissures are present but sulci are lacking.

Schizencephaly

The essential component of schizencephaly is a complete hemispheric cleft from pia to ependyma with both sides of the cleft lined by gray matter. The condition is rare, and there are no reliable data regarding its incidence. It is postulated to result from an intrauterine ischemic or other insult prior to or during neuronal migration probably in the first half of the second trimester. The cleft is bilateral in about 35% and is most often frontal (44%) or frontoparietal (30%). In type I schizencephaly the pial-ependymal walls of the cleft are in apposition (closed lip), whereas in type II the cleft is filled with CSF. Affected patients manifest seizures, contralateral hemiparesis, and developmental delay. The best prognosis correlates with unilaterality, closed lip configuration, and frontal lobe sparing.

Primary Abnormalities

- Gray matter lined cleft, usually near sylvian fissure, extending from pial surface to ependymal lining of the lateral ventricle
- Cleft may be unilateral or bilateral and open (type II, filled with CSF) or fused (type I)
- Dimple in wall of ventricle where it connects with cleft

Ancillary Findings

- Gray matter heterotopias
- Polymicrogyria
- Pachygyria
- Absence of septum pellucidum in 80–90%
- Hypoplastic optic nerves (septo-optic dysplasia)
- Partial absence of corpus callosum

Gray Matter Heterotopia

Heterotopic gray matter is the hallmark of all of the migrational disorders. This section describes those conditions in which ectopic gray matter is the primary abnormality. These patients present most often with seizures. They may possess normal intelligence or manifest varying degrees of developmental delay. Focal cortical dysplasia or agenesis of the corpus callosum may be present in the more severely affected patients.

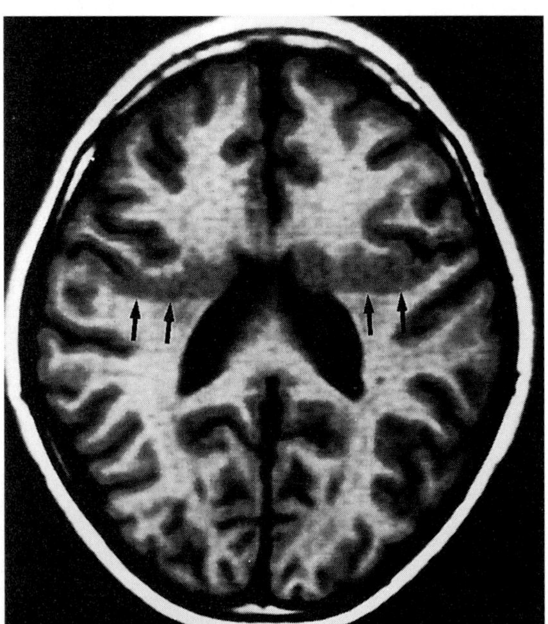

Figure 2–43. Closed lip schizencephaly. T1-weighted MR shows bifrontal seams of gray matter (arrows) extending from pia to ependyma.

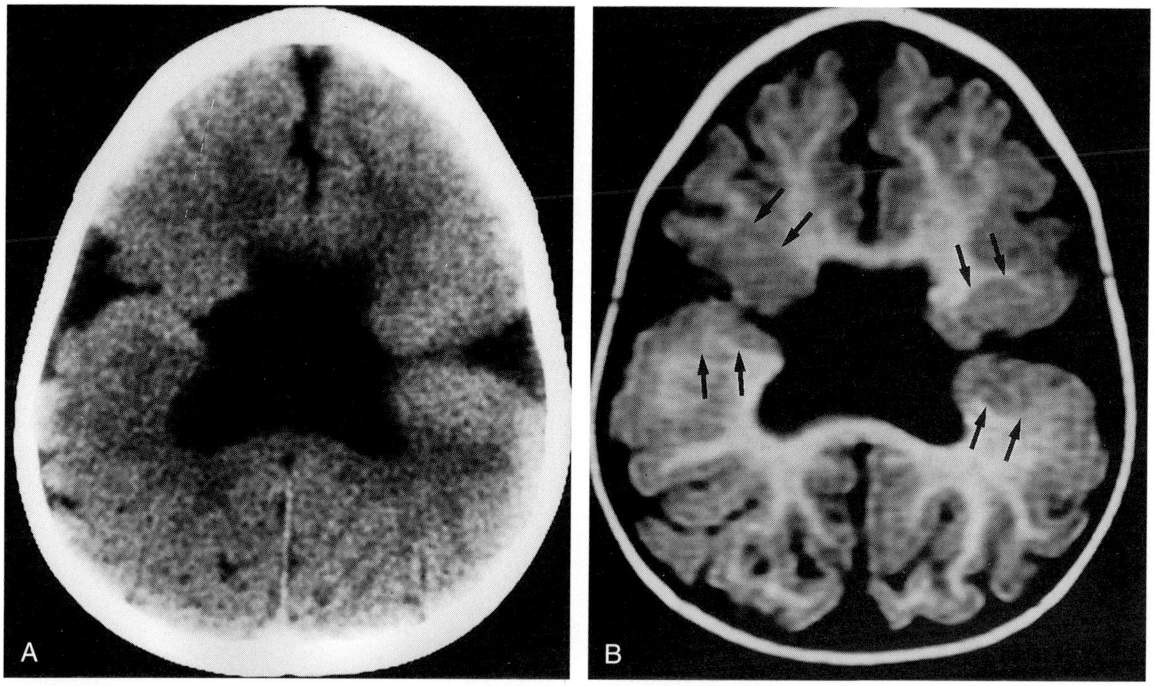

Figure 2–44. Open lip schizencephaly. **(A)** CT shows bifrontal transcortical clefts. **(B)** T1-weighted MR shows a continuous layer of gray matter (arrows) completely lining both sides of both clefts. The septum pellucidum is absent.

Primary Abnormality

- Ectopically located gray matter in the brain:
  - Usually diffuse and symmetric but may be focal and unilateral
  - Most often frontal or occipital poles of the lateral ventricles

Three forms have been described:

Nodular. Rests of gray matter in a subependymal distribution, typically bilateral and symmetric (most common and most associated with normal cognition)

Laminar. Rests of gray matter in a subcortical location that may extend from pial to ependymal surface

Band. Diffuse, bilaterally symmetric sheet of gray matter separated from both the cortex and ependyma by a layer of white matter

Ancillary Finding

- Increased incidence of agenesis of corpus callosum

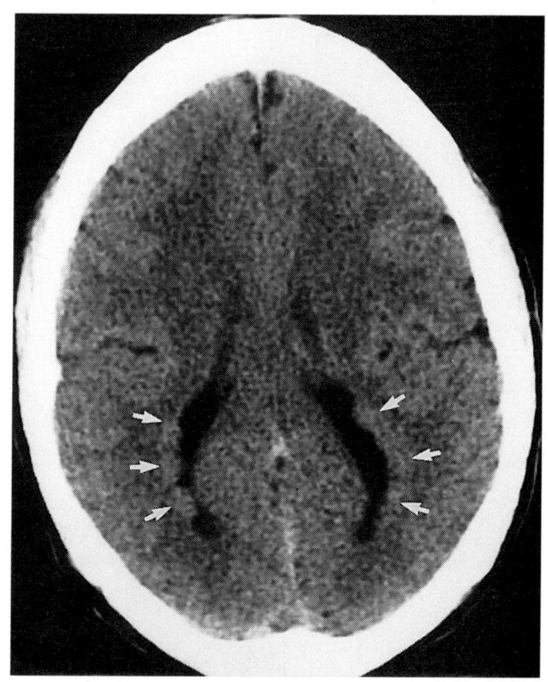

Figure 2–45. Nodular (subependymal) heterotopia. CT shows gray matter nodules (arrows) lining the lateral ventricles. The nodules are isodense with gray matter.

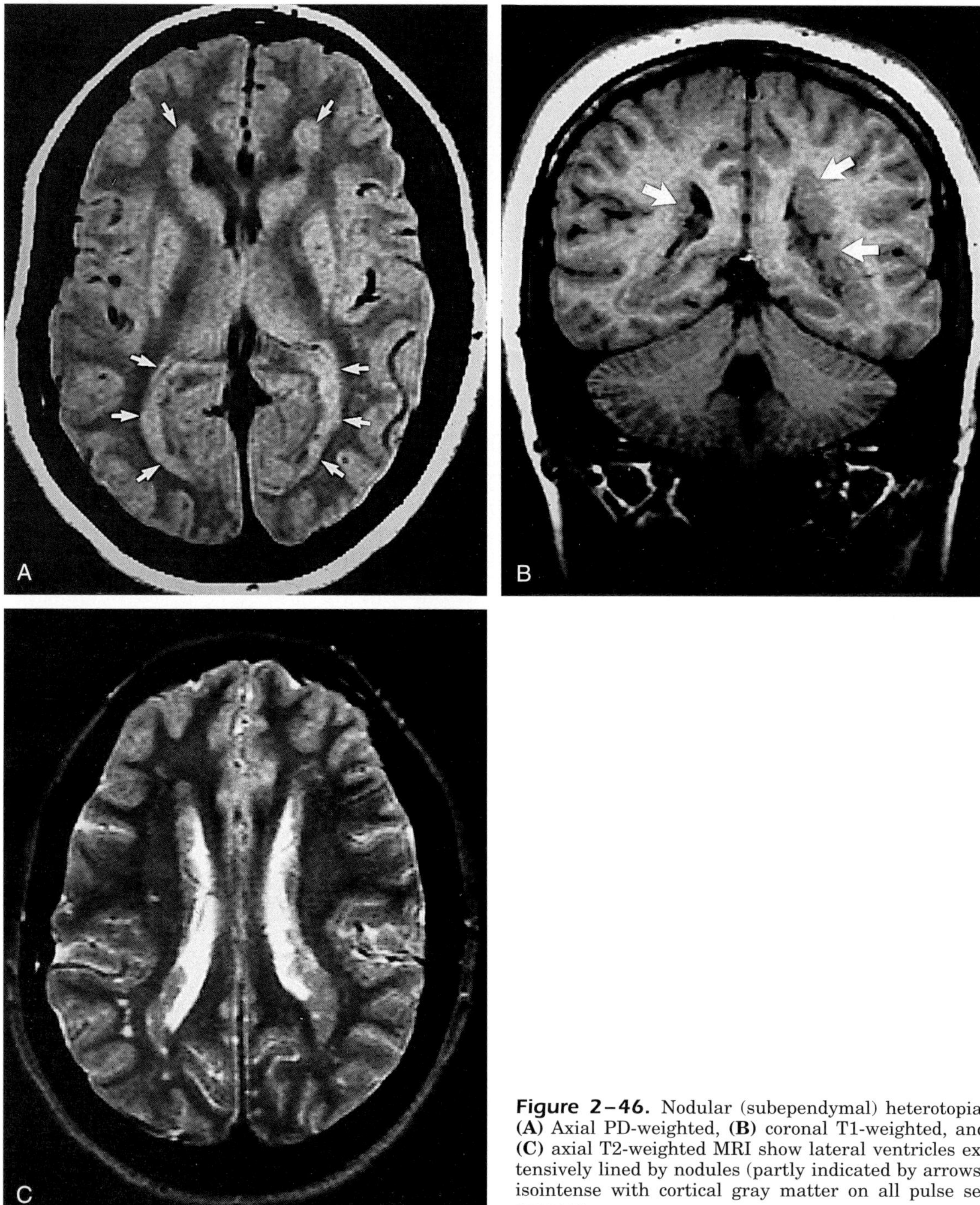

Figure 2–46. Nodular (subependymal) heterotopia. **(A)** Axial PD-weighted, **(B)** coronal T1-weighted, and **(C)** axial T2-weighted MRI show lateral ventricles extensively lined by nodules (partly indicated by arrows) isointense with cortical gray matter on all pulse sequences.

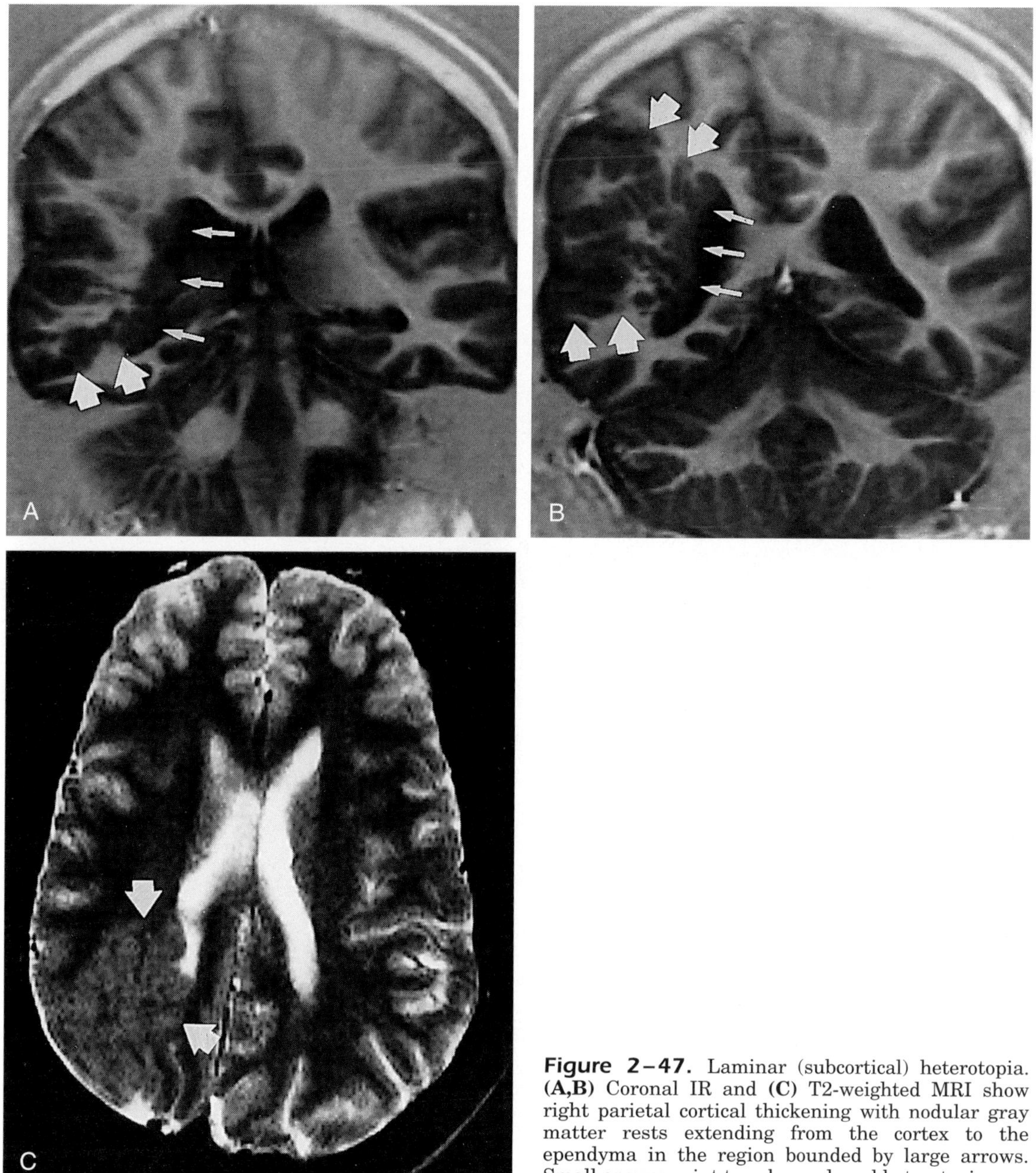

Figure 2–47. Laminar (subcortical) heterotopia. **(A,B)** Coronal IR and **(C)** T2-weighted MRI show right parietal cortical thickening with nodular gray matter rests extending from the cortex to the ependyma in the region bounded by large arrows. Small arrows point to subependymal heterotopias.

Focal Cortical Dysplasia

Maldevelopment of the cerebral gyri may result in complete absence (agyria); excessively broad, thick gyri (pachygyria); or a cluster of abnormally small, densely packed gyri (polymicrogyria). Diffuse cortical dysplasia correlates with severe neurologic disability and is seen in lissencephaly and hemimegalencephaly, following congenital cytomegalovirus (CMV) infection, and in association with many congenital syndromes. Focal dysplasia may present as a seizure disorder in developmentally normal individuals, who may benefit from surgical resection. It is believed that most cases arise from an insult at or after 26 weeks of gestation.

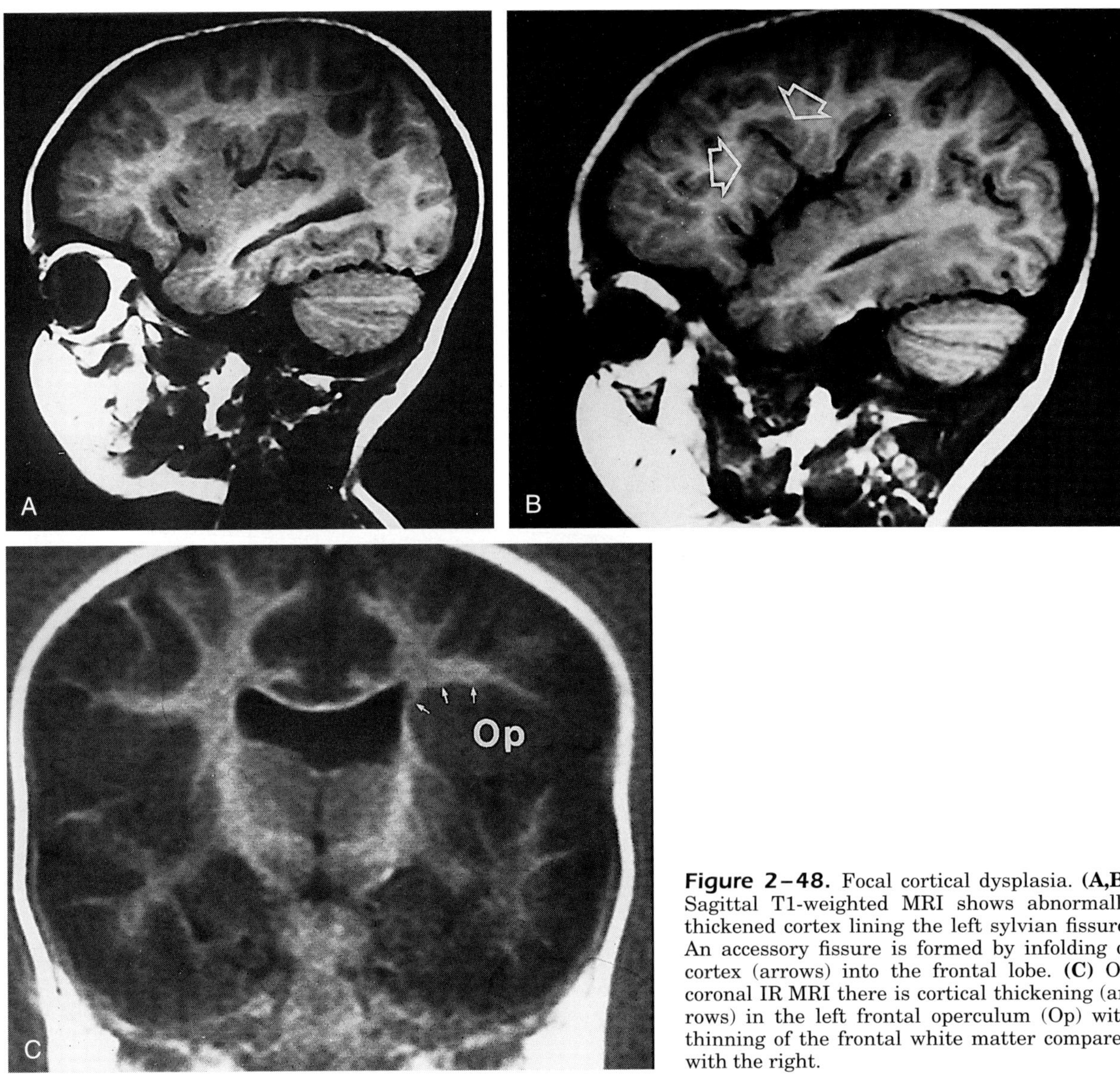

Figure 2–48. Focal cortical dysplasia. **(A,B)** Sagittal T1-weighted MRI shows abnormally thickened cortex lining the left sylvian fissure. An accessory fissure is formed by infolding of cortex (arrows) into the frontal lobe. **(C)** On coronal IR MRI there is cortical thickening (arrows) in the left frontal operculum (Op) with thinning of the frontal white matter compared with the right.

Primary Abnormalities

Polymicrogyria

- Small, excessively numerous convolutions of the cerebral cortex
- Typically found in opercular region (insula)
- Because either the sulci are extremely small or the gyri fuse, manifests MRI findings that in most instances are indistinguishable from pachygyria

Pachygyria

- Broad-based, thickened gyri with bumpy outer surface, thickened gray matter (normal thickness ≤5 mm), and reduced white matter digitations
- May be focal and unilateral or diffuse
- Frontal lobes most often and severely involved
- May appear as abnormally deep infolding of thickened gray matter

Focal Cortical Dysplasia

- Focal cortical thickening (>5 mm) with lumpy contours, broad gyri, and shallow sulci
- Involves sylvian fissure in over 50%
- May also appear as infolding of thickened cerebral cortex
- Hyperintensity may appear on T2-weighted MRI due to gliosis or CSF deep within abnormal fissure

Ancillary Findings

- Microcephaly
- Findings of congenital CMV infection (periventricular calcifications, white matter gliosis)

Associated Anomalies

- Chiari II malformation
- Schizencephaly

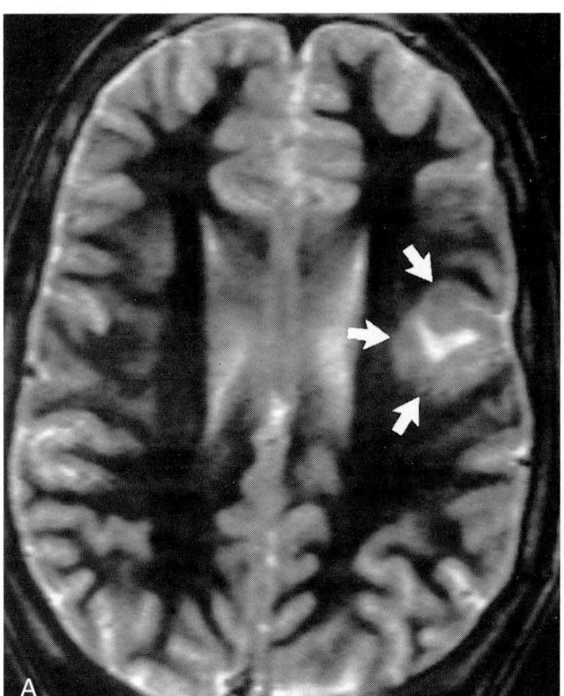
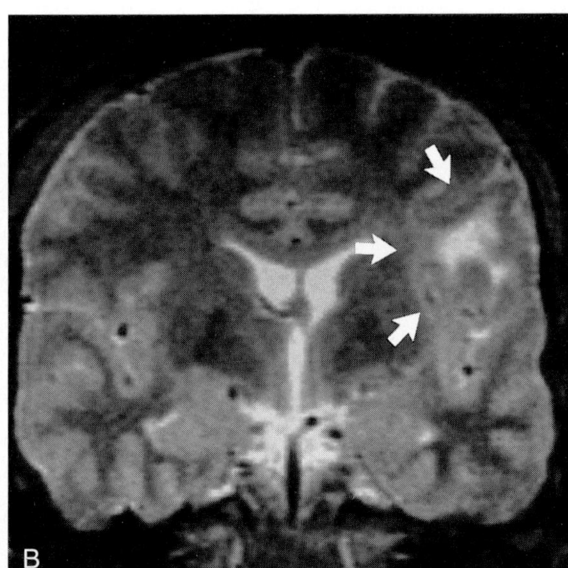

Figure 2-49. Focal cortical dysplasia. **(A)** Axial IR and **(B)** coronal T2-weighted MRI show an infolded area of thickened cortex (arrows) in the left frontal lobe. The pathologic basis for the central hyperintensity is unknown.

Dysgenesis of Corpus Callosum

The corpus callosum develops between the 12th and 20th weeks of gestation. The posterior genu is the first to form, with development proceeding in both anterior and posterior directions from there. The last areas to form are the posterior body, splenium, and rostrum, in that order. Callosal dysgenesis results when there is an arrest in its development, causing the absence of those areas last to develop. When it is present as an isolated anomaly, patients often remain asymptomatic throughout life. Up to 80% of cases, however, are associated with other major malformations.

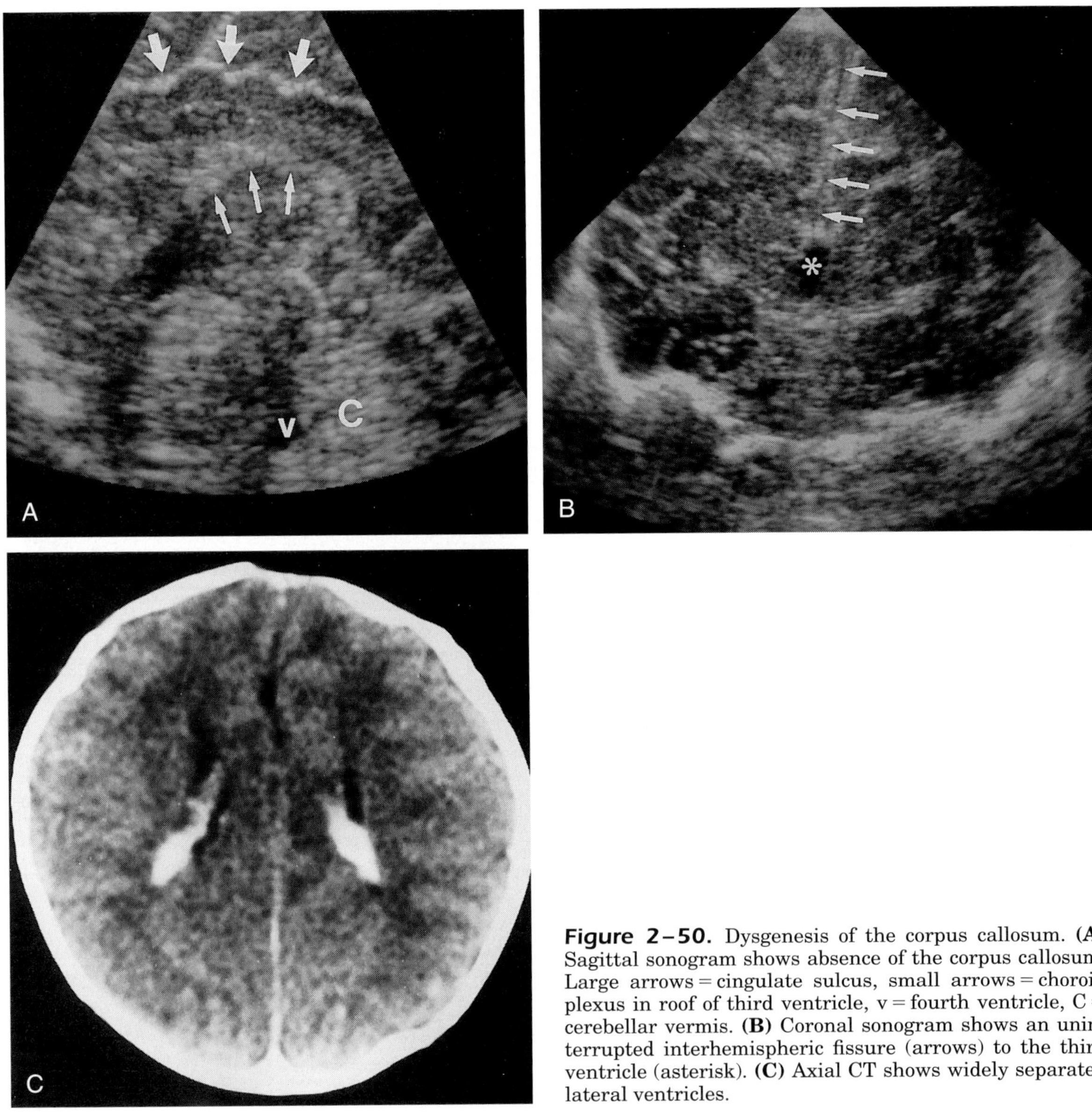

Figure 2–50. Dysgenesis of the corpus callosum. **(A)** Sagittal sonogram shows absence of the corpus callosum. Large arrows = cingulate sulcus, small arrows = choroid plexus in roof of third ventricle, v = fourth ventricle, C = cerebellar vermis. **(B)** Coronal sonogram shows an uninterrupted interhemispheric fissure (arrows) to the third ventricle (asterisk). **(C)** Axial CT shows widely separated lateral ventricles.

Primary Abnormalities

- Partial or complete absence of corpus callosum on coronal or sagittal imaging
- If partial, the more posterior portion fails to develop

Ancillary Findings

Cerebral Gyri

- Sunburst pattern of midline gyri radiating from third ventricle
- Failure of convergence of calcarine and parieto-occipital sulci
- Cingulate gyrus rotated out of midline sagittal plane

Vascular

- Elevated internal cerebral veins
- Wandering anterior cerebral artery branches

Ventricles

- Lateral ventricles widely separated
- Viking helmet deformity of lateral ventricles in coronal projections due to sharply angled lateral peaks of frontal horns
- Dilated third ventricle
- Arachnoid cyst or diverticulum of third ventricle in interhemispheric fissure in up to 30%
- Hypoplasia of limbic system (hippocampus, dentate nucleus) with dilated temporal horns
- Colpocephaly

Gray, White Matter

- Wide separation of thalami
- Hypoplastic anterior commissure
- Bundles of Probst, enlarged white matter tracts lying anteroposteriorly along the medial wall of the lateral ventricle

Associated Anomalies

- Commonly seen in association with a wide range of anomalies, especially midline cysts, Dandy-Walker malformations, and Chiari II malformations

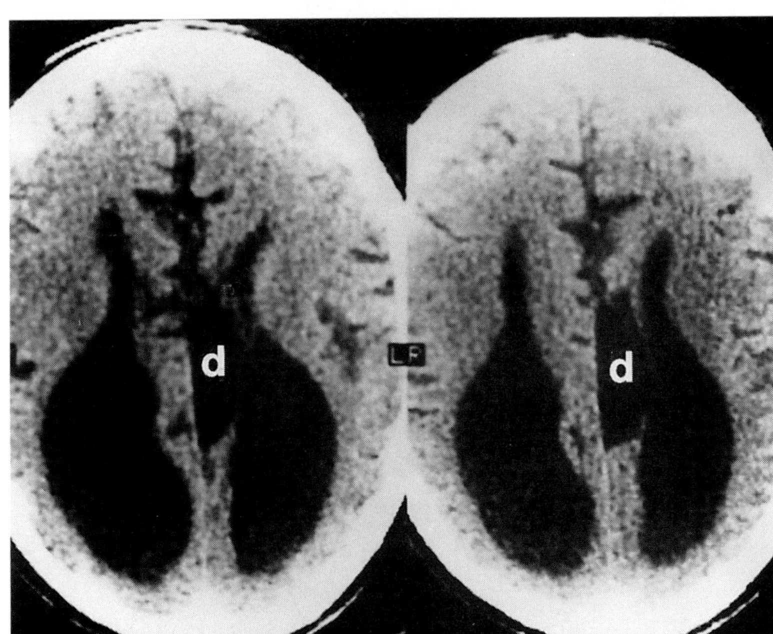

Figure 2–51. Dysgenesis of the corpus callosum. Axial CT shows marked colpocephaly and a diverticulum (d) of the third ventricle into the interhemispheric fissure. Note the widely separated frontal horns.

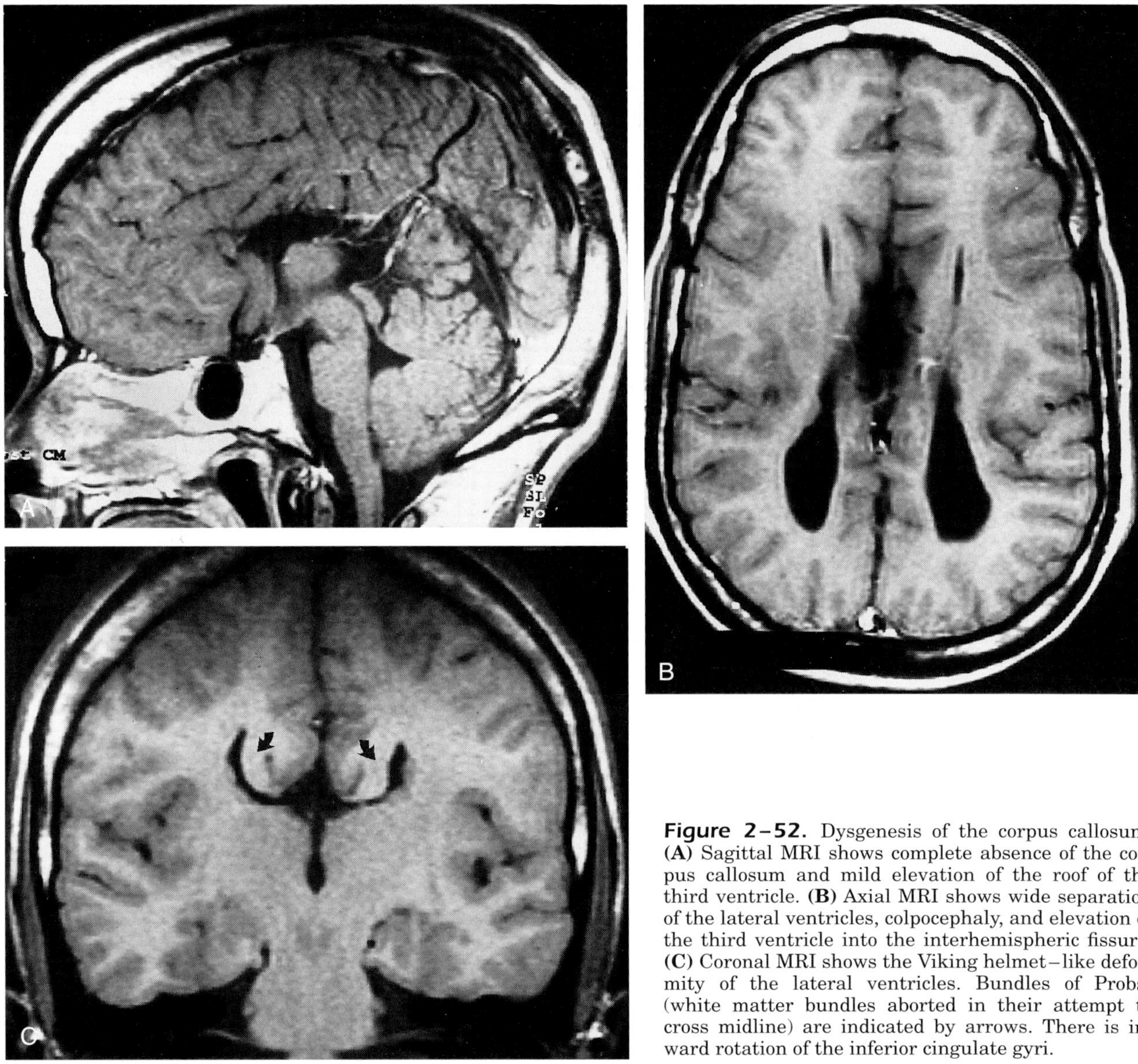

Figure 2–52. Dysgenesis of the corpus callosum. **(A)** Sagittal MRI shows complete absence of the corpus callosum and mild elevation of the roof of the third ventricle. **(B)** Axial MRI shows wide separation of the lateral ventricles, colpocephaly, and elevation of the third ventricle into the interhemispheric fissure. **(C)** Coronal MRI shows the Viking helmet–like deformity of the lateral ventricles. Bundles of Probst (white matter bundles aborted in their attempt to cross midline) are indicated by arrows. There is inward rotation of the inferior cingulate gyri.

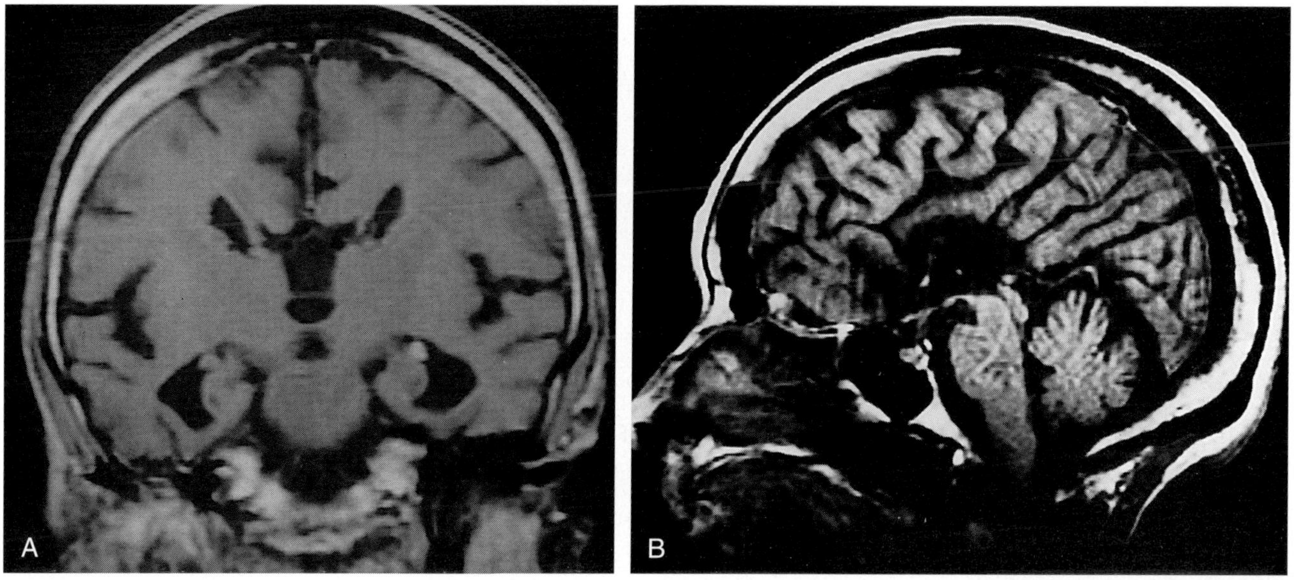

Figure 2–53. Dysgenesis of the corpus callosum. **(A)** Coronal MRI shows wide separation of the thalami with a wide third ventricle. The temporal horn dilatation results from hypoplasia of the limbic system. **(B)** Sagittal MRI shows the sunburst-like pattern of gyri radiating from the third ventricle and the nonconvergence of the calcarine and parieto-occipital fissures. (Courtesy of Dr. Alan Lovell, Birmingham, AL).

Destructive Lesions

Porencephaly

Porencephaly may describe any condition in which parenchymal destruction leads to a gross CSF-filled cavity. It may be applied to type II (open lip) schizencephaly but usually is used to describe cavities that are purely destructive in nature, unassociated with other anomalies, and not lined by gray matter (encephaloclastic porencephaly). This necessitates an insult after neuronal migration is complete. Possible etiologies include intrauterine arterial (especially middle cerebral) occlusion, hemorrhage, and infection. Clinically patients manifest seizures or spastic hemiparesis (cerebral palsy).

Primary Abnormality

- CSF-filled cavity of cerebral parenchyma, which may communicate with the ventricles or subarachnoid space and is not lined by a continuous layer of gray matter

Ancillary Findings

- Multiple in about 25% of cases
- Subarachnoid cysts in 20%
- Hydrocephalus in 35%
- Atrophy of involved hemisphere

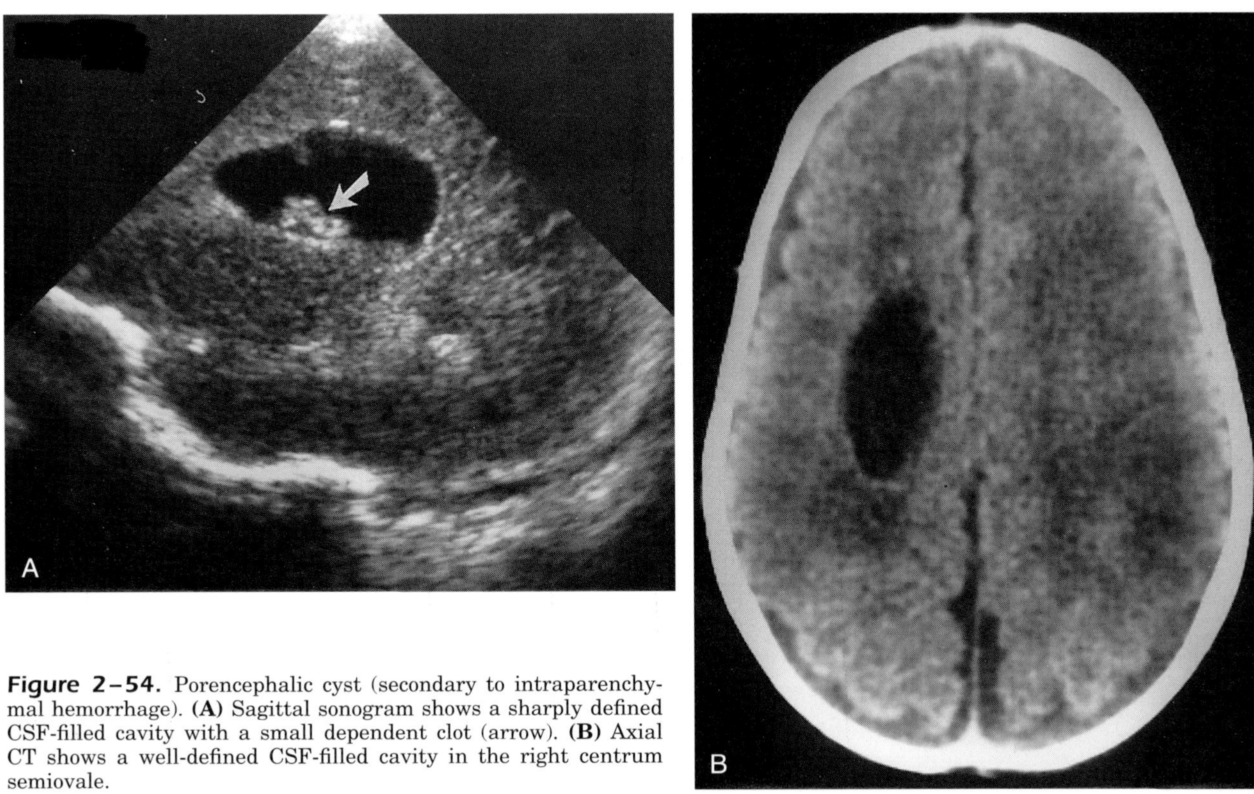

Figure 2–54. Porencephalic cyst (secondary to intraparenchymal hemorrhage). **(A)** Sagittal sonogram shows a sharply defined CSF-filled cavity with a small dependent clot (arrow). **(B)** Axial CT shows a well-defined CSF-filled cavity in the right centrum semiovale.

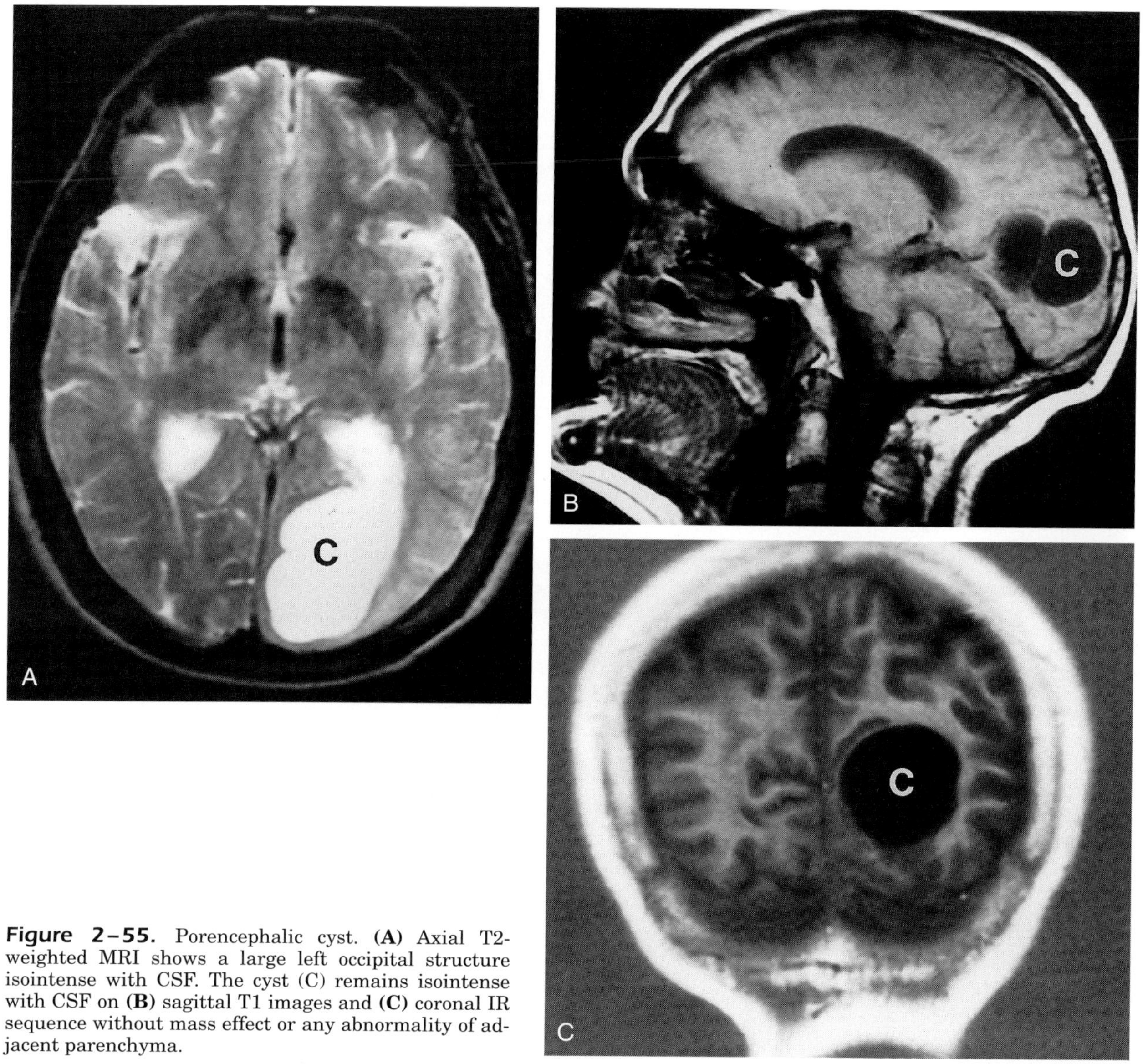

Figure 2–55. Porencephalic cyst. **(A)** Axial T2-weighted MRI shows a large left occipital structure isointense with CSF. The cyst (C) remains isointense with CSF on **(B)** sagittal T1 images and **(C)** coronal IR sequence without mass effect or any abnormality of adjacent parenchyma.

Hydranencephaly

Hydranencephaly is an uncommon but severe malformation in which there is partial or complete absence of the cerebral hemispheres, typically with intact thalami, brainstem, and cerebellum. It is attributed to in utero internal carotid occlusion during the early or middle second trimester, although some cases may be due to fulminant intrauterine cerebritis. There is normal formation of the skull and dura. The presence of an intact falx cerebri, unfused thalami, and normal facies serves to exclude alobar holoprosencephaly, which otherwise may be indistinguishable. In either case, however, the prognosis is uniformly dismal.

Primary Abnormality

- Subtotal or total absence of cerebral hemispheres with intact falx cerebri

Ancillary Findings

- Preservation of inferior and posterior temporal and occipital lobes
- Preservation of posterior fossa structures
- Brainstem atrophy
- Small, unfused remnants of thalami

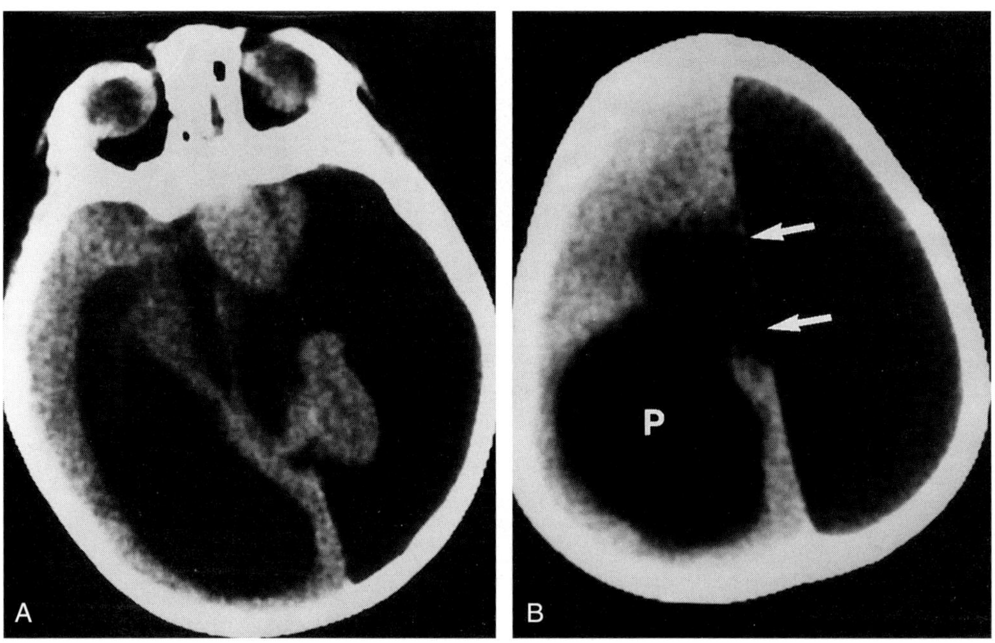

Figure 2–56. Unilateral hydranencephaly. **(A,B)** Axial CT shows absence of the left cerebral hemisphere with intact falx (arrows). The left hemicalvarium is hypoplastic. There is massive porencephaly (P) of the right hemisphere with a variable degree of residual cortical mantle, which is mostly frontal.

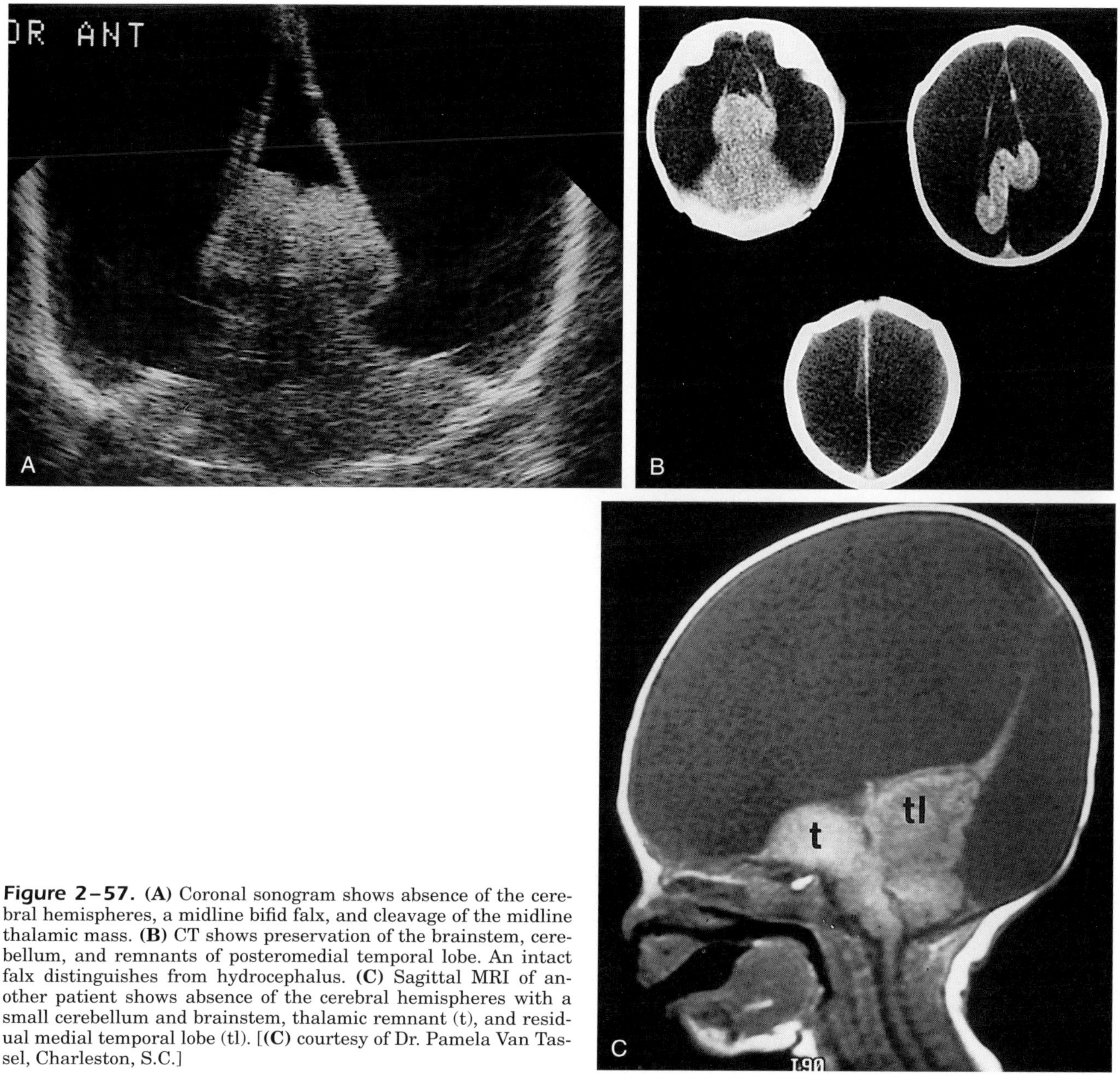

Figure 2–57. **(A)** Coronal sonogram shows absence of the cerebral hemispheres, a midline bifid falx, and cleavage of the midline thalamic mass. **(B)** CT shows preservation of the brainstem, cerebellum, and remnants of posteromedial temporal lobe. An intact falx distinguishes from hydrocephalus. **(C)** Sagittal MRI of another patient shows absence of the cerebral hemispheres with a small cerebellum and brainstem, thalamic remnant (t), and residual medial temporal lobe (tl). [**(C)** courtesy of Dr. Pamela Van Tassel, Charleston, S.C.]

Disturbances of Meningeal Development

Lipoma

Intracranial lipomas are neither neoplasms nor hamartomas but are congenital malformations resulting from faulty differentiation of the meninx primitiva, an embryonic tissue that gives rise to the meninges and, through its lysis, the subarachnoid space. Lipomas are usually encountered as an incidental finding on CT or MRI, and most patients are asymptomatic. About 50% occur around (not in) the corpus callosum, about 25% in the quadrigeminal and superior cerebellar cisterns, and the remainder in other cisternal spaces.

CT Findings. The usual CT finding is a mass of fatty attenuation (less than −50 HU) in the region of the corpus callosum. Lipomas may be quite large. Direct extension into the choroid plexus is present in 40–75%, with the higher frequency in the largest lesions. Peripheral calcifications are frequent. Callosal dysgenesis proportionate to the size of the lipoma is present in most pericallosal lipomas. The septum pellucidum may be absent.

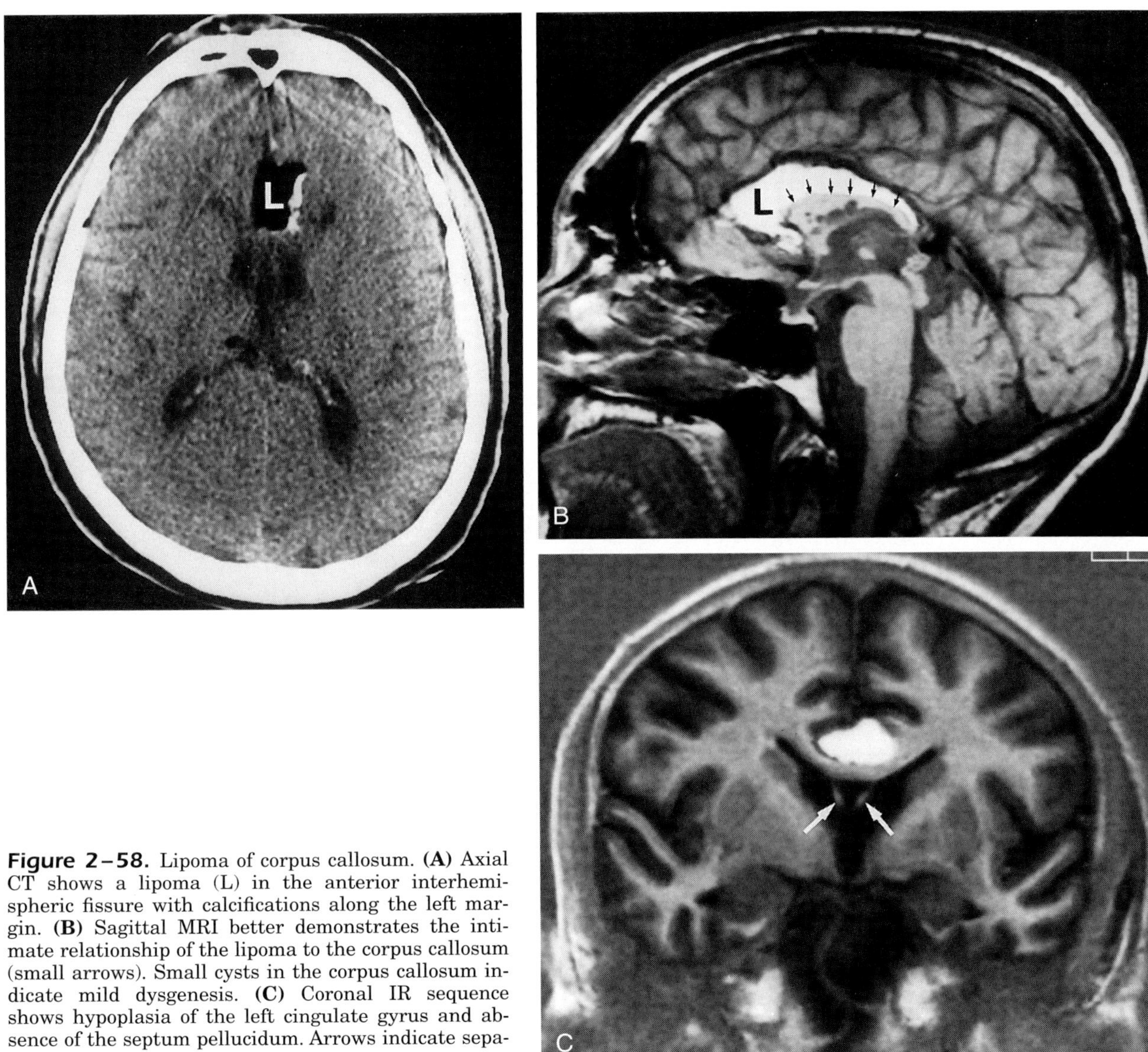

Figure 2–58. Lipoma of corpus callosum. **(A)** Axial CT shows a lipoma (L) in the anterior interhemispheric fissure with calcifications along the left margin. **(B)** Sagittal MRI better demonstrates the intimate relationship of the lipoma to the corpus callosum (small arrows). Small cysts in the corpus callosum indicate mild dysgenesis. **(C)** Coronal IR sequence shows hypoplasia of the left cingulate gyrus and absence of the septum pellucidum. Arrows indicate separation of the columns of the fornix.

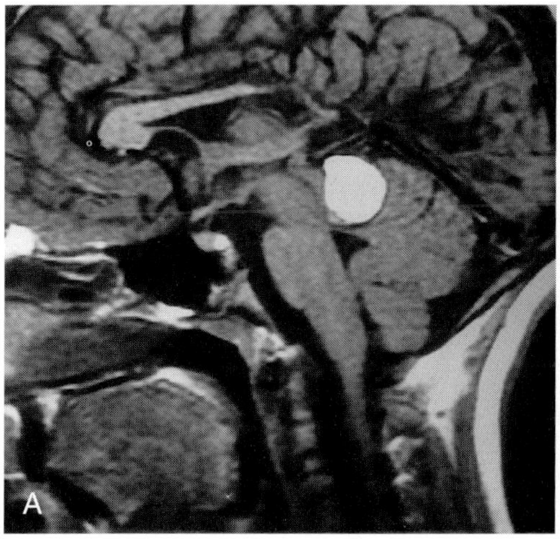
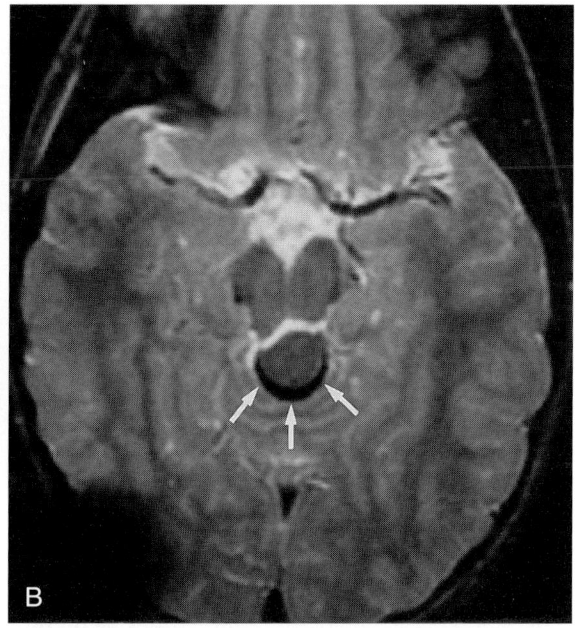

Figure 2–59. Lipoma of quadrigeminal cistern. **(A)** Sagittal T1-weighted MRI shows a lipoma of the quadrigeminal cistern. There is a beaking deformity of the tectum and dysgenesis of the posterior body and splenium of the corpus callosum. **(B)** Axial T2-weighted sequence shows the chemical shift artifact (arrows), which can establish the fatty nature of the mass and exclude other causes of hyperintensity on T1 images.

MRI Findings. The mass exhibits typical signal characteristics of fat, namely, marked hyperintensity on T1-weighted images and hypointensity on T2-weighted images. Chemical shift artifact may cause dark or bright bands along the edges. MRI provides better contrast with adjacent CSF than does CT, and callosal dysgenesis is more easily recognized. Nearby cerebral vessels are incorporated rather than displaced by the lipoma and may be identified by their signal voids. Lipomas occurring in other regions are also associated with hypoplasia of the adjoining neural structures.

Differential Diagnosis

Fat may occur in dermoids and teratomas and rarely in meningiomas. These are distinguished by the presence of mass effect and additional nonfatty components, their differing distribution, and the absence of hypoplastic changes in the neighboring brain.

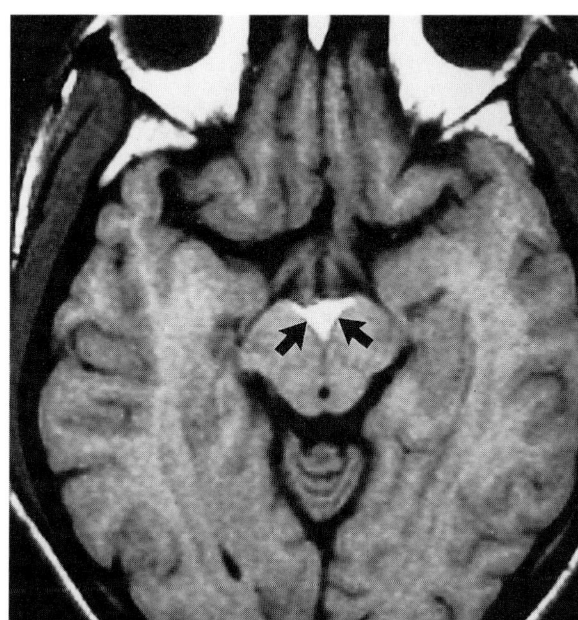

Figure 2–60. Lipoma of interpeduncular cistern. Axial MRI shows a lipoma of the interpeduncular cistern (arrows), which is a rare location.

RECOMMENDED READINGS

General References

Babcock,DS. Sonography of Congenital Malformations of the Brain. *Neuroradiology* 28:428–439, 1986.

Barkovich,AJ, Norman,D. Absence of the Septum Pellucidum: A Useful Sign in the Diagnosis of Congenital Brain Malformations. *AJR* 152:353–360, 1989.

Funk,KC, Siegel,MJ. Sonography of Congenital Midline Brain Malformations. *Radiographics* 8:11–25, 1988.

Poe,LB, Coleman,LL, Mahmud,F. Congenital Central Nervous System Anomalies. *Radiographics* 9:801–826, 1989.

van der Knapp,MS, Valk,J. Classification of Congenital Abnormalities of the CNS. *AJNR* 9:315–326, 1988.

Chiari I

Barkovich,AJ, Wippold,FJ, Sherman,JL, Citrin,CM. Significance of Cerebellar Tonsillar Position on MR. *AJNR* 7:795–799, 1986.

Elster,AD, Chen,MYM. Chiari I Malformations: Clinical and Radiologic Reappraisal. *Radiology* 183:347–353, 1992.

Chiari II

El Gammal,T, Mark,EK, Brooks,BS. MR Imaging of Chiari II Malformation. *AJR* 150:163–170, 1988.

McLone,DG, Naidich,TP. Developmental Morphology of the Subarachnoid Space, Brain Vasculature, and Contiguous Structures, and the Cause of the Chiari II Malformation. *AJNR* 13:463–484, 1992.

Wolpert,SM, Anderson,M, Scott,RM, Kwan,ESK, Runge,VM. Chiari II Malformation: MR Imaging Evaluation. *AJR* 149:1033–1042, 1987.

Encephalocele

Castillo,M, Quencer,RM, Dominguez,R. Chiari III Malformations: Imaging Features. *AJNR* 13:107–113, 1992.

Naidich,TP, Altman,NR, Braffman,BH, McLone,DG, Zimmerman,RA. Cephaloceles and Related Malformations. *AJNR* 13:655–690, 1992.

Holoprosencephaly

Byrd,SE, Osborn,RE, Radkowski,MA, McArdle,CB, Prenger,EC, Naidich,TP. Disorders of Midline Structures: Holoprosencephaly, Absence of Corpus Callosum, and Chiari Malformations. *Semin Ultrasound CT MR* 9:201–215, 1988.

Castillo,M, Bouldin,TW, Scatliff,JH, Suzuki,K. Radiologic-Pathologic Correlation: Alobar Holoprosencephaly. *AJNR* 14:1151–1156, 1993.

Fitz,CR. Holoprosencephaly and Related Entities. *Neuroradiology* 25:225–238, 1983.

Fitz,CR. Holoprosencephaly and Septo-optic Dysplasia. *Neuroimaging Clin N Am* 2:263–282, 1994.

Oba,H, Barkovich,AJ. Holoprosencephaly: An Analysis of Callosal Formation and Its Relation to Development of the Interhemispheric Fissure. *AJNR* 16:453–460, 1995.

Septo-optic Dysplasia

Barkovich,AJ, Fram,EK, Norman,D. Septo-Optic Dysplasia: MR Imaging. *Radiology* 171:189–192, 1989.

Fitz,CR. Holoprosencephaly and Septo-optic Dysplasia. *Neuroimaging Clin North Am* 2:263–282, 1994.

Kuban,KCK, Teele,RL, Wallman,J. Septo-optic-dysplasia-schizencephaly. *Pediatr Radiol* 19:145–150, 1989.

Dandy-Walker Malformation and Variant

Altman,NR, Naidich,TP, Braffman,BH. Posterior Fossa Malformations. *AJNR* 13:691–724, 1992.

Barkovich,AJ, Kjos,BO, Norman,D, Edwards,MS. Revised Classification of Posterior Fossa Cysts and Cystlike Malformations Based on the Results of Multiplanar MR Imaging. *AJNR* 10:977–988, 1989. *AJR* 153:1289–1300, 1989.

Sturge-Weber Syndrome

Braffman,B, Naidich,TP. The Phakomatoses: Part II. von Hippel-Lindau Disease, Sturge-Weber Syndrome, and Less Common Conditions. *Neuroimaging Clin North Am.* 4:325–348, 1994.

Elster,AD, Chen,MYM. MR Imaging of Sturge-Weber Syndrome: Role of Gadopentetate Dimeglumine and Gradient-Echo Techniques. *AJNR* 11:685–689, 1990.

Smirniotopoulos,JG, Murphy,FM. The Phakomatoses. *AJNR* 13:725–746, 1992.

Tuberous Sclerosis

Bell,DG, King,BF, Hattery,RR, et al. Imaging Characteristics of Tuberous Sclerosis. *AJR* 156:1081–1086, 1991.

Braffman,BH, Bilaniuk,LT, Naidich,TP, et al. MR Imaging of Tuberous Sclerosis: Pathogenesis of This Phakomatosis, Use of Gadopentetate Dimeglumine, and Literature Review. *Radiology* 183:227–238, 1992.

Braffman,B, Naidich,TP. The Phakomatoses: Part I. Neurofibromatosis and Tuberous Sclerosis. *Neuroimaging Clin North Am* 4:299–324, 1994.

Shepherd,CW, Houser,OW, Gomez,MR. MR Findings in Tuberous Sclerosis Complex and Correlation with Seizure Development and Mental Impairment. *AJNR* 16:149–155, 1995.

Smirniotopoulos,JG, Murphy,FM. The Phakomatoses. *AJNR* 13:725–746, 1992.

Neurofibromatosis

Aoki,A, Barkovich,AJ, Nishimura,K, et al. Neurofibromatosis Types 1 and 2: Cranial MR Findings. *Radiology* 172:527–534, 1989.

Braffman,B, Naidich,TP. The Phakomatoses: Part I. Neurofibromatosis and Tuberous Sclerosis. *Neuroimaging Clin North Am* 4:299–324, 1994.

Itoh,T, Magnaldi,S, White,RM, et al. Neurofibromatosis Type 1: The Evolution of Deep Gray and White Matter MR Abnormalities. *AJNR* 15:1513–1519, 1994.

Shu,HH, Mirowitz,SA, Wippold,FJ. Neurofibromatosis: MR Imaging Findings Involving the Head and Spine. *AJR* 160:159–164, 1993.

Smirniotopoulos,JG, Murphy,FM. The Phakomatoses. *AJNR* 13:725–746, 1992.

Aqueductal Stenosis

Atlas,SW, Mark,AS, Fram,EK. Aqueductal Stenosis: Evaluation with Gradient-Echo Rapid MR Imaging. *Radiology* 169: 449–453, 1988.

Barkovich,AJ, Newton,TH. MR of Aqueductal Stenosis: Evidence of a Broad Spectrum of Tectal Distortion. *AJNR* 10:471–476, 1989.

Lapras,C, Tommasi,M, Bret,P. Stenosis of the aqueduct of Sylvius. *Handbook of Clinical Neurology* 6(50):301–322, 1987.

Hemimegalencephaly

Barkovich,AJ, Chuang,SH. Unilateral Megalencephaly: Correlation of MR Imaging and Pathologic Characteristics. *AJNR* 11:523–531, 1990.

Kalifa,GL, Chiron,C, Sellier,N, et al. Hemimegalencephaly: MR Imaging in Five Children. *Radiology* 165:29–33, 1987.

Wolpert,SM, Cohen,A, Libenson,MH. Hemimegalencephaly: A Longitudinal MR Study. *AJNR* 15:1479–1482, 1994.

Lissencephaly

Byrd,SE, Bohan,TP, Osborn,RE, Naidich,TP. The CT and MR Evaluation of Lissencephaly. *AJNR* 9:923–927, 1988.

Dobyns,WB, McCluggage,CW. Computed Tomographic Appearance of Lissencephaly Syndromes. *AJNR* 6:545–550, 1985.

Rhodes,RE, Hatten,HP, Ellington,KS. Walker-Warburg Syndrome. *AJNR* 13:123–126, 1992.

Schizencephaly

Barkovich,AJ, Kjos,BO. Schizencephaly: Correlation of Clinical Findings with MR Characteristics. *AJNR* 13:85–94, 1992.

Barkovich,AJ, Norman,D. MR Imaging of Schizencephaly. *AJR* 150:1391–1396, 1988. *AJNR* 9:297–302, 1988.

Barth,PG. Schizencephaly and Nonlissencephalic Cortical Dysplasias. *AJNR* 13:104–106, 1992.

Bird,CR, Gilles,FH. Type I Schizencephaly: CT and Neuropathologic Findings. *AJNR* 8:451–454, 1987.

Gray Matter Heterotopia

Barkovich,AJ, Jackson,DE, Boyer,RS. Band Heterotopias: A Newly Recognized Neuronal Migration Anomaly. *Radiology* 171:455–458, 1989.

Barkovich,AJ, Kjos,BO. Gray Matter Heterotopias: MR Characteristics and Correlation with Developmental and Neurologic Manifestations. *Radiology* 182:493–499, 1992.

Smith,AS, Ross,JS, Blaser,SI, Weinstein,MA. Magnetic Resonance Imaging of Disturbances in Neuronal Migration: Illustration of an Embryologic Process. *Radiographics* 9:509–522, 1989.

Focal Cortical Dysplasia

Barkovich,AJ, Kjos,BO. Nonlissencephalic Cortical Dysplasias: Correlation of Imaging Findings with Clinical Deficits. *AJNR* 13:95–103, 1992.

Barkovich,AJ, Rowley,HA, Andermann,F. MR in Partial Epilepsy: Value of High-Resolution Volumetric Techniques. *AJNR* 16:339–343, 1995.

Titelbaum,DS, Hayward,JC, Zimmerman,RA. Pachygyriclike Changes: Topographic Appearance at MR Imaging and CT and Correlation with Neurologic Status. *Radiology* 173: 663–667, 1989.

Dysgenesis of Corpus Callosum

Atlas,SW, Zimmerman,RA, Bilaniuk,LT, et al. Corpus Callosum and Limbic System: Neuroanatomic MR Evaluation of Developmental Anomalies. *Radiology* 160:355–362, 1986.

Babcock,DS. The Normal, Absent, and Abnormal Corpus Callosum: Sonographic Findings. *Radiology* 151:449–453, 1984.

Barkovich,AJ, Lyon,G, Evrard,P. Formation, Maturation, and Disorders of White Matter. *AJNR* 13:447–461, 1992.

Gebarski,SS, Gebarski,KS, Bowerman,TA, Silver,TM. Agenesis of the Corpus Callosum: Sonographic Features. *Radiology* 151:443–448, 1984.

Porencephaly and Hydranencephaly

Dublin,AB, French,BN. Diagnostic Image Evaluation of Hydranencephaly and Pictorially Similar Entities, with Emphasis on Computed Tomography. *Radiology* 137:81–91, 1980.

Kolawole,TM, Patel,PJ, Mahdi,AH. Porencephaly: Computed Tomography (CT) Scan Findings. *Computerized Radiology* 11:53–58, 1987.

Raybaud,C. Destructive Lesions of the Brain. *Neuroradiology* 25:265–291, 1983.

Rorke,LB, Zimmerman,RA. Prematurity, Postmaturity, and Destructive Lesions in Utero. *AJNR* 13:517–536, 1992.

Lipoma

Truwit,CL, Williams,RG, Armstrong,EA, Marlin,AE. MR Imaging of Choroid Plexus Lipomas. *AJNR* 11:202–204, 1990.

Truwit,CL, Barkovich,AJ. Pathogenesis of Intracranial Lipoma: An MR Study in 42 Patients. *AJNR* 11:665–674, 1990, *AJR* 155:855–864, 1990.

Uchino,A, Hasuo,K, Matsumoto,S, Masuda,K. Solitary Choroid Plexus Lipomas: CT and MR Appearance. *AJNR* 14:116–118, 1993.

CHAPTER THREE

Infectious and Inflammatory Diseases

The rapid spread of AIDS during the past decade has led to a sizable increase in the incidence of many infectious diseases of the CNS. The leading AIDS-related disorders are described in this chapter, along with the classic CNS inflammatory processes that are still commonly encountered. No specific features allow consistent and easy differentiation of inflammatory processes from various neoplastic, vascular, and degenerative disorders that may manifest similar imaging findings. The differential diagnoses offered herein do not aspire to be comprehensive. Still, one should always proceed with the axiom that common things occur commonly, and the few disorders presented in this chapter account for the overwhelming majority of CNS inflammatory diseases seen in most practices.

Bacterial Infections

Bacterial Meningitis

Bacterial meningitis is a pyogenic infection of the meninges and subarachnoid space. The major predisposing factors are otomastoiditis (25%), immunosuppression (19%), ethanol abuse (18%), pneumonia (15%), and sinusitis (12%). Meningitis is usually acute in onset and fulminant in its course. The leading causative organisms include *Haemophilus influenzae*, *Neisseria meningitidis*, and *Streptococcus pneumoniae*. Since the availability of a *Haemophilus* vaccine, pneumococcus has become the leading organism and pneumonia is a more common predisposing condition. Most cases of bacterial meningitis are diagnosed using CSF, and patients respond well to antibiotic treatment. Neuroimaging plays a diagnostic role when the initial clinical presentation is not straightforward or when complications arise.

CT Findings. CT often shows sinusitis or mastoiditis but no intracranial abnormalities on initial presentation. Hydrocephalus develops in most patients during the course of disease but is usually self-limited. Less frequent findings include obliteration and enhancement of the basal cisterns and meningeal enhancement. Ventriculitis may develop secondary to meningitis or by direct extension of a brain abscess. Enhancement of the ventricular walls is caused by, and a sign of, ventriculitis. Infarcts may develop secondary to arterial or venous thrombosis. Middle cerebral territory infarcts are highly suggestive of tuberculous meningitis.

MRI Findings. Sinusitis or mastoiditis is commonly present, with thickening and enhancement of adjacent meninges. Pial enhancement extends deep into fissures and sulci and conforms to the brain surface. Dural-arachnoid enhancement is linear and conforms to the inner table and skull base. Subarachnoid enhancement is enhancement of the cisterns proper and tends to be thicker and more diffuse. Unenhanced studies are insensitive for the meningeal abnormalities. MRI can effectively detect the complications of meningitis, such as subdural empyema, brain abscess, cerebritis, ventriculitis, venous sinus thrombosis, infarct, and hydrocephalus.

Differential Diagnosis

The most common forms of meningitis and the differential diagnosis of meningeal enhancement are given in Tables 3–1 and 3–2.

TABLE 3–1 **Differential Diagnosis of Meningitis**

	Bacterial	Tuberculous	Cryptococcal	Viral
Mastoiditis/sinusitis	Usually present	No	No	No
Meningeal enhancement	Adjacent to infected sinus	Usually present, especially basal cisterns	Infrequent, often nodular	Infrequent
Abscesses	Common	Infrequent	Infrequent	No
Cerebral granulomas	No	Common	Infrequent	No
Parenchymal hyperintensity on T2-weighted MRI	Occasional: infarcts in middle cerebral territory	Common: infarcts in basal ganglia and brainstem	Infrequent: gelatinous pseudocysts in basal ganglia	No, but may have parenchymal edema with coexistent encephalomyelitis
Hydrocephalus	Frequent	Frequent	Infrequent	Infrequent
Clinical course	Acute	Subacute to chronic	Subacute to chronic	Acute
CSF	↑↑ neutrophils ↑↑ protein ↓ glucose	↑ lymphocytes ↑ protein ↓ glucose	↑ lymphocytes ↑ protein ↓ glucose + India ink stain	↑ lymphocytes ↑ protein Normal glucose

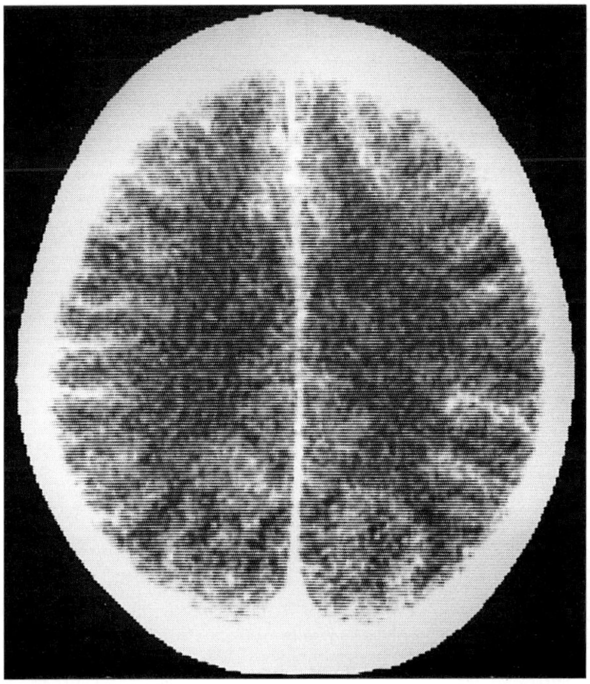

Figure 3–1. *Haemophilus influenzae* meningitis. Contrast-enhanced CT shows diffusely increased enhancement in the cortical fissures.

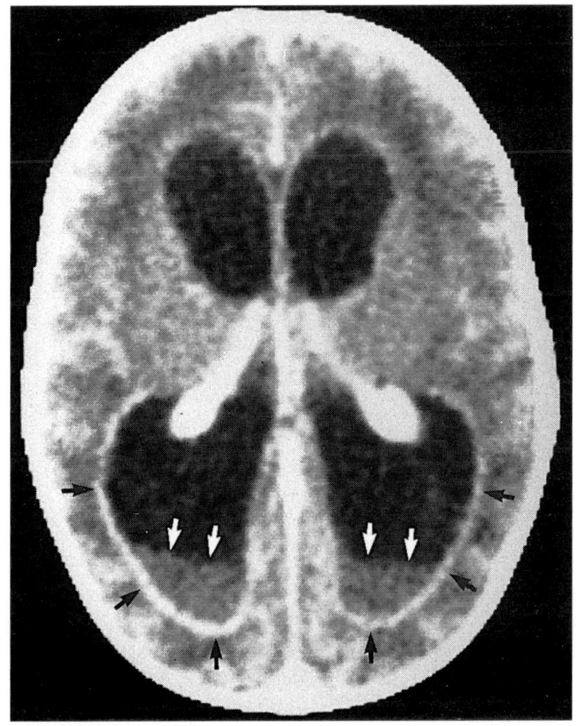

Figure 3–2. Ventriculitis. Contrast-enhanced CT shows enhancement of the ependyma (black arrows), hydrocephalus, and debris-fluid levels (white arrows) in the occipital horns.

TABLE 3–2 Differential Diagnosis of Meningeal Enhancement

Common
Meningitis
Bacterial
Tuberculous
Viral
Fungal
Chemical
Meningioma
Craniotomy
Metastases
Cerebral Infarct
Less Common
Sinus thrombosis
Subarachnoid hemorrhage
Sarcoidosis
Histiocytosis
Chronic ventricular shunting
Sturge-Weber syndrome
Postlumbar puncture

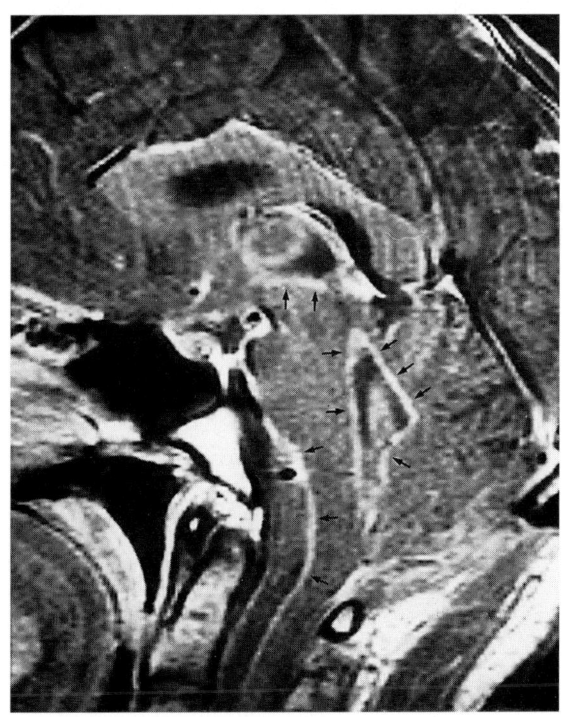

Figure 3–3. Viral meningitis. Contrast-enhanced MRI demonstrates pial, arachnoid, and ependymal enhancement (arrows).

Pyogenic Cerebritis and Brain Abscess

The meninges normally provide an effective barrier against bacteriologic contamination of the CNS. Parenchymal brain infection may occur by hematogenous spread from a remote infection, retrograde thrombophlebitis from sinusitis or mastoiditis, or congenital or traumatic meningeal defects. Once established, the infection evolves over a period of days to weeks. The initial stage of cerebritis consists of a local inflammatory response, edema, and disruption of the blood-brain barrier. Central necrosis begins to develop in late cerebritis. After about 2 weeks, a fibrogliotic capsule forms around the zone of necrosis, finally resulting in a mature abscess. Patients present with symptoms of a rapidly enlarging mass lesion, such as headaches, seizures, and focal deficits. Therapy usually consists of a combination of antibiotics and surgical drainage. The mortality rate is usually under 5%.

CT Findings. The CT findings depend on the age of the abscess. Early cerebritis appears as a focal area of low attenuation (edema) with a small central focus of solid enhancement. Thick, irregular ring enhancement typifies late cerebritis. A moderate amount of vasogenic edema is consistently present. In a mature abscess, the central necrotic zone appears hypodense relative both to the capsule and surrounding edema. The capsule is usually visible without contrast and enhances as a smooth, relatively thin ring. The ring tends to be thicker on the cortical side and thinner toward the ventricles. An abscess may be bilocular or multilocular, and satellite lesions are common.

MRI Findings. Acute cerebritis appears as a small area of vasogenic edema. A distinctive feature is the presence of a central hypointense zone on T2-weighted images, which enhances with contrast. As the abscess matures, the developing rim is isointense to hyperintense on T1-weighted images and hypointense on T2-weighted images. Ring enhancement is a consistent finding, and morphologic features described for CT also apply to MRI. On T2-weighted images, the central necrotic zone is hyperintense, and concentric rings or bands may be present within. Vasogenic edema is consistently present. On T1-weighted images, the cavity is intermediate in intensity between white matter and CSF.

Differential Diagnosis

Abscess must be distinguished from other cystic intracerebral mass lesions and other causes of ring enhancement. The subacute onset of symptoms helps to distinguish between vascular events (acute onset) and tumor (more insidious onset). (See also Tables 3–3, 4–6, and 4–8.)

TABLE 3–3 | Brain Abscess Versus Neoplasm

	Abscess	Tumor
Vasogenic edema	Moderate but consistent	Highly variable
Rim	Hypointense on T2 Smooth and thin Mesial thinning	Hyperintense on T2 Nodular and thick
Hemorrhage	Rare	Common
Satellite lesions	Common	Rare with metastases Occasionally with GBM
Multiple lesions	Rare	Common with metastases

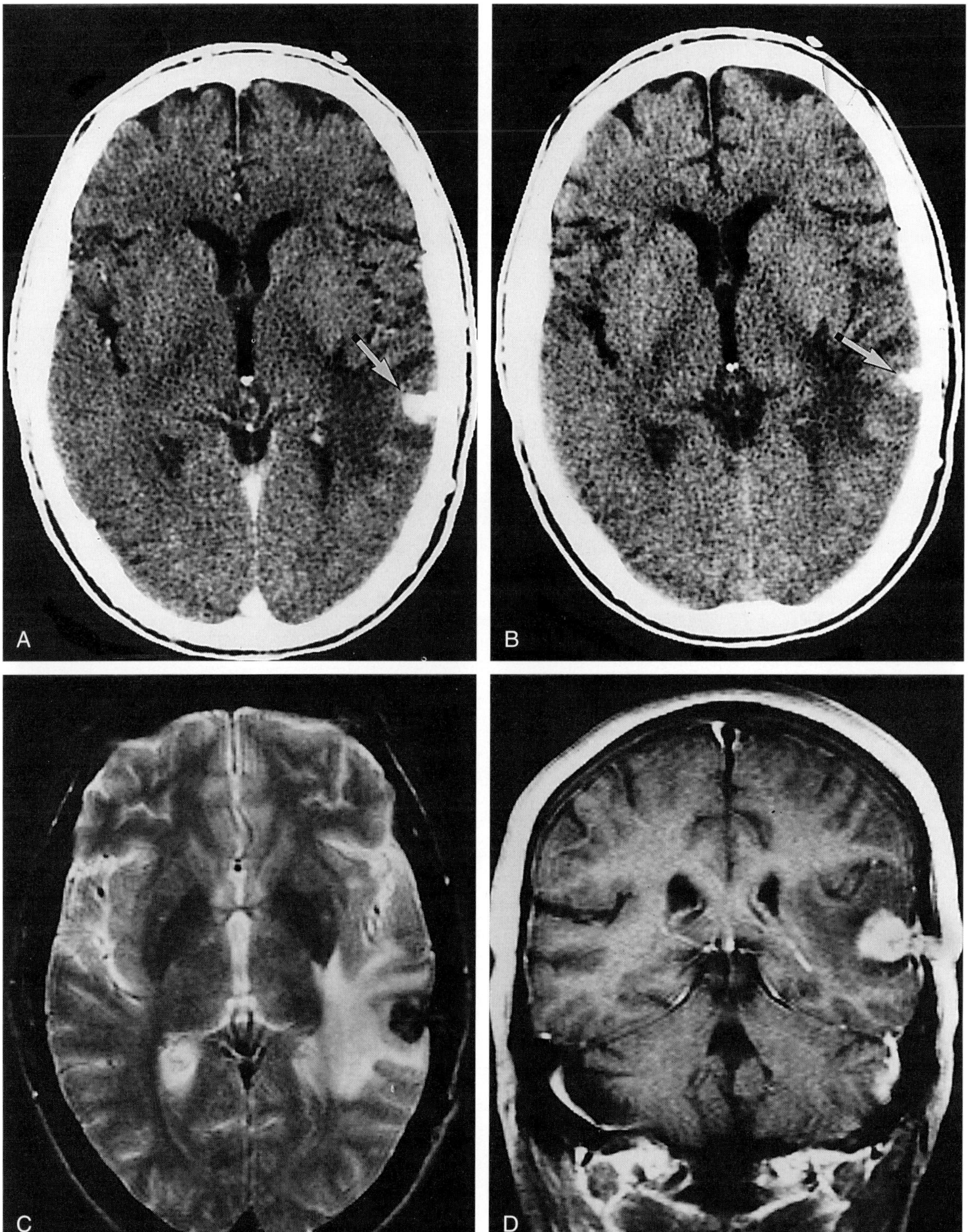

Figure 3–4. Cerebritis due to penetrating trauma. **(A)** Contrast-enhanced CT shows an area of solid cortical enhancement (arrow) surrounded by vasogenic edema. **(B)** Noncontrast CT shows a depressed bone fragment (arrow) caused by placement of a halo device. **(C)** Axial T2-weighted MRI shows a markedly hypointense mass with prominent vasogenic edema. **(D)** Coronal contrast-enhanced MRI shows solid enhancement and discontinuity of the calvarium.

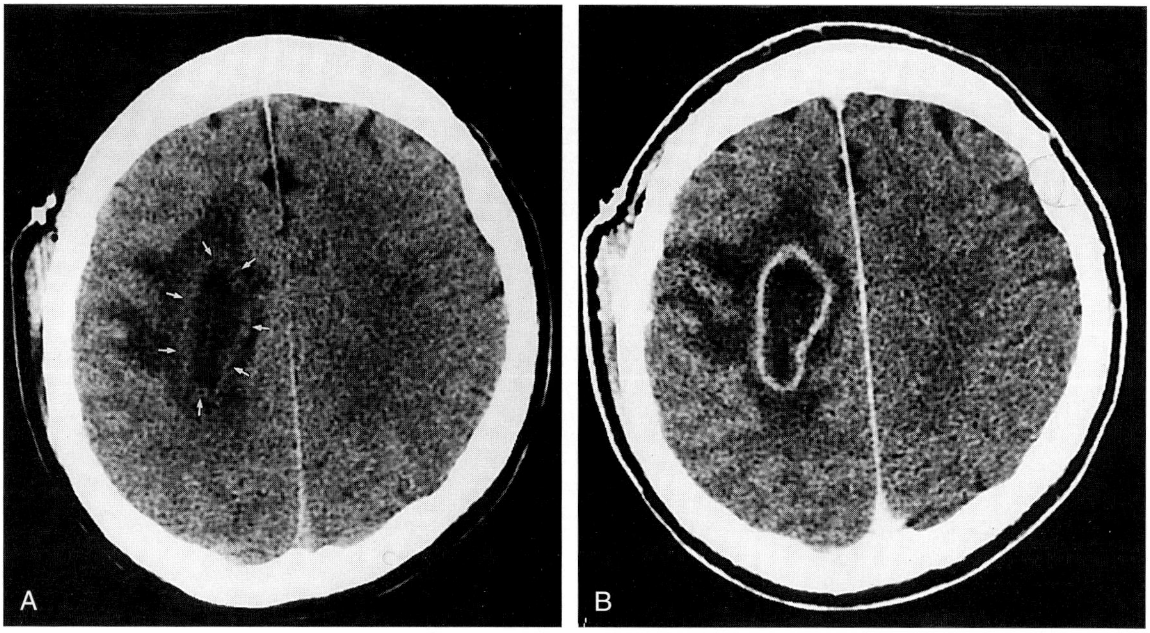

Figure 3–5. Abscess. **(A)** On unenhanced CT, the central necrotic zone is hypointense relative to the capsule (arrows) and surrounding edema. **(B)** Smooth, thin rim enhancement is seen after intravenous contrast.

Empyema

Extracerebral abscesses may be subdural (also called empyema) or epidural. The leading cause of both is spread from an adjacent infection, usually sinusitis or otomastoiditis. Postcraniotomy infection and secondary infection of extracerebral hematoma account for most other cases. Subdural empyema may lead to extensive venous and dural sinus thrombosis, resulting in venous infarction.

CT Findings. CT shows a hypodense fluid collection conforming to the subdural or epidural space with a concave or convex medial border. An epidural abscess tends to be sharply limited with a convex inner border, whereas subdural empyema is more often diffuse and inwardly concave and may extend into the interhemispheric fissure. Enhancement occurs at the interface with the cerebral cortex. Underlying cortex may also exhibit thickening and increased attenuation or enhancement. Early empyemas are often small and very subtle. Predisposing factors (sinusitis, previous craniotomy, hematoma) are usually present.

MRI Findings. MRI shows an extracerebral fluid collection slightly hyperintense relative to CSF on T1-weighted images and hyperintense on proton-density and T2-weighted images. An additional feature of epidural abscess is visualization of a hypointense medial border representing the displaced dura. Marked enhancement is seen on both inner and outer borders of subdural abscess, whereas epidural abscess may only enhance on the parenchymal side. Secondary findings may include edema, mass effect, and infarction.

Differential Diagnosis

The primary differential consideration is sterile subdural effusion. Sterile effusions are much more common than is empyema. Features of subdural effusion include isodensity with CSF on CT, isointensity with CSF on MRI, and little or no meningeal enhancement.

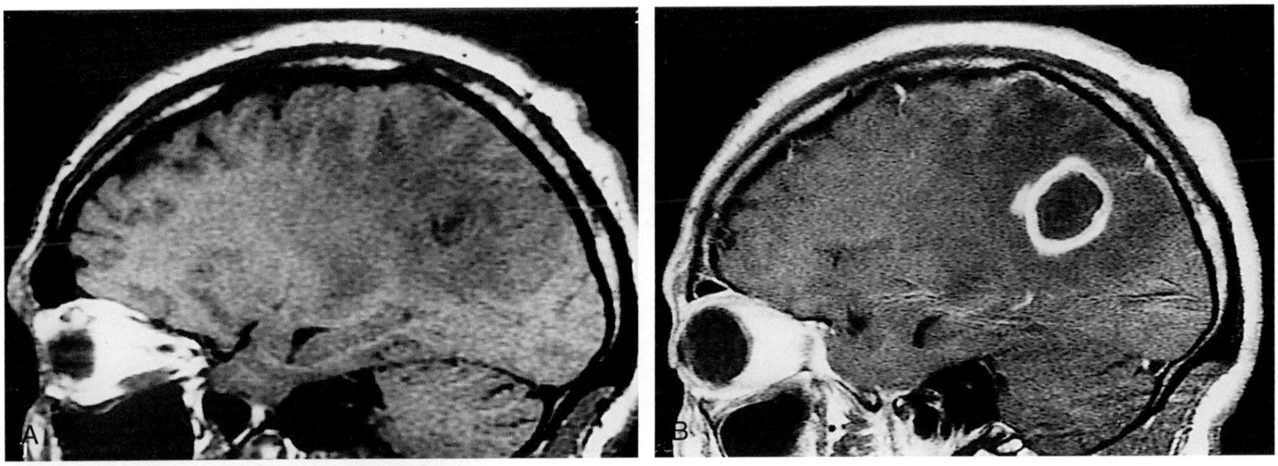

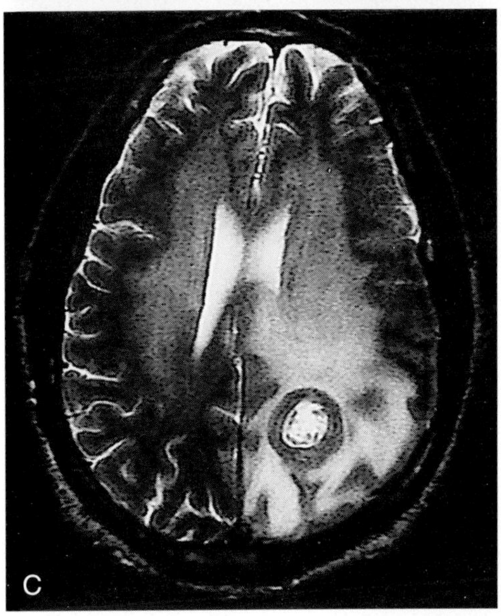

Figure 3–6. Abscess. **(A)** Sagittal T1-weighted MRI shows a hypointense mass with marked edema. The capsule is isointense to brain. **(B)** Sagittal contrast-enhanced MRI shows smooth and relatively thin rim enhancement. **(C)** On axial T2-weighted MRI, the capsule is hypointense with hyperintense central necrosis and surrounding edema. Some partial concentric rings can be seen within the cavity.

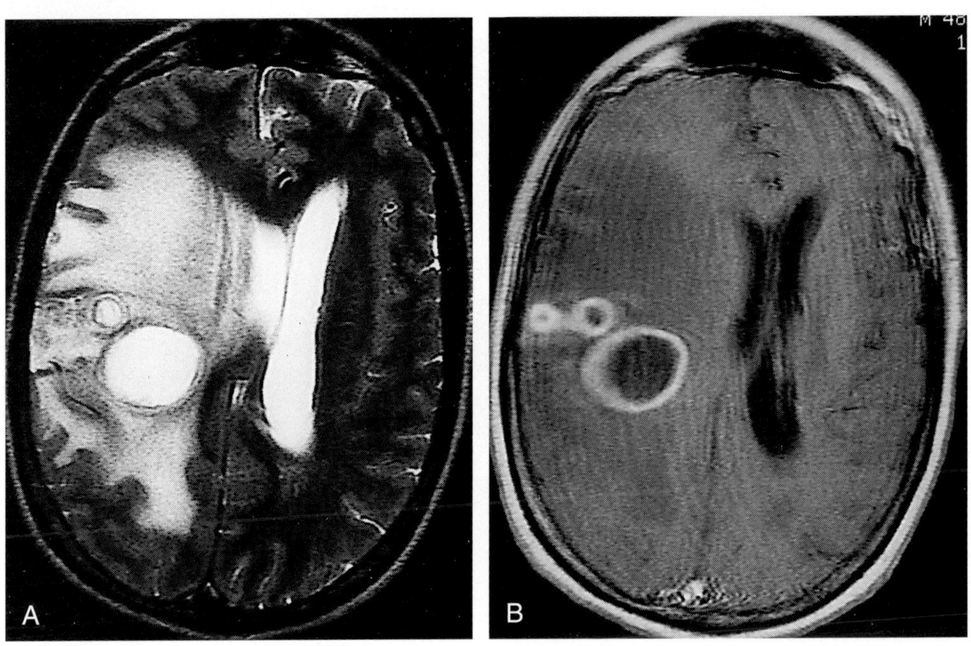

Figure 3–7. Abscess with satellite lesions. **(A)** Axial T2-weighted MRI shows a large brain abscess with satellite lesions. The central necrosis is hyperintense. The rim is hyperintense but demarcated by hypointense inner and outer boundaries. **(B)** Contrast-enhanced MRI shows smooth ring enhancement of both primary and satellite lesions.

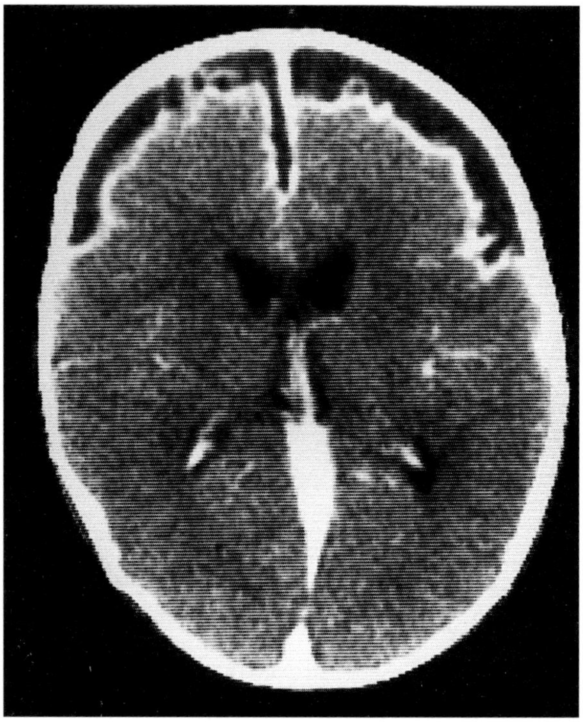

Figure 3–8. Subdural empyema complicating *Haemophilus influenzae* meningitis. Contrast-enhanced CT shows bilateral subdural fluid collections with marked enhancement at the interface with cerebral cortex. The empyema extends into the right interhemispheric fissure.

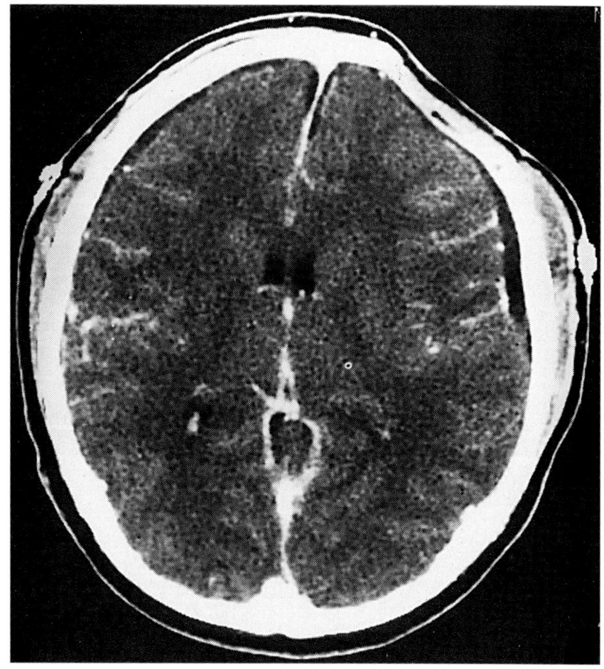

Figure 3–9. Postoperative empyema. Contrast-enhanced CT shows bifrontal subdural fluid collections with inward displacement of cortical veins and minimal meningeal enhancement.

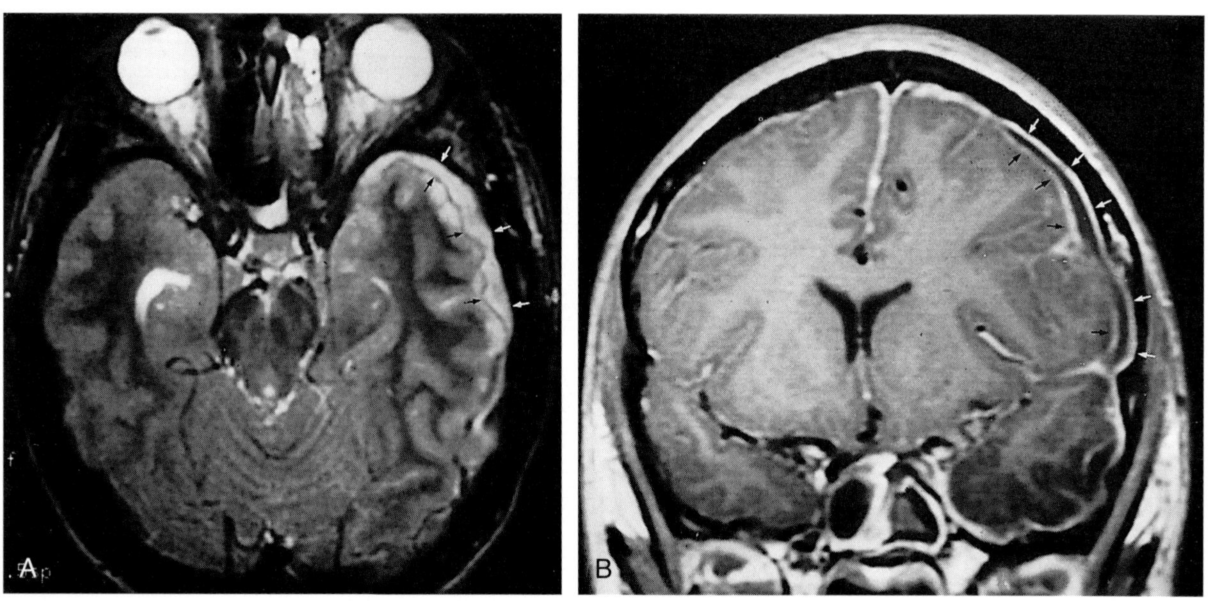

Figure 3–10. Subdural empyema. **(A)** Axial T2-weighted MRI shows left ethmoid sinusitis and a hyperintense left subdural fluid collection (arrows). **(B)** Coronal contrast-enhanced MRI shows a left subdural fluid collection with enhancement of both outer dural (white arrows) and inner arachnoid (black arrows) walls. (Courtesy of Dr. Pamela Van Tassel, Charleston, SC.)

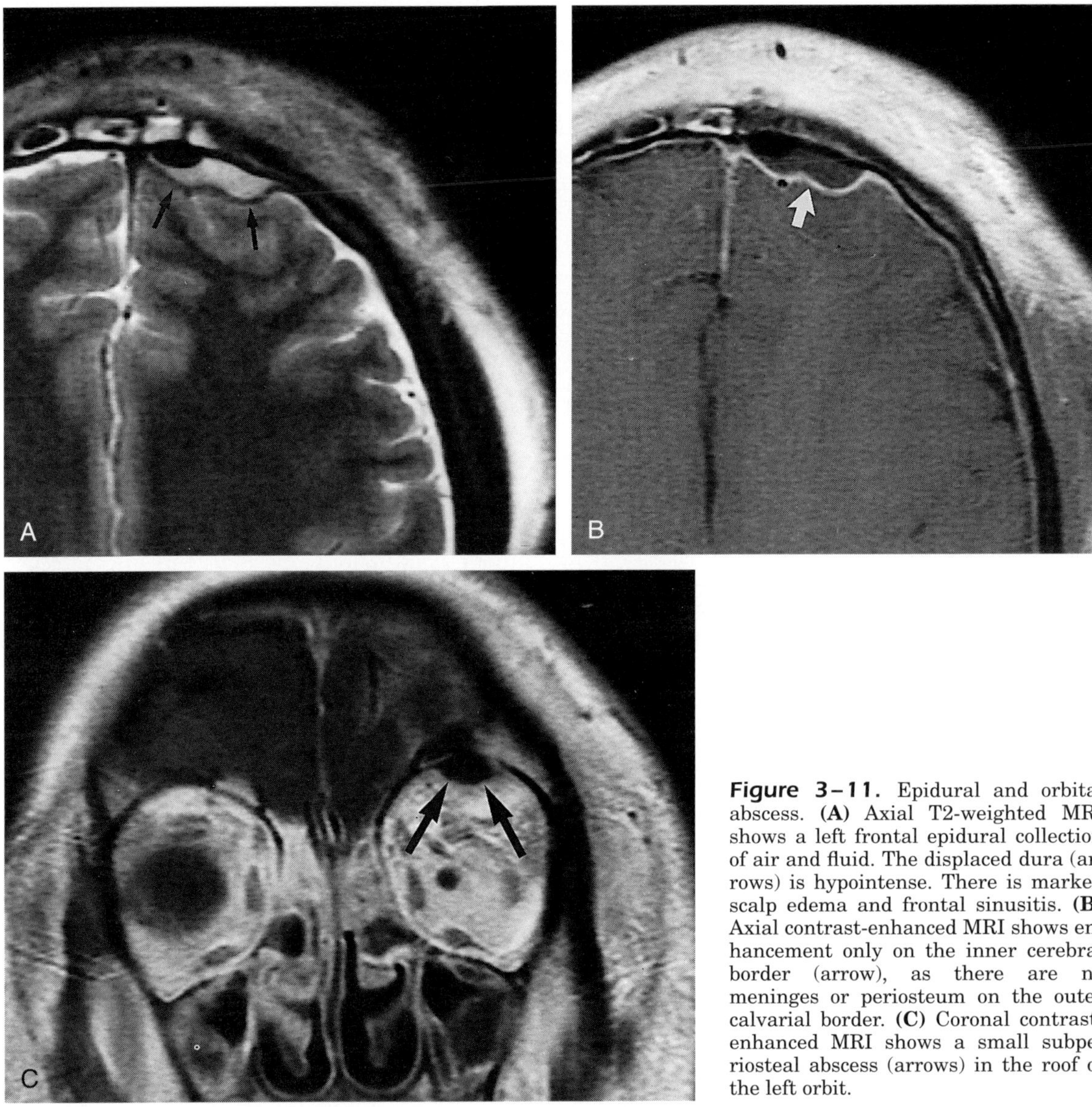

Figure 3–11. Epidural and orbital abscess. **(A)** Axial T2-weighted MRI shows a left frontal epidural collection of air and fluid. The displaced dura (arrows) is hypointense. There is marked scalp edema and frontal sinusitis. **(B)** Axial contrast-enhanced MRI shows enhancement only on the inner cerebral border (arrow), as there are no meninges or periosteum on the outer calvarial border. **(C)** Coronal contrast-enhanced MRI shows a small subperiosteal abscess (arrows) in the roof of the left orbit.

Tuberculosis

Mycobacterium tuberculosis has been a major human pathogen for millennia. Although developed countries have experienced a decline in pulmonary tuberculosis, it has remained a common condition in less developed nations. Because of AIDS, tuberculosis is now on the upswing in the United States. Within the CNS, meningitis is the most common manifestation of tuberculosis, followed by parenchymal granulomas (tuberculomas). All age groups are affected. Tuberculous brain abscess and encephalitis are rare conditions.

CT Findings. Tuberculous meningitis primarily affects the basal cisterns, with dense enhancement after intravenous contrast. Hydrocephalus is very common. Secondary parenchymal involvement may ensue. Vasculitis of the supraclinoid internal carotid and proximal middle cerebral arteries is common, resulting in middle cerebral territory infarctions. Dense meningeal calcifications may appear late in the course.

CT of tuberculoma typically shows a hyperdense mass that enhances in a solid or ringlike pattern with surrounding edema. Necrosis may be present. Calcification may occur late in the course.

MRI Findings. MRI of tuberculous meningitis typically shows intense enhancement of the basal cisterns. Hydrocephalus and ischemic changes in the middle cerebral territory are common. Ventriculitis and secondary parenchymal tuberculomas may be present.

Tuberculomas tend to be isointense to gray matter on T1-weighted images and isointense to hypointense on T2-weighted images with surrounding edema. Necrosis may cause central hyperintensity on T2-weighted images. The detection of lesions is greatly improved with contrast, which results in solid or ring enhancement.

Differential Diagnosis

The findings of dense enhancement of the basal cisterns and middle cerebral infarcts are highly suggestive of tuberculosis. The primary differential diagnosis of basal cistern enhancement includes other forms of meningitis, metastasis, and sarcoidosis.

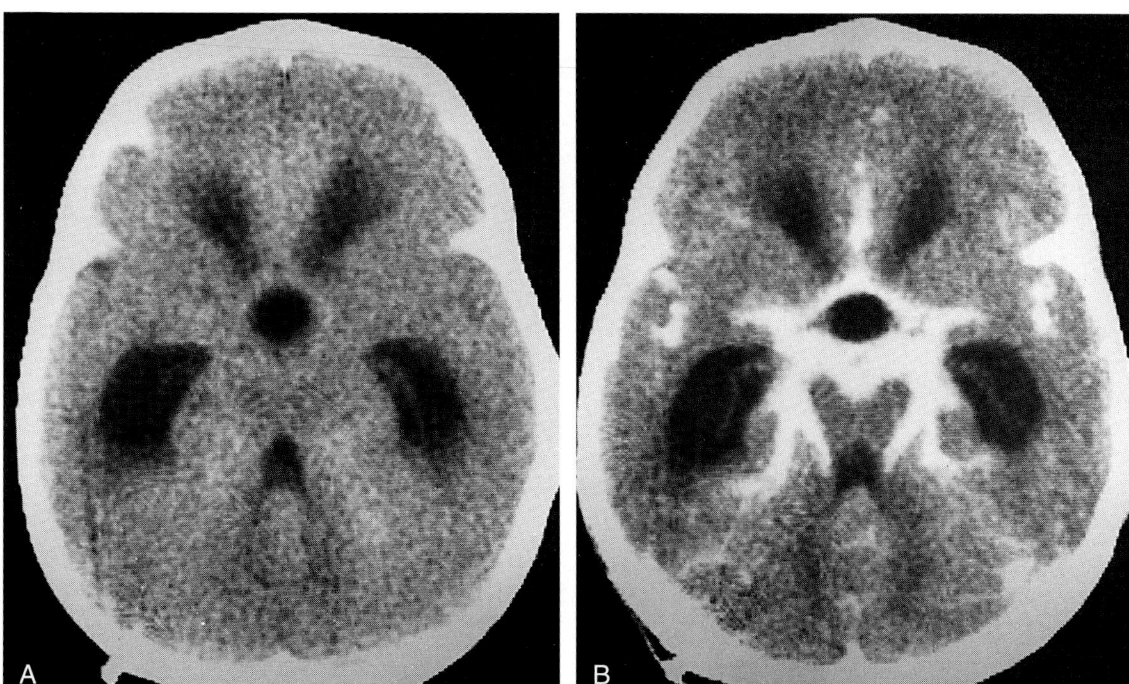

Figure 3–12. TB meningitis. CT **(A)** before and **(B)** after contrast shows hydrocephalus and intense enhancement in the basal cisterns and sylvian fissures.

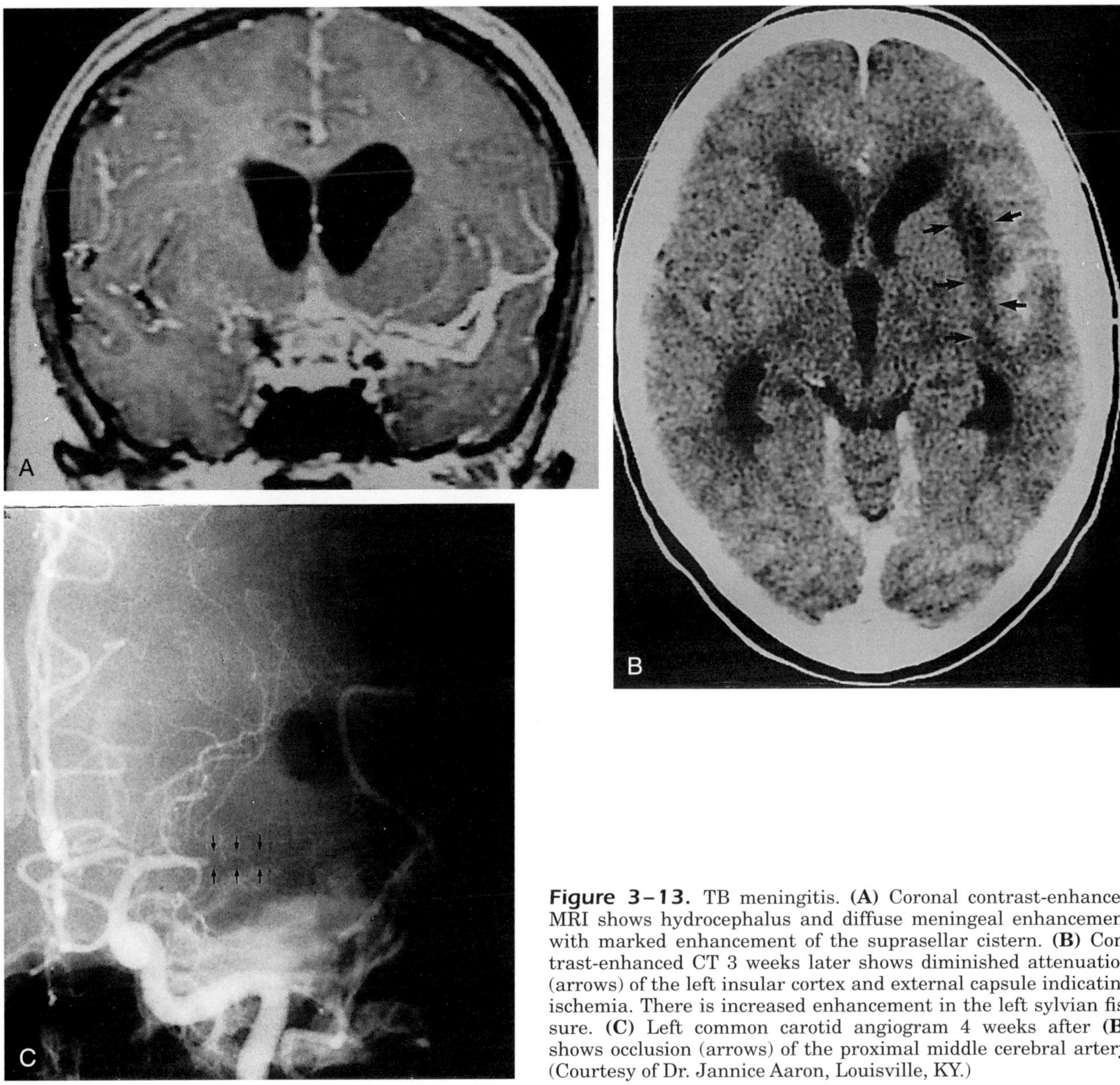

Figure 3–13. TB meningitis. **(A)** Coronal contrast-enhanced MRI shows hydrocephalus and diffuse meningeal enhancement with marked enhancement of the suprasellar cistern. **(B)** Contrast-enhanced CT 3 weeks later shows diminished attenuation (arrows) of the left insular cortex and external capsule indicating ischemia. There is increased enhancement in the left sylvian fissure. **(C)** Left common carotid angiogram 4 weeks after **(B)** shows occlusion (arrows) of the proximal middle cerebral artery. (Courtesy of Dr. Jannice Aaron, Louisville, KY.)

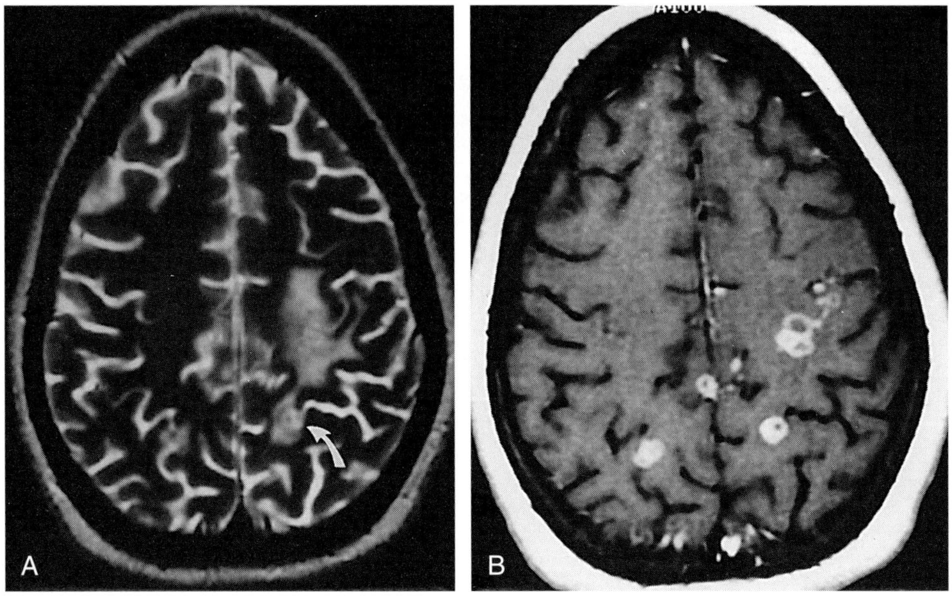

Figure 3–14. Tuberculomas in case of miliary tuberculosis. **(A)** Axial T2-weighted MRI shows vasogenic edema in the left convexity with a small target lesion (curved arrow). **(B)** Contrast-enhanced MRI shows multiple small solid and ring-enhancing granulomas.

Viral Infections

Herpes Simplex 1 Encephalitis

Herpes simplex virus type 1 is the most common sporadic cause of fatal encephalitis. It is believed to arise from retrograde spread along cranial nerves, especially the trigeminal. Herpes encephalitis has a distinct predilection for structures of the limbic system. Patients present with fever, declining mental status, and neurologic deficits. Neuroimaging, especially MRI, serves to localize the disease and suggest the diagnosis, which is usually confirmed by biopsy.

CT Findings. CT is usually normal the first few days. Subsequently, areas of low attenuation may develop in the temporal lobes, insular cortex, and subfrontal regions. Hemorrhage occurs infrequently but if present is relatively specific for this form of encephalitis. Calcifications may appear late in the course.

MRI Findings. T2-weighted images show hyperintensity in the temporal lobes, insular cortex, gyrus rectus, and sometimes cingulate gyrus. The basal ganglia are usually spared. Signal abnormalities often begin unilaterally with later and less severe contralateral spread. Leptomeningeal or gyriform enhancement may develop during the course of the illness. Other manifestations may include enhancement of the trigeminal nerve (neuritis) and involvement of the pons (rhombencephalitis).

Differential Diagnosis

The clinical presentation and laboratory findings are most helpful in excluding other etiologies. Similar imaging findings may be seen with temporal lobe astrocytoma; however, this would not tend to spare the basal ganglia. The differential diagnosis would also include progressive multifocal leukoencephalopathy (PML) (which usually spares gray matter) and other viral encephalitides. (See Table 3–4.)

TABLE 3–4 | Common Forms of Encephalitis

	Herpes Encephalitis	Herpes Encephalitis (Infants)	Progressive Multifocal Leukoencephalopathy	HIV Encephalitis	Acute Disseminated Encephalomyelitis
Organism	Herpes simplex 1	Herpes simplex 2	Papovavirus	HIV	Immune mediated(?)
Clinical	Headaches, fever, and disorientation	Irritability, seizures and rash	Focal neurologic deficits in immunocompromised patients	Progressive dementia	Fever, headaches, and neurologic deficits following prodromal viral infection
Location	Temporal lobes Gyrus rectus Insular cortex	Diffuse cerebral involvement Open or closed cleft	Parietal and occipital white matter	Periventricular white matter, diffuse, and bilateral	Multifocal, supratentorial, and infratentorial
Gray matter involvement	Usual	Common, may become hyperdense on CT and hypointense on T2 MRI	Uncommon	Uncommon	Occasional
White matter involvement	Usual	Usual	Usual	Usual; atrophy is predominant finding	Usual
Contrast enhancement	Gyral enhancement in subacute stages	Meningeal enhancement in early course and minimal gyral enhancement in later stages	Rare	No	Present in about 25%
Calcifications	Occasional, late in course	Frequent, punctate, or gyral	No	No	No
Hemorrhage	Specific but uncommon	Rare	No	No	Present in fulminant cases

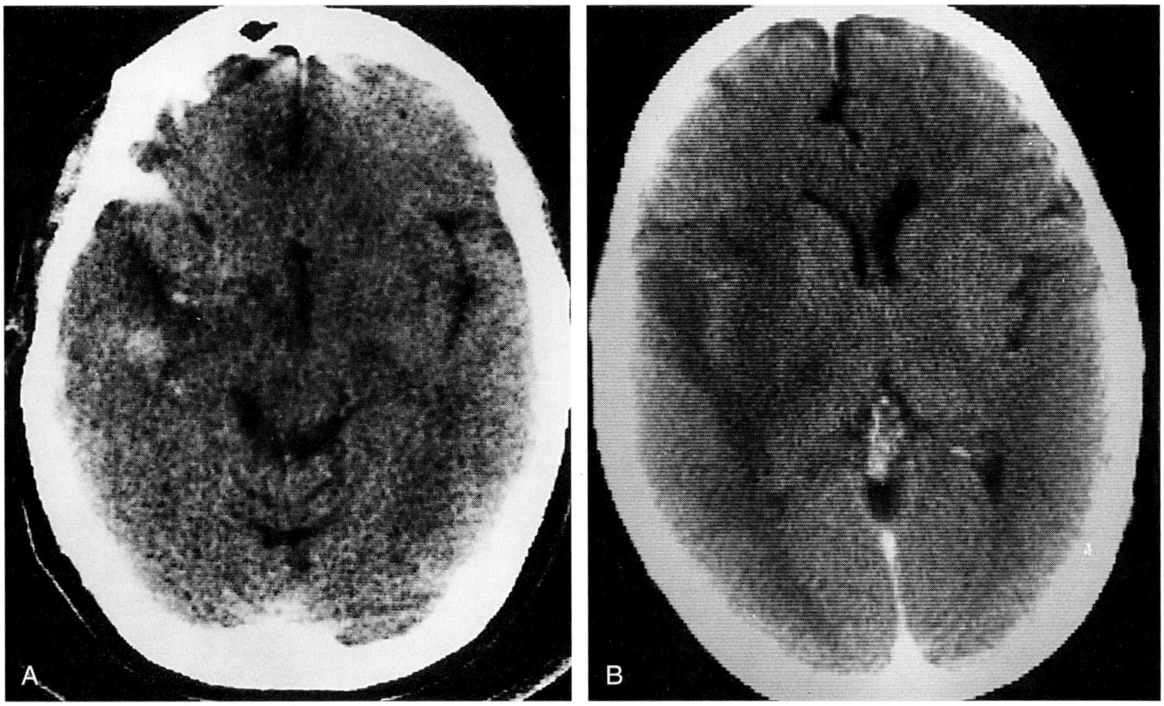

Figure 3–15. Herpes encephalitis. **(A)** CT 2 days after presentation shows diminished attenuation and patchy hemorrhage in the right temporal lobe. **(B)** CT 12 days later shows diminished attenuation in the right deep frontal white matter, insular cortex, and temporal lobe.

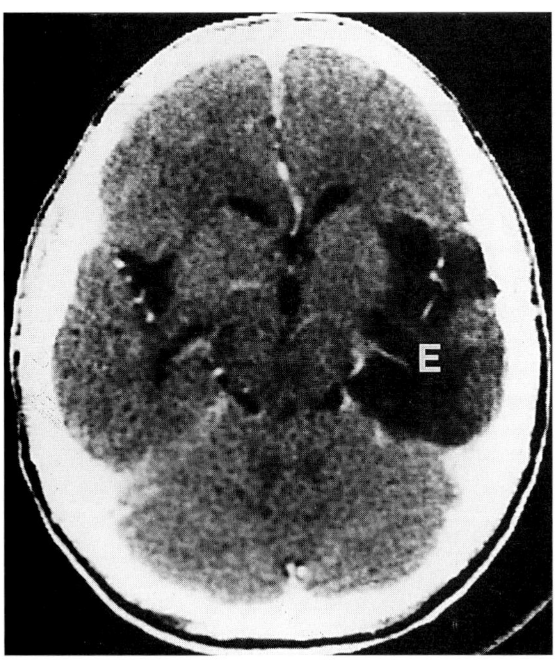

Figure 3–16. Herpes simplex encephalitis. CT shows encephalomalacia (E) of the left temporal lobe and insular cortex following recovery from herpes encephalitis.

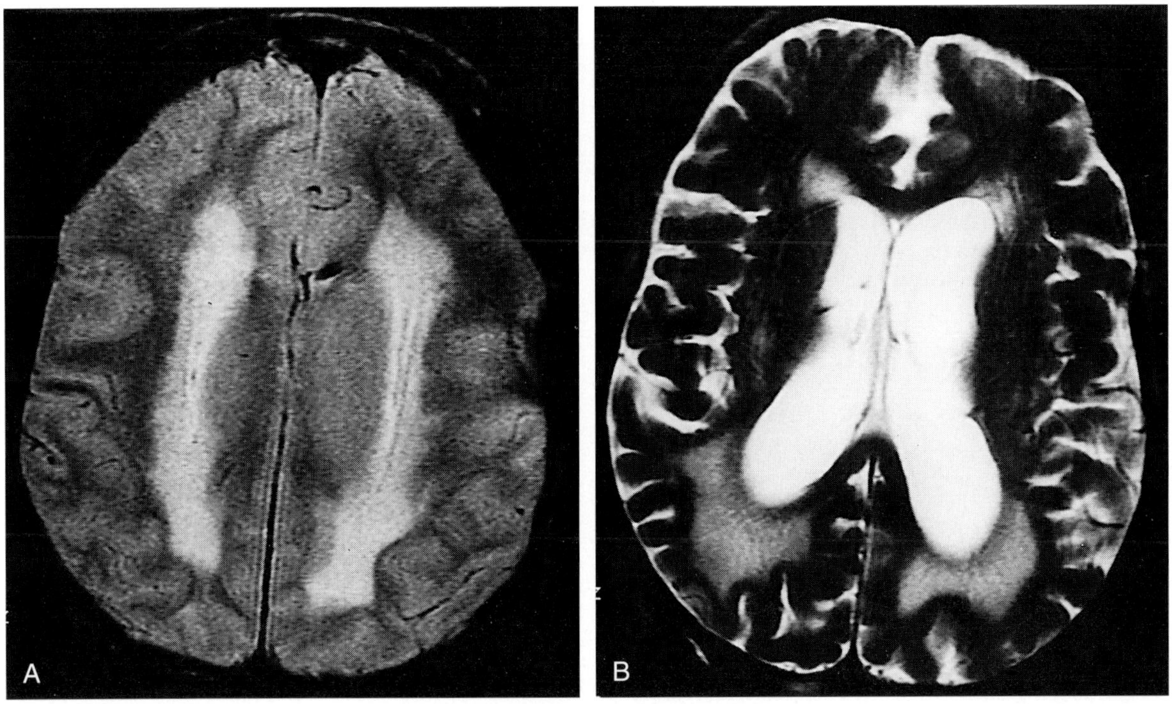

Figure 3–18. HIV encephalitis. Axial **(A)** PD-weighted and **(B)** T2-weighted MRI show extensive and symmetric hyperintensity in the periventricular white matter. The ventricles and sulci are enlarged, indicating atrophy.

Progressive Multifocal Leukoencephalopathy

PML is a papovavirus infection of oligodendrocytes, resulting in progressive demyelination within the CNS. Affected individuals exhibit progressive cognitive decline accompanied by motor and speech deficits, leading to death within 9 months of onset. Most patients are immunocompromised, with AIDS now the most common predisposing condition.

CT Findings. CT shows multiple areas of low attenuation in the white matter accentuating the gray-white junction. Mass effect and contrast enhancement are rare.

MRI Findings. T2-weighted MRI typically reveals multiple focal, well-defined areas of hyperintensity anywhere white matter is present with a propensity for subcortical white matter. Nearby gray matter is involved in up to 50%. Asymmetry between the hemispheres is typical. The early lesions are round or oval, becoming confluent with disease progression. Absence of mass effect helps to distinguish PML from tumor. Faint peripheral enhancement occurs in less than 10%, and enhancement when present strongly suggests an alternative diagnosis such as lymphoma or toxoplasmosis.

Differential Diagnosis

As most cases of PML now occur in AIDS patients, the primary differential consideration is HIV encephalitis. PML usually shows more pronounced signal abnormalities, especially on T1-weighted images, and has a greater propensity for subcortical white matter.

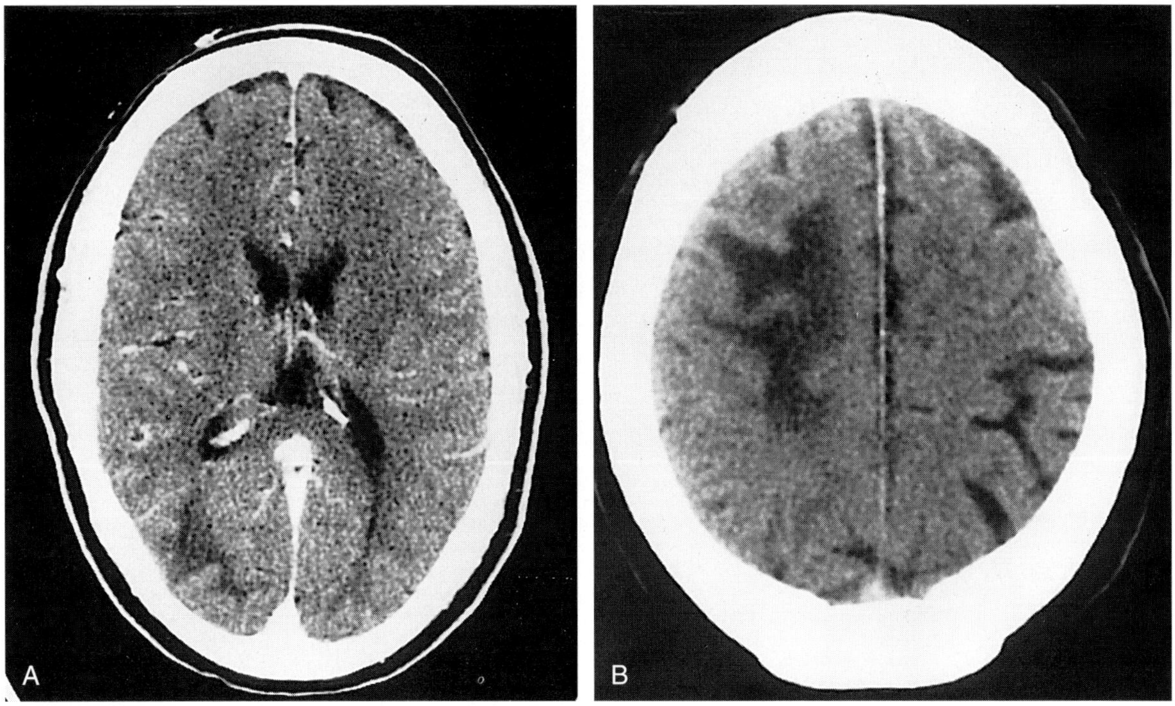

Figure 3–19. Progressive multifocal leukoencephalopathy. **(A,B)** Contrast-enhanced CT shows areas of diminished attenuation mostly within white matter without enhancement or mass effect.

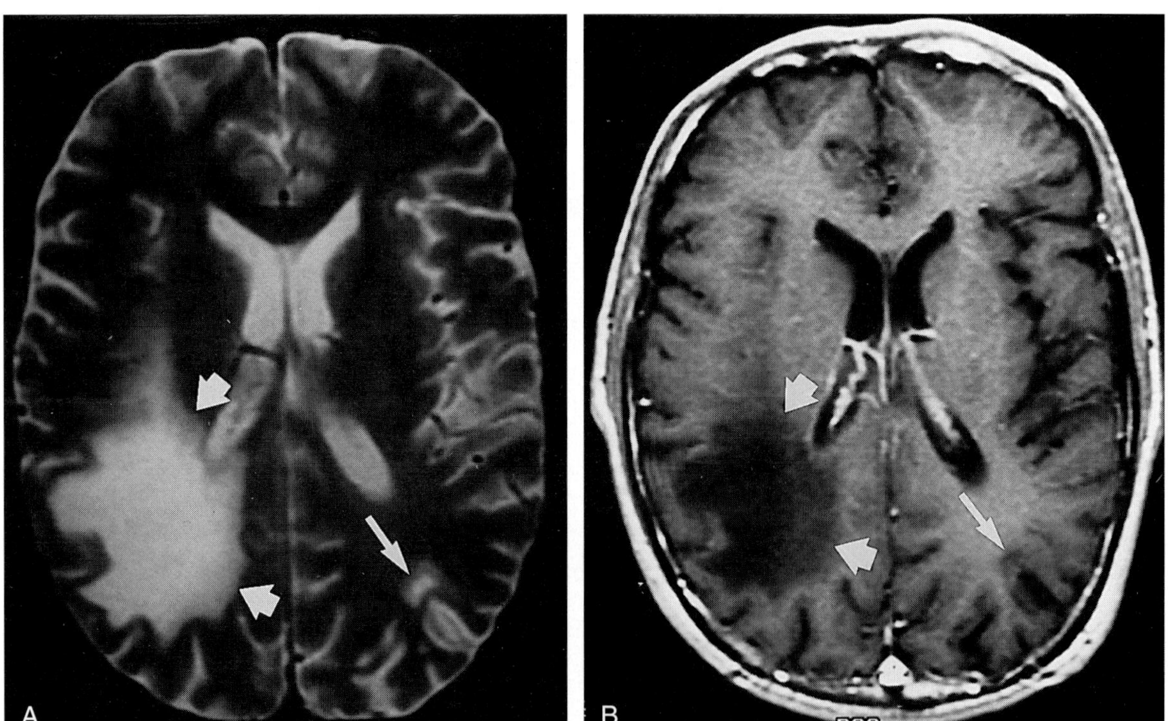

Figure 3–20. Progressive multifocal leukoencephalopathy. **(A)** Axial T2-weighted MRI shows bilateral and asymmetric hyperintensity (arrows) concentrated in the subcortical white matter. There was no mass effect. **(B)** Contrast-enhanced MRI shows no enhancement.

Creutzfeldt-Jakob Disease

Creutzfeldt-Jakob disease is a condition of rapidly progressive dementia, upper motor neuron dysfunction, and myoclonic seizures leading to death within 2 years. Most cases are sporadic without identified risk factors, and patients present between ages 40 and 80 years. It is thought to be caused by a viruslike particle called a prion. Pathology reveals marked neuronal loss and gliosis with spongiform degeneration of the neuropil.

CT Findings. CT is usually normal at presentation. Rapidly progressive atrophy develops over a period of months. No attenuation abnormality or enhancement has been observed.

MRI Findings. No mass or enhancement is observed. Initially, MRI may reveal atrophy or areas of hyperintensity on T2-weighted images. Gray matter is preferentially involved, and signal abnormalities have been seen in the thalamus, basal ganglia, and cerebral gyri. Progressive atrophy ensues, becoming severe within 2 years of presentation.

Differential Diagnosis

Because of the clinical presentation and paucity of imaging findings, the differential diagnosis includes other dementing diseases of the CNS, which are discussed in Chapter 5. The EEG is most specific, but a definitive diagnosis requires biopsy.

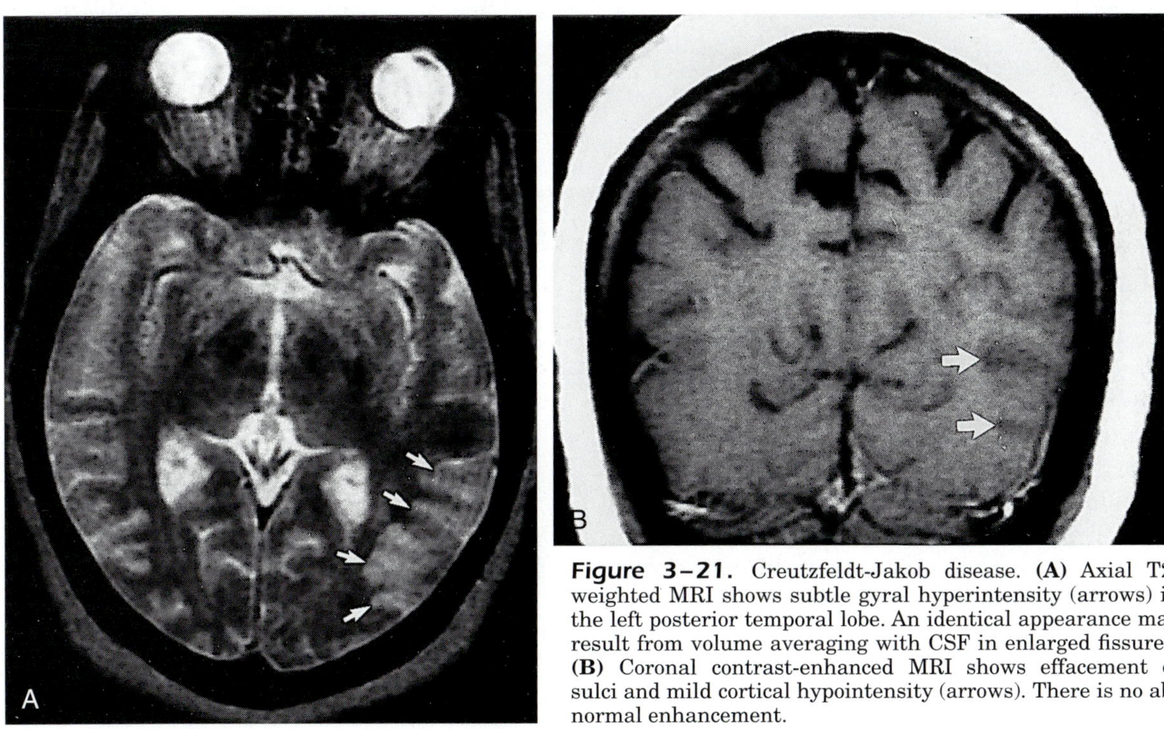

Figure 3–21. Creutzfeldt-Jakob disease. **(A)** Axial T2-weighted MRI shows subtle gyral hyperintensity (arrows) in the left posterior temporal lobe. An identical appearance may result from volume averaging with CSF in enlarged fissures. **(B)** Coronal contrast-enhanced MRI shows effacement of sulci and mild cortical hypointensity (arrows). There is no abnormal enhancement.

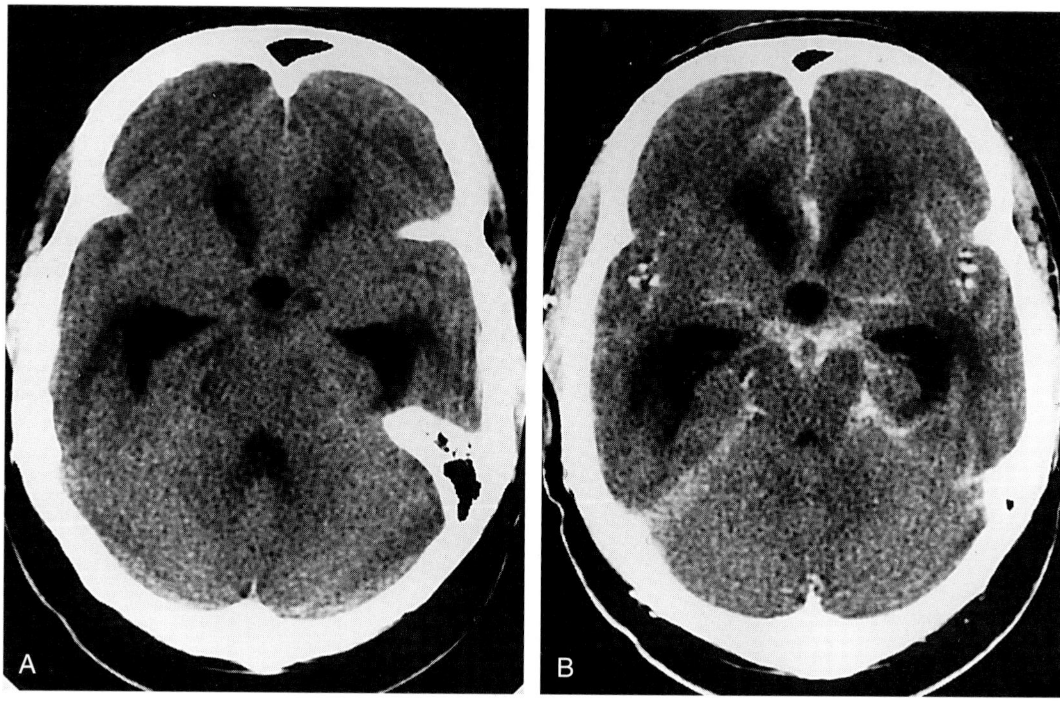

Figure 3–22. Cryptococcal meningitis (HIV-negative patient). CT **(A)** before and **(B)** after contrast shows hydrocephalus and moderate meningeal enhancement, especially in the interpeduncular cistern.

Fungal/Parasitic Infections

Cryptococcosis

Cryptococcus neoformans is the third most common CNS pathogen to infect the CNS in AIDS patients, after the HIV virus and toxoplasma. It is also a common pathogen in other immunocompromised states and is not altogether rare in normal hosts. An indolent meningitis is the usual manifestation; however, the organism may proliferate within the Virchow-Robin spaces forming gelatinous pseudocysts or within the brain parenchyma forming cryptococcomas.

CT Findings. CT is most often normal with uncomplicated meningitis. CNS cryptococcosis may present as enhancing granulomas, ring-enhancing abscesses, or focal or diffuse meningeal enhancement. Small, nonenhancing hypodense lesions in or around the basal ganglia represent cryptococcomas in the perivascular spaces (gelatinous pseudocysts). Hydrocephalus may be present.

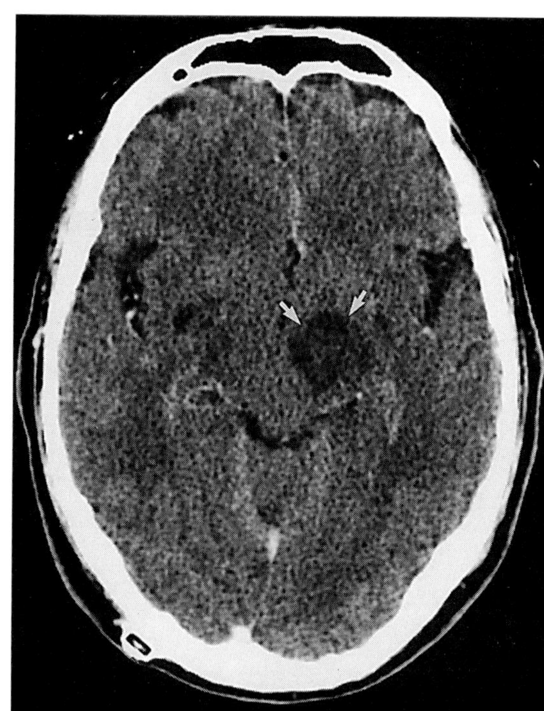

Figure 3–23. Cryptococcal meningitis (AIDS related). Contrast-enhanced CT shows a typical nonenhancing hypodensity (arrows) in the left basal ganglia consistent with gelatinous pseudocysts.

MRI Findings. Cryptococcal infection of the CNS occurs primarily as meningitis with secondary parenchymal involvement via the Virchow-Robin spaces. MRI may reveal the following alone or in any combination:

- Meningeal enhancement. In non-AIDS patients, meningeal enhancement is the most common finding. It has been observed in AIDS patients that cryptococcus elicits little inflammatory response, and as a result contrast enhancement is infrequent.
- Parenchymal cryptococcoma. MRI shows a mass nearly isointense to brain on T1- and T2-weighted images with vasogenic edema and solid or ring enhancement. Enhancement may be absent in AIDS patients.
- Gelatinous pseudocysts. MRI shows hyperintense foci in the basal ganglia, thalamus, or midbrain on T2-weighted images that are isointense or slightly hypointense on T1-weighted images and do not enhance. This is the most common finding in patients with AIDS.
- Miliary infection. Miliary cortical and/or leptomeningeal-enhancing nodules representing hematogenous dissemination.

Differential Diagnosis

In AIDS patients, the major differential considerations are toxoplasmosis and lymphoma, both of which enhance fairly consistently. In non-AIDS patients, the appearance may resemble other forms of meningitis or sarcoid. The diagnosis is made by CSF analysis, especially cryptococcal antigen titers.

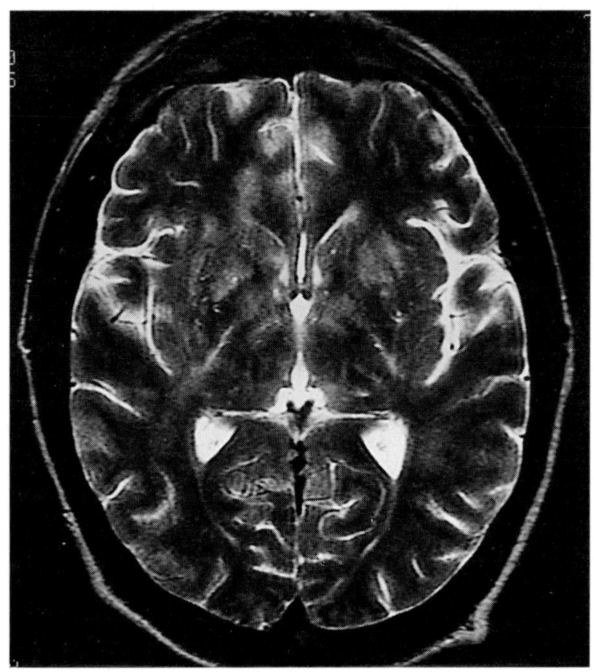

Figure 3–24. Cryptococcal meningitis (AIDS related). Axial T2-weighted MRI shows typical bilateral hyperintensities in the basal ganglia consistent with gelatinous pseudocysts.

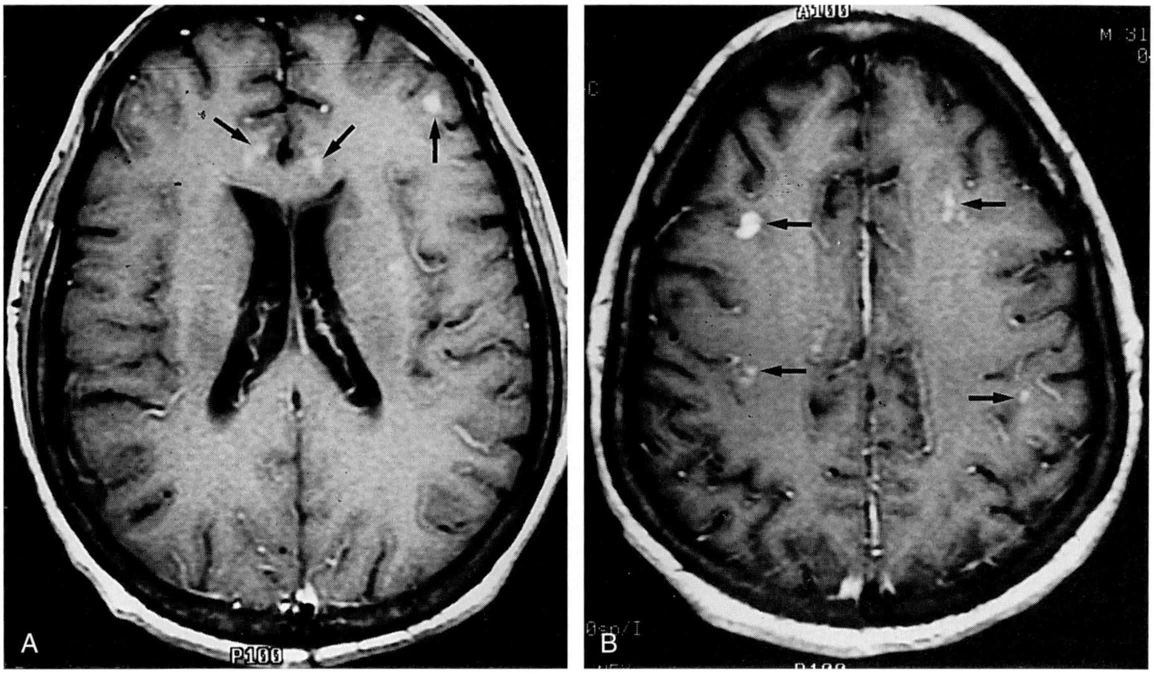

Figure 3–25. Cryptococcomas (AIDS related). Axial contrast-enhanced MRI **(A)** and **(B)** above lateral ventricles shows multiple small solidly enhancing lesions (arrows). (Courtesy of Dr. Pamela Van Tassel, Charleston, SC.)

Toxoplasmosis

Infection by *Toxoplasma gondii* is both the leading CNS infection and the number one cause of cerebral mass lesions in AIDS patients. Fever, headache, neurologic deficits, and seizures are the usual presenting complaints.

CT Findings. CT shows multiple low attenuation lesions in the basal ganglia and corticomedullary junction with mild vasogenic edema and mass effect. Either ring or nodular enhancement may occur. Residual findings of treated disease include atrophy, encephalomalacia, and punctate calcifications.

MRI Findings. MRI shows multiple masses that are hypointense on T1-weighted images and hypointense to hyperintense on T2-weighted images with surrounding edema. The basal ganglia and gray-white junction are favored locations. Thin rim enhancement is typical but not invariable.

Differential Diagnosis

Most cases occur as enhancing mass lesions in AIDS patients. The main differential diagnostic consideration is primary lymphoma. Factors favoring toxoplasmosis include multiplicity of lesions, thin rim enhancement, and corticomedullary and basal ganglia involvement. Factors favoring lymphoma include a solitary lesion, periventricular location, subependymal spread, hyperdensity on unenhanced CT, thick ring enhancement, and corpus callosum involvement. Sometimes a trial course of antitoxoplasma therapy is initiated; if toxoplasmosis is the correct diagnosis, improvement should be seen in 2 to 4 weeks. Definitive diagnosis currently requires biopsy.

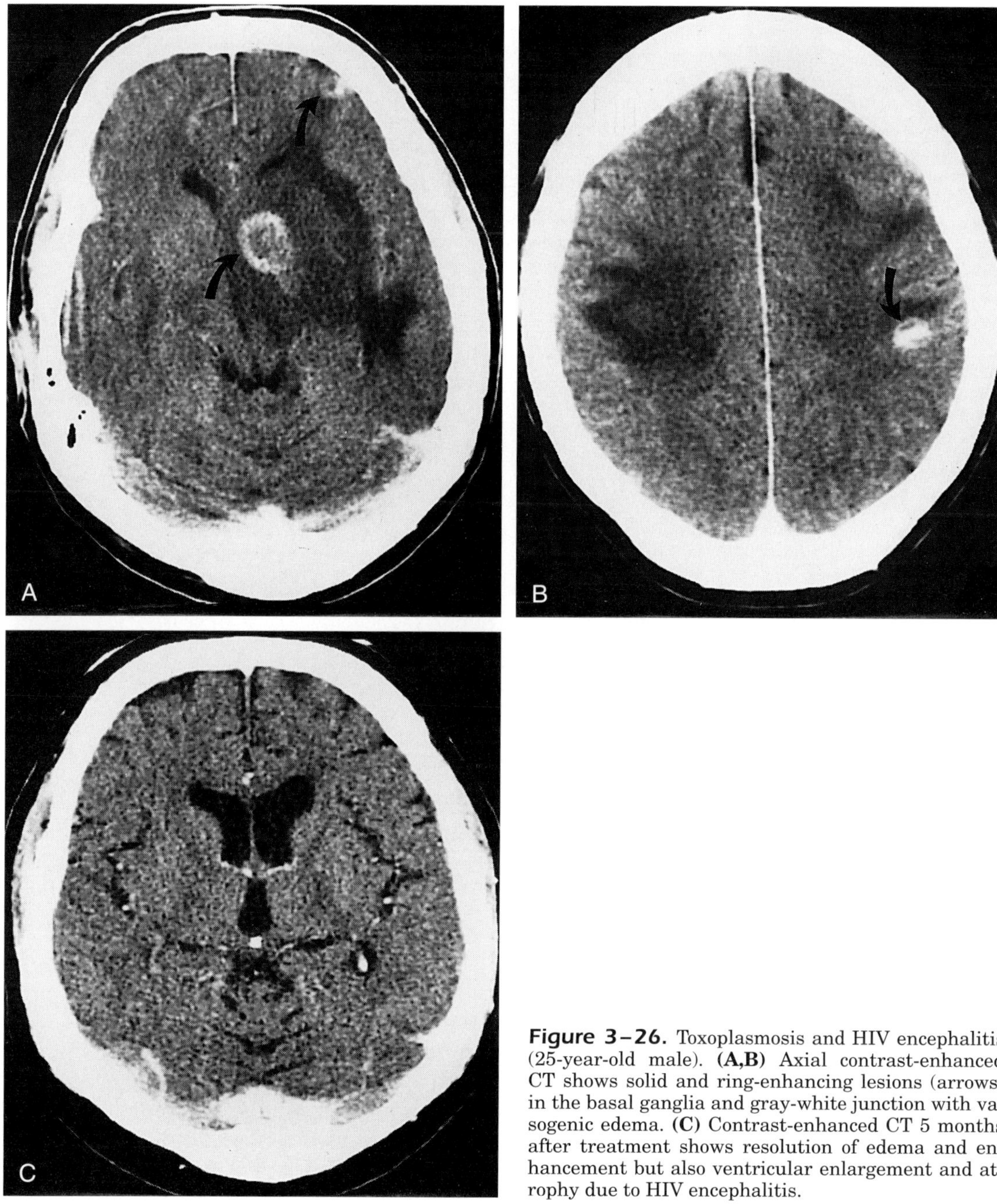

Figure 3–26. Toxoplasmosis and HIV encephalitis (25-year-old male). **(A,B)** Axial contrast-enhanced CT shows solid and ring-enhancing lesions (arrows) in the basal ganglia and gray-white junction with vasogenic edema. **(C)** Contrast-enhanced CT 5 months after treatment shows resolution of edema and enhancement but also ventricular enlargement and atrophy due to HIV encephalitis.

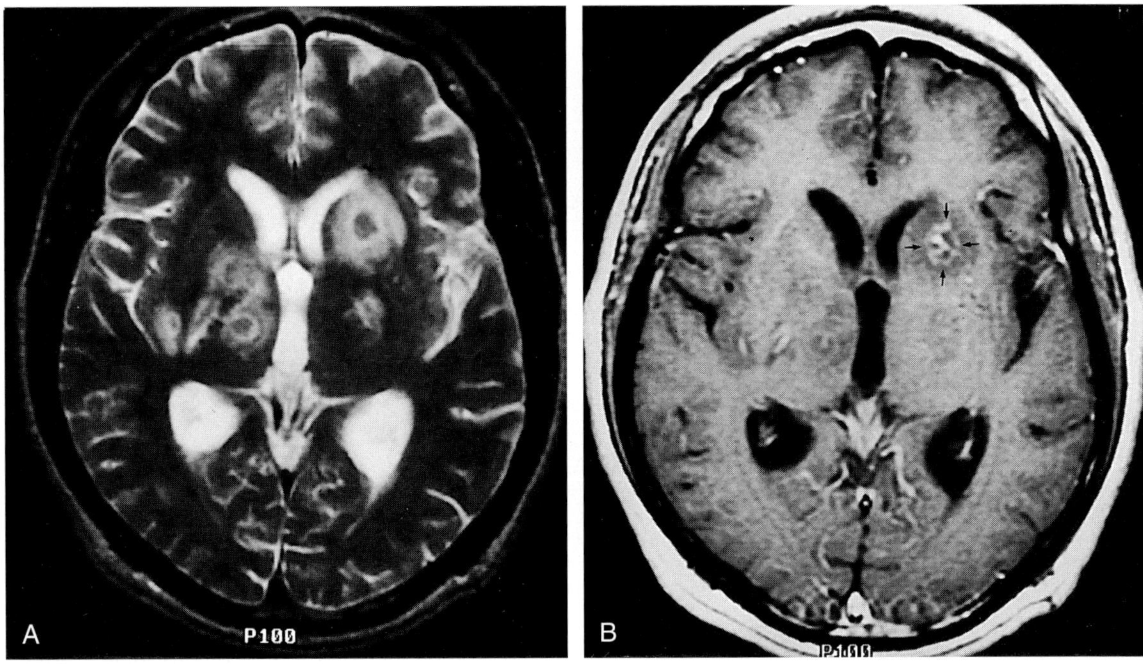

Figure 3–27. Toxoplasmosis. **(A)** Axial T2-weighted MRI shows multiple hypointense lesions in the basal ganglia with surrounding vasogenic edema. **(B)** Contrast-enhanced MRI shows both ring and central enhancement in the left caudate lesion (arrows) but minimal enhancement of the other lesions. (Courtesy of Dr. Pamela Van Tassel, Charleston, SC.)

Cysticercosis

Neurocysticercosis is an infestation of the CNS by the larvae of *Taenia solium*, the pork tapeworm. Although rare in the United States, it is one of the most common causes of cerebral mass lesions in endemic areas of Mexico, Central and South America, Africa, and East Asia. Most cases in the United States are diagnosed in immigrants from those regions. Following ingestion of the eggs, the larvae enter the bloodstream and disseminate throughout the body. The CNS is involved in 60–90% of infections, leading to seizures, increased intracranial pressure, and neurologic deficits.

CT and MRI Findings. The neuroimaging findings are related to the stage of infection. Various stages of infection may be and often are present in the same patient.

Vesicular Stage. In the vesicular stage, there is a viable larva within a small cyst; there is little or no inflammatory response. This stage is manifested by one or more cysts 0.1 to 1.0 cm in diameter at the gray-white junction, within the ventricles, or in the cisterns. These cysts exhibit CSF characteristics on CT and MRI and do not enhance. A small mural nodule (the scolex) may be visible. A unique and pathognomonic feature of the intraventricular cysts is that they may migrate or shift with patient position.

Colloidal Stage. Over several years, the larva dies, the cyst contents become more proteinaceous, and an inflammatory response develops. In the colloidal stage, the cysts become unequal to CSF (increased attenuation on CT and greater intensity on MRI) and surrounded by vasogenic edema. Ringlike enhancement develops, and the scolex may be visible as a small mural nodule. As in the previous stage, lesions may be present in parenchyma, cisterns, and ventricles.

Granular Nodular Stage. In this stage, the cyst has begun to involute. The scolex is no longer visible. Solid nodular enhancement is seen on both CT and MRI, possibly with a central calcification hyperdense on CT (target sign).

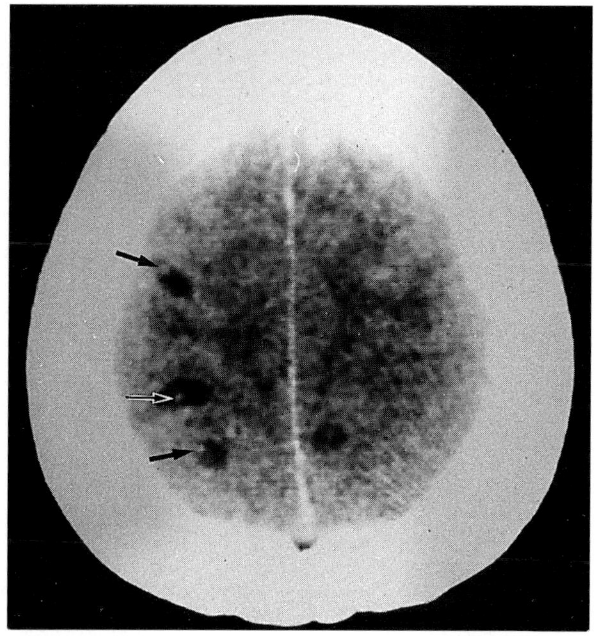

Figure 3–28. Cysticercosis (vesicular stage). CT shows multiple cysts isodense with CSF and without enhancement. Small scoleces (arrows) are visible in several cysts. (Courtesy of Dr. Alexia Abuhid, Belo Horizonte, Brazil.)

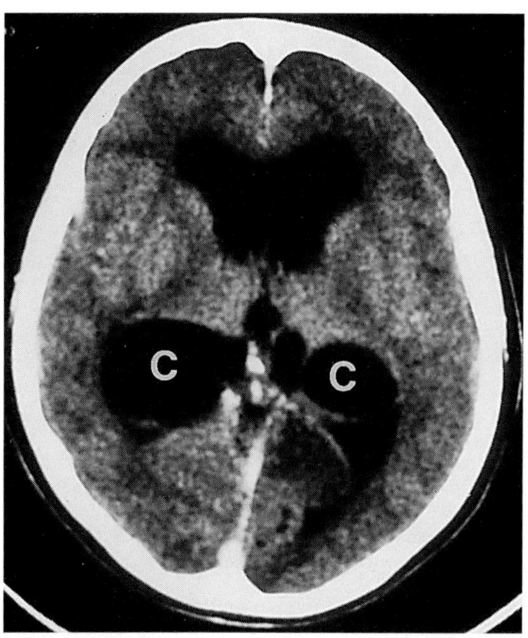

Figure 3–29. Cysticercosis (intraventricular cysts). Axial CT through the lateral ventricles shows hydrocephalus and bilateral intraventricular cysts (C). (Courtesy of Dr. Alexia Abuhid, Belo Horizonte, Brazil.)

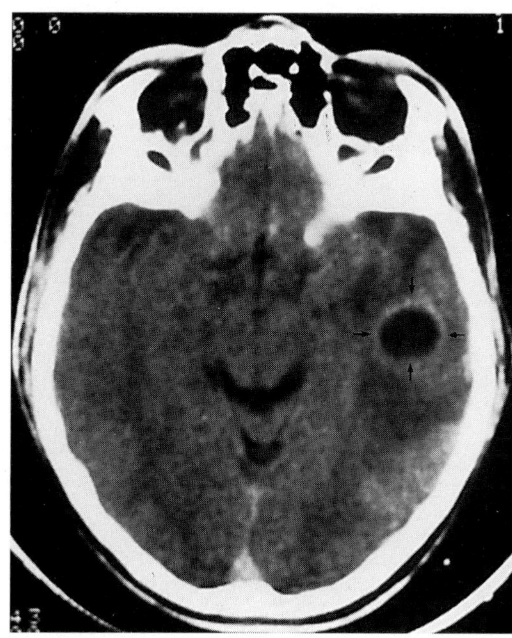

Figure 3–30. Cysticercosis (colloidal stage). Contrast-enhanced CT shows a left temporal lobe cyst with moderate ring enhancement (arrows) and vasogenic edema. (Courtesy of Dr. Alexia Abuhid, Belo Horizonte, Brazil.)

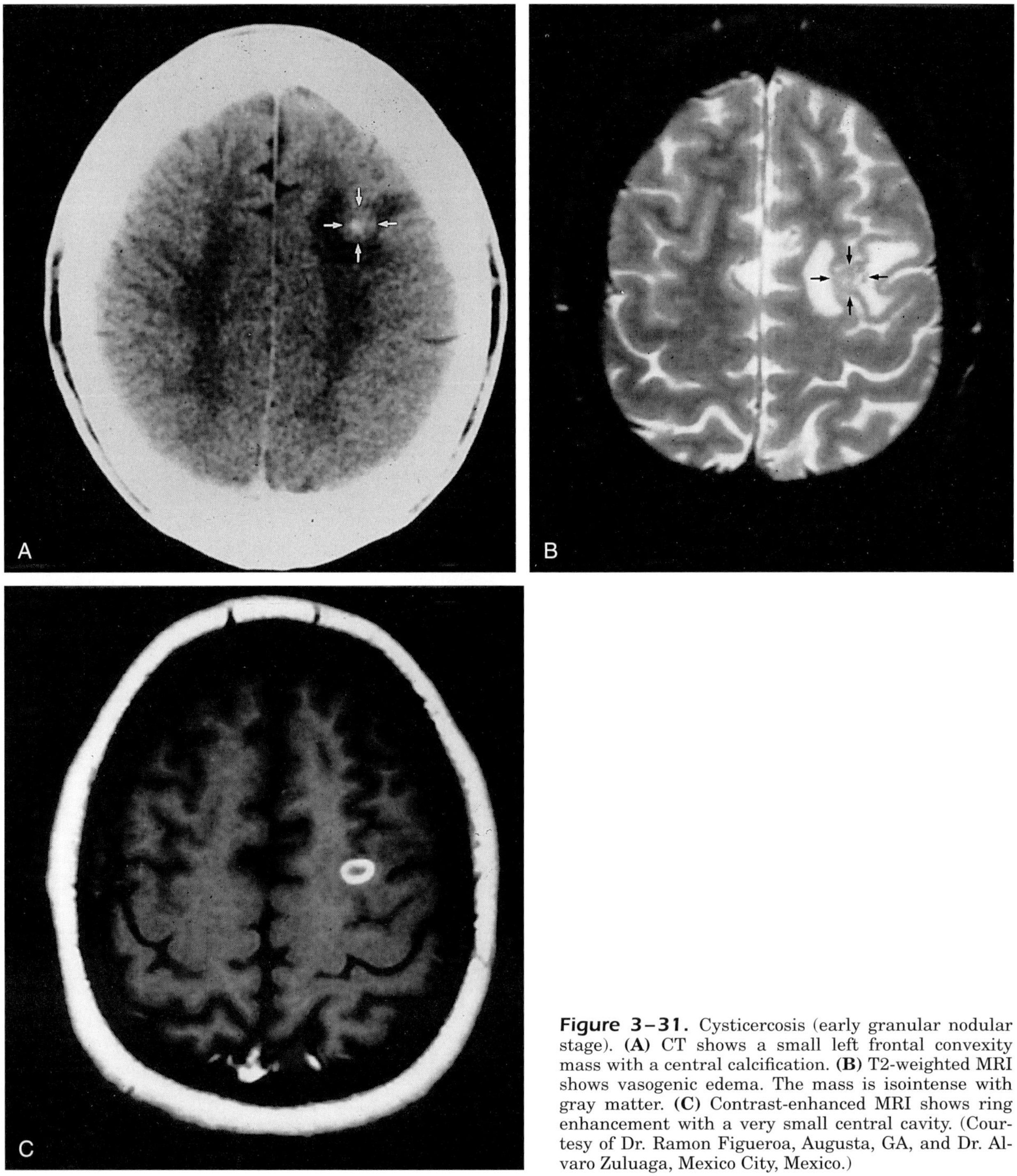

Figure 3–31. Cysticercosis (early granular nodular stage). **(A)** CT shows a small left frontal convexity mass with a central calcification. **(B)** T2-weighted MRI shows vasogenic edema. The mass is isointense with gray matter. **(C)** Contrast-enhanced MRI shows ring enhancement with a very small central cavity. (Courtesy of Dr. Ramon Figueroa, Augusta, GA, and Dr. Alvaro Zuluaga, Mexico City, Mexico.)

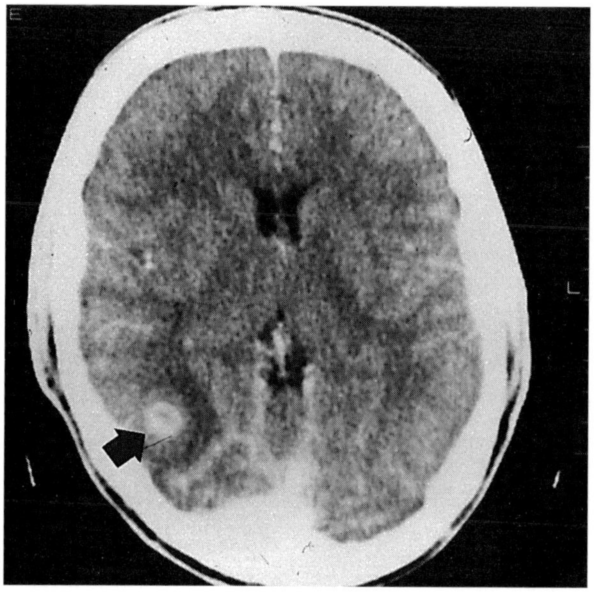

Figure 3–32. Cysticercosis (granular nodular stage). Contrast-enhanced CT shows a small, solidly enhancing right temporal lesion (arrow) with mild edema. (Courtesy of Dr. Alexia Abuhid, Belo Horizonte, Brazil.)

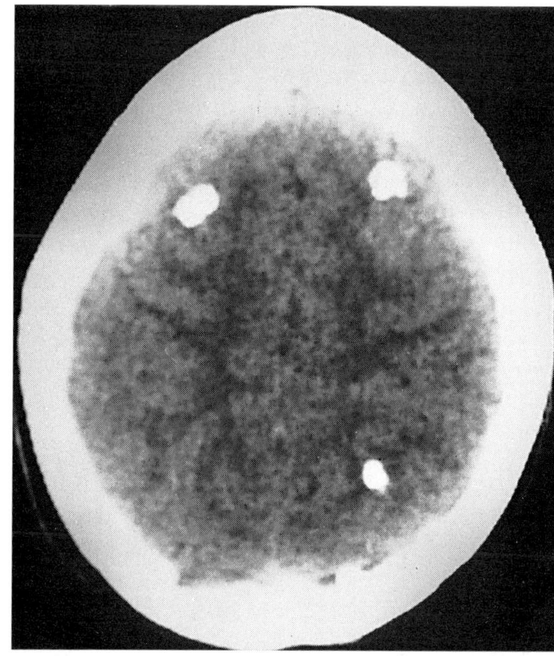

Figure 3–33. Cysticercosis (nodular calcified stage). CT shows multiple small, densely calcified masses.

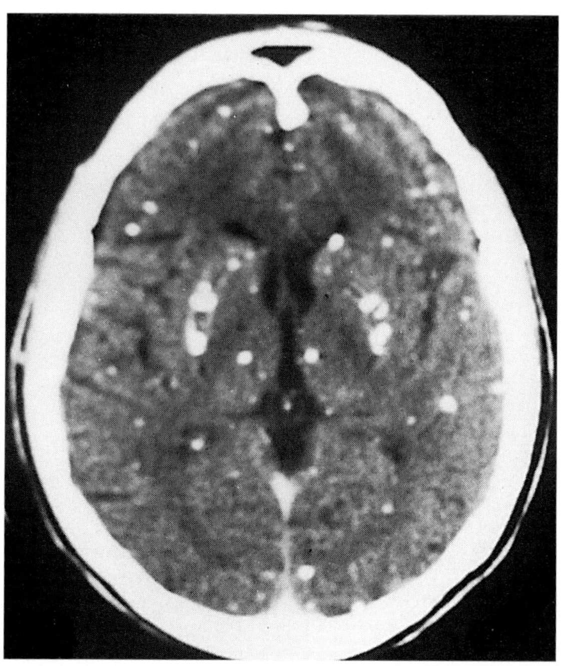

Figure 3–34. Cysticercosis (nodular calcified stage). CT shows multiple small, densely calcified masses. (Courtesy of Dr. Alexia Abuhid, Belo Horizonte, Brazil.)

Nodular Calcified Stage. This is the end stage of the inflammatory response. One or more coarse, 2 to 6-mm calcific nodules remain and are best seen on CT.

Other Findings. Arachnoiditis is common with meningeal enhancement on MRI. Hydrocephalus is common due to intraventricular cysts, periaqueductal lesions, or arachnoid adhesions. Racemose cysts are larger, lack scoleces, and may spread extensively through the basal cisterns or sylvian fissure.

Differential Diagnosis

An exhaustive differential diagnosis would be quite lengthy because of the varied appearance according to stage. Since multiple lesions are nearly always present, see Table 4–2. This gives the differential diagnosis of multiple cerebral mass lesions. Meningeal cysticercosis may resemble other forms of meningitis, whereas racemose cysts may resemble arachnoid cysts or epidermoid. Intraventricular cysticercosis must be differentiated from epidermoid and neuroepithelial cysts.

Noninfectious Processes

Sarcoidosis

Sarcoidosis is a multisystem disease characterized by noncaseating granulomas of idiopathic origin. It is most common in black females ages 20 to 40 years. The lungs, lymph nodes, skin, and orbits are most commonly affected, and the CNS is involved in only 5%. CNS sarcoidosis is primarily a disease of the leptomeninges, affecting in particular the basal cisterns, optic chiasm, hypothalamus, and infundibulum. Parenchymal involvement is less common but may occur anywhere within the brain, with a propensity for periventricular white matter. CNS sarcoidosis responds well to corticosteroids.

CT Findings. Hydrocephalus is perhaps the most common finding. Parenchymal granulomas appear as slightly hyperdense masses with surrounding edema and homogeneous contrast enhancement. Meningeal disease exhibits focal or diffuse contrast enhancement, especially in the basal cisterns.

MRI Findings. T1-weighted images may show thickening of the dura, infundibulum, or chiasm. On T2-weighted images, there may be hyperintensities in the hypothalamus, pons, and subcortical or periventricular white matter. Contrast-enhanced MRI typically shows arachnoid or pial thickening and enhancement with solid enhancement of parenchymal lesions. Mass effect may be significant. Hydrocephalus is often present, usually due to fourth ventricular obstruction. Spinal involvement is infrequent, with intramedullary and meningeal disease about equal in incidence.

Differential Diagnosis

The parenchymal lesions may bear a striking resemblance to multiple sclerosis, whereas meningeal involvement may resemble infectious meningitis, meningeal metastases, or meningioma. (See Table 3–2.)

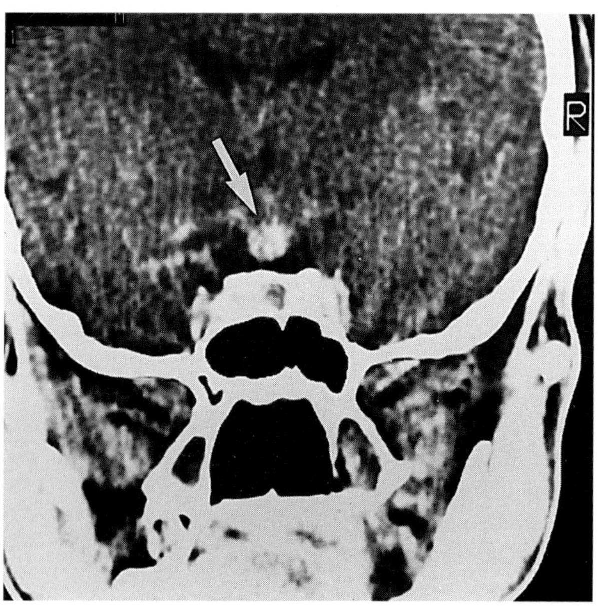

Figure 3–35. Sarcoidosis. Coronal contrast-enhanced CT shows enlargement and marked enhancement of the hypothalamus and pituitary infundibulum (arrow).

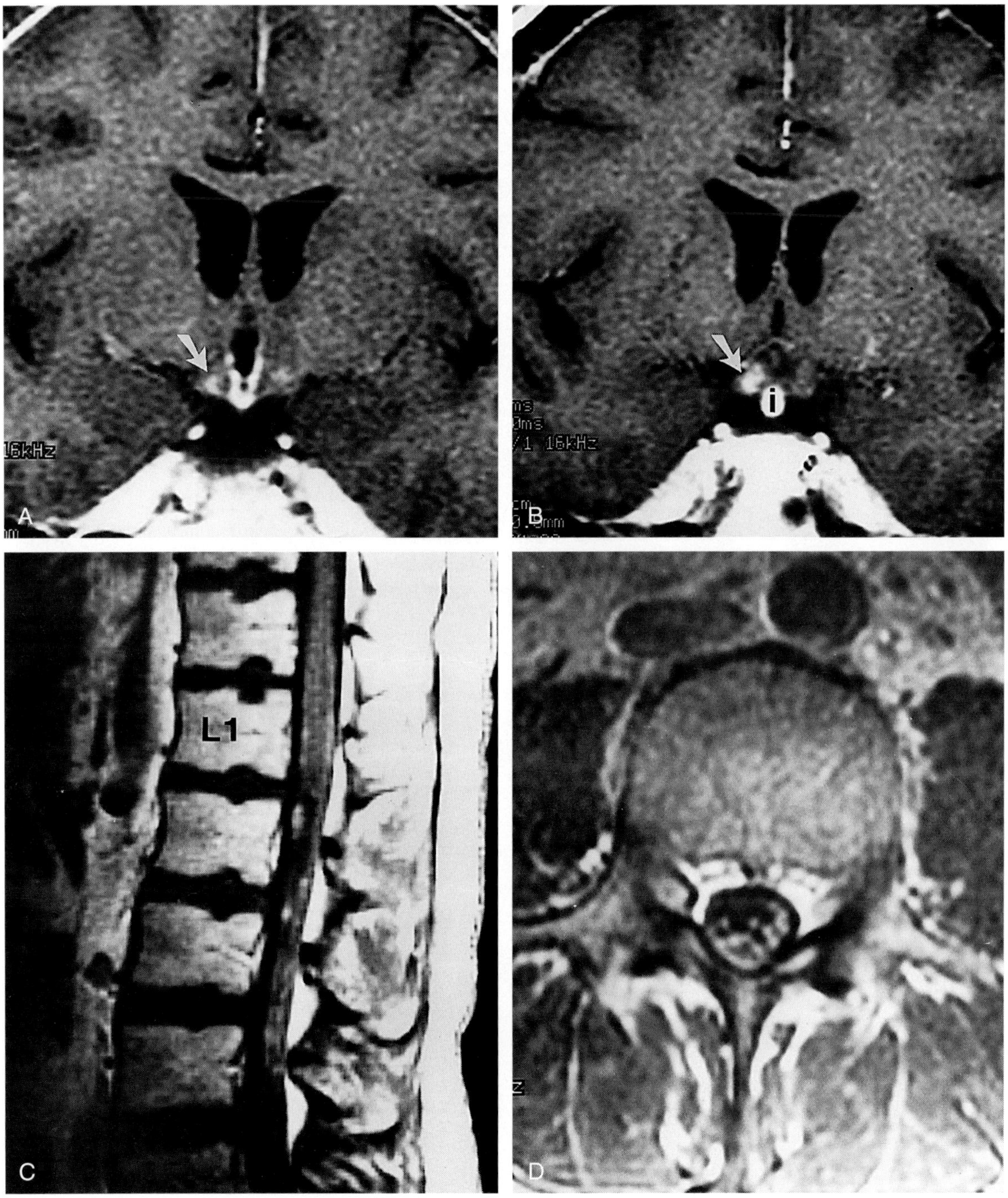

Figure 3–36. Sarcoidosis. **(A,B)** Coronal contrast-enhanced MRI shows enhancement of the right optic nerve (arrow), hypothalamus, infundibulum (i), and ependyma of the third ventricle. **(C)** Sagittal and **(D)** axial contrast-enhanced MRI of the upper lumbar spine shows nodular enhancement of multiple nerve roots.

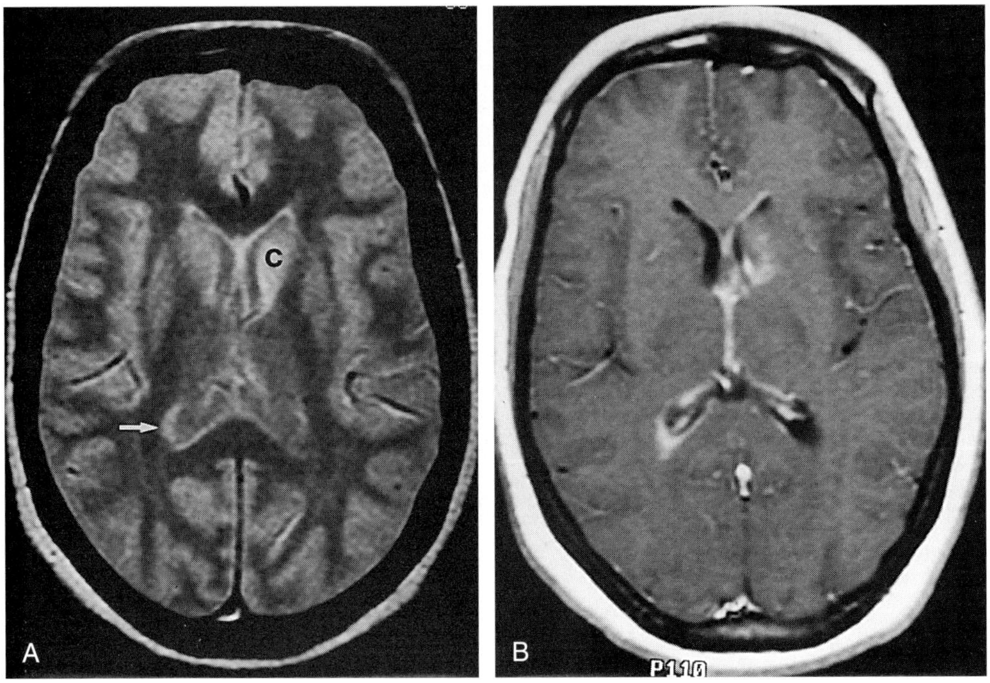

Figure 3–37. Sarcoidosis. **(A)** Axial PD-weighted MRI shows hyperintensity of the left caudate head (c) and mild periventricular hyperintensity (arrow) abutting the right trigone. **(B)** Post-contrast scan shows left caudate and right periventricular enhancement.

Congenital and Neonatal Infections

Herpes Simplex 2 Encephalitis

Neonatal herpes infection is acquired when a newborn infant is exposed to the herpes simplex virus type 2 during passage through the birth canal. Seizures are often the first clinical manifestation. Diffuse brain involvement is the rule, in contrast to the orbitotemporal and insular localization seen in older children and adults. Progressive parenchymal destruction may occur, leading to multicystic encephalomalacia.

CT Findings. The initial CT is usually normal, soon followed by the appearance of diffuse, patchy gray and white matter hypodensities. Increased gyral density and minimal meningeal enhancement subsequently appear, and possibly hemorrhagic infarction. CT in end-stage disease may show atrophy, multicystic encephalomalacia, and parenchymal calcifications.

MRI Findings. The initial MRI may reveal gray matter edema, causing a loss of gray-white contrast on both T1- and T2-weighted scans. Diffuse meningeal enhancement is observed after intravenous contrast. In the intermediate stage, marked hypointensity of the gray matter is seen corresponding to the gyral hyperdensity on CT. In the late stages, parenchymal destruction results in multicystic encephalomalacia.

Differential Diagnosis

Similarly devastating diseases in the newborn period include varicella-zoster encephalitis and fulminant meningitis.

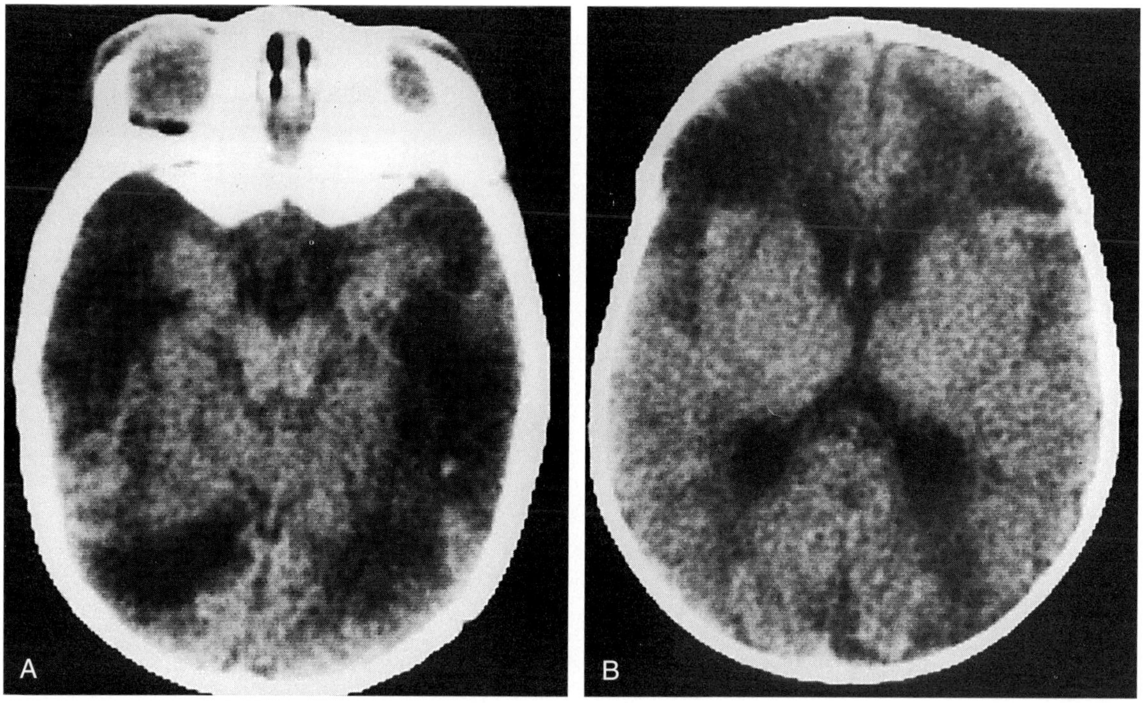

Figure 3–38. Neonatal herpes encephalitis (early) **(A,B)**. Noncontrast CT shows multiple areas of diminished attenuation affecting gray and white matter of both hemispheres.

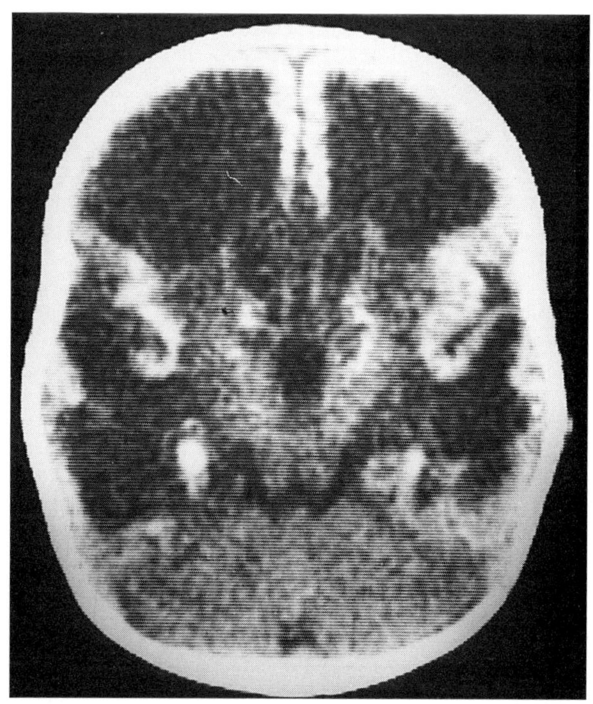

Figure 3–39. Neonatal herpes encephalitis (subacute). Axial CT shows increased gyral density with severely diminished attenuation of hemispheric white matter.

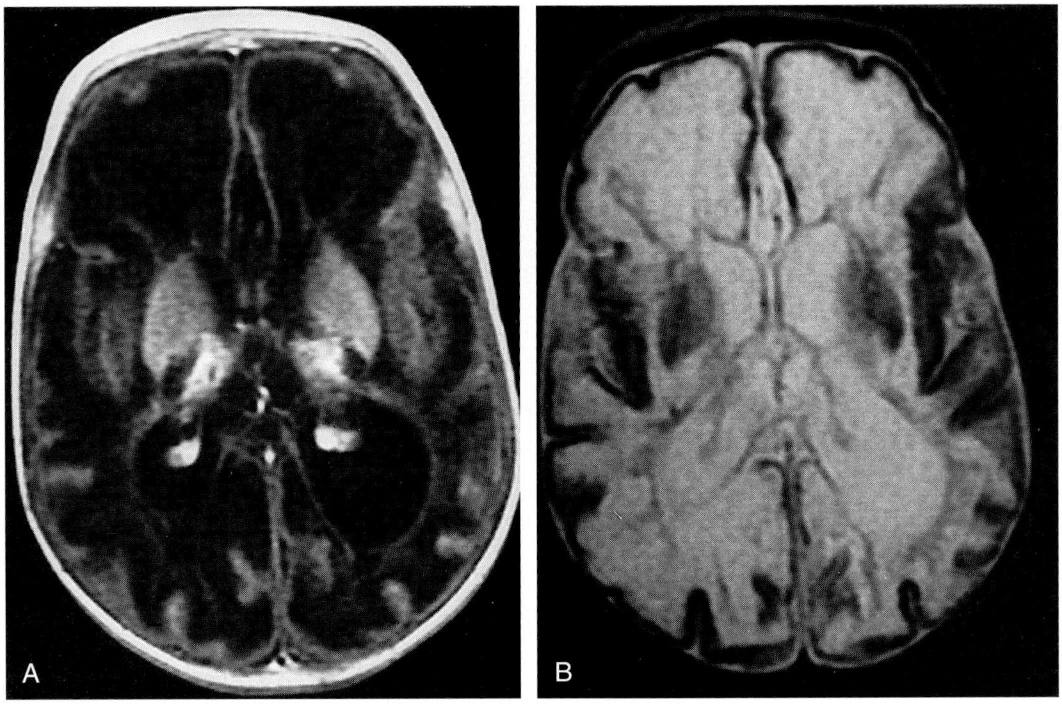

Figure 3–40. Neonatal herpes encephalitis (subacute). **(A)** Axial T1-weighted MRI shows ventricular enlargement, diffuse hypointensity of the white matter, and bilateral hemorrhage in the thalami. **(B)** T2-weighted MRI shows the characteristic marked hypointensity of the gray matter with marked hyperintensity of the white matter. (Courtesy of Dr. Pamela Van Tassel, Charleston, SC.)

Cytomegalovirus Encephalitis

Cytomegalovirus is a common virus with which most people are at some point infected. Prior to AIDS, it was the most common and serious fetal infection. Intrauterine transmission occurs when the mother is infected during pregnancy or when a latent infection is reactivated. Infected infants may manifest hepatosplenomegaly, jaundice, thrombocytopenia, deafness, and chorioretinitis.

CT Findings. CT shows parenchymal calcifications that are usually or mostly periventricular, but the distribution may overlap with that of toxoplasmosis. Destructive lesions (encephalomalacia, porencephaly, and hydranencephaly) are present in more severe cases. Other findings may include microcephaly, migration anomalies, cerebellar hypoplasia, and subependymal cysts in the occipital horns.

MRI Findings. MRI may be required to diagnose the subependymal cysts and migration anomalies but is much less sensitive for calcifications.

Differential Diagnosis

Toxoplasmosis is the major differential consideration. The definitive diagnosis is made by means of serology.

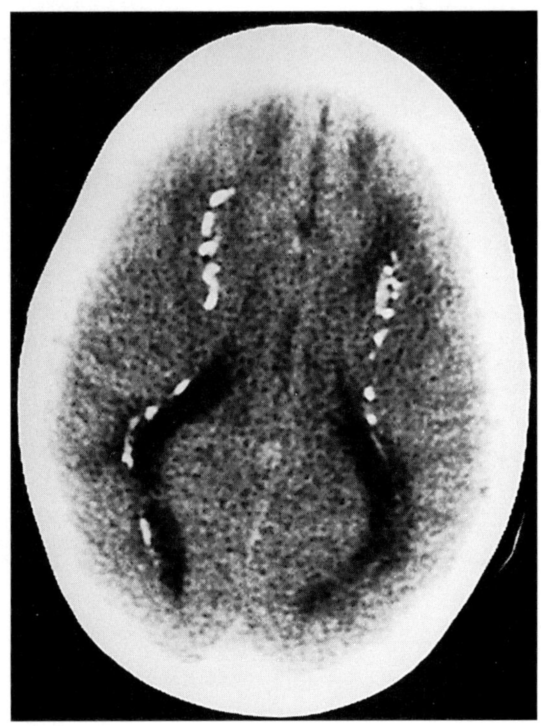

Figure 3–41. CMV encephalitis. Axial CT shows bilateral fine punctate calcifications, which are mostly periventricular.

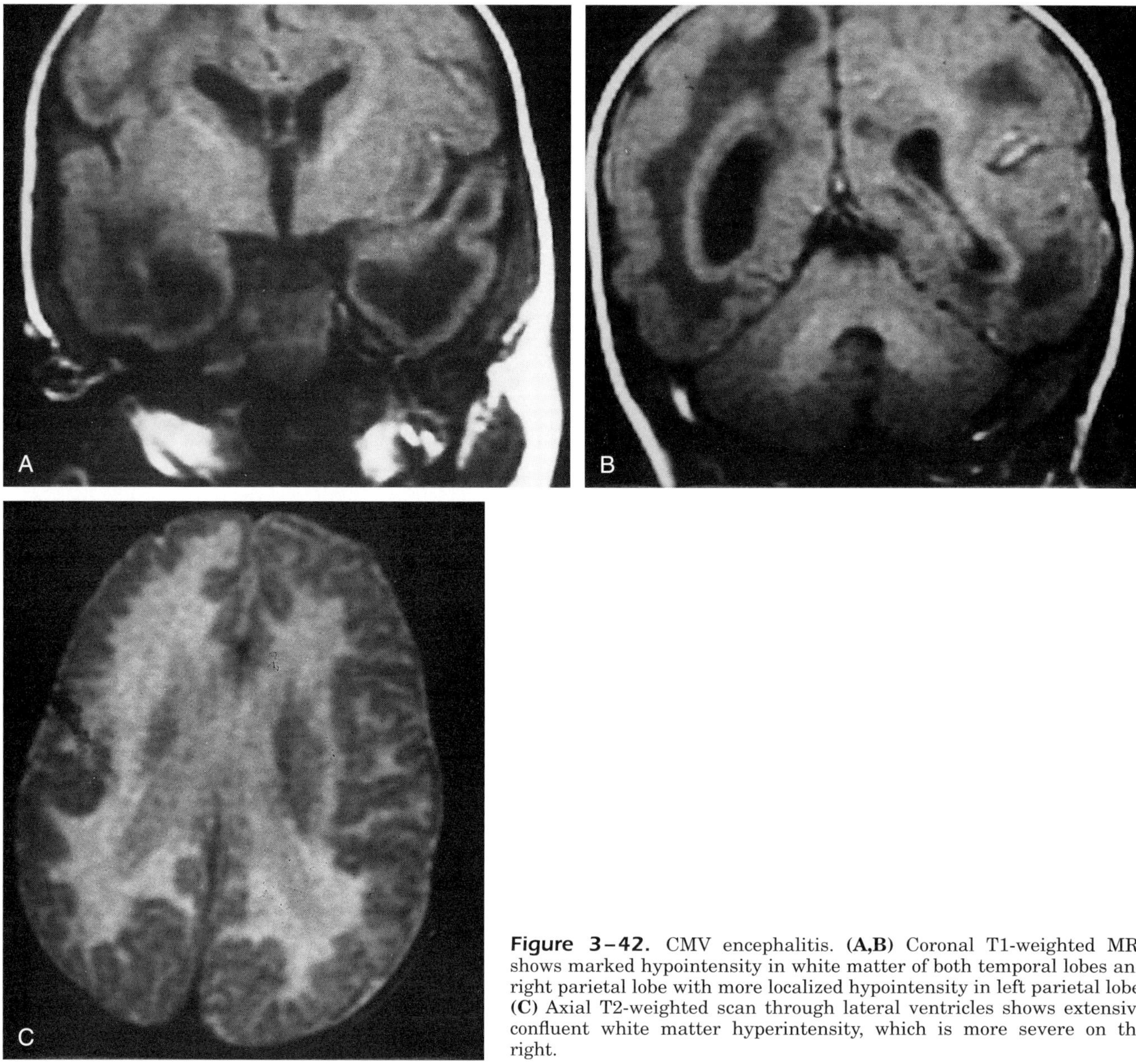

Figure 3–42. CMV encephalitis. **(A,B)** Coronal T1-weighted MRI shows marked hypointensity in white matter of both temporal lobes and right parietal lobe with more localized hypointensity in left parietal lobe. **(C)** Axial T2-weighted scan through lateral ventricles shows extensive confluent white matter hyperintensity, which is more severe on the right.

Toxoplasmosis

Toxoplasma gondii is passed to humans from cats, which are the primary host. A mother who becomes infected during pregnancy may pass on the infection to her child. Infected infants may present with chorioretinitis, seizures, and developmental delay.

CT Findings. CT is the preferred imaging modality because of its greater sensitivity for calcifications. Intracranial calcifications may be present in the basal ganglia, periventricular white matter, and cortex. Hydrocephalus due to acquired aqueductal stenosis is common. Destructive lesions (encephalomalacia, porencephaly, hydranencephaly) may be present, with the earliest (in gestation) infections causing the most severe damage.

MRI Findings. MRI may show migrational anomalies (pachygyria) unrecognized by CT. Delayed myelination may be observed in older patients.

Differential Diagnosis

Cytomegalovirus infection is the primary diagnostic consideration. The two lesions cannot be reliably differentiated on imaging findings alone.

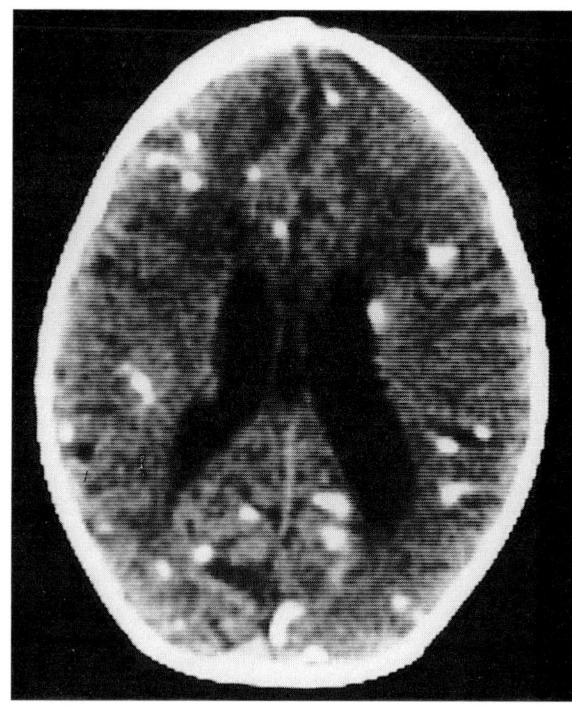

Figure 3–43. Toxoplasmosis. CT shows multiple course parenchymal calcifications dispersed throughout both hemispheres and atrophy or gliosis of frontal white matter.

RECOMMENDED READINGS

Bacterial Meningitis

Chang,KH, Han,MH, Kim,IO, Roh,JK, Han,MC, Kim,CW. Gd-DTPA Enhanced MR Imaging of the Brain in Patients with Meningitis: Comparison with CT. *AJNR* 11:69–76, 1990. *AJR* 154:809–816, 1990.

Harris,TM, Edwards,MK. Meningitis. *Neuroimaging Clin North Am* 1:39–56, 1991.

Phillips,ME, Ryals,TJ, Kambhu,SA, Yuh,WTC. Neoplastic vs. Inflammatory Meningeal Enhancement with Gd-DTPA. *J Comput Assist Tomogr* 14:536–541, 1990.

Pyogenic Cerebritis and Brain Abscess

Haimes,AB, Zimmerman,RD, Morgello,S, et al. MR Imaging of Brain Abscesses. *AJNR* 10:279–291, 1989. *AJR* 152: 1073–1085, 1989.

Zimmerman,RD, Weingarten,K. Neuroimaging of Cerebral Abscesses. *Neuroimaging Clin North Am* 1:1–16, 1991.

Empyema

Tsuchiya,K, Makita,K, Furui,S, Kusano,S, Inoue,Y. Contrast-Enhanced Magnetic Resonance Imaging of Sub- and Epidural Empyemas. *Neuroradiology* 34:494–496, 1992.

Weingarten,K, Zimmerman,RD, Becker,RD, Heier,LA, Haimes,AB, Deck,MD. Subdural and Epidural Empyemas: MR Imaging. *AJR* 152:615–621, 1989.

Zimmerman,RD, Leeds,NE, Danziger, A. Subdural Empyema: CT Findings. *Radiology* 150:417–422, 1984.

Tuberculosis

de Castro,CC, Hesselink,JR. Tuberculosis. *Neuroimaging Clin North Am* 1:119–139, 1991.

Chang,KH, Han,MH, Roh,JK, Kim,MC, Choi,KS, Kim,CW. Gd-DTPA Enhanced MR Imaging in Intracranial Tuberculosis. *Neuroradiology* 32:19–25, 1990.

Gupta,RK, Jena,A, Sharma,A, Guha,DK, Khushu,S, Gupta,AK. MR Imaging of Intracranial Tuberculomas. *J Comput Assist Tomogr* 12:280–285, 1988.

Herpes Simplex I Encephalitis

Jordan,J, Enzmann,DR. Encephalitis. *Neuroimaging Clin North Am* 1:17–38, 1991.

Tien,RD, Felsberg,GJ, Osumi,AK. Herpesvirus Infections of the CNS: MR Findings. *AJR* 161:167–176, 1993.

HIV Encephalitis

Balakrishnan,J, Becker,PS, Kumar,AJ, Zinreich,SJ, McArthur, JC, Bryan,RN. Acquired Immunodeficiency Syndrome: Correlation of Radiologic and Pathologic Findings in the Brain. *Radiographics* 10:201–215, 1990.

Chrysikipoulos,HS, Press,GA, Grafe,MR, Hesselink,JR, Wiley, CA. Encephalitis Caused by Human Immunodeficiency Virus: CT and MR Imaging Manifestations with Clinical and Pathologic Correlation. *Radiology* 175:185–191, 1990.

Progressive Multifocal Leukoencephalopathy

Mark,AS, Atlas,SW. Progressive Multifocal Leukoencephalopathy in Patients with AIDS: Appearance on MR Images. *Radiology* 173:517–520, 1989.

Olsen,WL, Longo,FM, Mills,CM, Norman,D. White Matter Disease in AIDS: Findings at MR Imaging. *Radiology* 169:445–448, 1988.

Whiteman,MLH, Post,MJD, Berger,JR, Tate,LG, Bell,MD, Limonte,LP. Progressive Multifocal Leukoencephalopathy in 47 HIV-seropositive Patients: Neuroimaging with Clinical and Pathologic Correlation. *Radiology* 187:233–240, 1993.

Creutzfeldt-Jakob Disease

Barboriak,DP, Provenzale,JM, Boyko,OB. MR Diagnosis of Creutzfeldt-Jakob Disease: Significance of High Signal Intensity of the Basal Ganglia. *AJR* 162:137–140, 1994.

Falcone,S, Quencer,RM, Bowen,B, Bruce,JH, Naidich,TP. Creutzfeldt-Jakob Disease: Focal Symmetrical Cortical Involvement Demonstrated by MR Imaging. *AJNR* 13: 403–406, 1992.

Uchino,A, Yoshinaga,M, Hata,H, Ohno,M. Serial MR Imaging in Creutzfeldt-Jakob Disease. *Neuroradiology* 33:364–367, 1991.

Cryptococcosis

Mathews,VP, Alo,PL, Glass,JD, Kumar,AJ, McArthur,JC. AIDS Related CNS Cryptococcosis: Radiologic-Pathologic Correlation. *AJNR* 13:1477–1486, 1992.

Tien,RD, Chu,PK, Hesselink,JR, Duberg,A, Wiley,C. Intracranial Cryptococcosis in Immunocompromised Patients: CT and MR Findings in 29 Cases. *AJNR* 12:283–289, 1991. *AJR* 156:1245–1251, 1991.

Wehn,SM, Heinz,ER, Burger,PC, and Boyko,OB. Dilated Virchow-Robin Spaces in Cryptococcal Meningitis Associated with AIDS: CR and MR Findings. *J Comput Assist Tomogr* 13:756–762, 1989.

Toxoplasmosis

Ciricillo,SF, Rosenblum,ML. Use of CT and MR Imaging to Distinguish Intracranial Lesions and to Define the Need for Biopsy in AIDS Patients. *J Neurosurg* 73:720–724, 1990.

Dina,TS. Primary Central Nervous System Lymphoma versus Toxoplasmosis in AIDS. *Radiology* 179:823–828, 1991.

Ransey,RG, Geremia,GK. CNS Complications of AIDS: CT and MR Findings. *AJR* 151:449–454, 1988.

Rovira,MJ, Post,MJD, Bowen,BC. Central Nervous System Infections in HIV-Positive Persons. *Neuroimaging Clin North Am* 1:179–200, 1991.

Cysticercosis

Chang,KH, Cho,SY, Hesselink,JR, Han,MH, Han,MC. Parasitic Diseases of the Central Nervous System. *Neuroimaging Clin N Am* 1:159–178, 1991.

Chang,KH, Lee,JH, Han,MH, Han,MC. The Role of Contrast-Enhanced MR Imaging in the Diagnosis of Neurocysticercosis. *AJNR* 12:509–512, 1991. *AJR* 157:393–396, 1991.

Kramer,LD, Locke,GE, Byrd,SE, Daryabagi,J. Cerebral Cysticercosis: Documentation of Natural History with CT. *Radiology* 171:459–462, 1989.

Teitelbaum,GP, Otto,RJ, Lin,M, et al. MR Imaging of Neurocysticercosis. *AJR* 153:857–866, 1989.

Sarcoidosis

Carmody,RF, Mafee,MF, Goodwin,JA, et al. Orbital and Optic Pathway Sarcoidosis: MR Findings. *AJNR* 15:775–783, 1994.

Hayes,WS, Sherman,JL, Stern,BJ, Citrin,CM, Pulaski,PD. MR and CT Evaluation of Intracranial Sarcoidosis. *AJR* 149:1043–1049, 1987.

Lexa,FJ, Grossman,RI. MR of Sarcoidosis in the Head and

Spine: Spectrum of Manifestations and Radiographic Response to Steroid Therapy. *AJNR* 15:973–982, 1994.

Seltzer,S, Mark,AS, Atlas,SW. CNS Sarcoidosis: Evaluation with Contrast-Enhanced MR Imaging. *AJNR* 12:1227–1233, 1991. *AJR* 158:391–398, 1992.

Sherman,JL, Stern,BJ. Sarcoidosis of the CNS: Comparison of Unenhanced and Enhanced MR Images. *AJNR* 11:915–923, 1990. *AJR* 155:1293–1301, 1990.

Congenital and Neonatal Infections

Barkovich,AJ, Lindan,CE. Congenital Cytomegalovirus Infection of the Brain: Imaging Analysis and Embryologic Considerations. *AJNR* 15:703–715, 1994.

Becker,LE. Infections of the Developing Brain. *AJNR* 13:537–549, 1992.

Enzmann,D, Chang,Y, Augustyn,G. MR Findings in Neonatal Herpes Simplex Encephalitis Type II. *J Comput Assist Tomogr* 14:453–457, 1990.

Fitz,CR. Inflammatory Diseases of the Brain in Childhood. *AJNR* 13:551–567, 1992.

Noorbehesht,B, Enzmann,DR, Sullender,W, Bradley,JS, Arvin,AM. Neonatal Herpes Simplex Encephalitis: Correlation of Clinical and CT Findings. *Radiology* 162:813–819, 1987.

Osborn,RE, Byrd,SE. Congenital Infections of the Brain. *Neuroimaging Clin North Am* 1:105–118, 1991.

CHAPTER FOUR

Brain Tumors

Approximately 17,500 new cases of primary brain tumors are diagnosed each year, and the estimated annual incidence of metastatic brain tumors ranges from 80,000 to 100,000 cases, many of which are only identified post mortem. Neuroimaging plays a crucial role in diagnosing brain neoplasia, planning treatment, and monitoring the effects of treatment. The main thrust of this chapter is the differential diagnosis of brain tumors. Because in clinical practice more scans tend to be performed for follow-up than for initial diagnosis, issues related to the follow-up of treated tumors are addressed in the final section.

Among children, approximately 1,500 new brain tumors are diagnosed annually (2.4 per 100,000). In children, brain tumors represent the most common solid malignant neoplasms and are only slightly less common than leukemia, the most common malignant disease.

Presenting symptoms of tumors are usually related to mass effect and include headaches (most common), visual changes, seizures, nausea and vomiting, and changes of personality or mental status. Localized seizures or focal deficits may point to the site of the lesion, but in general the presenting symptomatology has little correlation with the tumor type. Neuroimaging, however, can significantly narrow the differential diagnosis and occasionally even pinpoint the diagnosis with a high probability of accuracy.

Differential Diagnosis

When a new intracranial mass lesion is observed, several questions must be answered correctly to arrive at a reasonable differential diagnosis. It may be helpful to proceed according to the following sequence:

1. Is the mass intraaxial or extraaxial?
   This is probably the most critical factor in arriving at a correct diagnosis. Intraaxial masses are primary to brain parenchyma or arise in the ventricles. Extraaxial masses occur outside the brain, usually in the meninges or subarachnoid space. The distinction is not always obvious, and the criteria for making it are explored in Chapter 1.
2. Where is the site of origin?
   - Infratentorial versus supratentorial
   - Parenchymal versus intraventricular
   - Lobar versus basal ganglia
   - Cerebellar versus brainstem
   - Skull base versus calvarium

   Most tumors exhibit a known propensity toward certain locations. Once a mass is confidently localized, the differential diagnosis may be narrowed as indicated in Table 4–1.
3. Is the mass solitary or multiple?
   The finding of multiple lesions eliminates most

TABLE 4–1 Differential Diagnosis of Intracranial Mass Lesions

		Extraaxial	Intraaxial	Intraventricular
Adults	Supratentorial	Meningioma Aneurysm Pituitary adenoma Arachnoid cyst Craniopharyngioma Empyema Sarcoid	Glioblastoma Astrocytoma Ependymoma Lymphoma Oligodendroglioma Ganglioglioma Vascular malformation Metastasis Abscess/infection Demyelination Infarct	Giant cell astrocytoma Colloid cyst Neuroepithelial cyst Meningioma
	Infratentorial	Dermoid Epidermoid Acoustic neuroma Meningioma Arachnoid cyst Chordoma	Hemangioblastoma Metastasis Astrocytoma Vascular malformation Infarction Infection Demyelination	Epidermoid Papilloma Subependymoma
Children	Supratentorial	Craniopharyngioma Arachnoid cyst Chiasm glioma Leptomeningeal cyst	Pineal tumors Astrocytoma Teratoma PNET	Papilloma
	Infratentorial	Epidermoid Dermoid	Astrocytoma Medulloblastoma Ependymoma	Medulloblastoma Ependymoma

Note: Hematoma may be found in any compartment and at any age and should always be considered in the differential diagnosis of a cerebral mass lesion.

TABLE 4-2 Differential Diagnosis of Multiple Cerebral Mass Lesions

	Comments
Intraaxial	
Metastasis	Very common in the general older adult population and may be the initial manifestation of the underlying malignancy All detectable metastases enhance with contrast
Toxoplasmosis	Most common mass in AIDS patients
Lymphoma	Very common in AIDS patients and post-transplant patients on immunosuppression
Cysticercosis	Very common in endemic populations (Latin America) and very rare elsewhere
Tuberous sclerosis (tubers)	Must exhibit other evidence of the disease (see Chapter 2)
Neurofibromatosis	Must exhibit other evidence of the disease (see Chapter 2)
Progressive multifocal leukoencephalopathy	Enhancement very rare Usually AIDS patients or immunosuppressed
Multiple sclerosis	Rarely associated with mass effect Enhancement (ring or solid) only in active lesions
Multicentric glioma	About 5% of gliomas Usually glioblastomas
Gliomatosis cerebri	Diffuse infiltration of brain parenchyma Rare
Extraaxial	
Metastasis	May cause meningeal enhancement or focal masses CSF cytology usually confirmatory
Neurofibromatosis	Meningiomas, optic gliomas, or neuromas Must meet clinical criteria for diagnosis of NF type 1 or 2
Sarcoidosis	Usually more closely applied to pia than arachnoid Propensity to involve the basal cisterns
Meningiomas	Multiple in about 8% of cases

primary tumors from the differential diagnosis, although basically anything may appear as a solitary lesion. A differential diagnosis for multiple cerebral mass lesions is given in Table 4–2.

4. What is known about the patient?
   - Age of patient—With tumors, this is probably the most useful clinical information.
   - Sex of patient—Only a few tumors exhibit a significant sex difference, such as meningiomas in adult females and germ cell tumors in young males.
   - Duration of symptoms—This information is especially useful in distinguishing vascular (acute onset) from neoplastic and inflammatory disease.
   - Laboratory data—Germ cell neoplasms and pituitary tumors represent cases in which laboratory data can help to limit the differential diagnosis. The presence of HIV infection strongly favors toxoplasmosis or lymphoma.
   - Presenting symptoms and signs—The nature of the neurologic deficit is occasionally helpful, especially in the diagnosis of nerve sheath tumors. Fevers or sinusitis may suggest brain abscess.
   - CSF examination—This is primarily useful in the diagnosis of infections and meningeal tumor invasion.
5. Among the possibilities, which are most common?
   Tables 4–3, 4–4, and 4–5 indicate the relative frequency of various primary brain neoplasms. It is difficult to find data comparing the overall frequency of neoplastic with non-neoplastic processes in a general population. The relative incidence of various cerebral mass lesions changes considerably in certain populations, such as those who are immunocompromised, HIV infected, or from less developed nations.
6. What are its enhancement characteristics?
   Contrast enhancement reflects either the vascularity of the tumor or local alteration of the

TABLE 4-3 Relative Frequency of Adult Primary Brain Tumors

Glioma	
Glioblastoma	40%
Astrocytoma	16%
Oligodendroglioma } Medulloblastoma } Ependymoma }	3%
Meningiomas	18%
Pituitary adenomas	12%
Germ cell tumors	3%
Craniopharyngioma	
Chordoma	
Colloid cyst	
Lymphoma	3%
Hemangioblastoma	3%
Schwannoma	2%

TABLE 4-4 Adult Primary Brain Tumors

Rank	Frequency	Tumor Type	Type Location	Peak Age (yr)
1	40%	Glioblastoma	Frontal, temporal	50–55
2	18%	Meningioma	Parasagittal	50–60
3	16%	Astrocytoma	Frontal, temporal	35–40
4	12%	Adenoma	Pituitary	35–40
5	>3%	Lymphoma	Deep white matter	>60 (younger if HIV-positive)

TABLE 4-5 | **Pediatric Primary Brain Tumors**

Rank	Frequency	Tumor Type	Location	Peak Age (yr)
1	65%	Astrocytoma	Cerebral hemispheres, cerebellar hemispheres, brainstem	5–14
2	15%	Medulloblastoma	Vermis	1–10
3	8%	Craniopharyngioma	Suprasellar	6–13
4	4%	Ependymoma	Fourth ventricle	1–10
5	3%	Choroid plexus papilloma	Trigone of lateral ventricle	1–5
6	2%	Germ cell tumor	Pineal region	11–20

Note: Teratoma is the most common intracranial tumor in the neonate.

blood-brain barrier and may manifest any of the following patterns:

- None
- Solid or nodular
- Thin or thick ring
- Irregular

Enhancement characteristics are sometimes helpful in distinguishing lower grade from higher grade glial neoplasms, identifying an active inflammatory process, or confirming the cystic nature of certain masses. Table 4–6 gives a differential diagnosis for ring-enhancing masses.

7. What are its attenuation and signal characteristics?

- Hypodense, hyperdense, isodense, or mixed on CT
- Hyperintense, hypointense, isointense, or mixed on MRI
- Presence of hemorrhage, fat, calcifications, cysts, or necrosis

These findings tend to be less useful because of considerable overlap between various tumors and variability among tumors of the same histology, although the findings of fat or calcifications may at times lead to a specific diagnosis. Tables 4–7, 4–8, and 4–9 provide differential diagnoses related to the observation of calcification, cysts, and hemorrhage.

TABLE 4-6 | **Differential Diagnosis of Ring-Enhancing Lesion**

Vascular
Hematoma
Infarct
Thrombosed giant aneurysm
Inflammatory
Abscess (pyogenic, toxoplasmosis, tuberculosis)
Acute demyelination
Neoplastic
Gliomas (ependymoma, glioblastoma, juvenile pilocytic astrocytoma, anaplastic astrocytoma)
Hemangioblastoma
Craniopharyngioma
Lymphoma
Metastasis
Radiation necrosis

TABLE 4-7 | **Differential Diagnosis of Calcified Masses**

Extraaxial	Comments
Meningioma	Variable, ranging from focal to diffuse and fine to solid calcification of entire tumor
Dermoid	Rim calcification or dense focal calcifications within tumor (dental enamel)
Craniopharyngioma	Rim calcification or dense globular calcifications
Germinoma	Coarse and stippled
Teratoma	Variable, including fine, course, or very dense
Chordoma	Scattered, punctate, and present in up to 50%
Aneurysm	Rim calcification
Intraaxial	
Astrocytoma	Scattered and punctate in fibrillary and pilocytic astrocytomas. More globular in giant cell type
Oligodendroglioma	Calcifications present in 40% and denser and more globular than in astrocytomas
Ependymoma	Small, granular, and present in about 50%
Medulloblastoma	Clumplike and present in 20–50%
Primitive neuroectodermal tumor	Calcifications present in 60–70%
Ganglioglioma	Dense, globular, and present in 35%
Vascular malformations	Usually multiple and punctate
Hamartoma	Associated with tuberous sclerosis Calcifications punctate and often multiple
Metastases	Multiple masses Calcifications rare

TABLE 4-8 | Differential Diagnosis of Cystic Masses

Extraaxial
Arachnoid cyst
Epidermoid
Dermoid
Craniopharyngioma
Intraaxial
Abscess
Cysticercosis
Ependymoma
Pilocytic astrocytoma
Hemangioblastoma
Ganglioglioma
Glioblastoma

TABLE 4-9 | Differential Diagnosis of Hemorrhagic Tumors

Pituitary adenoma*
Metastasis
Choriocarcinoma
Melanoma
Lung
Renal
Thyroid
Gastrointestinal
Glioblastoma
Astrocytoma
Ependymoma
Choroid plexus papilloma
Sarcoma
Meningioma

*Highest frequency of spontaneous hemorrhage.

Extraaxial Tumors

Meningioma

Meningiomas are benign tumors of meningeal origin. They are the most common extraaxial neoplasm in adults and usually the easiest for which to make a specific diagnosis. The highest incidence is among middle-aged adult females. Multiple meningiomas are a hallmark of type 2 neurofibromatosis; however, meningiomas are multiple in about 8% of patients, most of whom do not have neurofibromatosis.

Meningiomas have traditionally been classified into meningothelial (syncytial), fibroblastic, transitional, and angioblastic types, but the current trend is to reclassify angioblastic meningiomas as hemangiopericytomas. Hemangiopericytomas exhibit more aggressive imaging characteristics and clinical behavior. Table 4–10 gives the diagnostic features of dural masses.

Location
In descending order of frequency:

1. Parasagittal
2. Falx
3. Convexity
4. Olfactory groove
5. Tuberculum sella
6. Sphenoid wing
7. Middle fossa
8. Cerebellopontine angle
9. Tentorium
10. Ventricles
11. Clivus and craniocervical junction

CT Findings. CT shows an isodense or hyperdense extraaxial mass with focal or diffuse calcification. Dense homogeneous contrast enhancement is seen in all but the most densely calcified tumors. Edema is common but variable in severity and may occasionally be severe. Hyperostosis occurs in approximately 5%, and invasion of adjacent bone is even less common.

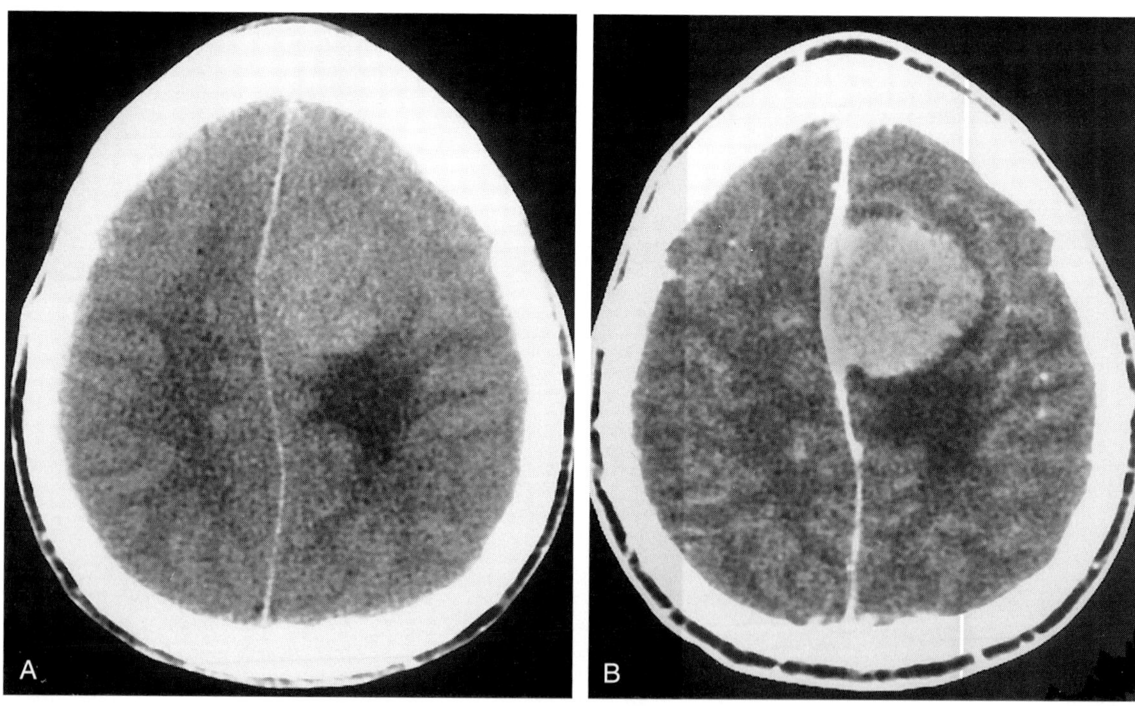

Figure 4–1. Parasagittal meningioma. **(A)** Precontrast CT shows a mildly hyperdense left parafalcine mass with vasogenic edema of the white matter. **(B)** After intravenous contrast, there is dense homogeneous enhancement of the tumor and enhancement of the thickened adjacent falx.

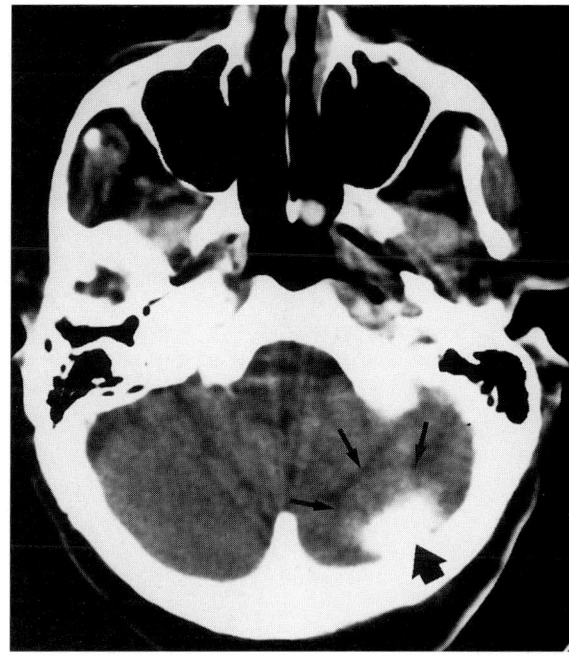

Figure 4–2. Calcified meningioma. Unenhanced CT shows a left posterior fossa meningioma (small arrows). A portion is densely calcified (large arrow).

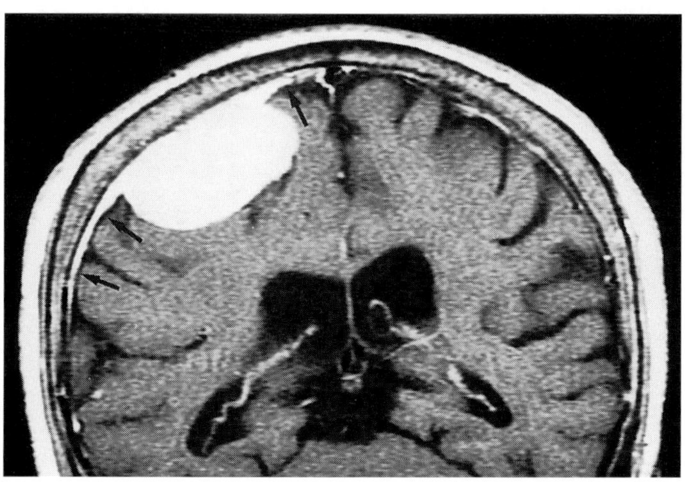

Figure 4–3. Convexity meningioma. Coronal contrast-enhanced MRI shows a classic convexity meningioma with dense solid enhancement and the dural tail sign (arrows).

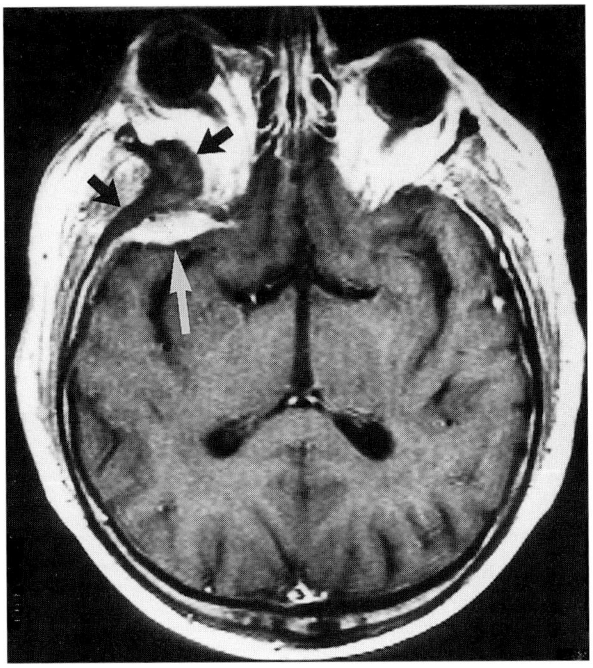

Figure 4–4. Sphenoid wing meningioma. Axial contrast-enhanced MRI shows an enhancing sphenoid wing meningioma (long white arrow) with hyperostosis of the sphenoid (short black arrows). En plaque growth is typical of sphenoid wing meningiomas.

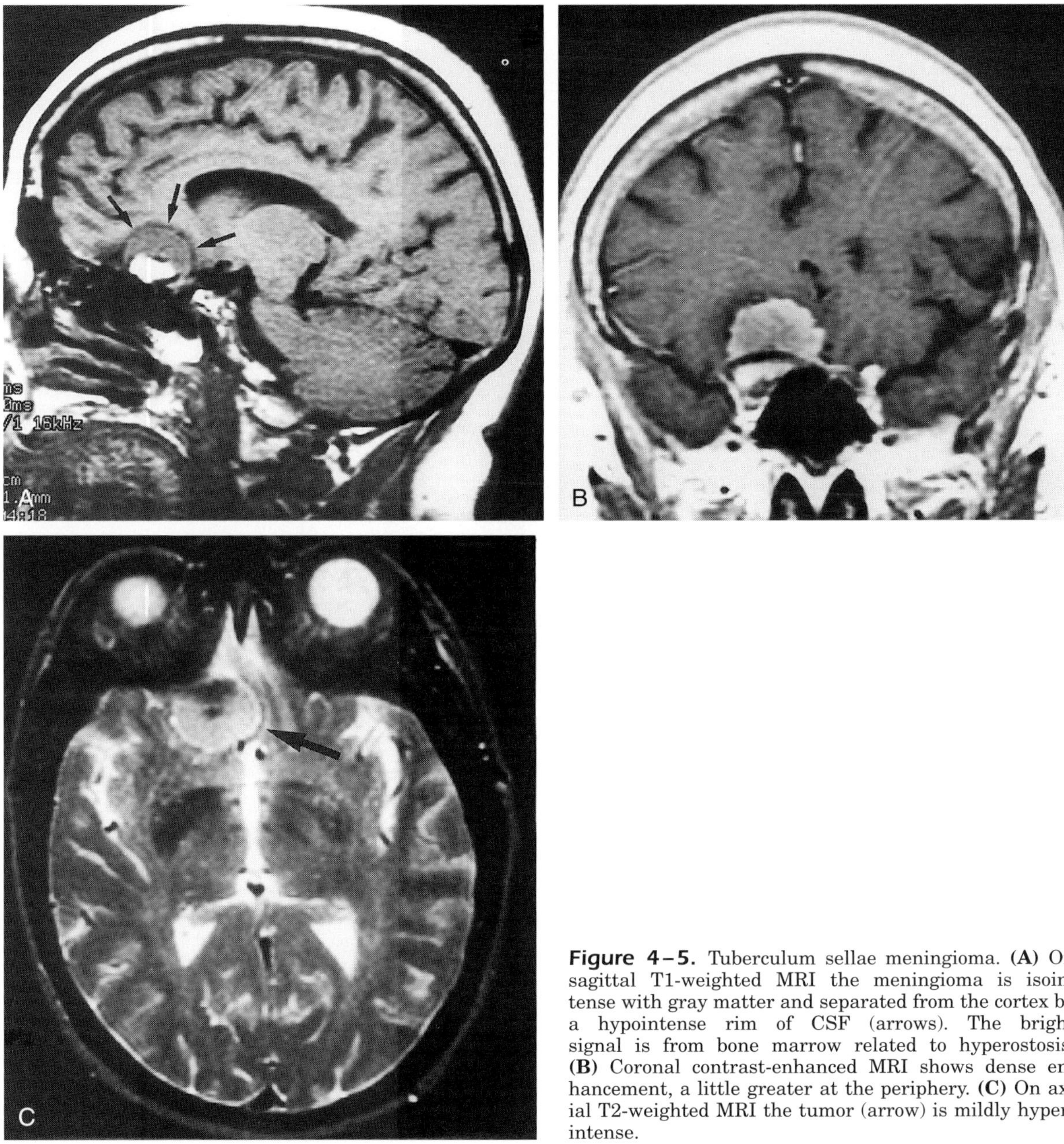

Figure 4–5. Tuberculum sellae meningioma. **(A)** On sagittal T1-weighted MRI the meningioma is isointense with gray matter and separated from the cortex by a hypointense rim of CSF (arrows). The bright signal is from bone marrow related to hyperostosis. **(B)** Coronal contrast-enhanced MRI shows dense enhancement, a little greater at the periphery. **(C)** On axial T2-weighted MRI the tumor (arrow) is mildly hyperintense.

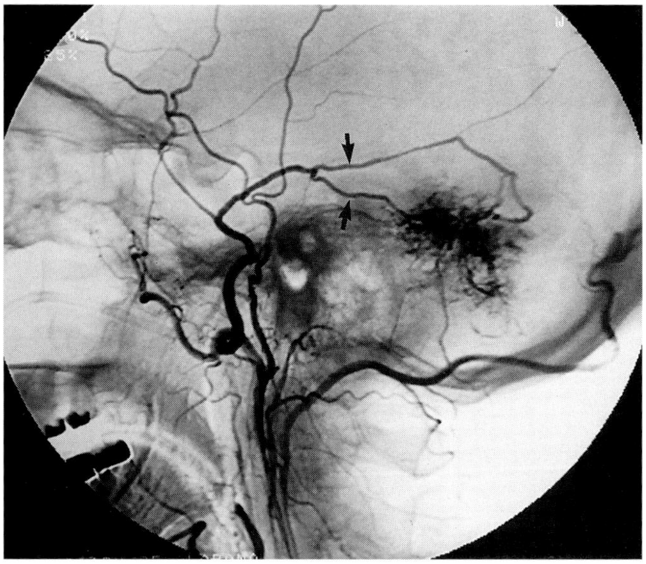

Figure 4–6. Meningioma. External carotid angiogram shows a meningioma supplied by the posterior division of the middle meningeal artery (arrows). Note the radial pattern of tumor vascularity.

MRI Findings. Meningiomas are usually isointense (60%) to hypointense (30%) relative to gray matter on T1-weighted MRI. On T2-weighted images, they are isointense (50%) to hyperintense (40%) relative to gray matter. MRI is quite insensitive for the detection of calcifications. All meningiomas enhance with intravenous contrast; enhancement of adjacent thickened dura (meningeal sign or dural tail) is a common and almost distinctive feature. This finding does not necessarily reflect tumor spread. Hyperostosis is manifest as thickening of the adjacent bone; the signal intensity of the bone varies markedly according to the marrow contents (cellular tumor versus fatty marrow). About 15% of meningiomas manifest atypical features, such as marked heterogeneity, fat, cysts, or necrosis. Meningiomas may cause occlusion of the major dural sinuses. This complication may be recognized by the loss of the normal flow void on unenhanced MRI.

Angiography. Meningiomas are preferentially supplied by meningeal arteries corresponding to the territory of the tumor, with recruitment of pial vessels by more advanced tumors. Feeding vessels form a radial pattern within the tumor, and dense staining persists late into the venous phase.

Differential Diagnosis

Lymphoma	Intraaxial but often has broad contact with pial surface of brain
Meningeal metastasis	Usually multiple but calcifications rare
Schwannoma	Parasellar (fifth cranial nerve) or cerebellopontine angle (eighth cranial nerve) Schwannomas brighter on T2-weighted MRI
Melanoma	Primary or metastatic; melanotic melanoma hyperintense on T1-weighted MRI
Pituitary adenoma	Enlargement of sella
Aneurysm	Exhibits flow or thrombus on MRI**See**

See Table 4–10.

TABLE 4–10 **Diagnostic Features of Dural Masses (Excluding Skull Base)**

Mass Lesion	CT Findings	MRI Findings	Angiographic Findings	Comments
Meningioma	Round, convex, or flat dural mass Intense contrast enhancement Bone changes common: hyperostosis, erosion	Isointense or hypointense to gray on T1-weighted images Highly variable signal intensity on T2-weighted images Intense enhancement Dural tail sign usually present Cerebral edema often present	Supplied by meningeal vessels with occasional pial recruitment Radial pattern of arterial feeders Dense staining persists late into venous phase	Most common meningeal neoplasm Usually occurs in middle-aged females
Metastasis	Enhancing dural mass Adjacent bone destruction common	Slightly brighter than CSF on T1-weighted images Intense enhancement	Usually hypovascular	Miliary seeding more common than isolated mass
Hematoma	Mass of increased or diminished attenuation Convex or concave inner border Enhancing wall or membranes in chronic stages	Signal intensity a function of age Subacute and chronic hematoma bright on T1-weighted images, almost specific	Avascular mass	History of trauma or acute onset of severe headache
Abscess/empyema	Low attenuation extraaxial mass with variable rim enhancement Sinusitis usually present	Slightly hyperintense relative to CSF on T1-weighted images Bright on T2-weighted images Marked rim enhancement	Avascular mass Possible early draining veins	Fevers, headaches, and meningismus History of sinusitis or surgery
Vascular malformation	Enhancing round or tubular structures Adjacent hematoma or subarachnoid hemorrhage Calcifications often present	Signal voids Areas of hemorrhage	Arteriovenous shunting Enlarged feeding vessels and draining veins	Acute onset of severe headache May present with seizures
Postoperative fibrosis	Craniotomy defects Dural abnormalities usually not seen	Thickened enhancing dura subjacent to a craniotomy site	No angiographic findings	History of previous surgery
Pachymeningitis	Thickened, enhancing tentorium or other dural regions	Hypointense dural thickening with marked enhancement	Occlusion of dural sinuses or carotid siphon	Headaches, cranial nerve deficits and elevated sedimentation rate
Hemangiopericytoma	Lobulated mass Intense homogeneous enhancement Bone erosion Possible narrow dural attachment	Intratumoral signal voids	Multiple irregular feeding vessels	Includes most tumors previously identified as angioblastic meningiomas
Capillary hemangioma	Slightly hyperdense mass with intense enhancement	Hyperintense on T2-weighted images Intense enhancement Draining veins	Enlarged meningeal feeders Intense staining Lobular architecture	Infants or very young children

Reprinted with permission from Willing,SJ, Faye-Petersen,O, Aronin,P, Faith,S. Radiologic-Pathologic Correlation: Capillary Hemangioma of the Meninges. *AJNR* 14:529–536, 1993.

Arachnoid Cyst

True arachnoid cysts are believed to be developmental anomalies of the meninges; with CT and especially MRI subclinical arachnoid cysts are frequently encountered. A minority of arachnoid cysts produce symptoms due to mass effect or hydrocephalus. Retrocerebellar arachnoid cysts represent the less severe spectrum of the Dandy-Walker complex.

Acquired arachnoid cysts may follow meningitis or trauma. Such pseudocysts result from adhesions of the arachnoid and entrapment of CSF and lack a complete arachnoid lining. They are more likely to present with mass effect but otherwise manifest imaging characteristics identical to true arachnoid cysts.

Location

In approximate descending order of frequency:

1. Middle fossa/sylvian fissure (about 50% of all arachnoid cysts)
2. Cerebellopontine angle
3. Quadrigeminal cistern
4. Suprasellar cistern
5. Retrocerebellar/cisterna magna

CT Findings. CT shows an extraaxial mass isodense with CSF, occurring in a characteristic location, and without fat, calcifications, or enhancement. The margins are consistently smooth and sharp; mass effect is variable. Remodeling of the overlying calvarium is common. Middle fossa cysts are typically associated with temporal lobe hypoplasia. Suprasellar cysts are associated with dilatation of prepontine cisterns and may invaginate into the third ventricle. On contrast cisternography, cysts usually do not communicate with the subarachnoid space or ventricles.

MRI Findings. MRI shows an extraaxial mass isointense with CSF on all pulse sequences although flow effects may cause deviation from this rule. In the middle fossa, the majority do not compress the temporal lobes but rather are associated with temporal lobe hypoplasia. Adjacent brain exhibits normal signal characteristics.

Differential Diagnosis
Tumor-associated cyst
Epidermoid

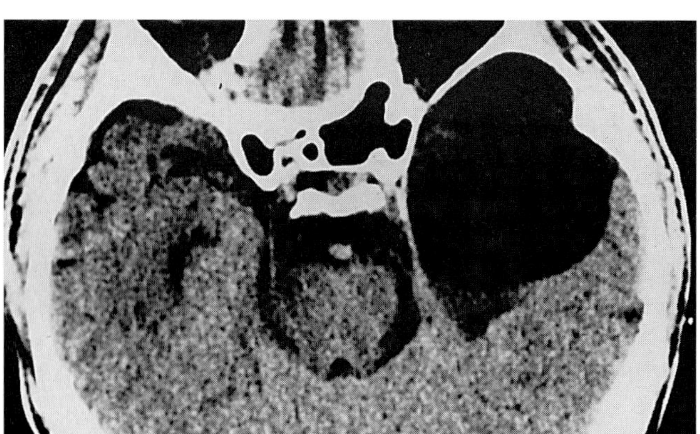

Figure 4–7. Arachnoid cyst. Unenhanced CT shows a typical arachnoid cyst of the left middle fossa. The cyst is isodense with CSF and has caused bony remodeling.

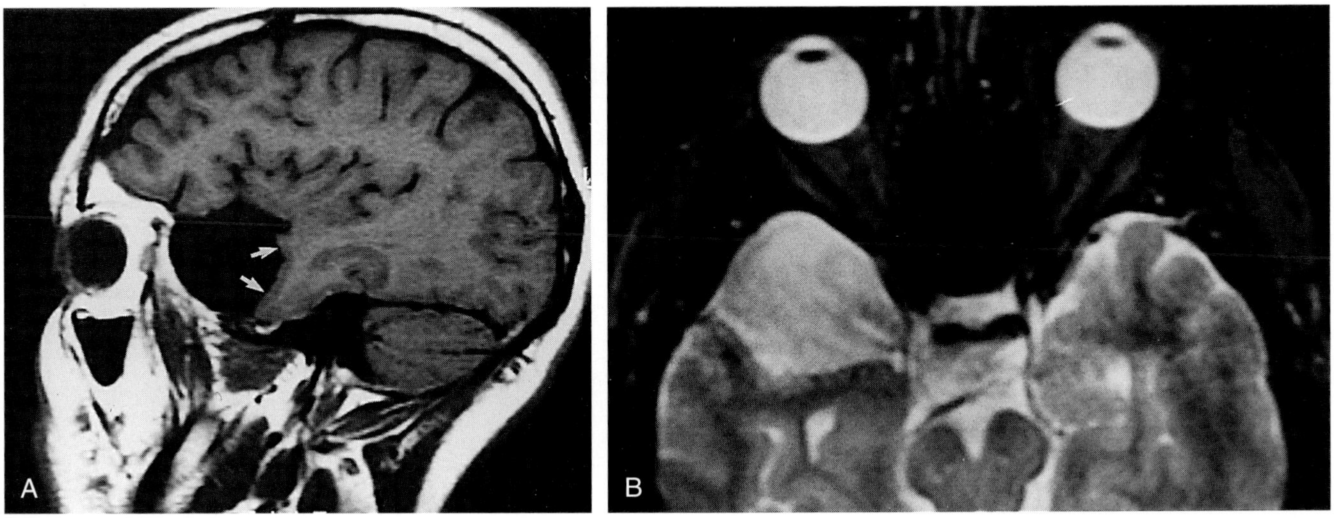

Figure 4–8. Congenital arachnoid cyst. **(A)** Sagittal T1-weighted and **(B)** axial T2-weighted MRI show isointensity with CSF, absence of mass effect, and temporal lobe hypoplasia. The cyst abuts cortical gray matter (arrows) of the temporal lobe establishing its extraaxial nature.

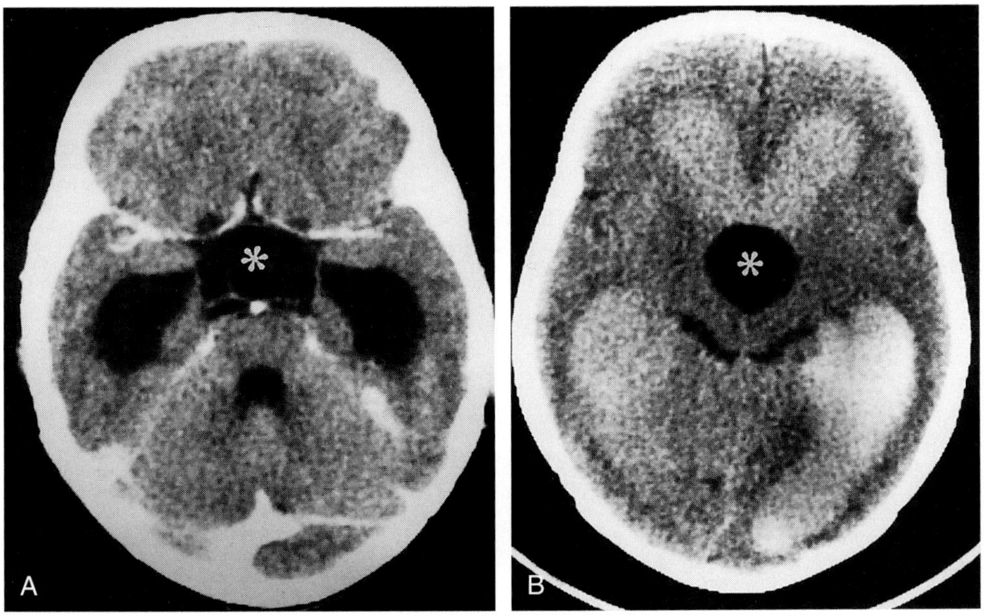

Figure 4–9. Suprasellar arachnoid cyst. **(A)** Contrast-enhanced CT and **(B)** contrast ventriculogram show a mass of water attenuation in the suprasellar cistern. Hydrocephalus is present. Nonfilling of the mass (asterisk) indicates the cyst has displaced the third ventricle and does not communicate with the ventricular system.

Dermoid

Dermoids are benign epithelial cysts thought to arise from ectodermal inclusions left behind at 3 to 5 weeks of gestation. They usually occur in or near the midline with a propensity for the posterior fossa followed by the parasellar area. Dermoids are distinguished from epidermoids by the presence of fat, hair, dental enamel, or sebaceous or sweat glands and their earlier presentation in the first two to three decades of life. Dermoids are slow growing with symptoms usually resulting from mass effect. The cysts may rupture spontaneously, provoking acute meningeal symptoms caused by the release of lipid debris into the ventricles and subarachnoid space.

Location
Midline, posterior fossa or parasellar.

CT Findings. CT shows a sharply marginated extraaxial mass near the midline skull base. It tends to be heterogeneous with areas of soft tissue, fat, and rim calcifications. When seen in conjunction with a mass in the appropriate location, the presence of fat is virtually pathognomonic for dermoid. Spontaneous rupture releases visible fat droplets into the ventricles and subarachnoid space. Intraventricular fat produces a fat-fluid level.

MRI Findings. MRI reveals a heterogeneous mass in a characteristic location. The fatty components are characterized by marked hyperintensity on T1-weighted images and low intensity on T2-weighted images. The solid components are hypointense on T1-weighted images and hyperintense on T2-weighted images. There typically is no edema in adjacent brain tissue. Enhancement is minimal and peripheral, reflecting enhancement of the tumor capsule and displaced meninges. Dermoids are sometimes associated with dermal sinus tracts, which appear as soft tissue bands extending from the mass through the skull to the dermis.

Rupture of a dermoid, not an uncommon occurrence, may release fat into the ventricles and subarachnoid space. The released fat is markedly hyperintense on T1-weighted images. Within the ventricles, fat-CSF levels are formed with the less dense fat floating above the CSF.

Differential Diagnosis	
Lipoma	Recognized by characteristic location, lack of mass effect, and encasement rather than displacement of cerebral vessels
Craniopharyngioma	Suprasellar location, sellar enlargement, and more prominent enhancement
Epidermoid	Usually homogeneous signal on T1-weighted MRI (slightly hyperintense relative to CSF), off-midline location, and older age groups
Teratoma	Most occur in pineal region
Intracranial pantopaque	Causes scattered hyperintensities in the subarachnoid space, which may suggest ruptured dermoid

Figure 4–10. Dermoid. **(A)** CT with contrast shows a large right hemisphere mass nearly isodense with CSF and with minimal peripheral enhancement. **(B)** On sagittal T1-weighted MRI the mass is moderately hyperintense relative to CSF with bright areas at the periphery due to fat. The margins are smooth and sharp. **(C)** Sagittal T1-weighted section through the left lateral ventricle shows a fat-fluid level in the frontal horn. This finding is pathognomonic for ruptured dermoid. **(D,E)** On T2-weighted sequence the mass is mostly hyperintense with streaky hypointensities related to fat. Fat in the left frontal horn (arrow) may be identified by the chemical shift artifact. **(F)** Contrast-enhanced scan shows minimal peripheral enhancement, probably arising from displaced meninges and the tumor capsule.

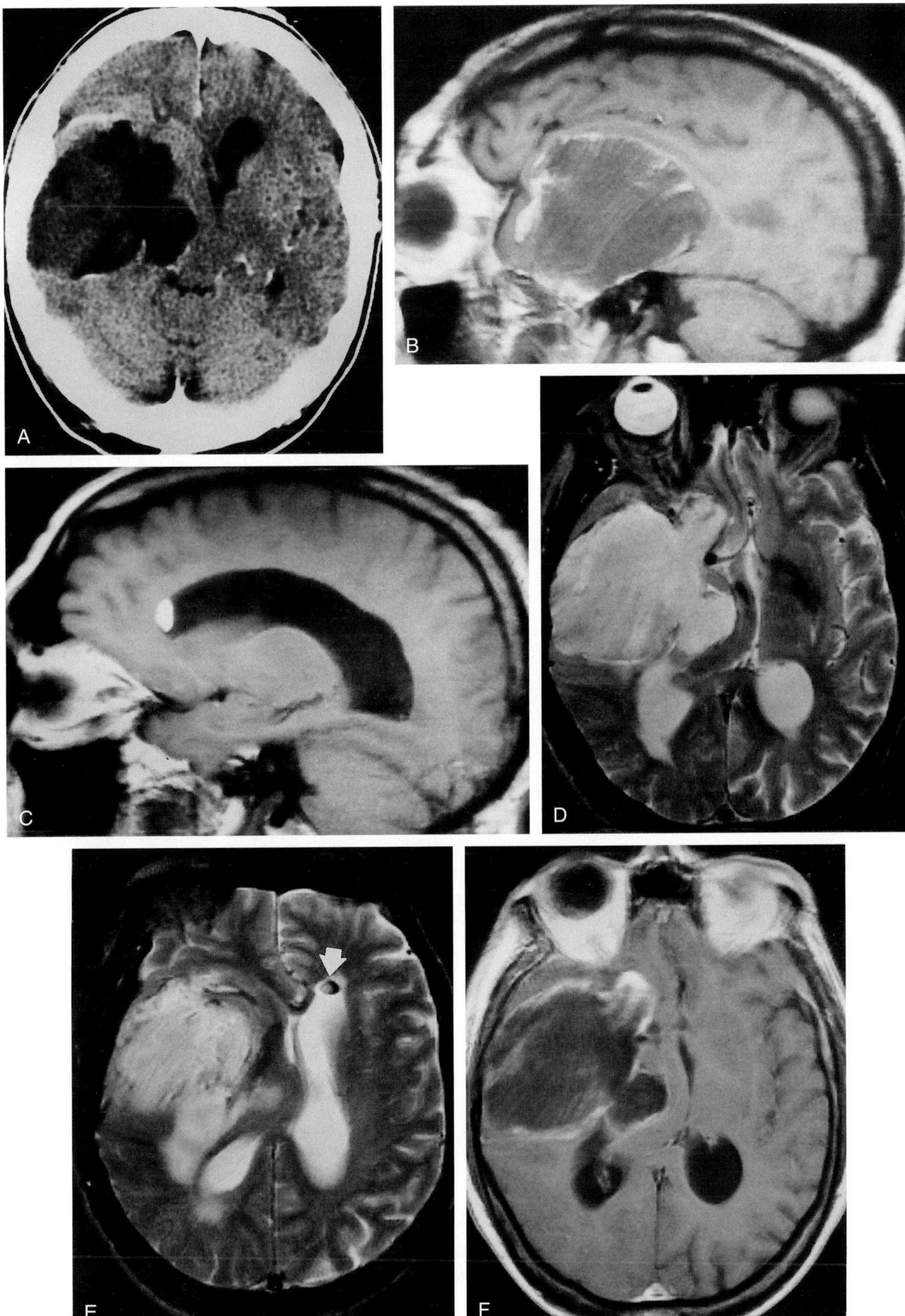
A
B
C
D
E
F

Epidermoid

Like dermoids, epidermoids result from congenital ectodermal inclusions. They are lined by stratified squamous epithelium and grow by the accumulation of keratinous debris and cholesterol crystals. Epidermoids are soft, pliable masses that insinuate into and around adjacent structures. They are the third most common mass of the cerebellopontine angle.

Location
Cerebellopontine angle (most common), parasellar/middle fossa, or intraventricular (15%), especially atria and fourth ventricle.

CT Findings. CT shows a low attenuation, multilobulated (in contrast with arachnoid cyst) mass without enhancement or edema. Marginal calcifications are infrequently encountered. Intrathecal contrast diffuses into the interstices of the tumor, giving a cauliflower like appearance on cisternography. Hydrocephalus is uncommon.

MRI Findings. Epidermoids manifest a slightly higher signal intensity than CSF on T1-weighted images. They become heterogeneous on proton-density images with a hyperintense rim and are markedly hyperintense on T2-weighted images. It is the slight difference in signal compared with CSF, especially on T1-weighted images, that allows differentiation from arachnoid cysts. Occasional epidermoids are encountered that may manifest more heterogeneity or even signal intensities directly opposite to the norm. Epidermoids do not enhance, although mild rim enhancement may be seen, probably arising from the meninges or tumor capsule.

Differential Diagnosis

Arachnoid cyst	Should be perfectly isointense with CSF, typical location in middle fossa, temporal lobe hypoplasia, and no mass effect
Dermoid cyst	(See Dermoid)
Craniopharyngioma	Enhancement usual, solid components, and heterogeneous texture
Cysticercosis	Usually multiple, intraaxial and calcifications common

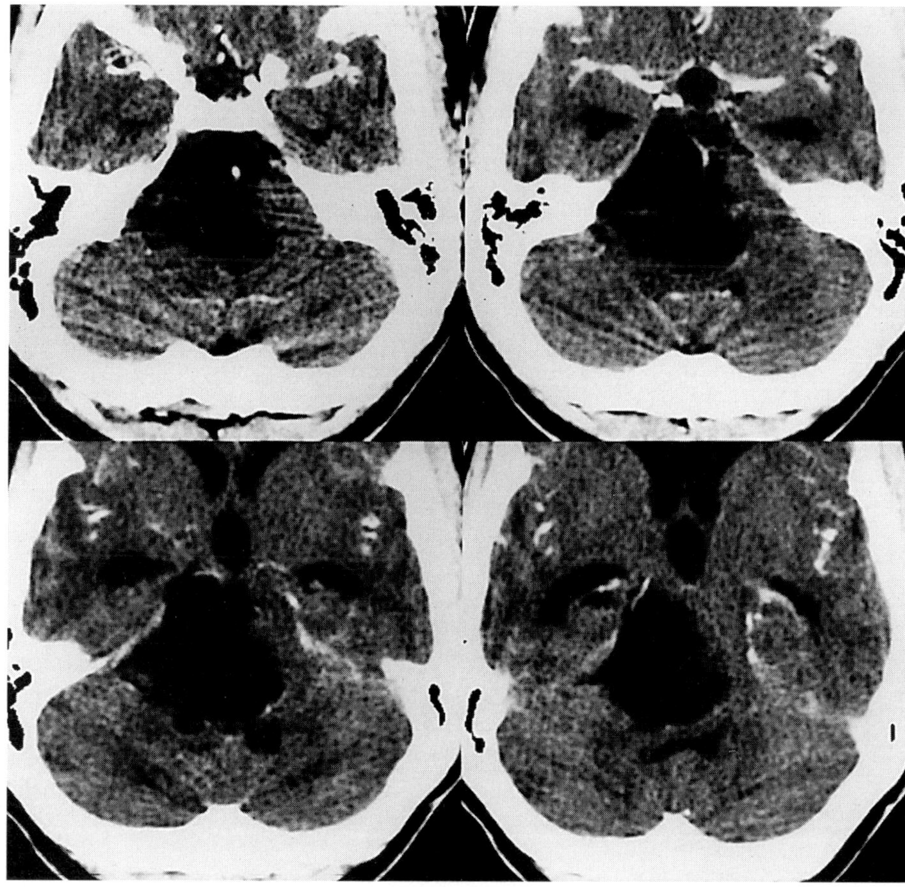

Figure 4–11. Epidermoid. Contrast-enhanced CT shows a large epidermoid of the prepontine cistern. The cyst is isodense with CSF and engulfs the basilar artery. Obstructive hydrocephalus is caused by mass effect upon the fourth ventricle.

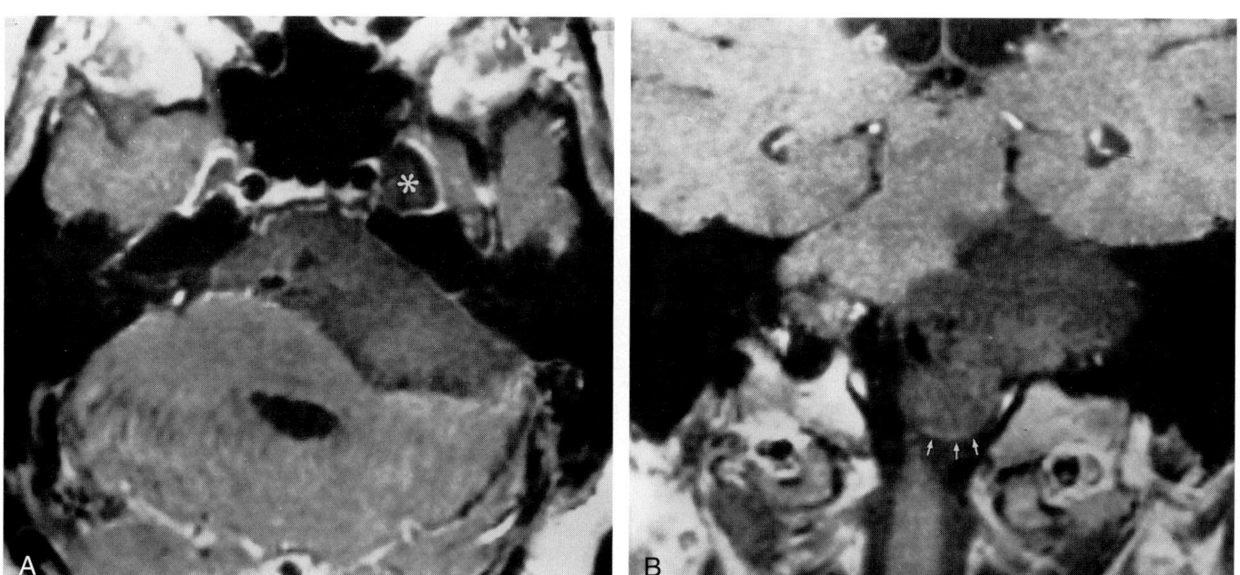

Figure 4–12. Epidermoid. **(A)** Axial contrast-enhanced MRI shows a large mass of the left cerebellopontine angle. The mass is slightly hyperintense relative to CSF and there is no enhancement. It infiltrates the prepontine cistern and left Meckel's cave (asterisk). **(B)** On coronal MRI the interface with CSF is clearly demarcated (arrows).

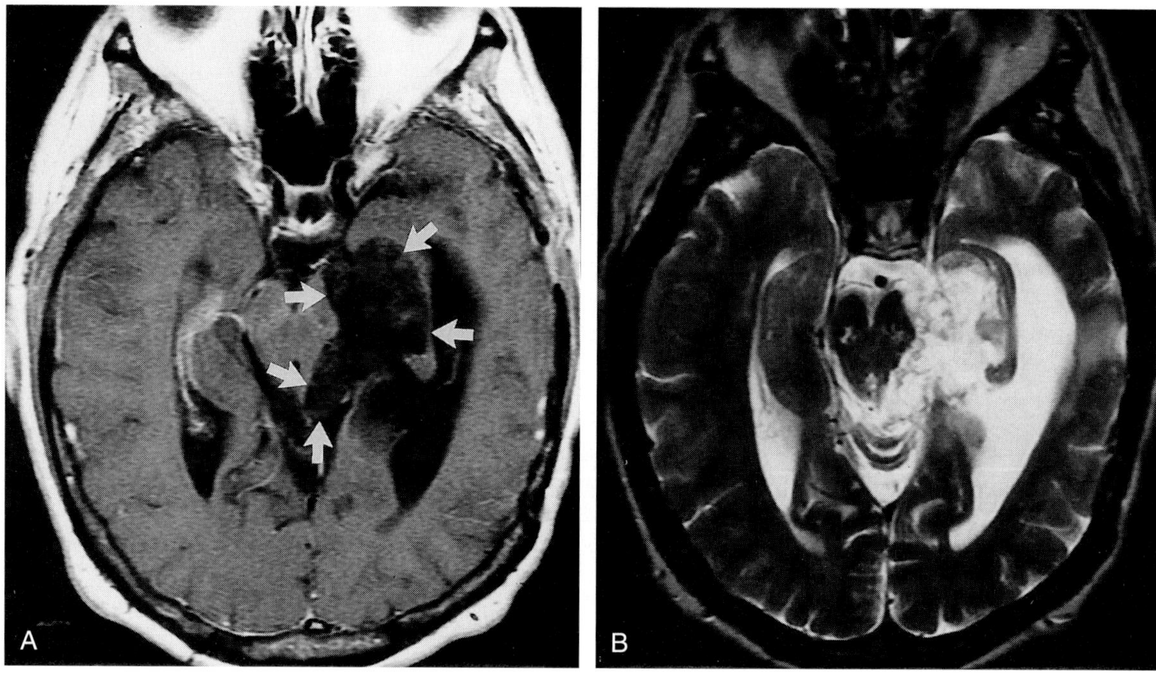

Figure 4–13. Epidermoid. **(A)** Axial contrast-enhanced MRI shows a mass (arrows) filling the left ambient cistern and choroidal fissure and compressing the brainstem. **(B)** On T2-weighted MRI the mass is nearly isointense with CSF but heterogeneous in texture.

Schwannoma

Synonyms: Neuroma, neurinoma, neurilemmoma.

Schwannomas are the most common tumors of the cerebellopontine angle, accounting for 80–90% of tumors in this location. They arise from the Schwann cells, which are responsible for the myelination of peripheral nerves. Most schwannomas originate from the vestibular division of the eighth cranial nerve and grow in the internal auditory canal and cerebellopontine angle. The fifth and seventh cranial nerves are the next most common nerves of origin. Any other cranial nerve may rarely give rise to a schwannoma. The finding of bilateral vestibular schwannomas is the primary diagnostic criterion for type 2 neurofibromatosis.

Location
See Table 4–11.

CT Findings. CT shows an isodense or hypodense mass in the internal auditory canal and cerebellopontine angle cistern. Hemorrhage and calcifications are rare. Associated arachnoid cysts are occasionally seen. Most cases exhibit enlargement or erosion of the internal auditory canal. Nearly all enhance, usually homogeneously and with sharp margins. The acute angle sign, where the tumor forms an acute angle at its junction with the temporal bone, is an important characteristic in differentiating neuroma from meningioma. Hydrocephalus may develop with the larger tumors. CT is very insensitive for tumors smaller than 1.5 cm, and MRI is the preferred modality for the detection of schwannomas.

MRI Findings. Schwannomas are usually hypointense on T1-weighted images and heterogeneously hyperintense on T2-weighted images. Most are readily detected without contrast. After intravenous contrast, they enhance intensely and usually homogeneously. Contrast is helpful in the detection of very small and intracanalicular tumors. Demonstration of enhancement within the internal auditory canal is highly specific for schwannoma but not pathognomonic.

TABLE 4–11 **Schwannomas**

Frequency	Nerve	Usual Site	Distinguishing Features
1	CN VIII	IAC, CP angle	Most common by far (>90% of total)
2	CN V	Gasserian ganglion	May cause dumbbell tumor encompassing middle and posterior fossa and expanding foramen ovale
3	CN VII	Geniculate ganglion	Typically expands facial canal within temporal bone
Rare	CN III, IV, VI	Basal cisterns	Present with ocular motility disturbance
Rare	CN IX, X, XI	Jugular foramen	Present with nerve deficits

CN = cranial nerve, IAC = internal auditory canal, CP = cerebellopontine.

Differential Diagnosis

Meningioma
Epidermoid
Aneurysm
Metastasis

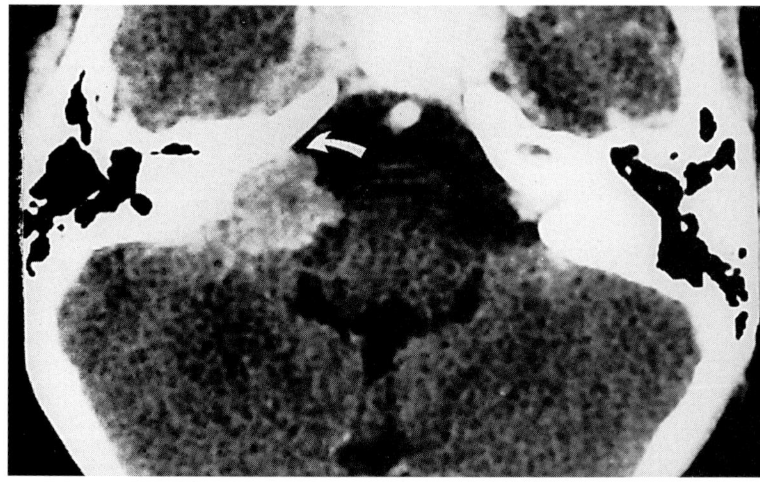

Figure 4–14. Schwannoma. CT with contrast shows a homogeneously enhancing mass in the right cerebellopontine angle. Note the acute angle formed (arrow) where the tumor abuts the temporal bone.

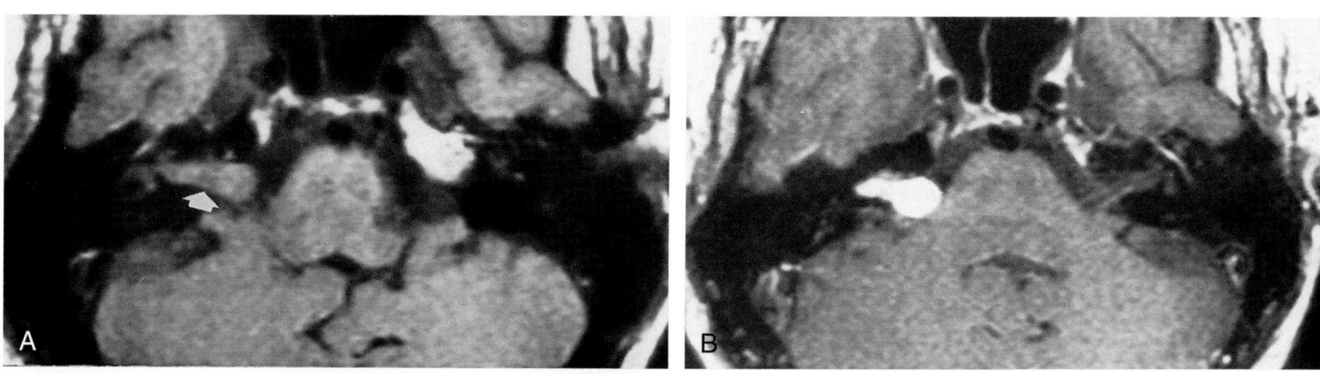

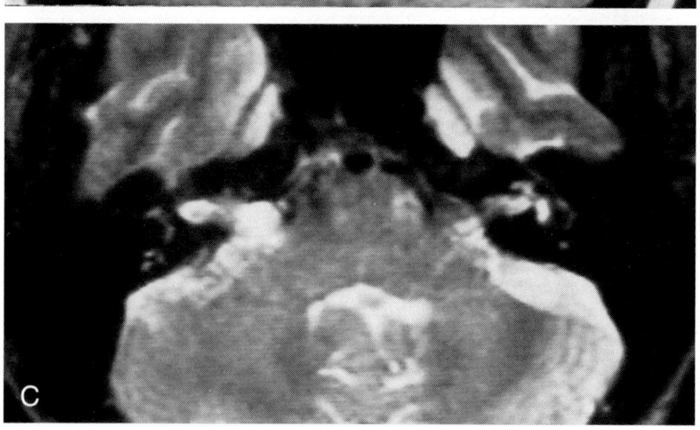

Figure 4–15. Acoustic schwannoma. **(A)** Axial T1-weighted image shows a fusiform mass (arrow) in the right internal auditory canal and cerebellopontine angle. **(B)** Following intravenous contrast there is intense homogeneous enhancement. (**C**) On T2-weighted images the tumor is hyperintense and difficult to distinguish from CSF.

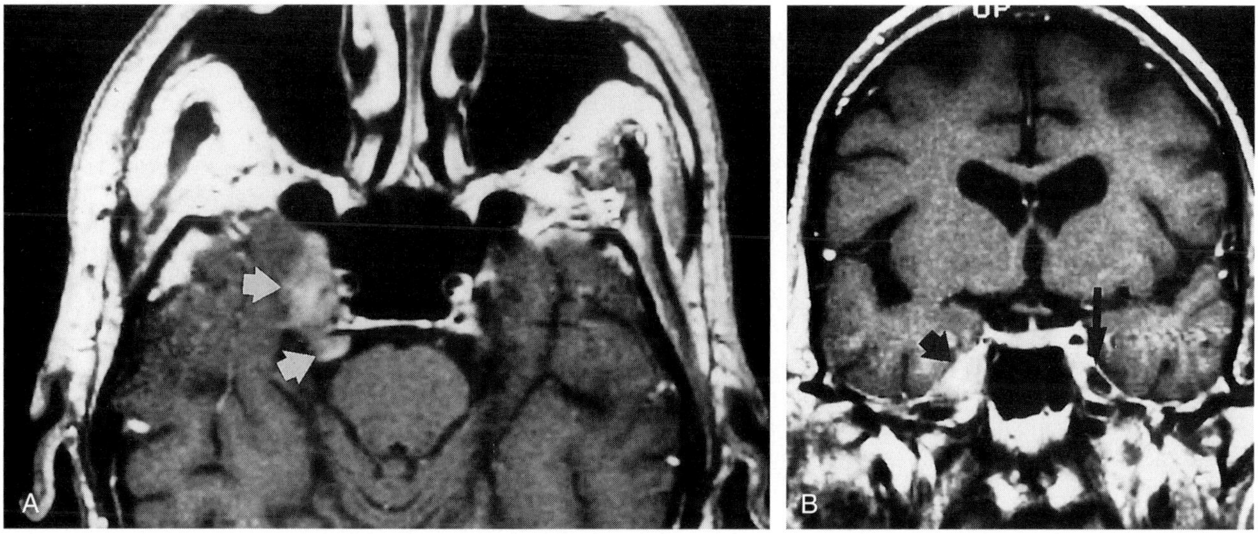

Figure 4–16. Trigeminal schwannoma. **(A)** Axial and **(B)** coronal contrast-enhanced MRI show an enhancing soft tissue mass (short arrows) in Meckel's cave and the cisternal segment of the trigeminal nerve. Long arrow indicates normal left Meckel's cave.

Pituitary Adenoma

Pituitary adenomas are common benign tumors that arise from active or inactive endocrinologic cells of the anterior pituitary. They are arbitrarily referred to as microadenomas if less than 1 cm and macroadenomas if greater than 1 cm in diameter. Microadenomas are much more common. The more common functional adenomas produce prolactin, adrenocorticotropic hormone (ACTH), or growth hormone, and patients present with somatic manifestations of hormonal overproduction. Patients with nonfunctioning adenomas present with symptoms of mass effect on adjacent structures and thus these tumors tend to be larger at the time of diagnosis. Of all intracranial neoplasms, pituitary adenomas have the highest incidence of spontaneous hemorrhage, and it is not rare for patients to present first with symptoms related to acute hemorrhage.

Location

Sella.

CT Findings

Microadenomas. With rapid, dynamic contrast scanning, microadenomas appear as areas of low attenuation within the pituitary gland. In practice, MRI should be performed whenever possible.

Macroadenomas. CT may show an isodense mass with marked enhancement and mass effect upon the optic chiasm and third ventricle. Bone destruction is common with the larger tumors, involving first the floor and dorsum of the sella.

MRI Findings

Microadenomas. The normal pituitary gland should not exceed 9 mm in height except in late pregnancy. A height of 10 mm or greater should raise strong suspicion for an adenoma. Asymmetric bulging of the top of the pituitary is a useful indirect finding. T2-weighted images are of little value. On noncontrast T1-weighted images, microadenomas most often appear as small areas of hypointensity in the pituitary gland that enhance less than the adjacent parenchyma after intravenous contrast. It is not unusual for microadenomas to be hyperintense, probably due to hemorrhage.

Macroadenomas. Macroadenomas are usually isointense with brain on T1-weighted images and hyperintense on T2-weighted images with uniform mild contrast enhancement. Marked hyperintensity or hypointensity may be present due to hemorrhage. Enlarging tumor typically elevates the optic chiasm and floor of the third ventricle. Invasion of the cavernous sinus can be diagnosed because the tumor enhances less intensely than the normal uninvolved cavernous sinus.

Differential Diagnosis

Rathke's cleft cyst produces an intrasellar mass of variable signal but does not enhance. Intrasellar craniopharyngioma is less common than adenoma and more likely to contain cysts or calcifications. Meningiomas are common in this location but nearly always off midline and unilateral (parasellar meningiomas) or anterior to the pituitary (tuberculum sella meningiomas). The pituitary gland is often heterogeneous, especially in the elderly, and focal signal abnormalities may be caused by fibrosis, infarction, or cysts of the pars intermedia. These changes cannot always be distinguished from microadenoma.

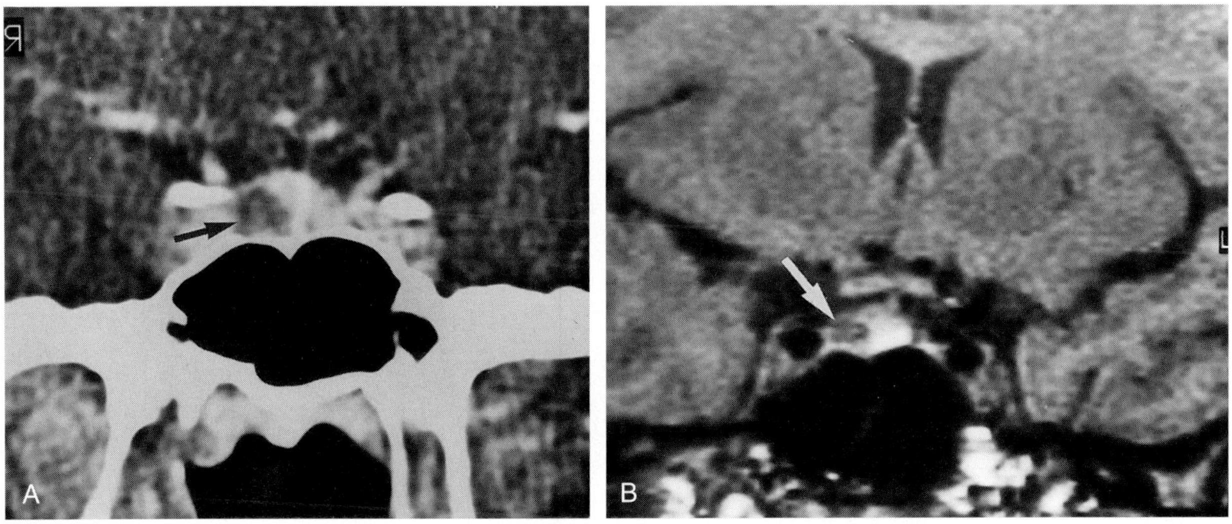

Figure 4–17. Microadenoma. **(A)** On dynamic contrast-enhanced coronal CT the adenoma (arrow) is of lower attenuation than enhancing pituitary parenchyma. The pituitary gland measures 9 mm in maximum height. **(B)** On coronal T1-weighted MRI the adenoma is hypointense relative to the pituitary. Bright signal in the pituitary is probably related to prior hemorrhage.

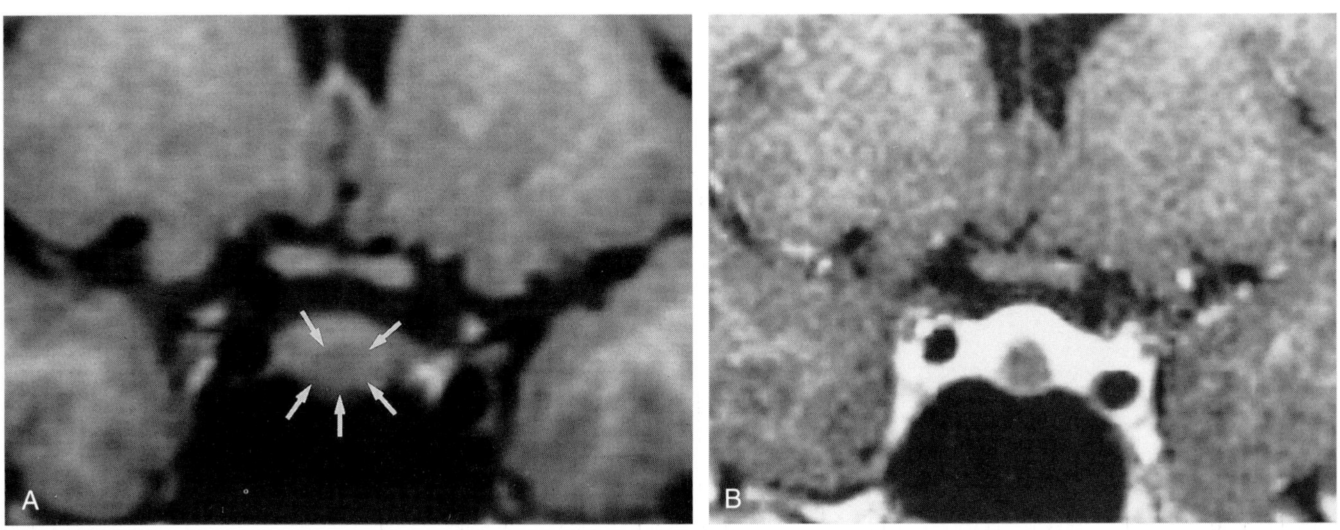

Figure 4–18. Microadenoma. **(A)** Coronal T1-weighted MRI shows a mildly hypointense mass (arrows) in the inferior pituitary gland. **(B)** Dynamic contrast-enhanced MR performed within 60 seconds of contrast injection affords striking contrast between adenoma and normal gland.

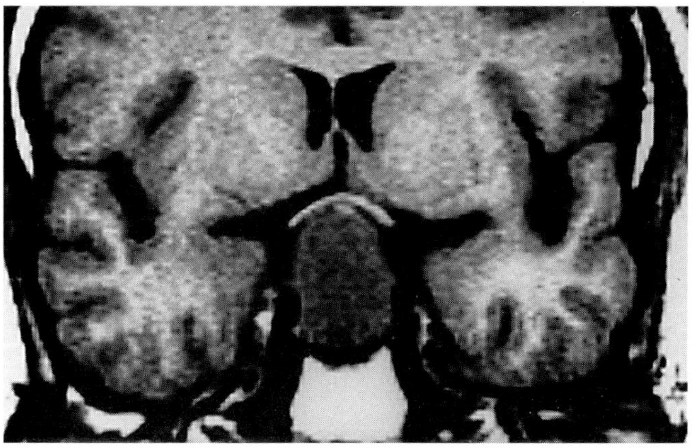

Figure 4–19. Macroadenoma. On coronal T1-weighted MRI the adenoma is isointense relative to cortical gray matter. The tumor protrudes into the suprasellar cistern with upward displacement of the optic chiasm.

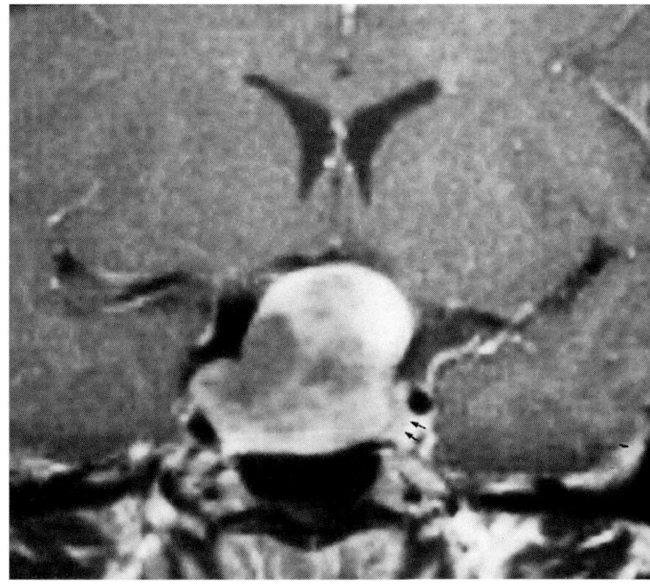

Figure 4–20. Macroadenoma. Coronal enhanced MRI shows a large pituitary adenoma with invasion of right cavernous sinus and suprasellar cistern. There is also probable invasion of the left cavernous sinus. Arrows indicate margin of tumor within left cavernous sinus.

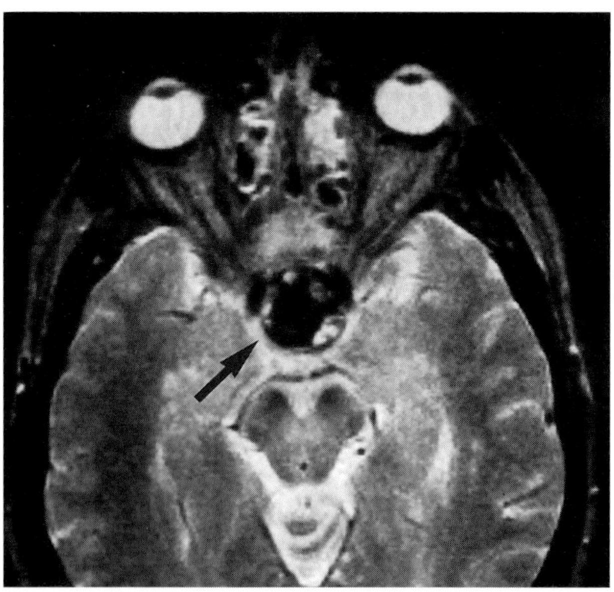

Figure 4–21. Hemorrhagic adenoma. Axial T2-weighted MRI shows marked hypointensity (arrow) due to intracellular hemoglobin breakdown products.

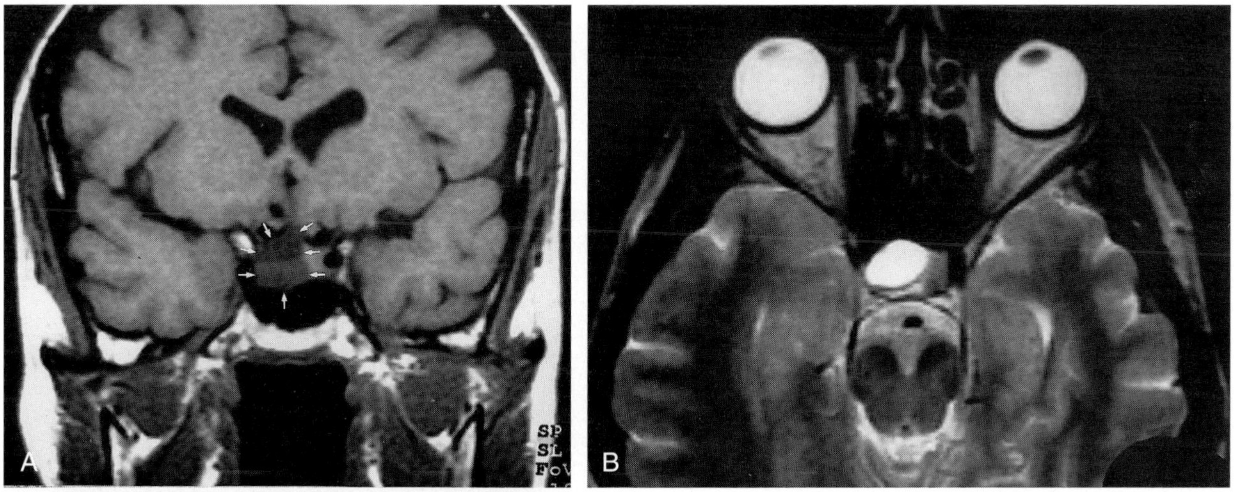

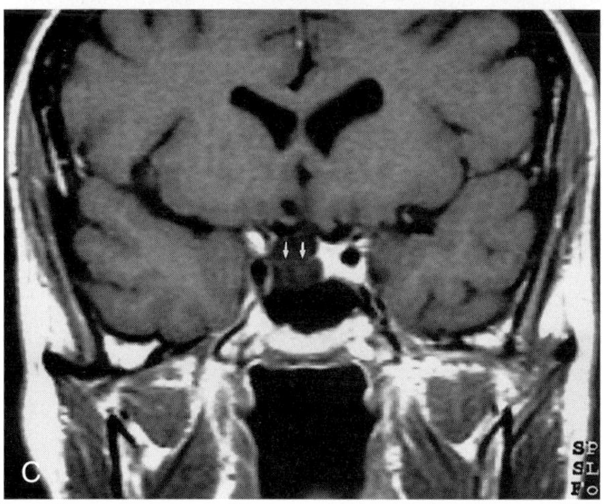

Figure 4–22. Rathke's cleft cyst. **(A)** Coronal T1-weighted MRI shows an intrasellar mass (arrows). Signal is higher than CSF but lower than normal pituitary. **(B)** On axial T2-weighted MRI the mass is extremely hyperintense. **(C)** Coronal contrast-enhanced MRI shows enhancement of the normal gland and a thin septum (arrows) but not within the mass.

Craniopharyngioma

Craniopharyngiomas are benign slow-growing tumors that arise from epithelial remnants of Rathke's pouch. Their age distribution is bimodal—with peaks during the first and second decades and the sixth decade. They constitute 50% of suprasellar tumors in children.

Location
Suprasellar with frequent extension into the sella; purely intrasellar craniopharyngiomas are rare.

CT Findings. CT shows a heterogeneous lobulated mass with dense calcifications in 80–90%. Craniopharyngiomas may range from completely cystic to completely solid but usually are composed of a combination of both. At least 70% contain some cystic component. Enhancement of the solid component occurs in 90%. CT is a helpful adjunct to MRI in the initial diagnosis of these tumors because of its greater sensitivity to calcium and the relative specificity of this finding for craniopharyngioma when seen in association with a suprasellar mass.

MRI Findings. The cystic portion of the tumor may range from hypointense to hyperintense on T1-weighted images. The solid portion manifests heterogeneous signal characteristics on T1-weighted images. The tumors are mostly hyperintense on T2-weighted images. Moderate heterogeneous enhancement of the solid component occurs following intravenous contrast. The optic chiasm and floor of the third ventricle are usually elevated. The tumor may invade overlying brain.

Differential Diagnosis

Pituitary adenoma
Optic glioma
Aneurysm

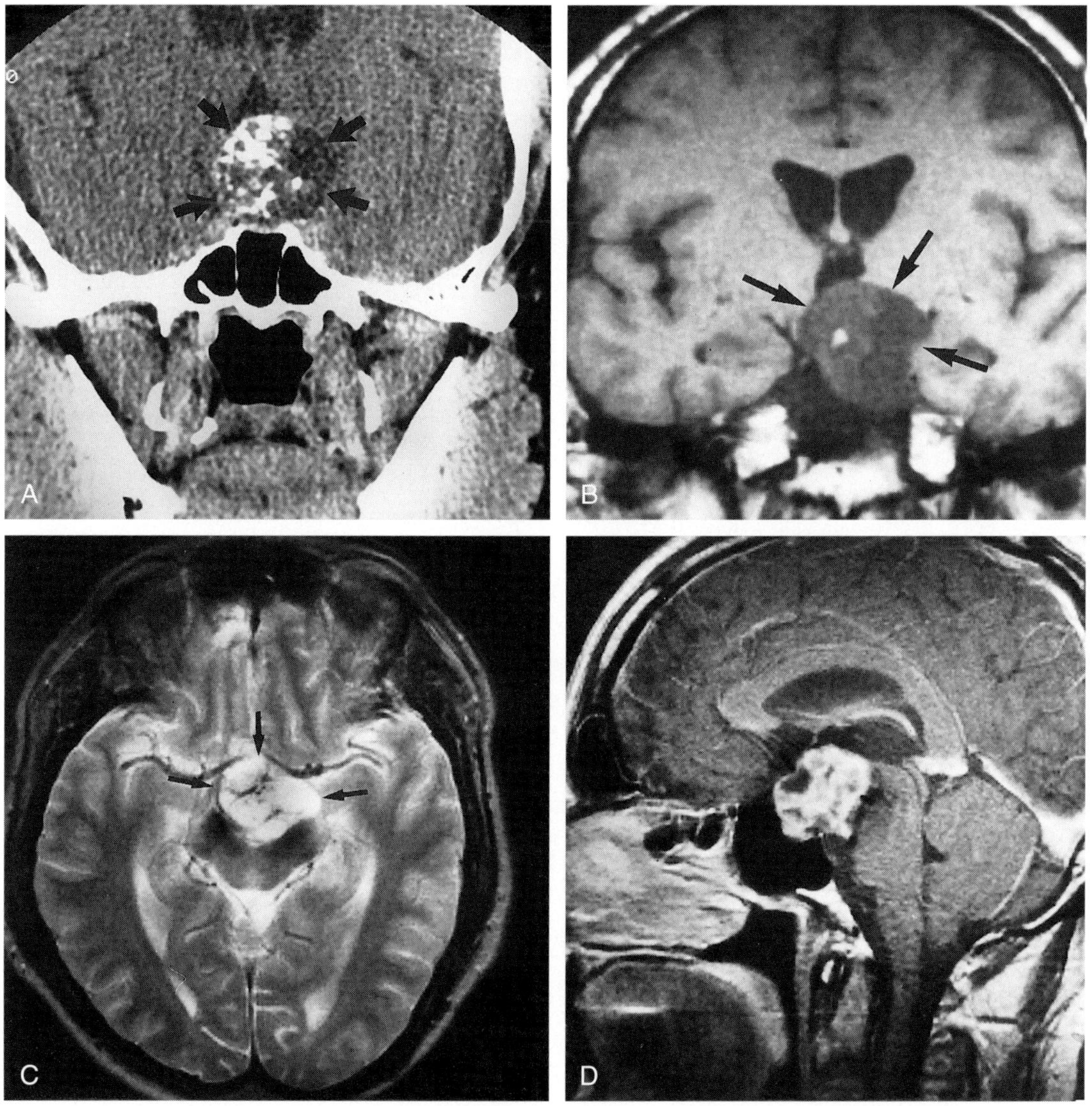

Figure 4–23. Craniopharyngioma. **(A)** Coronal CT shows a mass (arrows) with dense calcification on the right and hypodensity on the left. **(B)** Coronal T1-weighted MRI shows heterogeneous hypointensity in the mass (arrows). The focal hyperintensity may be due to calcium or hemorrhage. **(C)** On T2-weighted sequence the mass (arrows) is mostly hyperintense. The central hypointensities probably represent calcification. **(D)** Sagittal contrast-enhanced MRI shows diffuse intense enhancement with scattered small cystic areas. The mass is both intrasellar and suprasellar. There is marked elevation of the third ventricle.

Chordoma

Chordomas are rare slow-growing tumors of the primitive notochord. Notochordal cell rests may persist into adulthood usually in the midline anywhere from the dorsum sellae to the coccyx. Patients present over a wide age range with a median age in the late 30s.

Location
Nearly 50% arise from the sacrum. About 35–40% occur intracranially, arising from the clivus, basiocciput, or sella. The remainder arise in the vertebral column.

CT Findings. CT shows a clival or parasellar mass with bone destruction that is often extensive. Chordomas are hyperdense relative to brain. Nearly all enhance with contrast. Small punctate calcifications are present in up to 50%, and cystic areas may be seen in about 10%. Chordomas tend to invade the parasellar region, prepontine cistern, and nasopharynx.

MRI Findings. MRI shows a clival or parasellar mass with bone destruction. On T1-weighted images, chordomas are isointense to brain in 75% and hypointense in the remainder. Occasional bright foci are encountered due to hemorrhage or mucin. Chordomas are moderately to extremely hyperintense on T2-weighted images reflecting their cystic gelatinous nature. Most are also mildly to markedly heterogeneous on T2-weighted images. Chordomas usually appear lobulated with septations of low signal intensity and a hypointense pseudocapsule. Heterogeneous enhancement is seen following intravenous contrast. Extension into the parasellar regions, posterior fossa, and nasopharynx is common. They may also spread to the sphenoid and ethmoid sinuses, parapharyngeal and prevertebral spaces, and middle cranial fossa.

Differential Diagnosis

Destructive lesions of the clivus:
Chondroma, chondrosarcoma
Meningioma
Metastasis
Pituitary adenoma
Nasopharyngeal carcinoma

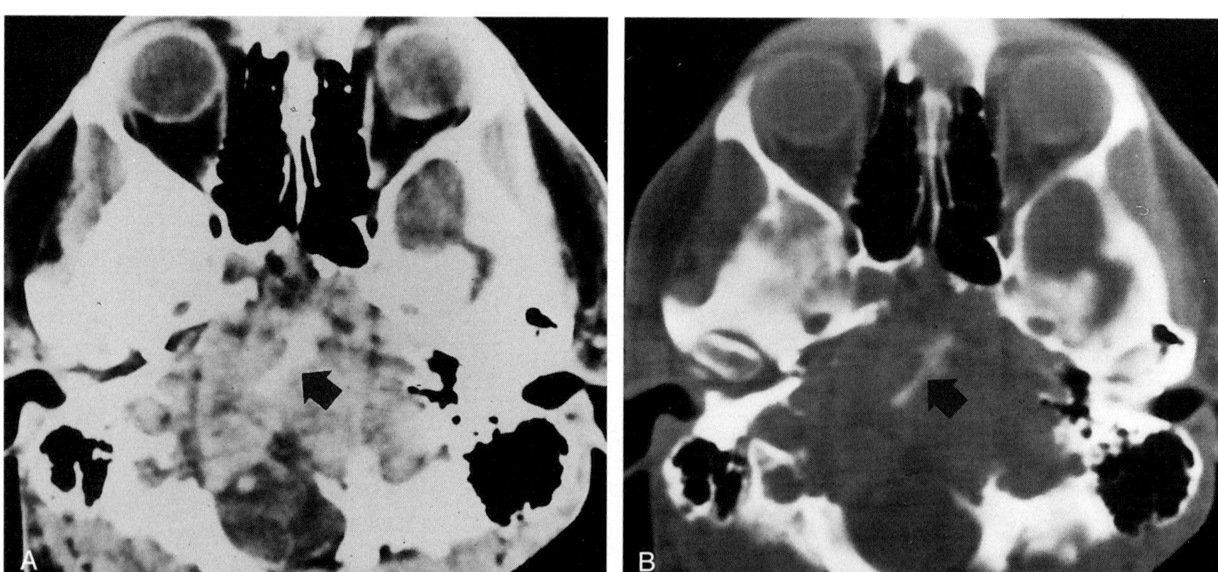

Figure 4–24. Chordoma. **(A)** Axial contrast-enhanced CT shows an enhancing mass of the clivus. **(B)** Bone window shows extensive destruction of the clivus, petrous apices, and sphenoid. Central high attenuation (arrow) represents tumor calcification or bone fragment. (Courtesy of Dr. Pamela Van Tassel, Charleston, SC.)

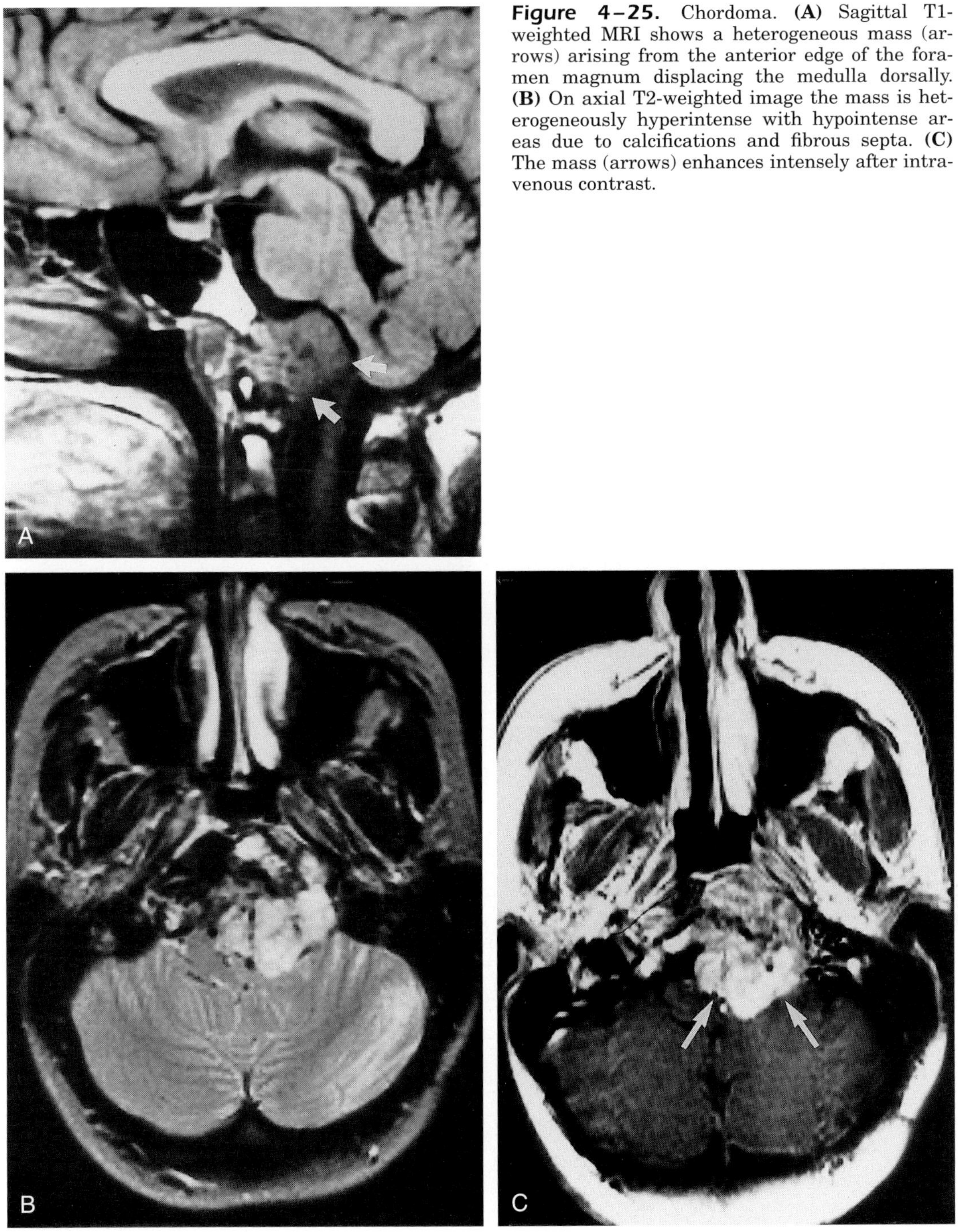

Figure 4–25. Chordoma. **(A)** Sagittal T1-weighted MRI shows a heterogeneous mass (arrows) arising from the anterior edge of the foramen magnum displacing the medulla dorsally. **(B)** On axial T2-weighted image the mass is heterogeneously hyperintense with hypointense areas due to calcifications and fibrous septa. **(C)** The mass (arrows) enhances intensely after intravenous contrast.

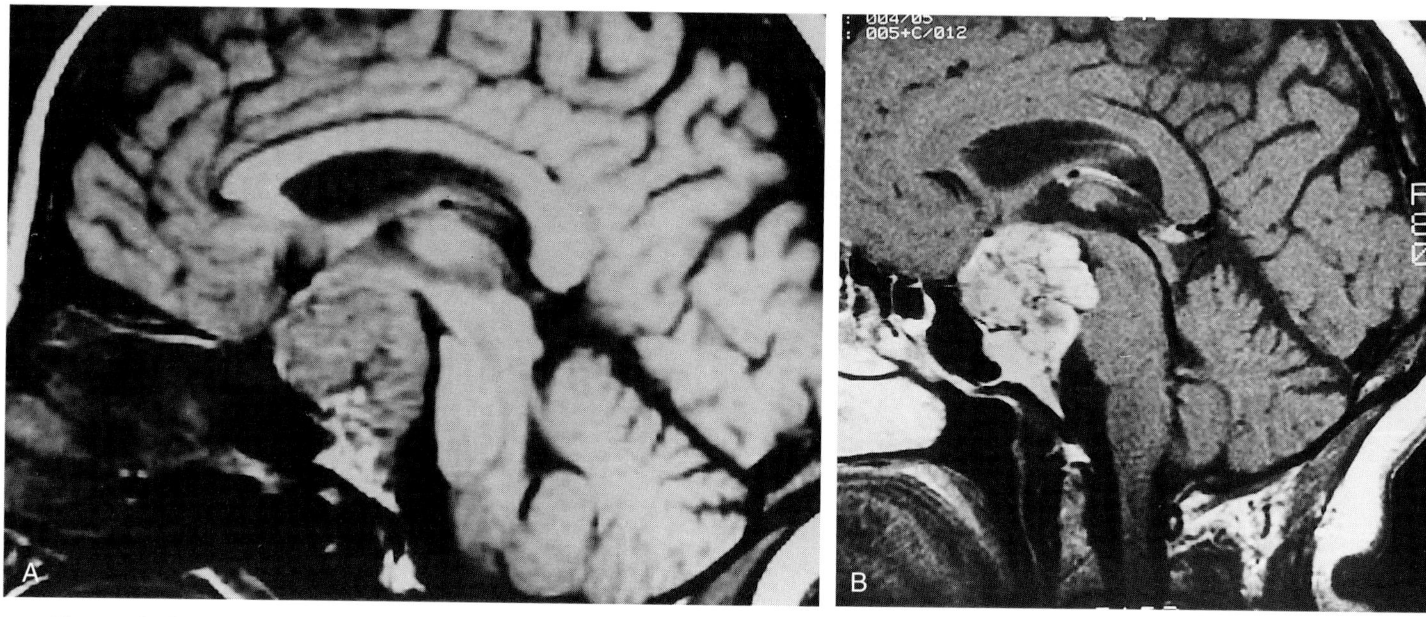

Figure 4–26. Chordoma. **(A)** Sagittal T1-weighted MRI shows a heterogeneous mass destoying the sella and upper clivus. **(B)** Diffuse enhancement is seen after intravenous contrast. Linear hypointensities in **B** indicate the fibrous septa typical of chordomas.

Meningeal Metastasis

Systemic malignancies may spread hematogeneously to the arachnoid and choroid plexus and once established may disseminate freely throughout the CSF. The brain may be secondarily invaded by meningeal tumor deposits. Neuroimaging, especially contrast-enhanced MRI, plays a complementary role to CSF cytology in the diagnosis of meningeal metastases. Tumors that disseminate within the CSF are listed in Table 4–12.

Location

Subarachnoid space, especially suprasellar cistern, ependyma of the lateral ventricles, cortical sulci, and virtually anywhere else that meninges are present or CSF circulates.

TABLE 4–12 | Tumors That Disseminate Within the CSF

Primary CNS tumors
Medulloblastoma (up to 80%)
Ependymoma (up to 30%)
Germinoma
Pinealoma
Glioblastoma
Primitive neuroectodermal tumor
Systemic neoplasms
Lymphoma
Leukemia
Lung carcinoma (especially small cell)
Breast carcinoma
Melanoma
Retinoblastoma

CT Findings. In the case of meningeal tumor seeding, intravenous contrast is essential for its detection. Four CT findings have classically been described: (1) obliteration and enhancement of cisterns and sulci, (2) ependymal enhancement, (3) thickened enhancing tentorium, and (4) communicating hydrocephalus. Overall, CT is quite insensitive for meningeal tumor involvement.

MRI Findings. Unenhanced MRI is rather insensitive in the detection of meningeal metastases, as the signal characteristics of the tumor deposits are often similar to CSF on both T1- and T2-weighted sequences. Larger deposits are of slightly higher intensity than CSF on T1-weighted images. After intravenous contrast, however, there may be mild to striking leptomeningeal, ependymal, or dural enhancement usually linear or finely nodular. Less commonly, meningeal metastases may present as bulky, single or multiple, extraaxial or intraventricular solid tumors.

Differential Diagnosis

Postoperative fibrosis
Subarachnoid hemorrhage
Sarcoidosis
Meningitis
Postinfarction gyral enhancement
Gliomatosis cerebri
Pachymeningitis

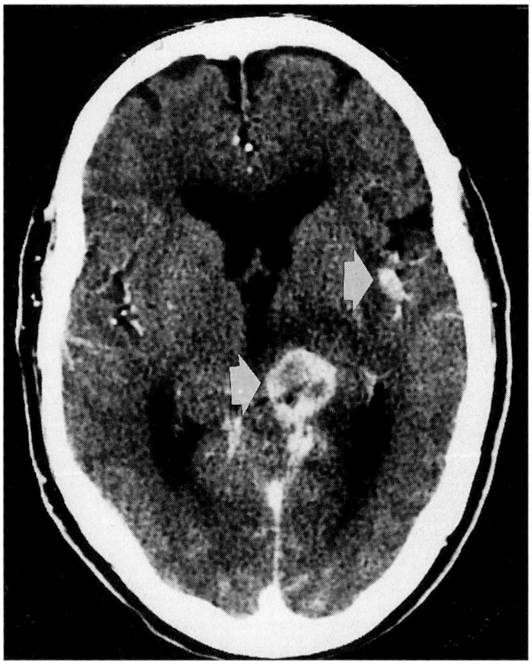

Figure 4–27. Meningeal metastases. CT shows enhancing masses (arrows) in the left sylvian fissure and the left quadrigeminal cistern and choroid fissure due to meningeal spread of systemic lymphoma.

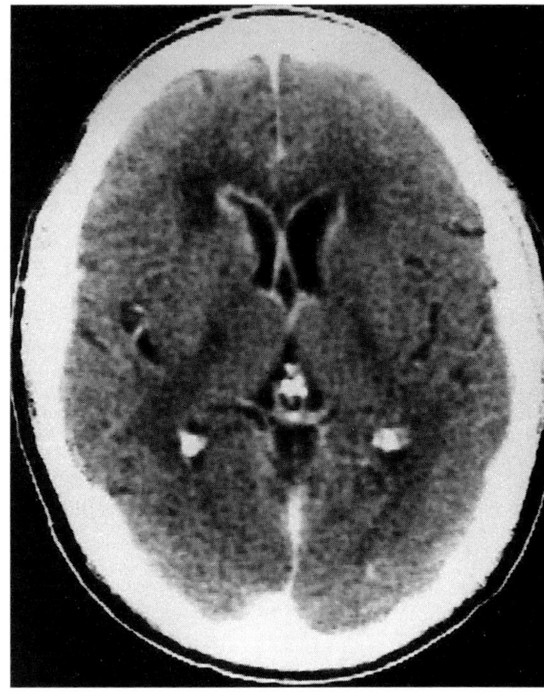

Figure 4–28. Subependymal metastases. Contrast-enhanced CT shows bilateral ependymal enhancement of the frontal horns due to metastatic oat cell carcinoma.

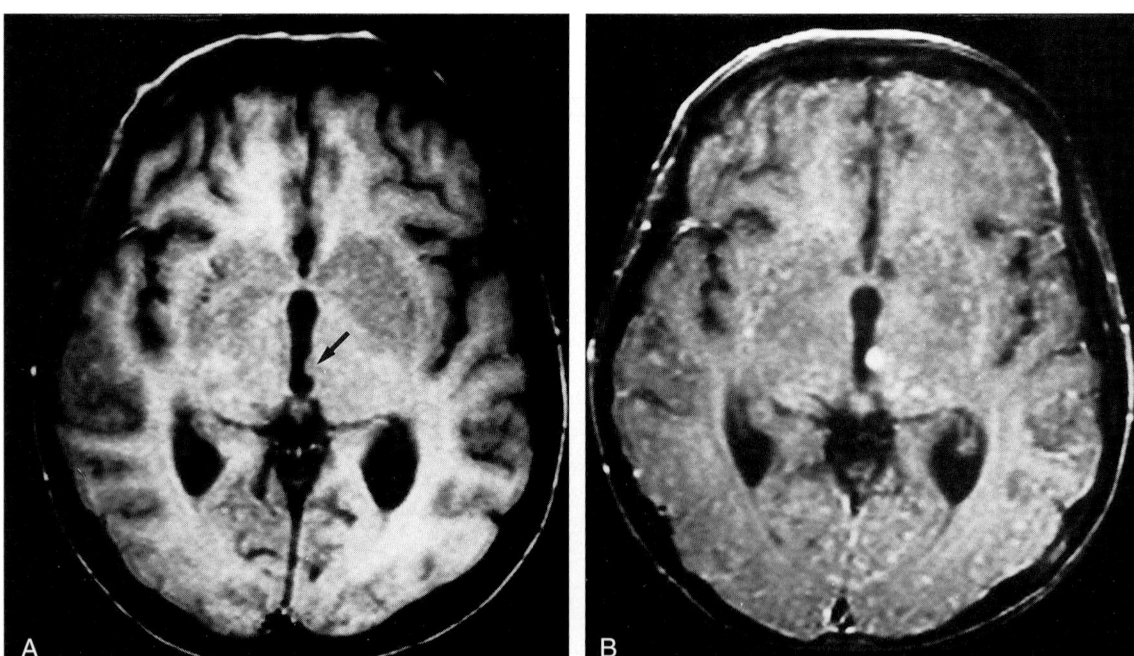

Figure 4–29. Meningeal metastases. **(A)** Axial T1-weighted image shows only a small subependymal nodule (arrow) in the third ventricle. **(B)** After intravenous contrast, there is diffuse finely nodular enhancement of pial surfaces of the brain and brain parenchyma.

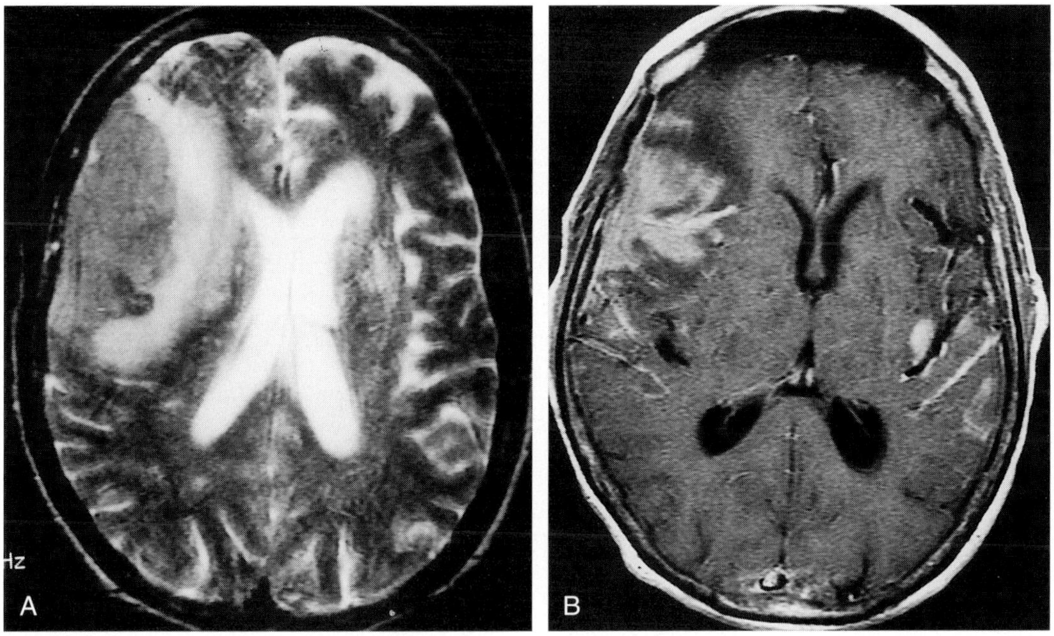

Figure 4–30. Meningeal metastases (lymphoma). **(A)** T2-weighted MRI shows a right frontal mass with broad pial interface and vasogenic edema. **(B)** Axial contrast-enhanced MRI shows an extensive enhancement in the subarachnoid spaces. The right side manifests secondary parenchymal invasion by meningeal lymphoma.

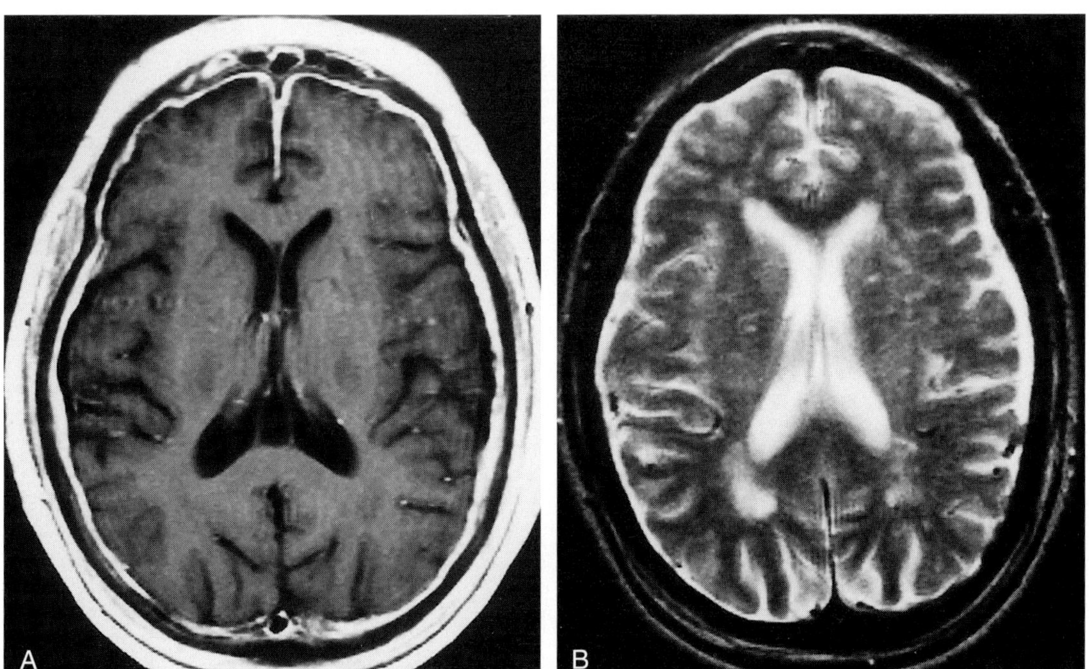

Figure 4–31. Dural-arachnoid carcinomatosis (metastatic adenocarcinoma). **(A)** Axial contrast-enhanced MRI shows bilateral diffuse enhancement of thickened arachnoid and/or dura (the two cannot be distinguished). **(B)** On T2-weighted sequence the hyperintense dura cannot be distinguished from subdural fluid.

Intraaxial Tumors

Gliomas

The glial cells of the brain include astrocytes, oligodendrocytes, and ependymal cells. Glioma is an all-encompassing term that applies to a neoplasm of any of these cell lines. Many individual tumors contain a mixture of various cell lines. Astrocytomas constitute 75–90% of all gliomas. It has been common to classify astrocytomas into one of four grades (I–IV) according to the degree of malignant transformation. A more current and practical classification system uses three stages: low grade (fibrillary) astrocytomas, anaplastic astrocytomas, and glioblastoma multiforme. Less common forms include pilocytic astrocytomas (juvenile and adult), protoplasmic astrocytomas, gemistocytic astrocytomas, and giant cell astrocytomas. Pure protoplasmic and gemistocytic astrocytomas are quite rare and are not discussed. Giant cell astrocytomas are almost unique to individuals affected with tuberous sclerosis and are discussed below and in Chapter 2. Table 4–13 presents a summary of tumors of astrocytic origin.

TABLE 4–13 | Tumors of Astrocytic Origin

	Pilocytic	Giant Cell	Fibrillary	Anaplastic	Glioblastoma
Peak age	1–20 years, mean 7	10–15 years	1–35 years	35–45 years	45–55 years
Location	Chiasm and cerebellum	Intraventricular	Variable	Frontal and parietal	Frontal and temporal
CT attenuation	Hypodense or isodense	Isodense or hyperdense	Hypodense	Hypodense	Mixed and hyperdense
MRI: T1	Isointense or hypointense	Mixed	Hypointense	Hypointense	Hypointense
MRI: T2	Hyperintense	Mixed	Hyperintense	Hyperintense	Hyperintense
Texture	Inhomogeneous	Homogeneous	Homogeneous	Variable	Inhomogeneous
Margins	Smooth and sharp	Sharp	Smooth	Smooth in 50%	Irregular
Enhancement	Nearly all	Intense and homogeneous	None	Present in 60%	Thick irregular ring
Cysts/necrosis	Cysts common	None	Rare	Common	Necrosis in nearly all
Calcifications	About 10%	Common	About 25%	10–20%	Less than 5%
Edema	Minimal or absent	None	Minimal	About 50%	Extensive

Glioblastoma Multiforme

Glioblastoma multiforme represents the most extreme malignant transformation of a glial cell line yet at the same time is the most common, comprising up to 60% of all gliomas and 40% of primary brain neoplasms. These tumors possess all the histologic features of a highly malignant tumor with marked hypercellularity and anaplasia, frequent mitotic figures, necrosis, and hypervascularity. They are rapidly growing tumors with a heterogeneous appearance usually including grossly visible areas of hemorrhage and necrosis. The prognosis is dismal with a mean survival after diagnosis of less than 1 year.

Location
Frontal lobes, followed by temporal lobes; spread through the corpus callosum and involvement of deeper structures is common.

CT Findings. Glioblastomas are heterogeneous before contrast with areas of both high and low attenuation. A complete or partial ring may be visible prior to intravenous contrast because of the almost invariable presence of necrotic foci. Calcifications are rare. Rim enhancement is always present in a unilocular or multilocular configuration. Edema tends to be prominent with a margin around the tumor usually exceeding 1 cm.

MRI Findings. MRI typically reveals a poorly defined mass with heterogeneous signal on T1- and T2-weighted images. Mass effect and edema are prominent. Both tumor extent and related edema show a marked preference for white matter. Hemorrhage occurs in a higher percentage than in the lower grade astrocytomas. The tumor may spread along white matter tracts (especially the corpus callosum), disseminate through the cerebral parenchyma, or spread along the ependyma of the ventricles or leptomeninges on the brain surface.

Differential Diagnosis

Abscess
Radiation necrosis
Enhancing infarct
Ependymoma
Metastasis

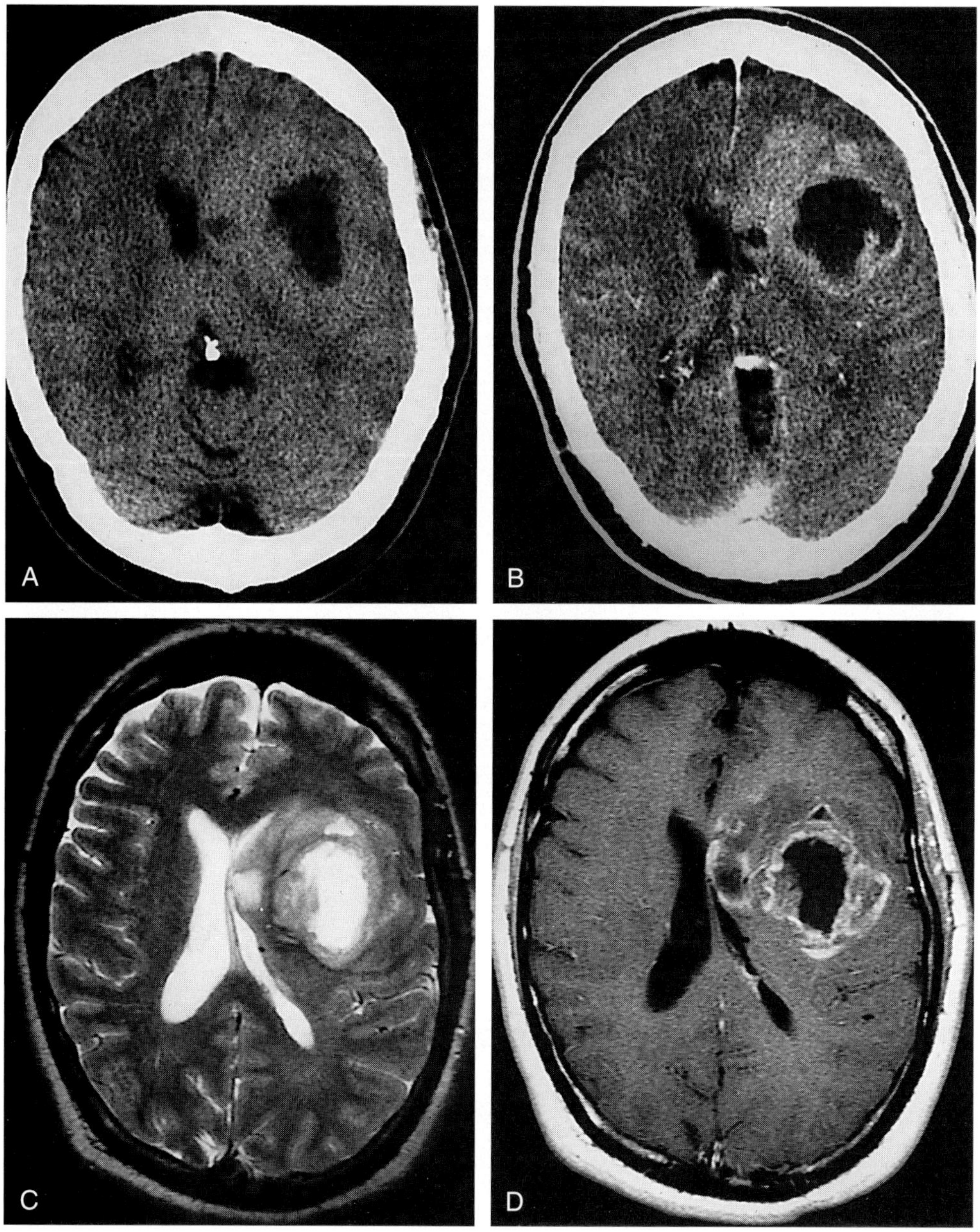

Figure 4–32. Glioblastoma multiforme. **(A)** Unenhanced CT shows a mildly hyperdense left frontal lobe mass with a large hypodense area of necrosis. The left lateral ventricle is compressed. **(B)** Postcontrast scan shows both solid enhancement anteriorly and irregular ring enhancement along the margins of the necrotic cavity. **(C)** T2-weighted MRI shows the hyperintense mass with very little edema. The necrotic cavity is isointense with CSF. **(D)** Postcontrast MRI shows thick irregular ring enhancement.

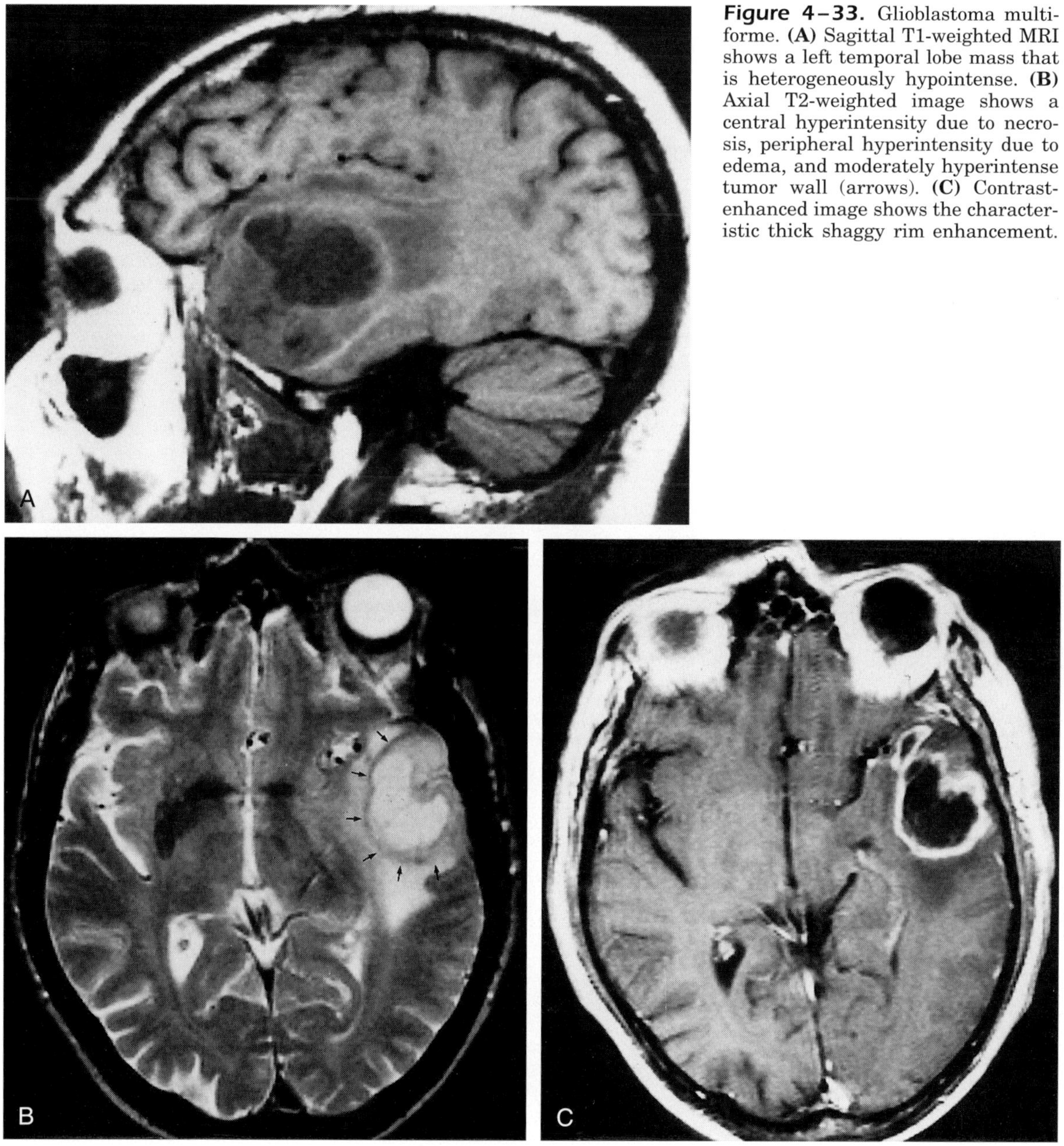

Figure 4–33. Glioblastoma multiforme. **(A)** Sagittal T1-weighted MRI shows a left temporal lobe mass that is heterogeneously hypointense. **(B)** Axial T2-weighted image shows a central hyperintensity due to necrosis, peripheral hyperintensity due to edema, and moderately hyperintense tumor wall (arrows). **(C)** Contrast-enhanced image shows the characteristic thick shaggy rim enhancement.

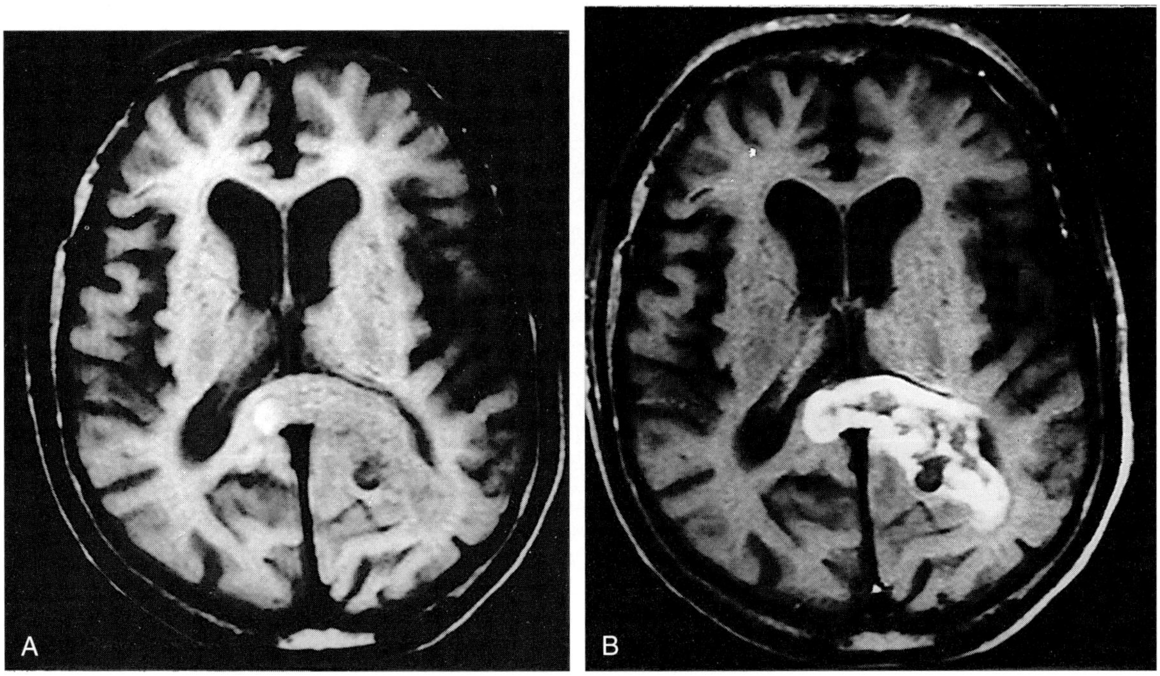

Figure 4–34. Glioblastoma multiforme. T1-weighted MRI **(A)** before and **(B)** after contrast shows markedly enhancing tumor crossing the midline via the splenium of the corpus callosum. Transcallosal spread is usually associated with malignant glial tumors but lymphoma may occasionally involve the corpus callosum.

Anaplastic Astrocytoma

Anaplastic astrocytomas probably arise from malignant transformation of low grade tumors and thus appear in a slightly older age group. Their pathology, clinical behavior, and imaging characteristics are intermediate between low-grade astrocytomas and glioblastomas. Pathology reveals hypercellularity and anaplasia; they are differentiated from glioblastomas by the absence of vascular proliferation, hemorrhage, and necrosis. The prognosis is poor with a median survival of 1 to 3 years.

Location
Frontal lobes (50%) and parietal lobes (25%), followed by temporal and occipital lobes.

CT Findings. These tumors exhibit CT characteristics intermediate between the low grade astrocytoma and the glioblastoma. Hence, mixed attenuation, edema, mass effect, and enhancement may all be present but not with the frequency or degree to which these are seen in glioblastoma. Its enhancement pattern may range from none to complex and ringlike.

MRI Findings. These tumors are homogeneously hypointense on T1-weighted and hyperintense on T2-weighted MRI. They may appear homogeneous or heterogeneous with equal frequency. The margins are smooth in 50%. Contrast enhancement occurs in 60%, which may be minimal to marked and solid or irregular. Edema with moderate mass effect is present in approximately 50%. Involvement of the corpus callosum is common.

Differential Diagnosis

Abscess
Radiation necrosis
Enhancing infarct
Ependymoma
Metastasis
Glioblastoma

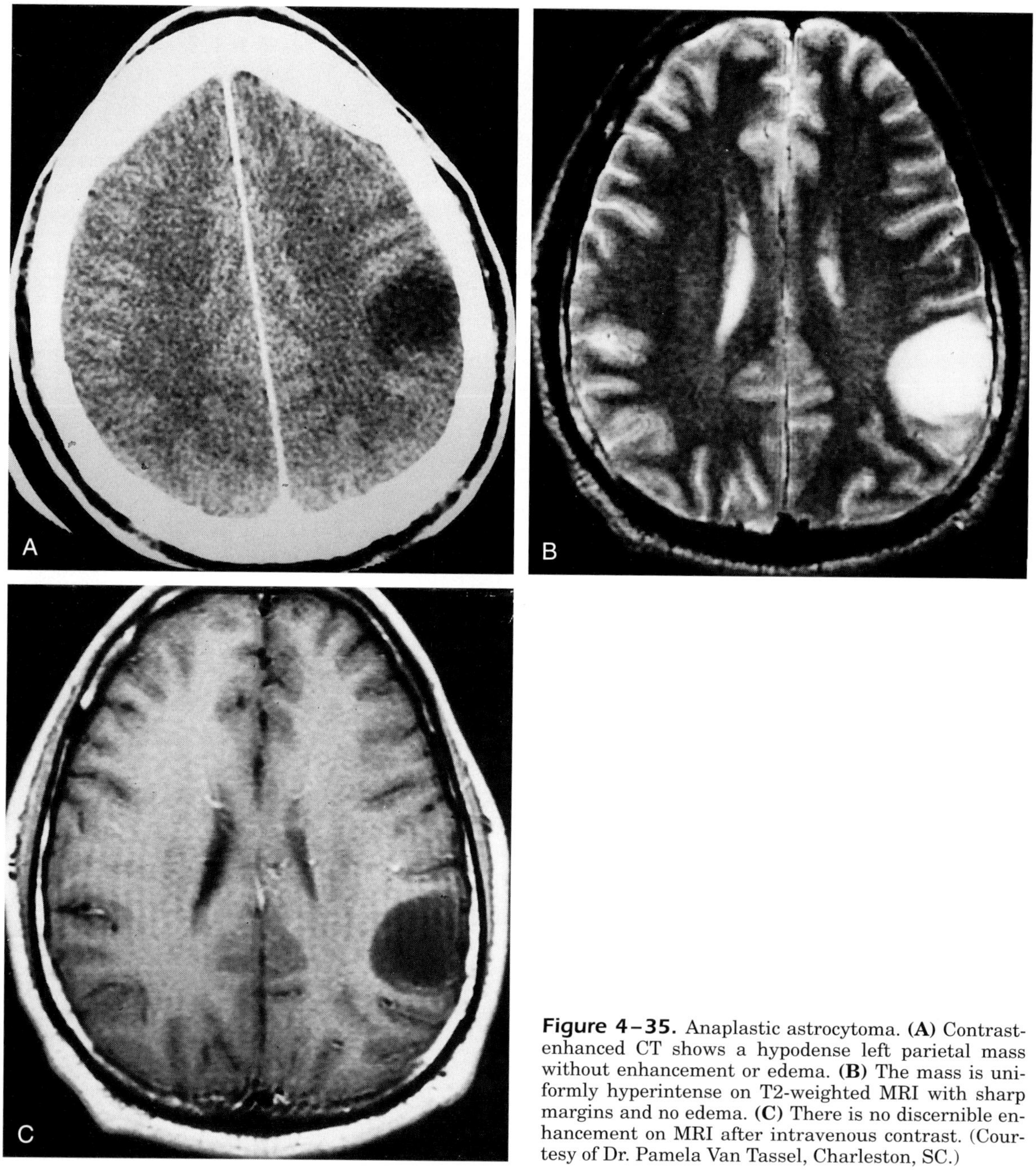

Figure 4–35. Anaplastic astrocytoma. **(A)** Contrast-enhanced CT shows a hypodense left parietal mass without enhancement or edema. **(B)** The mass is uniformly hyperintense on T2-weighted MRI with sharp margins and no edema. **(C)** There is no discernible enhancement on MRI after intravenous contrast. (Courtesy of Dr. Pamela Van Tassel, Charleston, SC.)

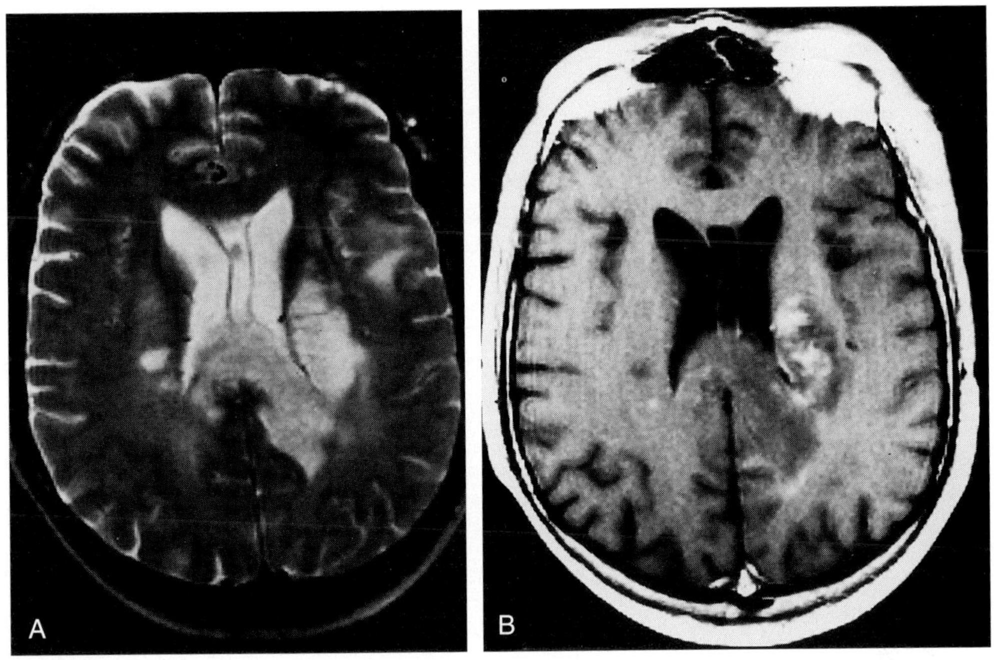

Figure 4–36. Anaplastic astrocytoma. **(A)** Axial T2-weighted MRI shows a hyperintense mass with irregular borders involving the left periventricular white matter and splenium of the corpus callosum. **(B)** Contrast-enhanced scan shows patchy irregular enhancement of the tumor.

Fibrillary Astrocytoma

Fibrillary astrocytes are the major supporting cell of the white matter from which most astrocytomas arise. Low-grade tumors of the fibrillary astrocytes are composed of a local proliferation of mostly normal-appearing astrocytes. Mitoses, necrosis, and vascular proliferation are absent. The margins are ill defined due to infiltration of adjacent brain, and tumor cellularity is often only minimally increased relative to normal white matter. Most patients survive for many years, although in some cases early malignant transformation occurs, leading to death within months.

Location
Cerebral hemispheres, brainstem.

CT Findings. CT shows a well-defined low attenuation mass without contrast enhancement. Calcifications occur in approximately 25%. Hemorrhage occurs in 10–15%. Cysts are unusual, although the uniformly low attenuation mass with smooth sharp margins may itself resemble a cyst. The attenuation of some solid masses may be almost equal to that of CSF.

MRI Findings. MRI shows a well-defined mass that is hypointense on T1-weighted images and homogeneously hyperintense on T2-weighted images with very little edema. The area of signal abnormality is typically larger on the T2-weighted scans. Cysts are atypical, and necrosis does not occur. Hemorrhage may be present in 10–15%.

Differential Diagnosis

The differential diagnosis includes other tumors that may lack enhancement, such as ganglioglioma, oligodendroglioma, hamartoma, and anaplastic astrocytoma.

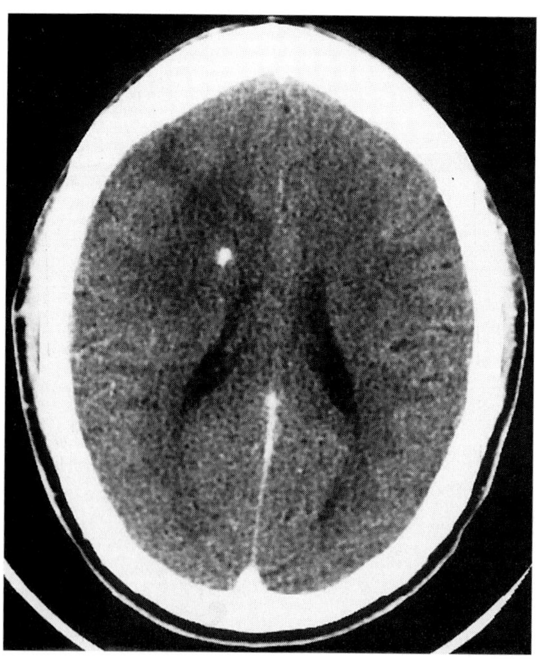

Figure 4–37. Fibrillary astrocytoma. Contrast-enhanced CT shows a hypodense right frontal lobe mass with focal calcification and absence of enhancement.

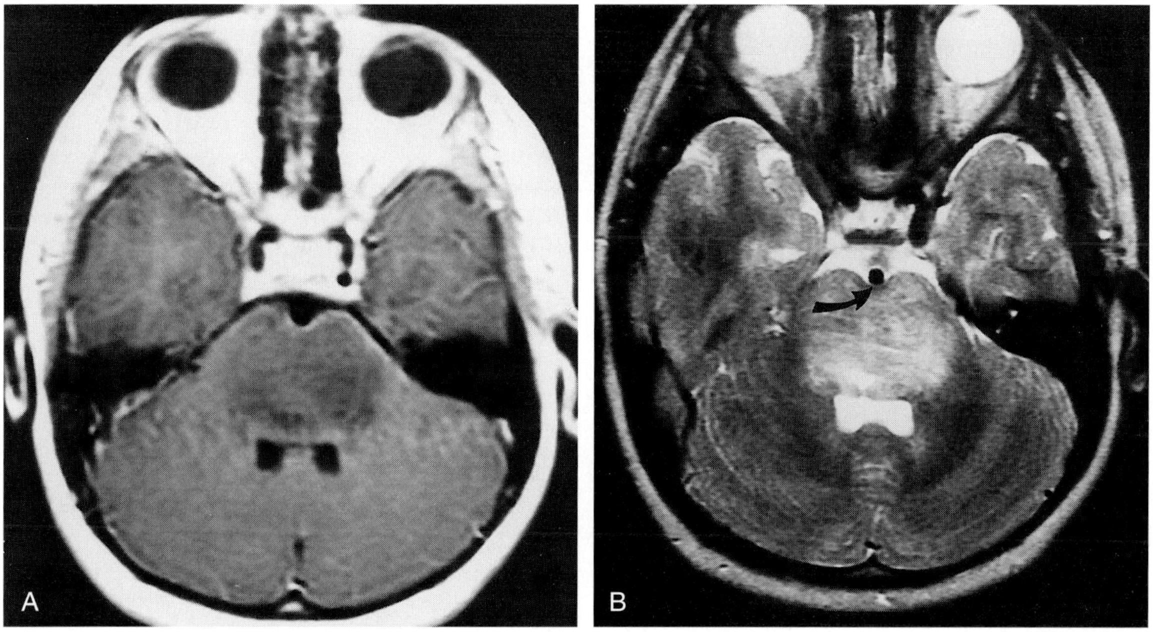

Figure 4–38. Brainstem glioma (probable fibrillary astrocytoma). **(A)** Axial contrast-enhanced MRI shows an enlarged pons without enhancement. **(B)** T2-weighted MRI shows hyperintensity within the enlarged pons. Anterior growth of these tumors tends to engulf the basilar artery (arrow).

Oligodendroglioma

Oligodendrogliomas are gliomas of the oligodendrocytes, which are responsible for the myelination of axons. They are most common from 35 to 40 years of age and are very slow growing. Histology reveals patternless sheets of cells with rare mitoses and absence of anaplastic changes. Calcification is present on histology in 70% or more. As many as 50% are actually mixed tumors with both oligodendroglial and astrocytic components. Postoperative survival averages 5 to 10 years.

Location

In decreasing order, the frontal, parietal, temporal, or occipital white matter.

CT Findings. CT commonly shows a large, round or oval, sharply defined mass of low or intermediate attenuation. Enhancement tends to be faint and heterogeneous and occurs in about 50%. Peripheral flecks or clumps of calcification may be seen in about 40%; it may be very extensive. Hemorrhage or cysts are each present in about 20%. Because the tumors are slow growing, calvarial erosion may occasionally occur.

MRI Findings. Oligodendrogliomas are mostly hypointense on T1-weighted images and hyperintense on T2-weighted images with marked heterogeneity due to cysts, calcification, or hemorrhage. The margins are usually sharp, and edema is mild or absent. As with CT, contrast enhancement is mild or absent.

Differential Diagnosis

Ganglioglioma
Low-grade astrocytomas

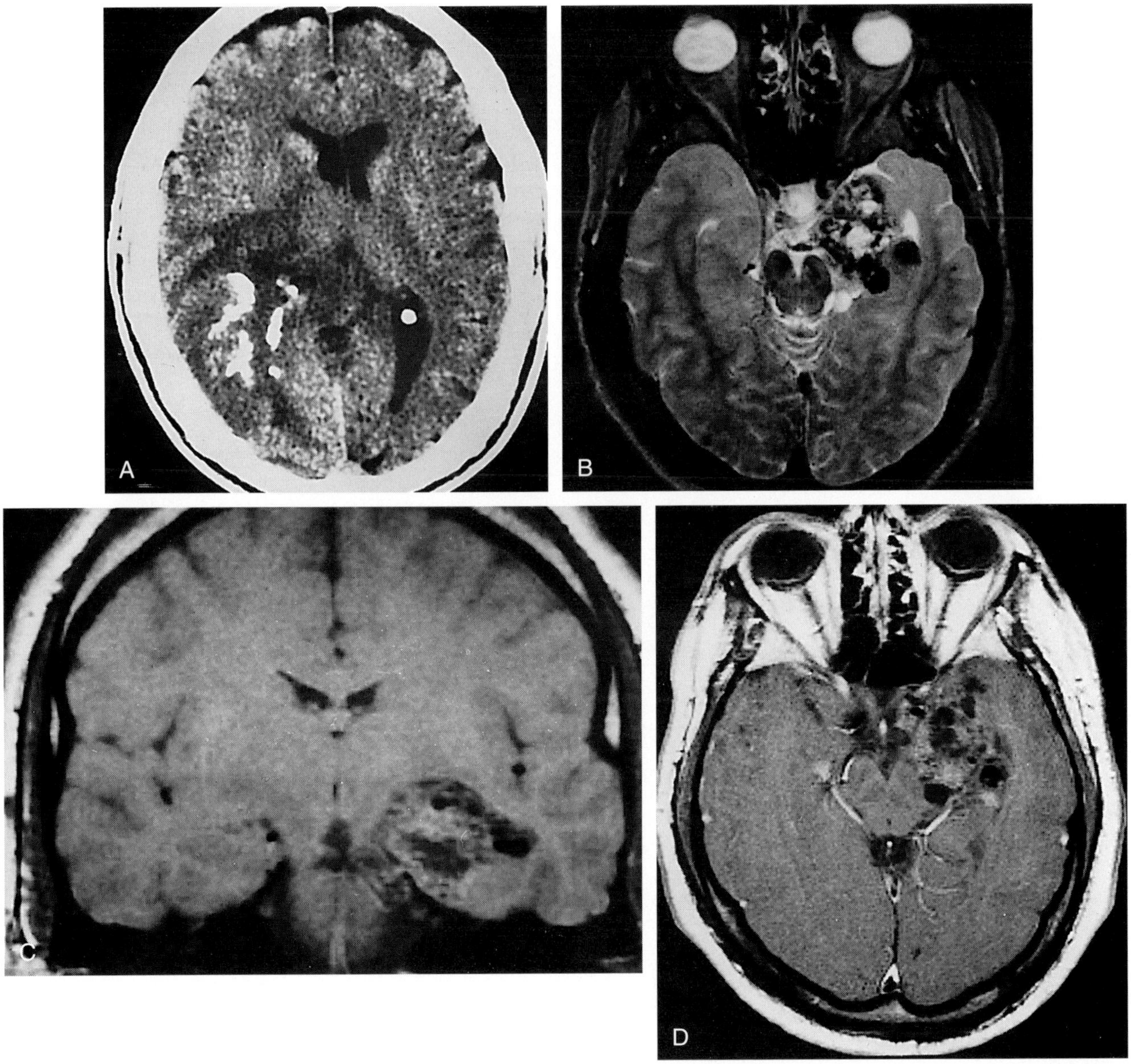

Figure 4–39. Oligodendroglioma. **(A)** CT without contrast shows a predominantly hypodense right parietal mass with dense nodular and confluent calcification. There was no significant enhancement after contrast (not shown). **(B)** Axial T2-weighted MRI shows a heterogeneous mass of the left temporal lobe. Marked hypointensities are due to dense calcification, and the uncalcified portions are hyperintense. **(C)** On coronal T1-weighted MRI the mass remains heterogeneous with both hyperintense and hypointense areas. **(D)** Axial contrast-enhanced MRI shows very mild enhancement within uncalcified portions of the tumor.

Ganglioglioma

Synonym: Neuroastrocytoma.

The ganglioglioma is an unusual low-grade neoplasm composed of both neuronal (ganglionic) and glial cell lines. It typically occurs in the second decade of life with a progressive seizure disorder. These tumors are indolent with a survival time of years; some cases may be cured by surgical resection. Ganglioneuromas (gangliocytomas) are similar tumors composed exclusively of neuronal elements.

Location

Temporal lobes most common but may occur anywhere in the CNS.

CT Findings. CT usually reveals a well-circumscribed isodense or hypodense mass with calcifications in 35% and enhancement in 50%. The calcifications may be quite solid and dense. At times, calcification may be the only finding. Cysts are present in about 30% and may predominate. Edema is not usually seen.

MRI Findings. The solid components have a variable appearance on T1-weighted images with low, intermediate, or high signal intensity. These tumors are usually hyperintense on T2-weighted images. The cystic components are hypointense on T1-weighted images and hyperintense on T2-weighted images. Enhancement after intravenous contrast may occur. Edema and mass effect are minimal or absent.

Differential Diagnosis

Oligodendroglioma
Low-grade astrocytoma
Ependymoma

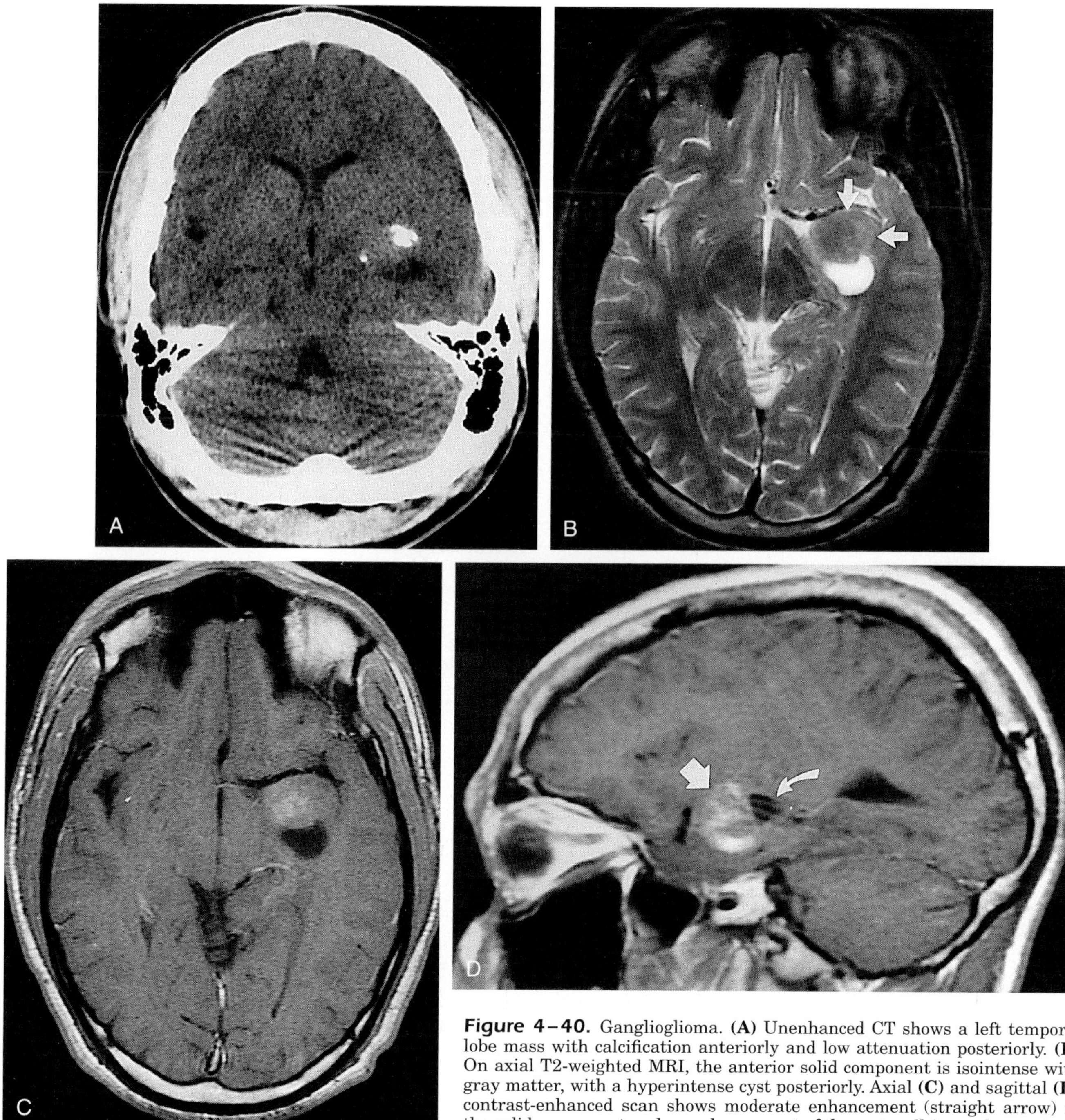

Figure 4–40. Ganglioglioma. **(A)** Unenhanced CT shows a left temporal lobe mass with calcification anteriorly and low attenuation posteriorly. **(B)** On axial T2-weighted MRI, the anterior solid component is isointense with gray matter, with a hyperintense cyst posteriorly. Axial **(C)** and sagittal **(D)** contrast-enhanced scan shows moderate enhancement (straight arrow) in the solid component and no enhancement of the cyst wall (curved arrow).

Lymphoma

Synonyms: Microglioma, reticulum cell sarcoma.

Lymphoma of the CNS may be primary or secondary. Primary CNS lymphoma is usually the diffuse large cell type of B cell origin and accounts for about one half of CNS lymphoma cases. It is most common in patients over 60 years of age. Lymphoma is the second most common intracranial mass lesion in AIDS patients, and its incidence is increasing in both AIDS and non-AIDS patients. The median survival is approximately 2 years after diagnosis.

Post-transplant lymphoproliferative disorder represents a neoplastic proliferation of lymphocytes in transplant recipients on immunosupression. It differs from true lymphoma in being of polyclonal origin. This disorder responds to the cessation of immunosuppressive therapy.

Location

Parenchymal mass nearly always in contact with the ependyma or meninges. Approximately one third to one half arise in deep structures (thalamus, basal ganglia, corpus callosum), and the rest in lobar white matter or vermis.

CT Findings. CT reveals an isodense or hyperdense mass usually with marked homogeneous enhancement, mild mass effect, and minimal edema. About one half of patients present with multiple lesions, although generally not more than four. The lesions tend to abut ventricular or pial surfaces and in the latter case may be confused with meningiomas. Lymphoma may occasionally cause extensive gyral enhancement. Calcifications are not seen.

AIDS-related lymphoma is more often multiple (frequently exceeding four lesions) and more often ring enhancing with areas of necrosis.

MRI Findings. Lymphoma appears on MRI as a sharply defined round or oval mass, slightly hypointense on T1-weighted images and hypointense to slightly hyperintense (relative to gray matter) on T2-weighted images with mild surrounding edema. Moderate to intense solid enhancement occurs after intravenous contrast.

Differential Diagnosis

Metastasis
Abscess
Glioma
Meningioma
Enhancing infarct

Note: **Because lymphoma tends to present with multiple lesions in an older patient, it is most often mistaken for metastases.**

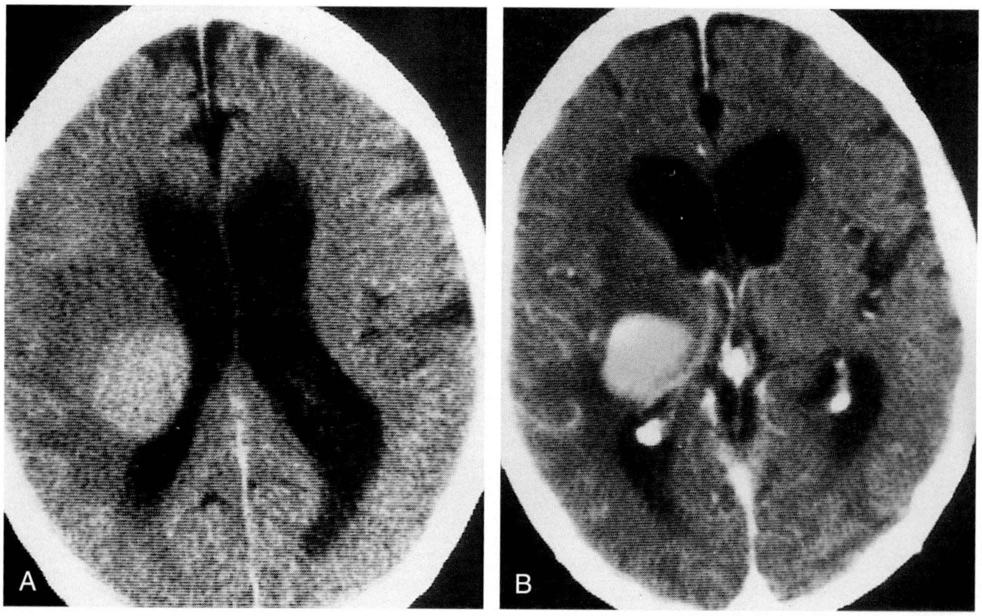

Figure 4–41. Lymphoma. **(A)** Unenhanced CT shows a uniformly hyperdense mass abutting the ependymal surface of the right lateral ventricle. **(B)** After intravenous contrast there is solid homogeneous enhancement.

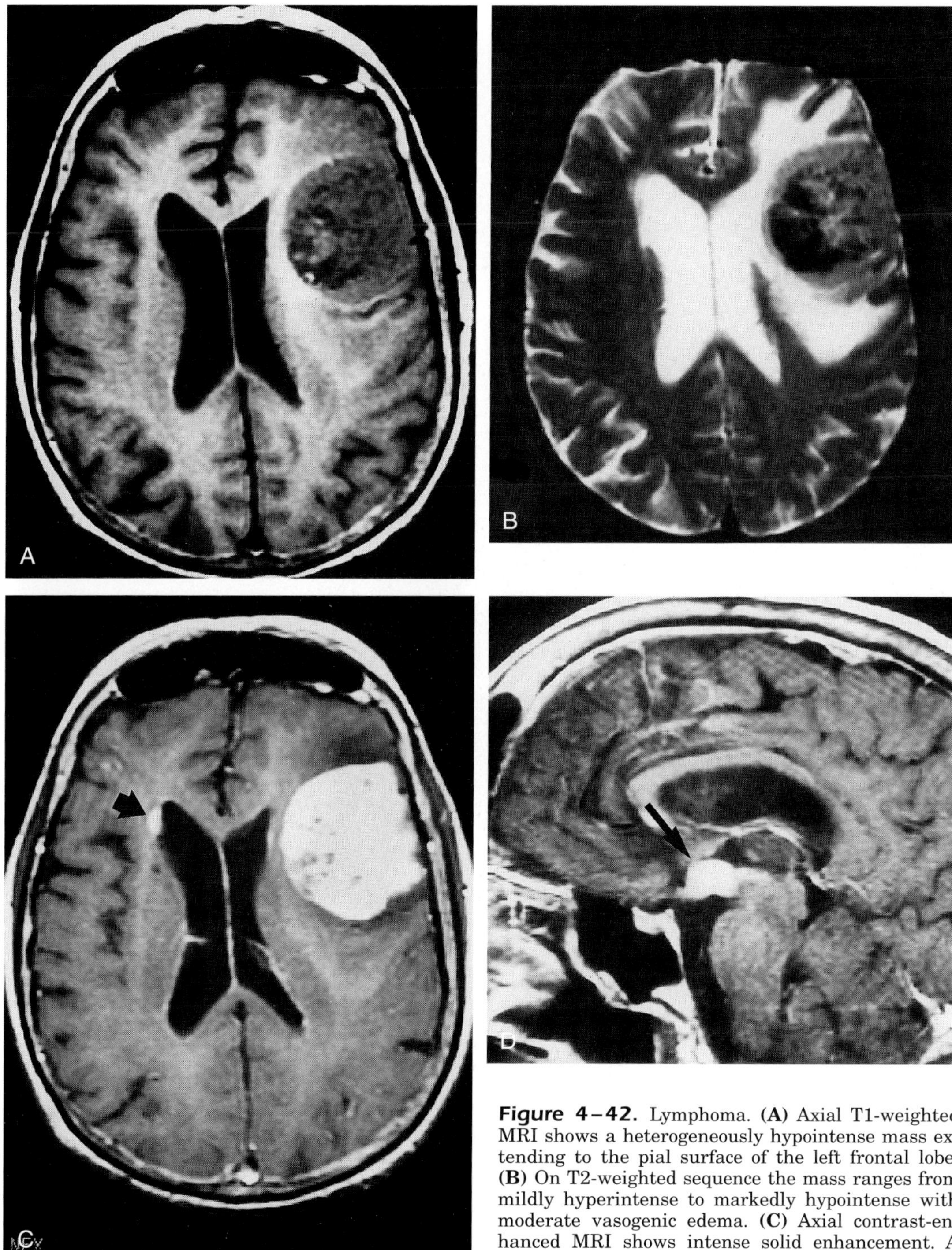

Figure 4–42. Lymphoma. **(A)** Axial T1-weighted MRI shows a heterogeneously hypointense mass extending to the pial surface of the left frontal lobe. **(B)** On T2-weighted sequence the mass ranges from mildly hyperintense to markedly hypointense with moderate vasogenic edema. **(C)** Axial contrast-enhanced MRI shows intense solid enhancement. A second lesion (arrow) abuts the surface of the right frontal horn. **(D)** Sagittal postcontrast MRI shows a third enhancing mass in the hypothalamus and floor of the third ventricle (arrow).

Hemangioblastoma

Hemangioblastomas are the most common primary neoplasms of the posterior fossa in adults with a peak incidence in the fourth decade. They are highly vascular and histologically benign. Although multiple hemangioblastomas strongly suggest the diagnosis of von Hippel-Lindau disease, this condition accounts for fewer than 20% of patients with hemangioblastomas. Complete surgical resection is usually curative.

Location
Usually cerebellar hemispheres. Less common in vermis, medulla, and spinal cord and rare in cerebral hemispheres.

CT Findings. CT usually reveals a well-defined cystic (60–70%) mass in a cerebellar hemisphere with an isodense mural nodule adjacent to the pial surface that enhances intensely. Prominent enhancing vessels may lead to or from the tumor. Multiple lesions may be present in 5–20%.

MRI Findings. MRI shows a sharply marginated mass with smooth borders. The solid component (solid tumor or mural nodule) tends to be isointense relative to gray matter on T1-weighted images and hyperintense on T2-weighted images. The cystic component is typically isointense or hyperintense relative to CSF on T1-weighted images and hyperintense on T2-weighted images. Signal voids due to tumor vessels are usually present. Evolving hemorrhage may be present. Mass effect leads to hydrocephalus and tonsillar herniation.

Angiography. Selective angiography demonstrates intense homogeneous or mottled tumor stain, arteriovenous shunting, and enlarged feeding arteries and veins.

Differential Diagnosis

The juvenile pilocytic astrocytoma may present a nearly identical appearance but without the intense staining on angiography. Hemangiopericytoma is a highly vascular tumor on imaging and angiography but is usually extraaxial. The most common cerebellar mass in an adult is metastasis, which should lead the differential but also usually lacks the intense staining on angiography.

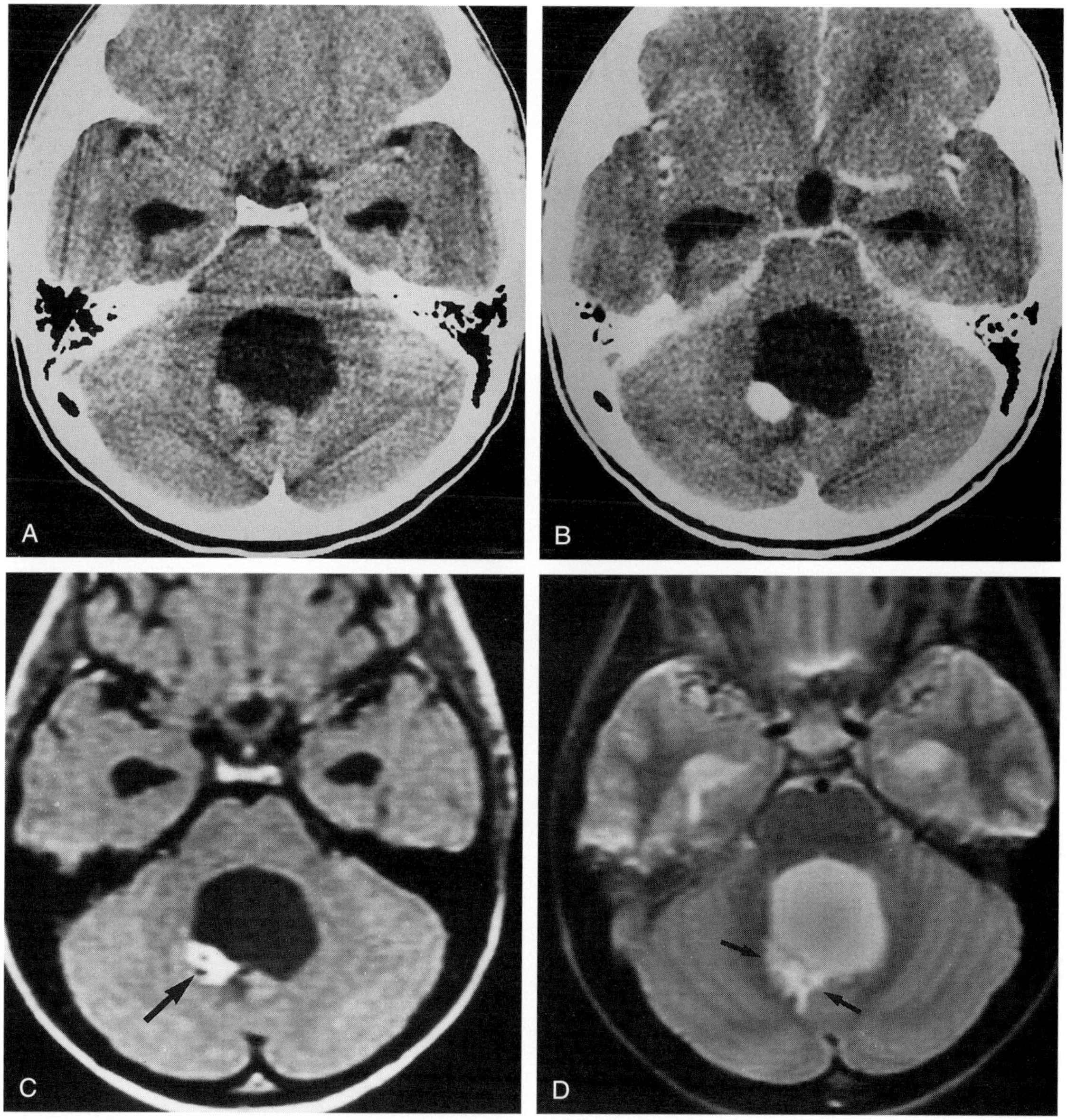

Figure 4–43. Hemangioblastoma. CT **(A)** before and **(B)** after contrast shows a midline cystic mass of the vermis with an intensely enhancing mural nodule. The temporal horns are dilated due to hydrocephalus. **(C)** Contrast-enhanced MRI shows the midline cystic mass with enhancing mural nodule. Flow voids within the nodule (arrow) indicate its hypervascular nature. **(D)** On T2-weighted MRI the nodule (arrows) is hyperintense relative to CSF and the cyst contents.

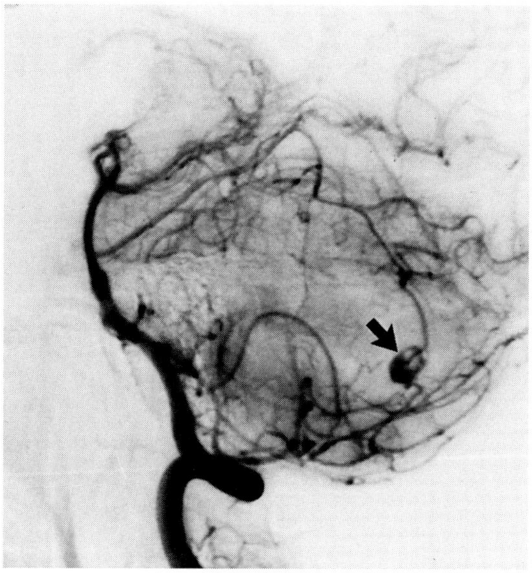

Figure 4–44. Hemangioblastoma. Lateral vertebral angiogram shows a hypervascular tumor nodule (arrow) in a case similar to the previous figure.

BRAIN TUMORS IN CHILDREN

The types and locations of tumors in children and teens differ substantially from those in adults. Between birth and age 3, supratentorial tumors are more common. From ages 4 to 11, the classic posterior fossa tumors of childhood (cerebellar astrocytomas, medulloblastomas, and ependymomas) predominate. From age 12 to early adulthood, the proportion of supratentorial and infratentorial tumors is about equal. Most astrocytomas in children are of the juvenile pilocytic or fibrillary type and consequently of benign histology.

Juvenile Pilocytic Astrocytoma

Juvenile pilocytic astrocytomas (JPAs) are one of the most benign tumors of glial origin. They form well-defined lobular masses and commonly contain cysts, and there is frequently a vascular tumor nodule in the cyst wall. Astrocytomas are the most common tumor of the cerebellum in children and usually are of the juvenile pilocytic type; brainstem astrocytomas, however, are usually fibrillary. Most optic pathway gliomas in childhood are also of the juvenile pilocytic type. The chance for complete cure of JPA is excellent following successful surgical resection. There is an increased incidence of JPAs in type 1 neurofibromatosis.

Location

Cerebellum, optic nerves or chiasm, and thalamus.

CT Findings. CT typically shows a round or an oval, smooth, sharply marginated mass hypodense or isodense relative to brain. Nearly all enhance either as a solid mass or mural nodule accompanying a cyst. The latter appearance is especially common among the cerebellar tumors. Necrosis may occur within solid tumors, in which case more extensive and heterogeneous enhancement is observed. Calcifications are seen in about 10%, and cysts (either macrocysts or microcysts) in about 70%. Edema is usually absent. JPAs arising in the optic pathways typically assume a fusiform or dumbbell configuration.

MRI Findings. JPAs are typically isointense or hypointense relative to brain on T1-weighted images and hyperintense on T2-weighted images. The cystic components are isointense to hyperintense relative to CSF on both sequences. Homogeneous enhancement of the solid component occurs with intravenous contrast.

Differential Diagnosis

Suprasellar
- Craniopharyngioma
- Germinoma
- Metastasis
- Pituitary adenoma

Posterior fossa
- Medulloblastoma
- Ependymoma
- Hemangioblastoma

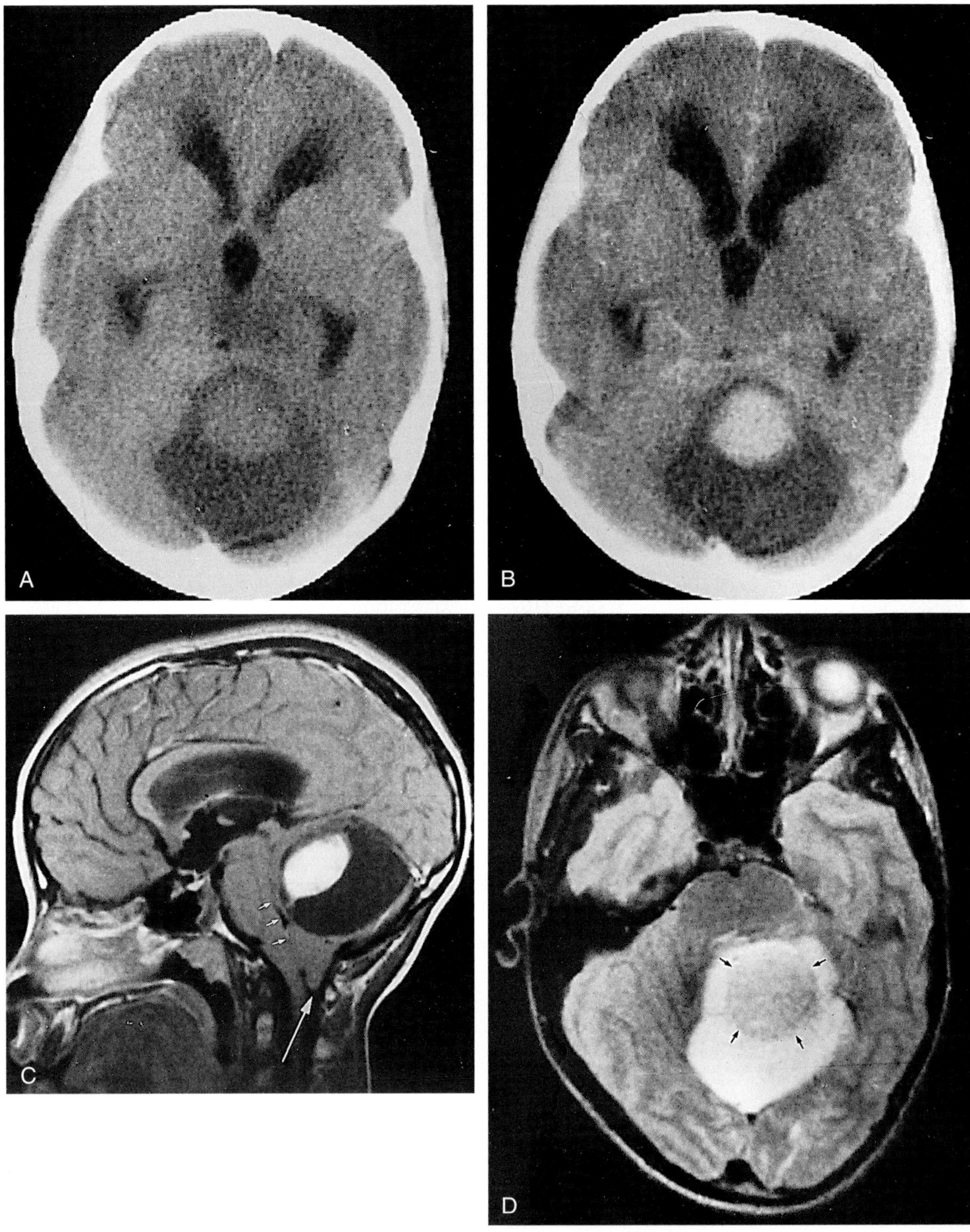

Figure 4–45. Juvenile pilocytic astrocytoma. CT **(A)** before and **(B)** after contrast shows a smoothly marginated hypodense mass with a large enhancing mural nodule. Hydrocephalus is present. **(C)** Sagittal contrast-enhanced MRI shows a cystic vermian mass with a large enhancing nodule. Note the tonsillar herniation (long arrow), compression of the fourth ventricle (short arrows), and hydrocephalic alterations of the third ventricle. **(D)** On axial T2-weighted MRI the cystic portion is more hyperintense than the solid mural nodule (arrows).

Medulloblastoma

According to contemporary thought, the medulloblastoma is a primitive neuroectodermal tumor of the posterior fossa that arises from neuroepithelial cells in the roof of the fourth ventricle. It is the second most common neoplasm of the posterior fossa in childhood. Over 50% occur in the first decade of life. About one third occur between 15 and 35 years of age, which indicates they may appear in adulthood. Up to 50% long-term survival may occur with combination therapy.

Location

Medulloblastomas arise in the mid and lower vermis in over 90% of cases and spread into the fourth ventricle. They tend to occur more laterally (cerebellar hemispheres) in older patients.

CT Findings. The usual CT appearance is a well-defined, round to oval, moderately hyperdense mass of the vermis with a mild rim of edema. It displaces the fourth ventricle anteriorly and usually causes hydrocephalus. Contrast-enhanced scans show mild homogeneous contrast enhancement, although up to 10% do not enhance on CT. Cysts are present in more than 25%, and calcifications are present in up to 50%. Evidence of CSF spread is sometimes present at diagnosis but commonly encountered in follow-up (see Leptomeningeal metastases, Chapters 4 and 12).

MRI Findings. MRI typically reveals a well-circumscribed mass in the inferior vermis. Medulloblastomas are hypointense relative to white matter on T1-weighted images. On T2-weighted images, they are usually hyperintense relative to white matter and mildly to markedly heterogeneous. Enhancement tends to be mild and heterogeneous and involves a variable portion of the tumor. Small cysts are frequent. The majority disseminate throughout the CNS in both the parenchyma and subarachnoid space. Tumoral seeding of the spinal axis commonly occurs. Contrast-enhanced MRI is the examination of choice for the evaluation of tumor spread but is still fairly insensitive because of the limited enhancement seen with this tumor. Systemic metastases are common, especially to bone.

The larger tumors may manifest more heterogeneity in texture and enhancement characteristics, more calcification, and more cystic or necrotic changes.

Differential Diagnosis	
Ependymoma	More calcification About one fourth as common
Juvenile pilocytic astrocytoma	Usually lateral in hemispheres Large cystic component

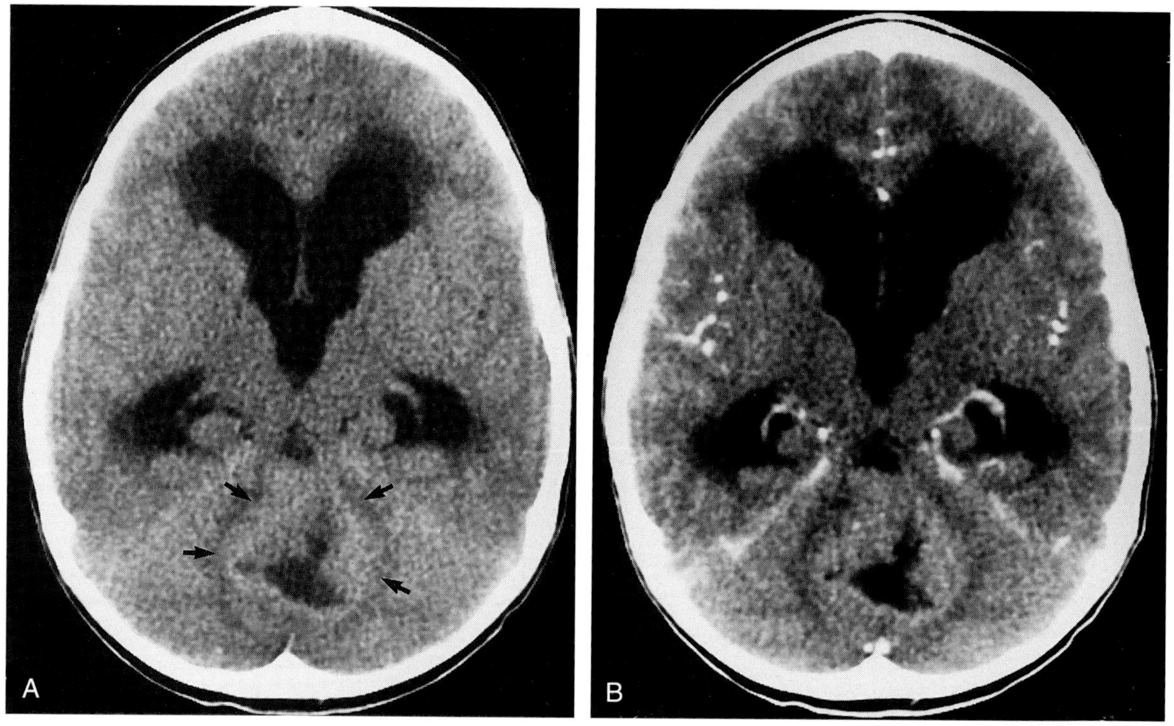

Figure 4–46. Medulloblastoma. (A) Unenhanced CT shows a midline vermian mass (arrows) isodense with gray matter and with an area of hypodensity reflecting cyst or necrosis. (B) Minimal enhancement is seen after contrast. There is severe hydrocephalus.

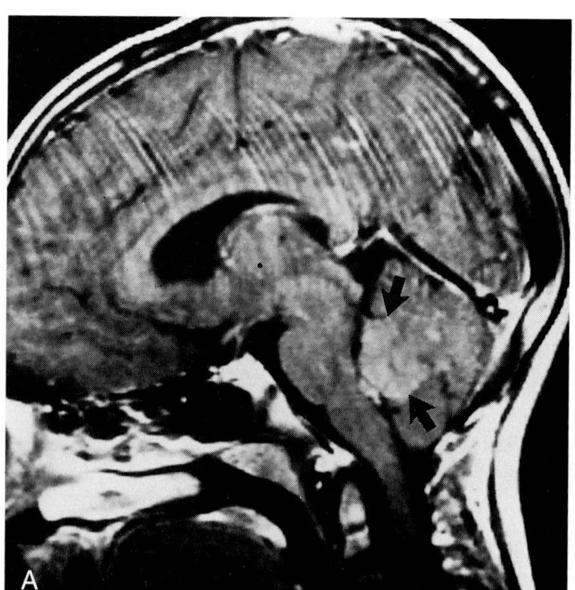

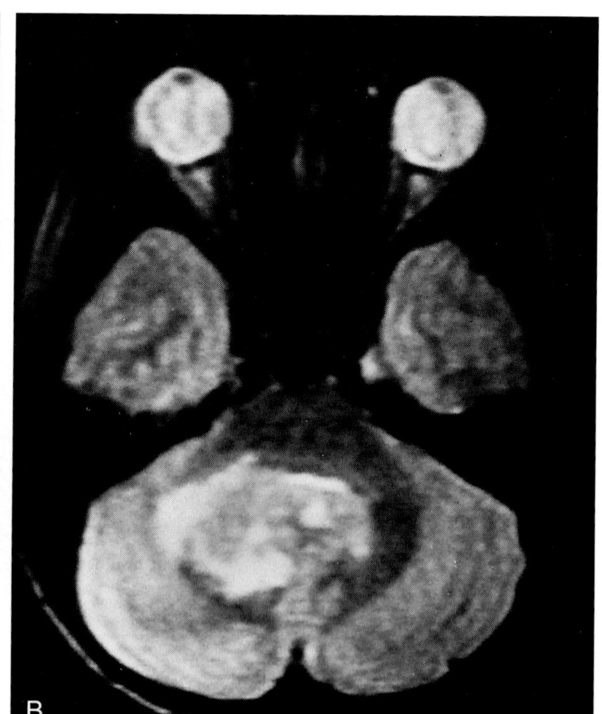

Figure 4–47. Medulloblastoma. (A) Sagittal contrast-enhanced MRI shows a midline vermian mass (arrows) invading the fourth ventricle and showing minimal enhancement. (B) On T2-weighted images the mass is heterogeneously hyperintense with irregular margins.

Supratentorial Primitive Neuroectodermal Tumor

Synonyms: Primary or primitive cerebral neuroblastoma, cerebral medulloblastoma, undifferentiated small cell neoplasm, PNET with neuronal differentiation.

The term primitive neuroectodermal tumor (PNET) applies to a group of pediatric brain tumors believed to arise from undifferentiated neuroepithelial precursors of the germinal matrix (neuroectoderm). Pineoblastomas, medulloblastomas, retinoblastomas, and systemic neuroblastomas are all placed in this category by some authorities. Various subtypes may manifest early differentiation along neuronal or glial cell lines.

In the cerebral hemispheres, most PNETs manifest early neuronal differentiation. These tumors present in early childhood (before age 5) with large intracranial masses. The 5-year survival rate is less than 30%.

Location

Frontal lobes are the most frequent but PNETs exhibit great diversity in their site of origin.

CT Findings. CT usually shows a well-circumscribed heterogeneous mass with a mean diameter of 7 cm. Areas of high attenuation are present in 75%, and discreet calcifications are seen in 60–70%. Cystic areas due to necrosis or hemorrhage are common. Edema is typically mild or absent, but hydrocephalus is often present. Postcontrast scans show heterogeneous, solid, or ring enhancement. Seeding of the subarachnoid space occurs commonly. These tumors may grow directly through the falx or tentorium, a feature unique among intraaxial neoplasms.

MRI Findings. MRI shows a large mass that is markedly heterogeneous on both T1- and T2-weighted images due to the presence of solid tumors, cysts, blood products, and calcifications. The enhancement patterns are as described for CT. Contrast-enhanced MRI is much more sensitive than CT in the detection of satellite nodules and leptomeningeal spread.

Differential Diagnosis	
Extraventricular ependymomas	Usually smaller at time of diagnosis
Teratomas	Most common mass in a neonate

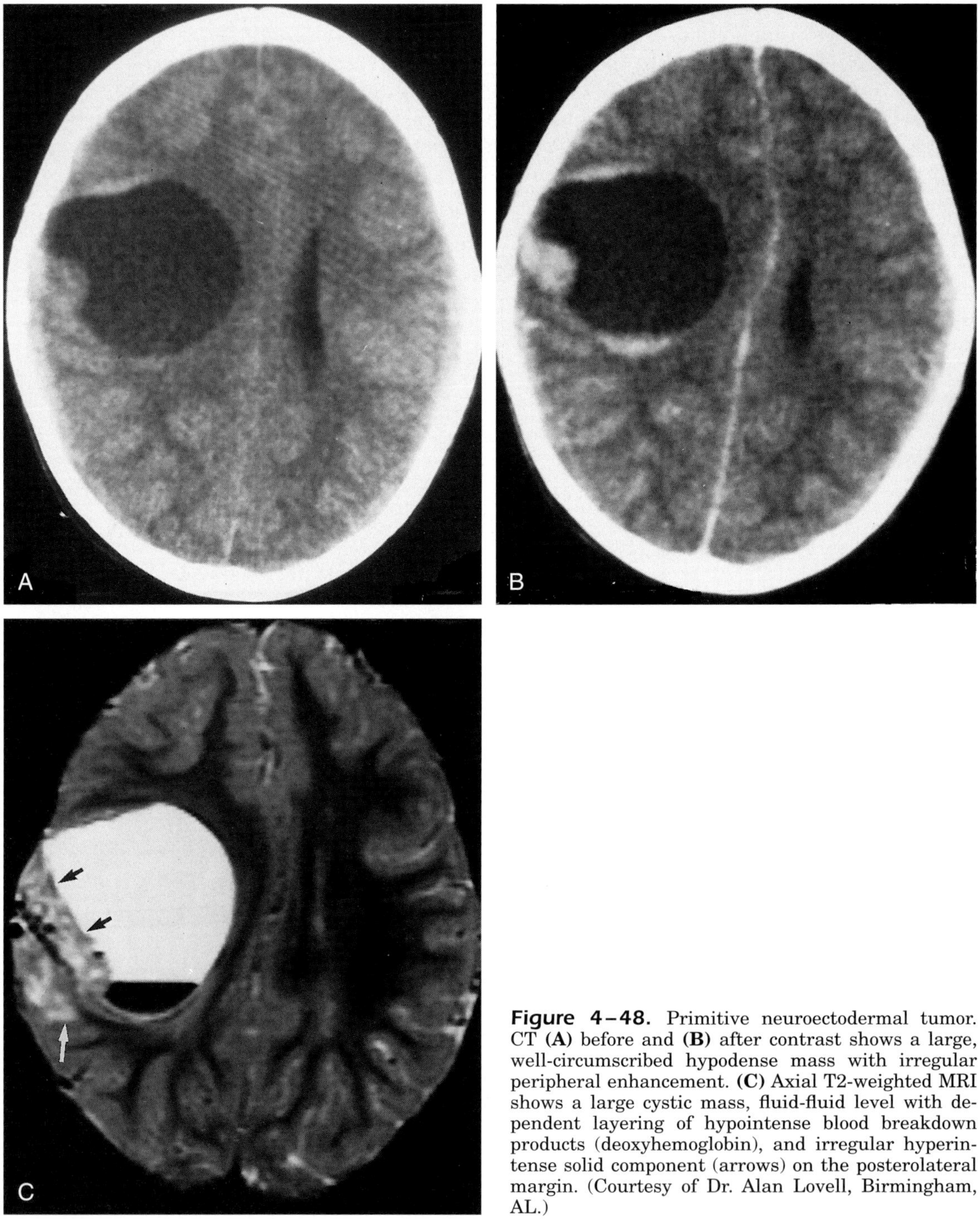

Figure 4–48. Primitive neuroectodermal tumor. CT **(A)** before and **(B)** after contrast shows a large, well-circumscribed hypodense mass with irregular peripheral enhancement. **(C)** Axial T2-weighted MRI shows a large cystic mass, fluid-fluid level with dependent layering of hypointense blood breakdown products (deoxyhemoglobin), and irregular hyperintense solid component (arrows) on the posterolateral margin. (Courtesy of Dr. Alan Lovell, Birmingham, AL.)

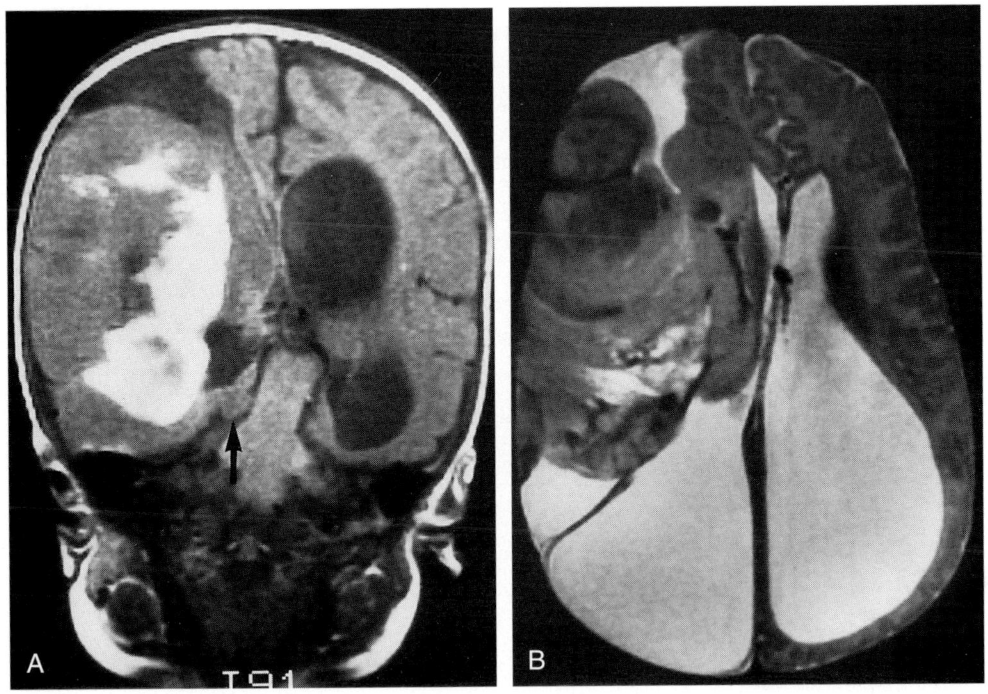

Figure 4–49. Primitive neuroectodermal tumor. **(A)** Coronal T1-weighted MRI shows a large solid right hemispheric mass with hyperintensity due to subacute hemorrhage. There is right uncal herniation (arrow) along with marked shift of the midbrain. **(B)** Axial T2-weighted scan shows severe hydrocephalus due to both transtentorial herniation and mass effect at the foramina of Monro. The large tumor mass exhibits markedly heterogeneous signal characteristics. (Reprinted with permission from Figueroa,RE, El Gammel,T, Brooks,BS, Holgate,R, Miller,W. MR Findings on Primitive Neuroectodermal Tumors. *J Comput Assist Tomogr* 13:773–778, 1989.)

Hamartoma

Synonym: Hypothalamic hamartoma.

Hamartomas of the tuber cinereum are congenital masses composed of mature neuronal ganglionic tissue and usually 1 to 2 cm in diameter. They typically present with precocious puberty, often before 2 years of age. Others are sometimes discovered incidentally. Surgical resection of symptomatic lesions is curative, whereas asymptomatic patients do not require treatment.

Location

Hypothalamus between mammillary bodies and infundibulum; may be suspended by a thick stalk.

CT Findings. CT reveals a spherical, isodense, homogeneous mass posterior to the infundibulum and anterior to the mammillary bodies extending into interpeduncular, prepontine, and suprasellar cisterns. Calcification, fat, and cysts are rarely seen. They do not enhance with intravenous contrast.

MRI Findings. Hypothalamic hamartomas are isointense with gray matter on T1-weighted images and usually hyperintense (but may be isointense) relative to brain on T2-weighted images. They do not enhance with intravenous contrast.

Differential Diagnosis

The typical location, absence of enhancement, and signal characteristics nearly identical to those of gray matter make the MRI appearance virtually pathognomonic.

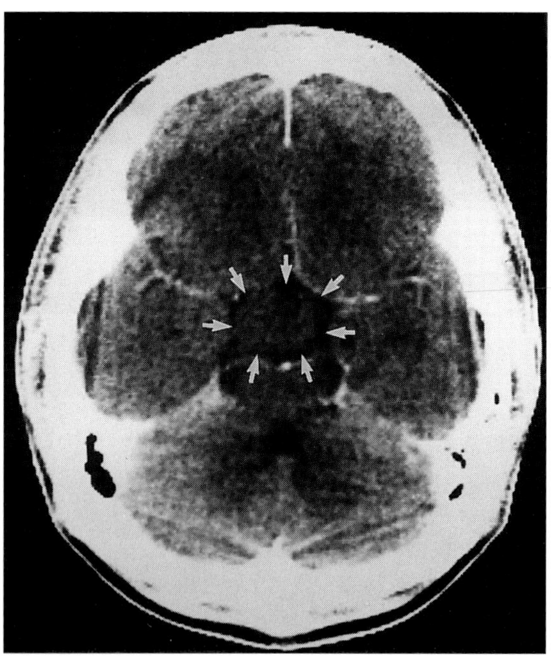

Figure 4–50. Hamartoma. CT with contrast shows an unenhancing mass (arrows) in the suprasellar cistern isodense with brain parenchyma.

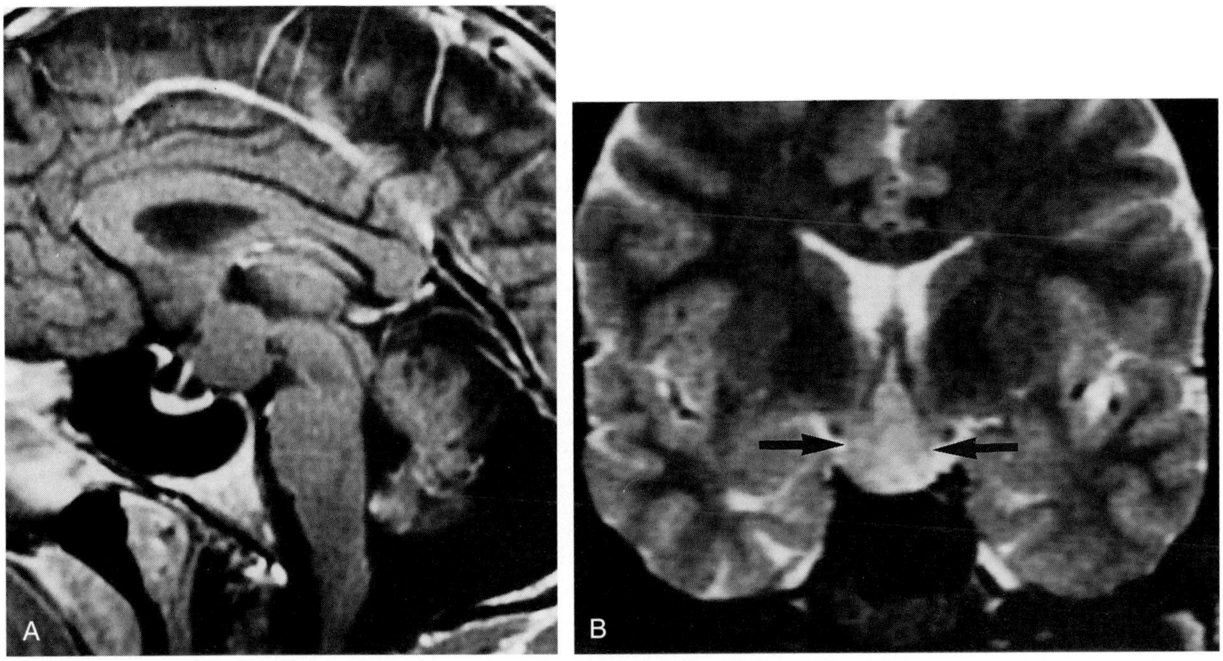

Figure 4–51. Hamartoma. **(A)** Sagittal contrast-enhanced MRI shows an unenhancing mass of the hypothalamus isointense with brain. **(B)** On coronal T2-weighted image the mass (arrows) is slightly hyperintense relative to gray matter.

Parenchymal Brain Metastasis

Brain metastases from systemic malignancies represent the most common cerebral neoplasm, although this may not be the case in all practice settings. Many metastases are diagnosed post mortem or in the terminal stages of disease and are neither followed nor treated. Hence in many published series, the incidence of metastases seems to approximate more closely the incidence of malignant glial tumors. The prognosis is generally grim, although improved survival may follow surgical resection of solitary lesions. Tables 4–14 and 4–15 list the major sources of brain metastasis and effects of systemic malignancy on the CNS.

Location

About 80% are supratentorial—most often the frontal lobes followed by the parietal lobes; 20% are in the posterior fossa—most often the cerebellum. Brainstem metastases are rare.

> In any adult patient with a newly diagnosed brain mass, a chest x-ray should always be obtained!

CT Findings. CT most often reveals multiple (average 4 to 5) foci of low or mixed attenuation with prominent vasogenic edema. The degree of edema may not correlate with the size of the mass. Nearly all enhance; this is usually ringlike but may be solid. Common variations include solitary lesions (15–30% of patients), high attenuation on unenhanced scans, or hemorrhage. Less common variations include calcification (less than 2%) or a miliary pattern (carcinomatous encephalitis, less than 1%). Bone destruction may be caused by dural or osseous metastases. It is customary to review all slices using bone windows when searching for metastases.

MRI Findings. MRI findings generally parallel those for CT. Nonhemorrhagic metastases are typically isointense to hypointense on T1-weighted images and hyperintense on T2-weighted images. Ring or solid enhancement occurs after intravenous contrast, but solid nodular enhancement is seen more commonly. The larger lesions are more likely to manifest ring enhancement. MRI with contrast is marginally more sensitive than CT for the detection of parenchymal disease. As with CT, the important distinguishing features are the multiplicity of lesions, marked edema, and nearly inevitable contrast enhancement. The percentage of patients in which a solitary lesion is identified appears lower with enhanced MRI. Diagnostic sensitivity for small lesions may be increased with higher contrast dosage or delayed scanning. These methods are not routinely employed but might be considered prior to surgical resection of a solitary lesion.

TABLE 4–15 | Effects of Systemic Malignancy on CNS

Direct
Brain metastasis
Dural carcinomatosis
Leptomeningeal carcinomatosis
Bone metastasis
Tumor emboli
Aneurysm formation
Spinal cord metastasis (rare)
Spinal cord compression
Indirect
Subacute cerebellar degeneration

TABLE 4–14 | Sources of Brain Metastasis

Percentage of Metastasis	Primary Tumor
50	Lung carcinoma
15	Breast carcinoma
10	Primary unknown
8	Gastrointestinal adenocarcinoma
6	Melanoma
6	Genitourinary carcinoma
5	Other

Differential Diagnosis

Glioblastoma
Abscess
Lymphoma
Toxoplasmosis
Cysticercosis
Enhancing infarct

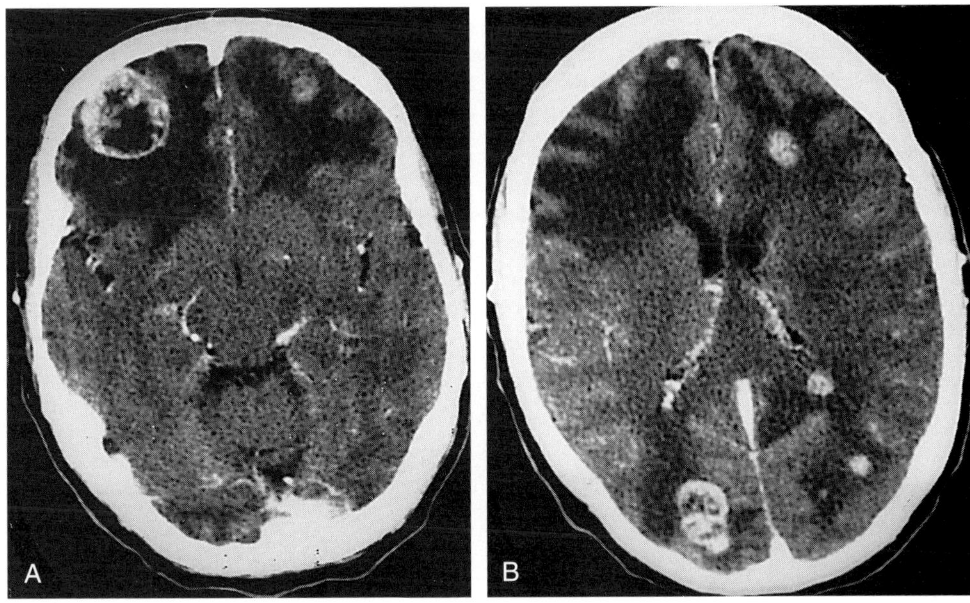

Figure 4–52. Brain metastases. **(A)** Enhanced CT shows a large irregular ring–enhancing mass of the right frontal lobe with marked vasogenic edema. **(B)** Higher section shows at least six enhancing nodules of variable size, mostly at the gray-white junction.

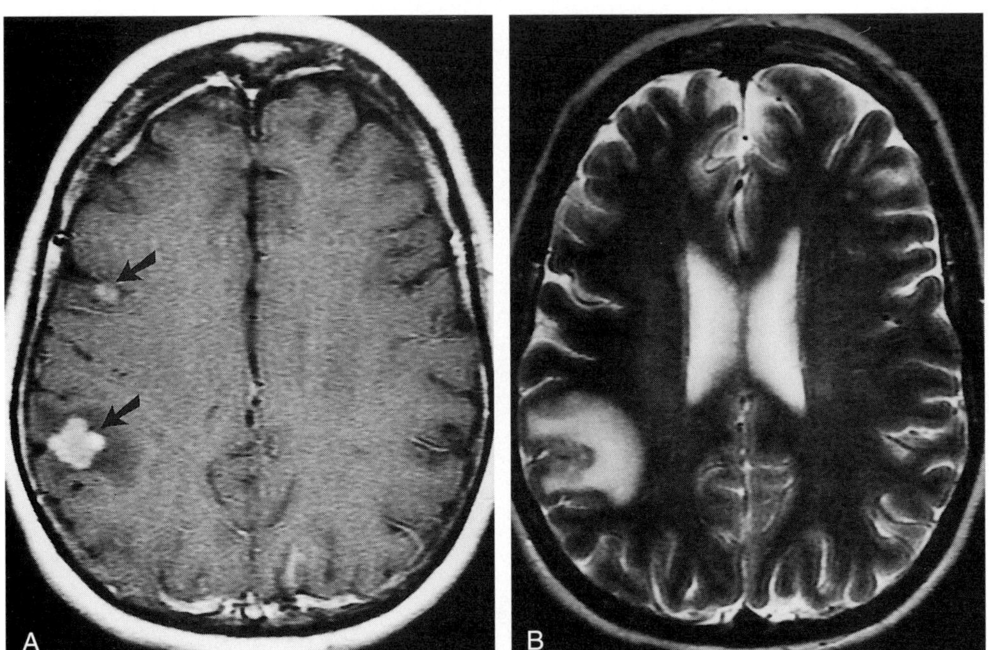

Figure 4–53. Brain metastases (breast carcinoma). **(A)** Axial contrast-enhanced MRI shows two solid enhancing lesions (arrows) involving gray matter on the right. **(B)** On T2-weighted image the larger mass shows mild hyperintensity and vasogenic edema; the smaller anterior metastasis cannot be seen.

Metastatic Melanoma

Melanoma represents the fourth most common cause of brain metastases. Its imaging features vary depending upon the presence of hemorrhage or melanin and in the case of melanotic melanoma may be sufficiently distinctive to allow a specific diagnosis. The prognosis is extremely poor.

Location
Frontal and parietal lobes.

CT Findings. CT shows multiple (60%) high attenuation masses with surrounding edema. Solid enhancement is seen in most.

MRI Findings. Signal intensities on MRI depend on whether the melanoma is melanotic, amelanotic, or hemorrhagic. Melanotic melanoma metastases are hyperintense on T1-weighted images and isointense to mildly hypointense on T2-weighted images. It is the appearance on T2-weighted images that may enable distinction between melanotic and hemorrhagic melanoma metastases. Amelanotic melanoma metastases are isointense to hypointense on T1-weighted images and mildly hyperintense on T2-weighted images (similar to other types of metastases). Hemorrhage is common and when present manifests the findings described for tumoral hemorrhage in general (see Chapter 1).

Differential Diagnosis

Fat-containing lesions (dermoids, teratomas, lipomas)
Hemorrhage

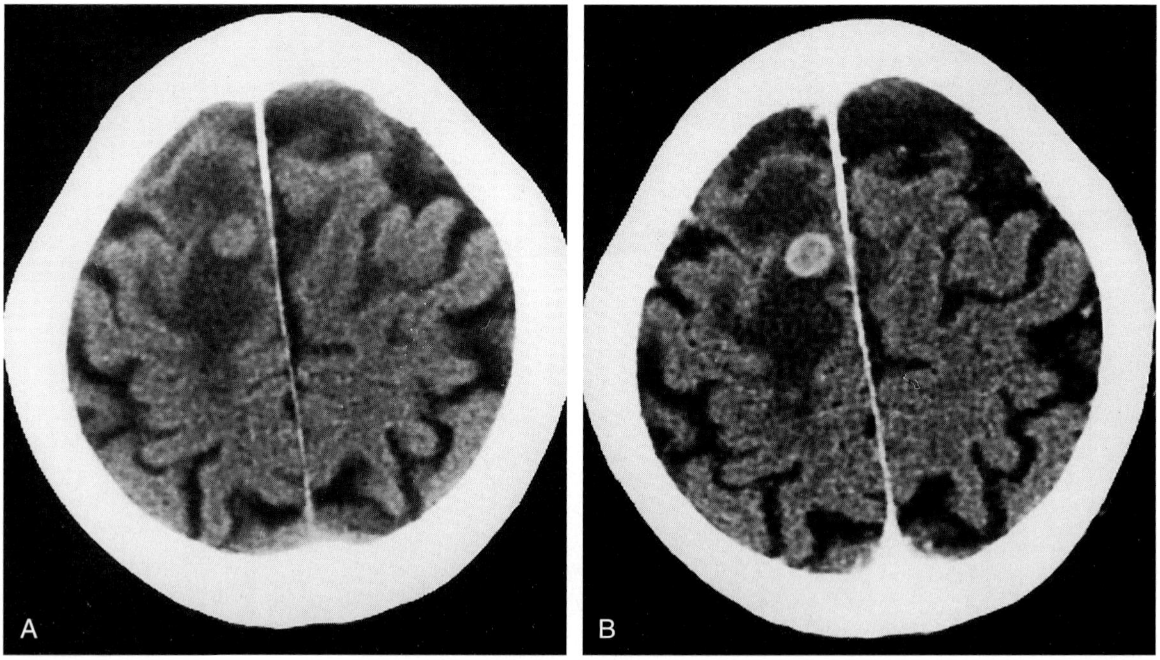

Figure 4–54. Metastatic melanoma. **(A)** Unenhanced CT shows a minimally hyperdense mass surrounded by vasogenic edema. **(B)** Solid enhancement, more intense at the periphery, is seen after contrast.

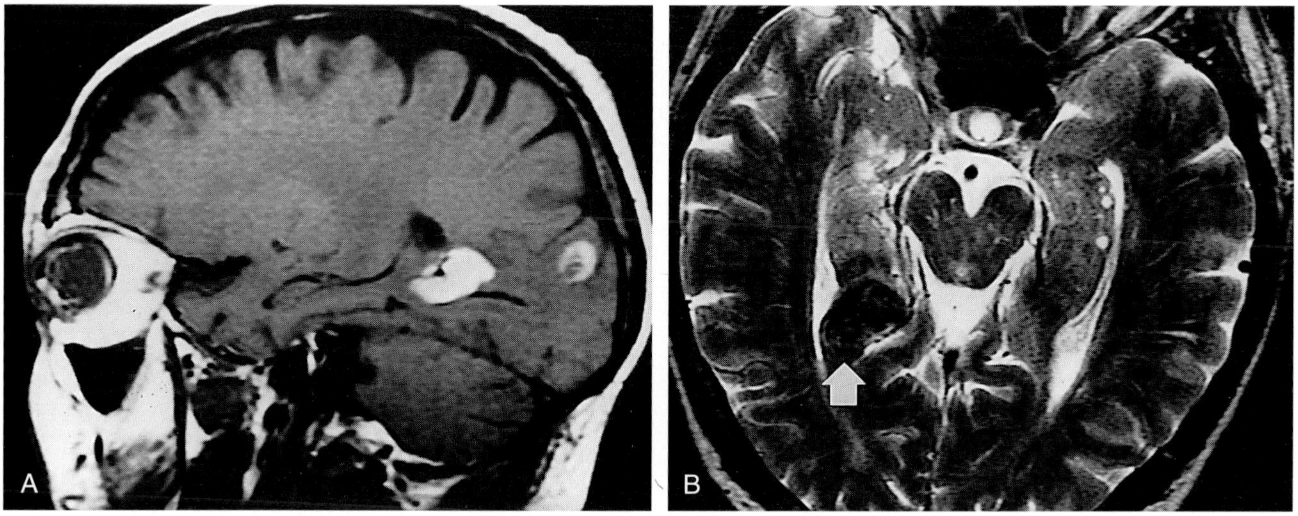

Figure 4–55. Metastatic melanotic melanoma. **(A)** Sagittal T1-weighted MRI shows hyperintense masses in the posterior right temporal and right occipital lobes. **(B)** On T2-weighted MRI the larger lesion (arrow) is minimally hypointense.

Intraventricular Tumors

Ependymoma

Ependymomas are gliomas arising from the ependymal cells that line the ventricular system. They are slow growing, relatively benign tumors that may become quite large. Ependymomas exhibit a bimodal age distribution with most occurring before age 5 but with a second peak in the fourth decade. From the wall of the ventricle they may grow into the ventricle (typical in children) or into adjacent parenchyma (more typical in adults). Although ependymomas are slow growing and histologically benign, most patients ultimately succumb to the tumors, sometimes after many years.

The subependymoma is a very slow-growing variant of the ependymoma that is more likely to occur in adults and often remains subclinical throughout life. It is nearly always intraventricular and most often found in the floor of the fourth ventricle. On imaging studies, it manifests findings similar to other ependymomas with a tendency to remain smaller and more homogeneous. Tables 4–16 and 4–17 provide the differential diagnosis and relative frequency of intraventricular masses.

Location

Fourth ventricle in children (60%) and parenchymal and supratentorial in young adults (40%). Also arise in the spinal cord.

CT Findings. CT usually shows a mass isodense with brain. Small, granular calcifications occur in about 50%. Ependymomas may enhance in either a uniform or heterogeneous pattern. Cysts are uncommon infratentorially (5%) but common supratentorially (up to 80%). About one half of the posterior fossa tumors extend into the cerebellopontine angle. Fourth ventricular ependymomas nearly always cause hydrocephalus. The supratentorial tumors tend to be larger, usually exceeding 4 cm in size at the time of presentation.

TABLE 4–16 Differential Diagnosis of Intraventricular Mass Lesions

Cystic
Ependymal cyst
Choroid plexus cyst
Colloid cyst
Epidermoid
Cysticercosis
Solid
Hyperplastic choroid plexus
Meningioma
Choroid plexus papilloma
Giant cell astrocytoma (tuberous sclerosis)
Ependymoma/subependymoma
Medulloblastoma
Oligodendroglioma
Metastasis

TABLE 4–17 Relative Frequency of Intraventricular Masses

Tumor	Frequency	Usual Site
Astrocytoma (usually giant cell)	20%	Frontal horns
Colloid cyst	14%	Nearly 100% occur in third ventricle
Meningioma	12%	Trigones
Ependymoma	10%	Fourth ventricle
Craniopharyngioma	7%	Third ventricle
Medulloblastoma	5%	Fourth ventricle
Cysticercosis	5%	Lateral ventricles
Choroid plexus papilloma (adults)	5%	Lateral ventricles (children) and fourth ventricle
Cysts*	4%	Trigones and choroidal fissure
Epidermoid	4%	Fourth ventricle
Dermoid	3%	Fourth ventricle
Subependymoma	3%	Fourth ventricle
Arteriovenous malformation	3%	Lateral ventricles
Miscellaneous	6%	—

*Use of MRI has resulted in improved detection of neuroepithelial cysts, which are probably more common than represented in this list.

Data derived from Morrison,G, Sobel,DF, Kelley,WM, Norman,D., Intraventricular Mass Lesions. *Radiology* 153:435–442, 1984.

MRI Findings. Ependymomas in children present as a fourth ventricular mass commonly invading adjacent parenchyma (a hallmark of this neoplasm) and growing out the fourth ventricular exit foramina. They are mostly solid tumors, isointense to hypointense to brain on T1-weighted images, and hyperintense on T2-weighted images. They are frequently quite heterogeneous due to blood products, calcifications (poorly seen on MRI), vessels, and necrosis. The margins are usually distinct on T2-weighted images. Ependymomas moderately and heterogeneously enhance with contrast. Leptomeningeal spread of tumor occurs in up to 30% of cases.

The supratentorial ependymomas are usually intraparenchymal (80%) and adjacent to the trigone but occasionally intraventricular (20%). Cystic changes are more common. The signal and enhancement characteristics otherwise parallel those of the infratentorial tumors.

Differential Diagnosis

- Choroid plexus papilloma
- Giant cell astrocytoma
- Intraventricular meningioma
- Metastasis
- Astrocytoma (especially juvenile pilocytic)
- Medulloblastoma

Text continued on page 205

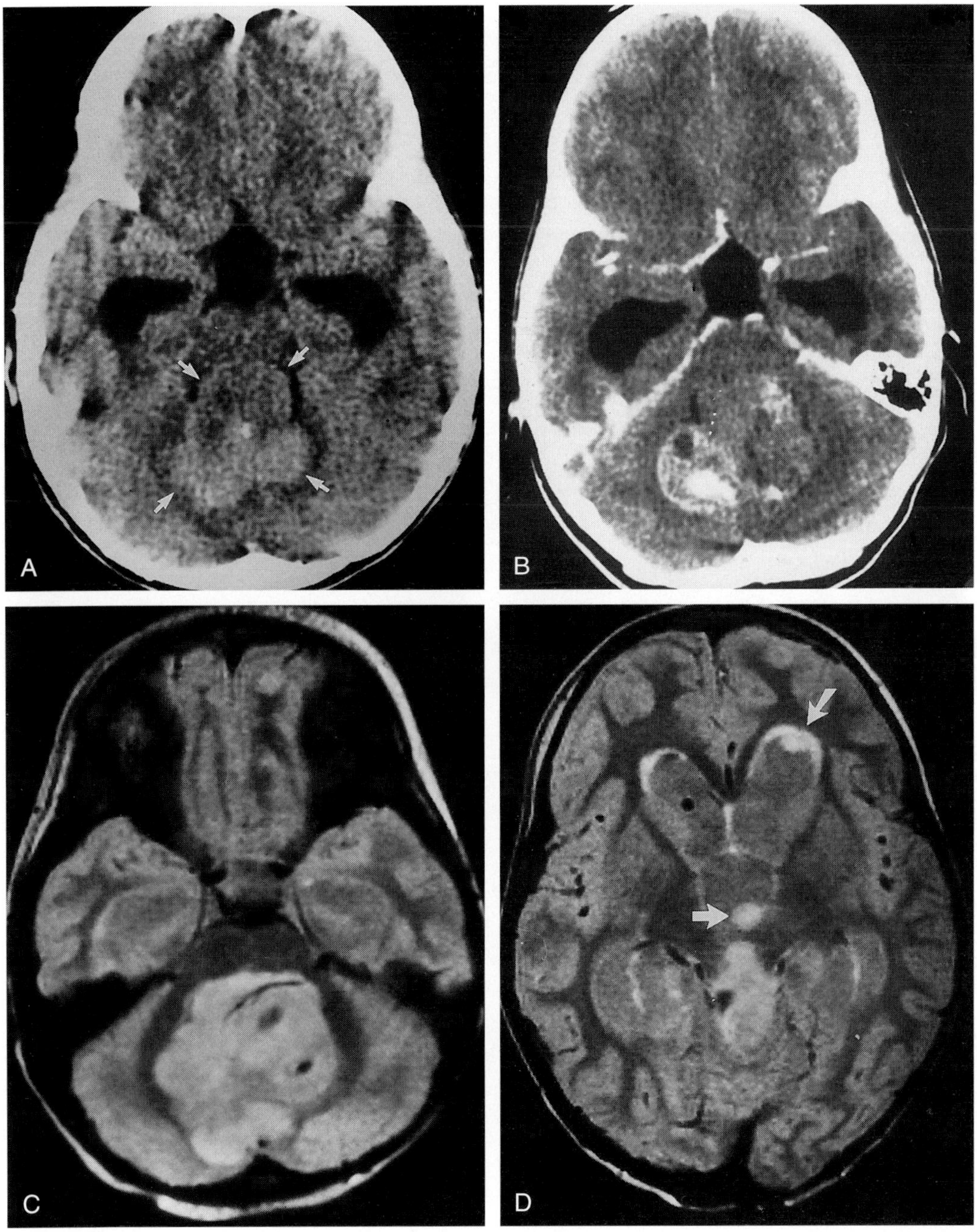

Figure 4–56. Ependymoma of fourth ventricle. **(A)** Unenhanced CT shows a partially hyperdense mass of the fourth ventricle (arrows) with a central calcification. Hydrocephalus is present. **(B)** Heterogeneous enhancement occurs following intravenous contrast. **(C)** Axial T2-weighted MRI shows a well-defined heterogeneously hyperintense mass. **(D)** Axial PD-weighted MRI through lateral ventricles shows ependymal metastases (arrows) and hydrocephalus.

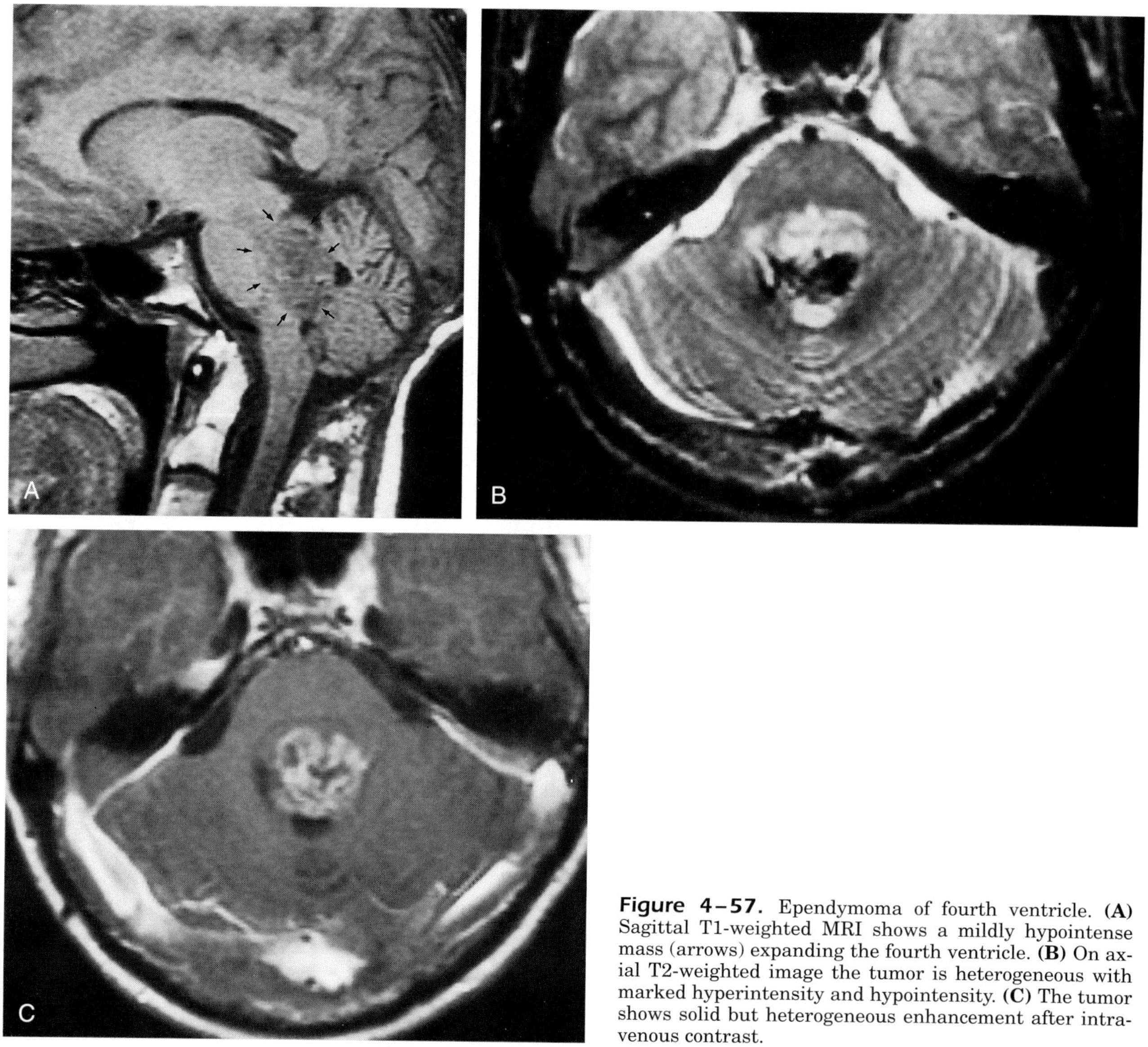

Figure 4–57. Ependymoma of fourth ventricle. **(A)** Sagittal T1-weighted MRI shows a mildly hypointense mass (arrows) expanding the fourth ventricle. **(B)** On axial T2-weighted image the tumor is heterogeneous with marked hyperintensity and hypointensity. **(C)** The tumor shows solid but heterogeneous enhancement after intravenous contrast.

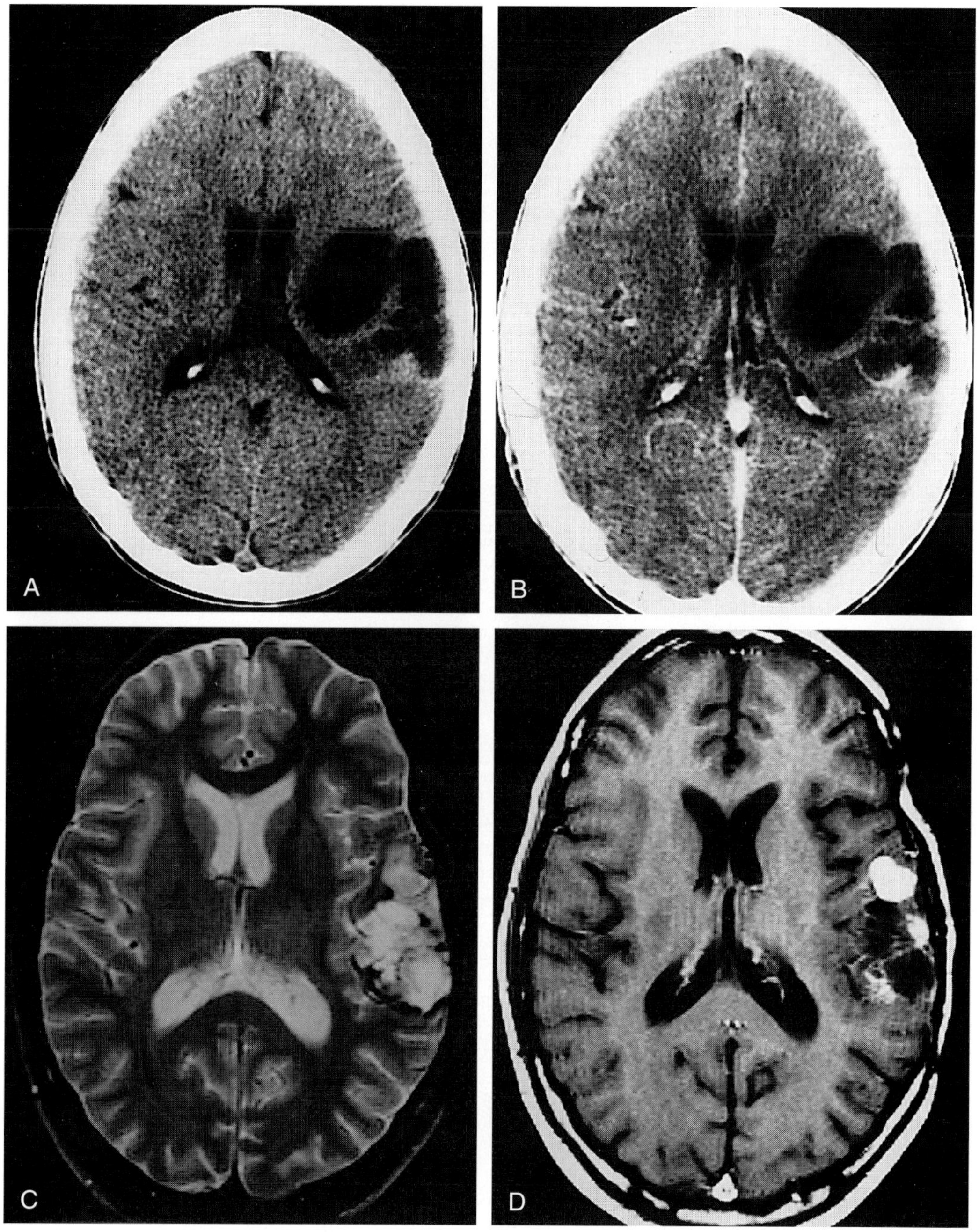

Figure 4–58. Ependymoma. CT **(A)** before and **(B)** after contrast shows a left frontal mass composed of multiple cysts with mild enhancement at the posterior margin. Following surgery, the tumor recurred locally. **(C)** T2-weighted MRI of recurrent tumor shows mildly hyperintense solid component and markedly hyperintense cystic portions. **(D)** The solid portions show dense enhancement after contrast.

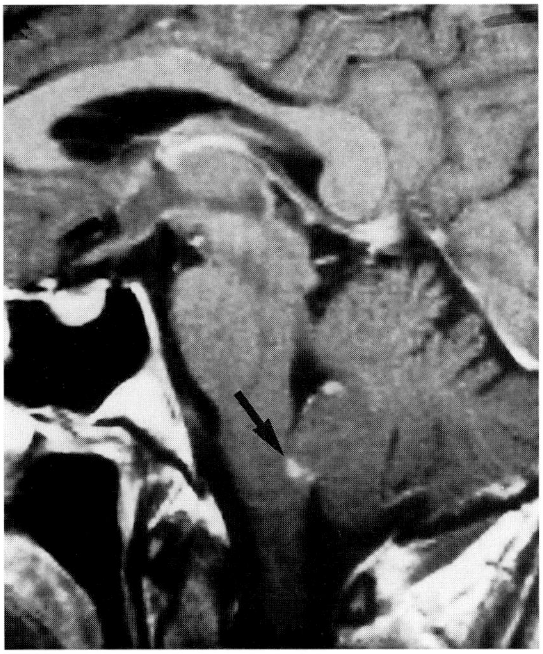

Figure 4–59. Subependymoma. Sagittal post-contrast MRI shows abnormal enhancement (arrow) on the posterior medulla near the foramen of Magendie. Enhancement in this region has been proposed as a normal variant, but this subependymoma was pathologically confirmed.

Choroid Plexus Papilloma

Choroid plexus papillomas (CPPs) arise from the epithelium of the choroid plexus. Because they possess the ability to produce CSF, overproduction of CSF ensues with resultant hydrocephalus. Most CPPs occur in the first 5 years of life. Surgical resection of benign papillomas is usually curative. About 10–20% undergo malignant transformation into choroid plexus carcinoma, which tends to invade cerebral parenchyma and prohibit total resection.

Location
In children, 80% arise in lateral ventricles. In adults, they arise in the fourth ventricle.

CT Findings. Unenhanced scans show an isodense to hyperdense well-marginated intraventricular mass, especially in the trigone of the lateral ventricle. Generalized hydrocephalus is usually present and even involves CSF spaces distal to and therefore not obstructed by the tumor. This pattern is not seen with any other neoplasm. Punctate calcifications are seen in about 25%. There is marked homogeneous contrast enhancement. The malignant choroid plexus carcinoma is characterized by greater heterogeneity and the presence of parenchymal invasion and vasogenic edema.

MRI Findings. Unenhanced MRI shows an intraventricular mass of low to intermediate signal intensity on T1-weighted images and heterogeneous signal intensity on T2-weighted images. Focal signal voids may be seen owing to calcifications or hypervascularity, and there is intense homogeneous enhancement following contrast injection. Choroid plexus carcinomas exhibit overall more heterogeneity in signal and enhancement characteristics with parenchymal invasion and vasogenic edema.

Differential Diagnosis

The association of hydrocephalus with a tumor that is not obstructive is virtually pathognomonic for CPP.

Papilloma

Ependymoma	Usually fourth ventricle in children and supratentorial in adults (opposite pattern of CPP)
Medulloblastoma	Vermian mass Less vascular and enhancing
Intraventricular meningioma	Rare Will not cause hydrocephalus if in lateral ventricle
Enlarged non-neoplastic choroid plexus	More homogeneous in texture Common in adults Usually multiple

Carcinoma

PNET	Little or no intraventricular component
Supratentorial ependymoma	Rare in childhood

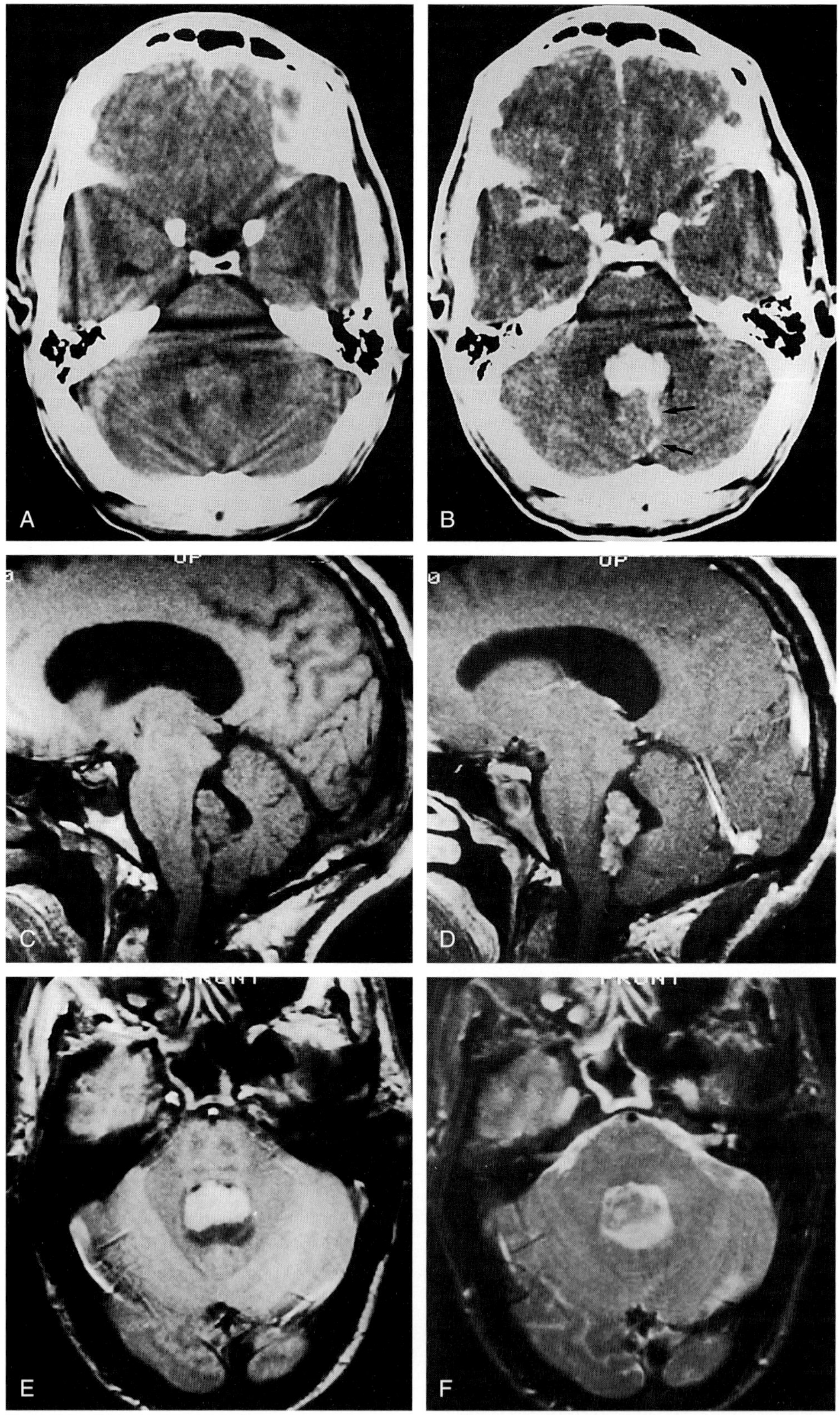

Figure 4–60. *See legend on opposite page*

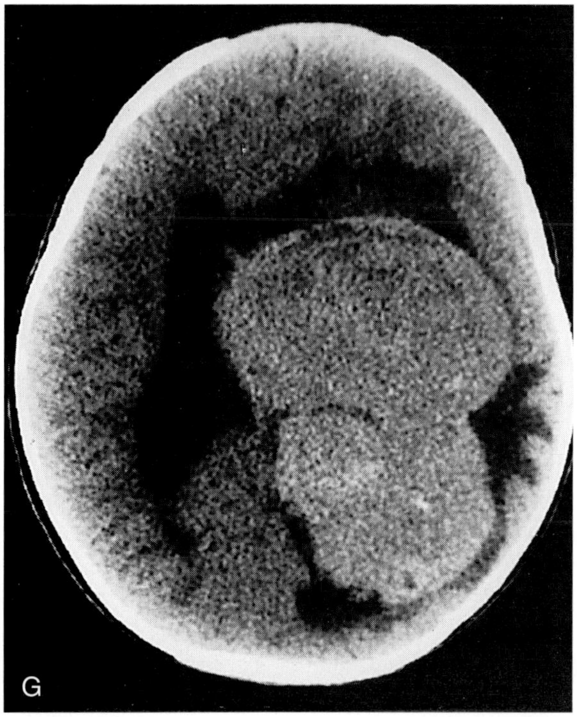

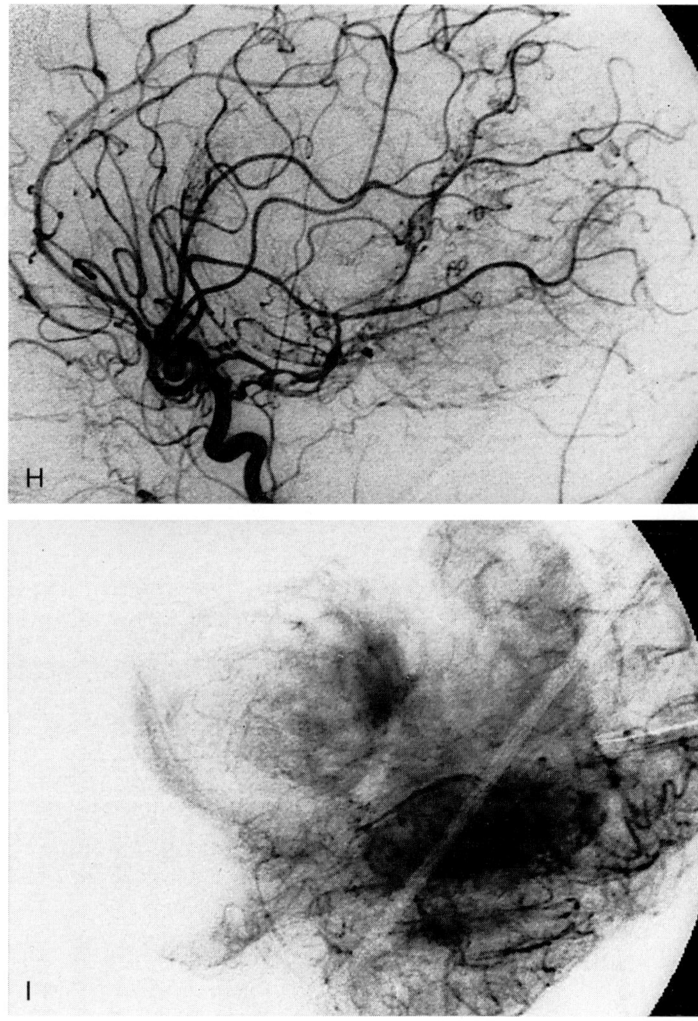

Figure 4–60. Choroid plexus papilloma. CT **(A)** before and **(B)** after contrast shows an isodense mass of the fourth ventricle with intense enhancement. Note enlarged vessel (arrows) leading to the tumor. On T1-weighted images **(C)** the mass is isointense with brain with **(D)** solid enhancement after intravenous contrast. There is hydrocephalus with upward bowing of the corpus callosum and dilatation of the fourth ventricle. The tumor is **(E)** hyperintense on PD-weighted images and **(F)** isointense with brain on T2-weighted images. **(G)** Unenhanced CT shows a huge left hemispheric mass with a few faint calcifications, vasogenic edema, severe left to right shift, and dilatation of the right lateral ventricle. Intraventricular location could not be proven from this examination. **(H)** Lateral internal carotid angiogram shows extensive neovascularity perfusing a hypervascular tumor. **(I)** Late arterial phase of lateral vertebral angiogram shows extensive tumor staining.

Colloid Cyst

Colloid cysts are rare developmental tumors with a marked predilection for the anterior third ventricle, where they commonly cause obstructive hydrocephalus. The cysts possess an epithelial lining and may contain dense mucoid material, fat, CSF, and cellular debris. They usually present in late adolescence and early adulthood. Surgical resection is usually curative.

Location
Anterosuperior third ventricle in nearly all cases.

CT Findings. CT shows a smooth, ovoid, or spherical mass in the anterior third ventricle at the level of the foramen of Monro. A colloid cyst is typically hyperdense (70–80%) and 10 to 20 mm in size and often shows mild contrast enhancement. Hydrocephalus, collapse of the posterior third ventricle, and thickening of the septum pellucidum are usually present. Some cysts may be isodense and thus difficult to detect. In such cases, the best indirect clue is the presence of dilated lateral ventricles with a small or collapsed third ventricle.

MRI Findings. Great diversity in the MRI characteristics of colloid cysts has been described. The usual appearance is a smooth round mass that is hyperintense on T1-weighted images and hypointense on T2-weighted images. However, colloid cysts may exhibit almost any possible signal intensity from hypointense to hyperintense on T1- and/or T2-weighted images. They are commonly heterogeneous with an outer layer exhibiting different signal characteristics from the center of the mass.

Differential Diagnosis

Basilar tip aneurysm
Meningioma
Ependymoma
Astrocytoma
Choroid plexus papilloma
Subependymal hamartoma (tuberous sclerosis)

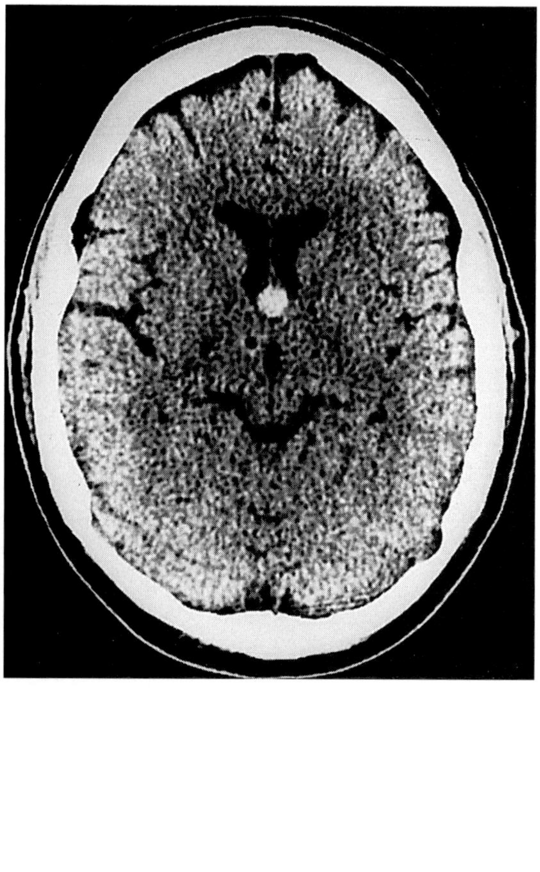

Figure 4–61. Colloid cyst. Unenhanced CT shows a characteristic round hyperdense mass in the anterior third ventricle near the foramina of Monro.

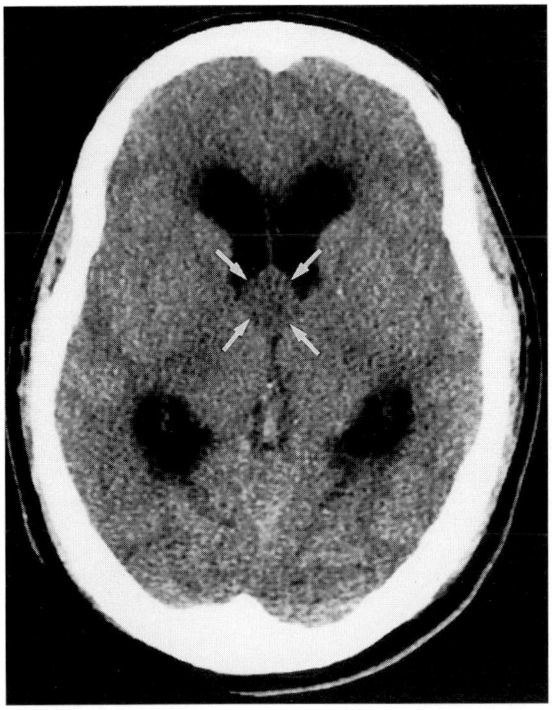

Figure 4–62. Colloid cyst. Unenhanced CT shows a 2-cm hypodense mass (arrows) in the anterior third ventricle occluding both foramina of Monro with resulting hydrocephalus.

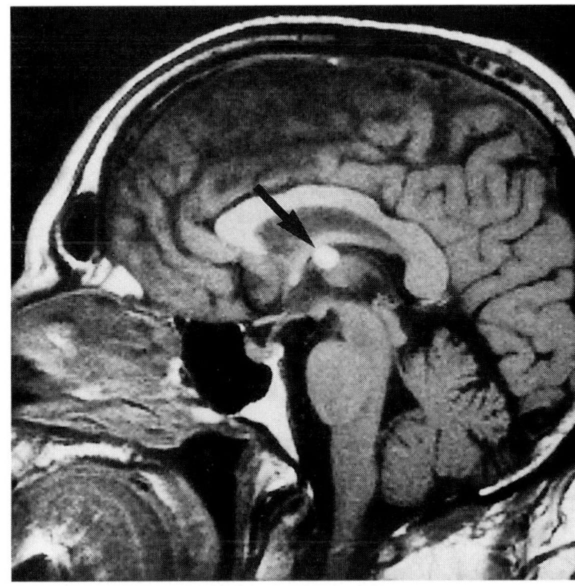

Figure 4–63. Colloid cyst. Sagittal T1-weighted MRI shows a round hyperintense mass (arrow) in the anterior third ventricle.

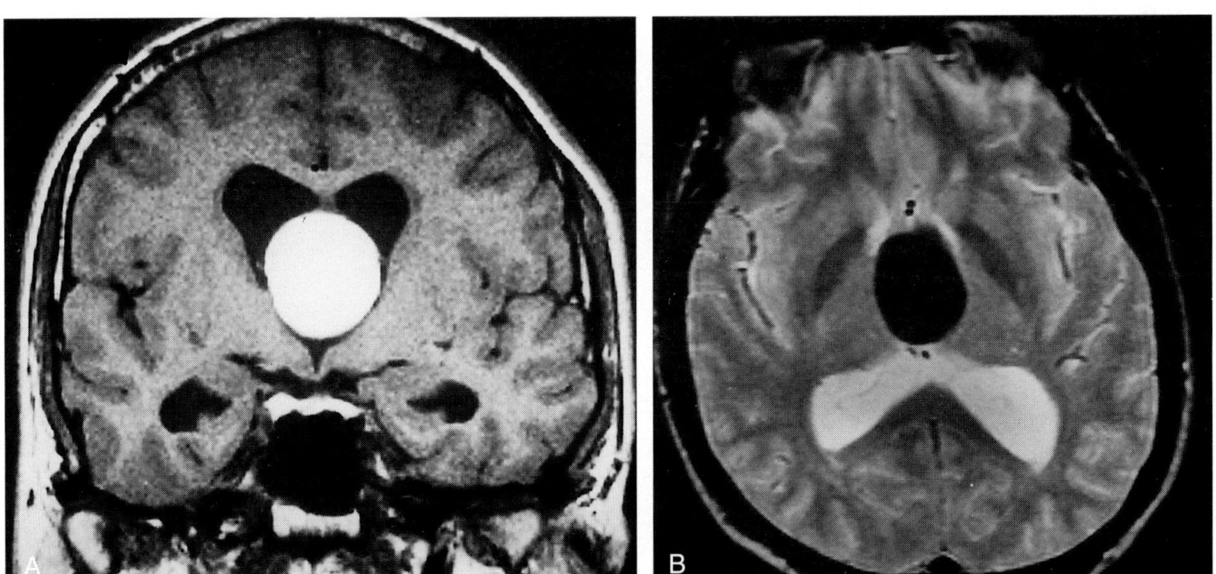

Figure 4–64. Colloid cyst. **(A)** Coronal T1-weighted MRI shows a round hyperintense mass of the third ventricle with hydrocephalus. This colloid cyst is unusually large. **(B)** Axial T2-weighted MRI shows near total absence of signal from the cyst.

Ependymal (Neuroepithelial) Cyst

The term neuroepithelial cyst applies to a spectrum of lesions, including the well-known colloid cysts, extremely common choroid plexus cysts, and ependymal cysts. Noncolloid neuroepithelial cysts (ependymal cysts) are lined by ependyma or fibrous connective tissue and contain clear serous fluid.

Location
Intraventricular in the atrium or choroidal fissure. Rarely may be parenchymal or extraaxial.

CT Findings. Because they are isodense with CSF and often intraventricular, the diagnosis may be difficult. The cyst wall usually cannot be resolved. CT shows enlargement of the ventricle around the cysts often at the trigone. The cyst may be outlined by intraventricular contrast, but this should be unnecessary with MRI available. Secondary findings include displacement of the septum pellucidum and choroid plexus. Parenchymal cysts are less common but more easily detected.

MRI Findings. Noncolloid neuroepithelial cysts should be isointense with CSF; however, with MRI, the cyst wall is more readily visualized, facilitating the diagnosis. The lack of pulsatile flow within the cyst may result in mild T1 and T2 prolongation relative to CSF. They do not enhance, and the adjacent brain parenchyma exhibits normal signal characteristics.

Differential Diagnosis
Porencephaly
Echinococcosis
Cysticercosis
Epidermoid

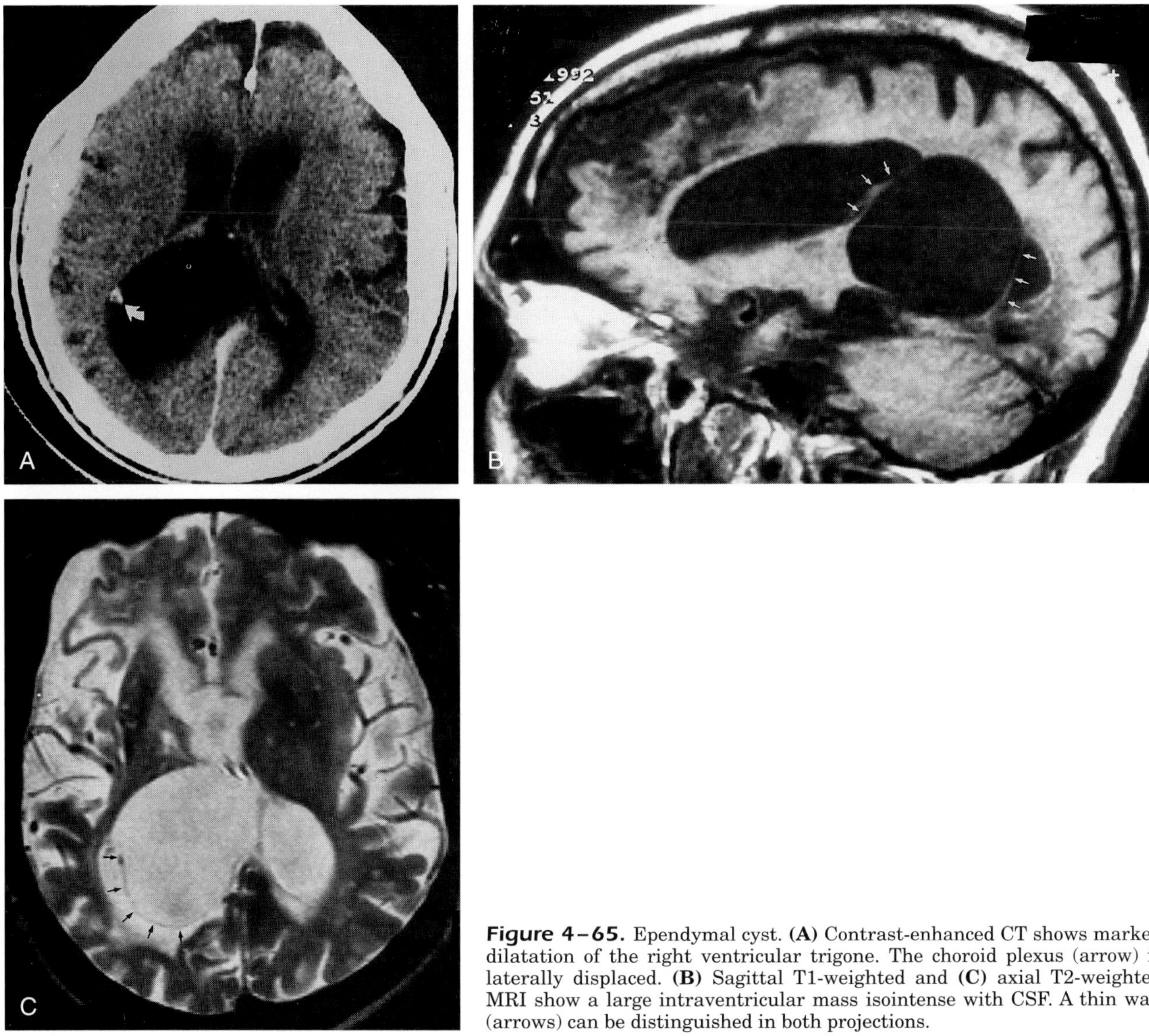

Figure 4–65. Ependymal cyst. **(A)** Contrast-enhanced CT shows marked dilatation of the right ventricular trigone. The choroid plexus (arrow) is laterally displaced. **(B)** Sagittal T1-weighted and **(C)** axial T2-weighted MRI show a large intraventricular mass isointense with CSF. A thin wall (arrows) can be distinguished in both projections.

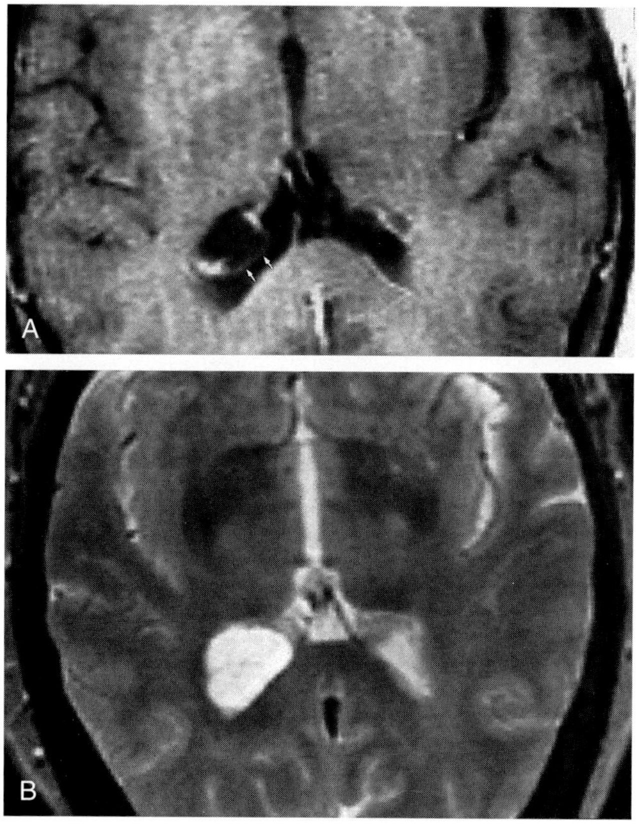

Figure 4–66. Choroid plexus cyst. **(A)** Contrast-enhanced MRI shows a cyst in the trigone of the right lateral ventricle surrounded by enhancing choroid plexus and a thin rim (arrows). **(B)** On T2-weighted MRI the cyst is brighter than free CSF due to the absence of flow.

Pineal Region Tumors

Germinoma

Germinomas account for up to 50% of all pineal region tumors. They occur during the first three decades of life with a peak in the middle of the second decade. Over 90% of pineal germinomas occur in males. As with most pineal tumors, they invade the posterior third ventricle, quadrigeminal plate, and aqueduct, resulting in the frequent presence of hydrocephalus at the time of diagnosis. The hypothalamus is the second most common primary site. Germinomas occasionally occur in the basal ganglia and thalamus. These tumors are extremely radiosensitive, and combined treatment may allow prolonged survival and even cure. However, dissemination throughout the CSF is common.

CT Findings. A germinoma characteristically appears as a hyperdense mass with intense homogeneous contrast enhancement. It commonly engulfs the calcified pineal gland, and coarse stippled tumoral calcification is frequent. Any calcification in the pineal region prior to 12 years of age merits close scrutiny. Meningeal and ependymal seeding are also frequent with enhancing foci in the ventricular walls and subarachnoid space. Germinomas of the basal ganglia tend to be more heterogeneous with cystic foci.

MRI Findings. Germinomas tend to be isointense or hypointense on T1-weighted images and slightly hyperintense on T2-weighted images with intense enhancement after intravenous contrast. The margins may be either sharp or irregular. Small cystic areas may be seen in about half of cases. Hydrocephalus may be present. Germinomas often invade the tectum and in 50% have already spread through the CSF at the time of diagnosis. Enhanced MRI is superior for the depiction of meningeal tumor seeding.

TABLE 4–18 Classification of Tumors in the Pineal Region

I. Tumors of germ cell origin
Germinoma
Teratoma
Teratocarcinoma
Embryonal cell carcinoma
Choriocarcinoma
Yolk sac tumor
Mixed tumor
II. Tumors of pineal origin
Pineocytoma
Pineoblastoma (PNET)
III. Other
Astrocytoma
Ependymoma
Meningioma

TABLE 4–19 Differential Diagnosis of Pineal Region Neoplasms

Tumor	Distinguishing Features
Common	
Germinoma	Most common (30–50% of total) CSF seeding Young males (10–25) Calcifications
Astrocytoma	Second most common Most arise from mesencephalon
Teratoma	Fat present Almost exclusively young male children
Pineocytoma	No sex predilection Older age group
Pineoblastoma	Produces large bulky masses Same as PNET
Rare	
Embryonal cell carcinoma	Elevated HCG and AFP in serum and CSF
Choriocarcinoma	Tumoral hemorrhage Elevated HCG
Endodermal sinus tumor	Elevated AFP
Teratocarcinoma	Large tumors Elevated HCG and AFP
Meningioma	Tentorial attachment
Mixed germ cell tumor	Contains elements of more than one of the above

Note: Pineal cyst is the most common mass of the pineal.

Differential Diagnosis

See Tables 4–18 and 4–19.

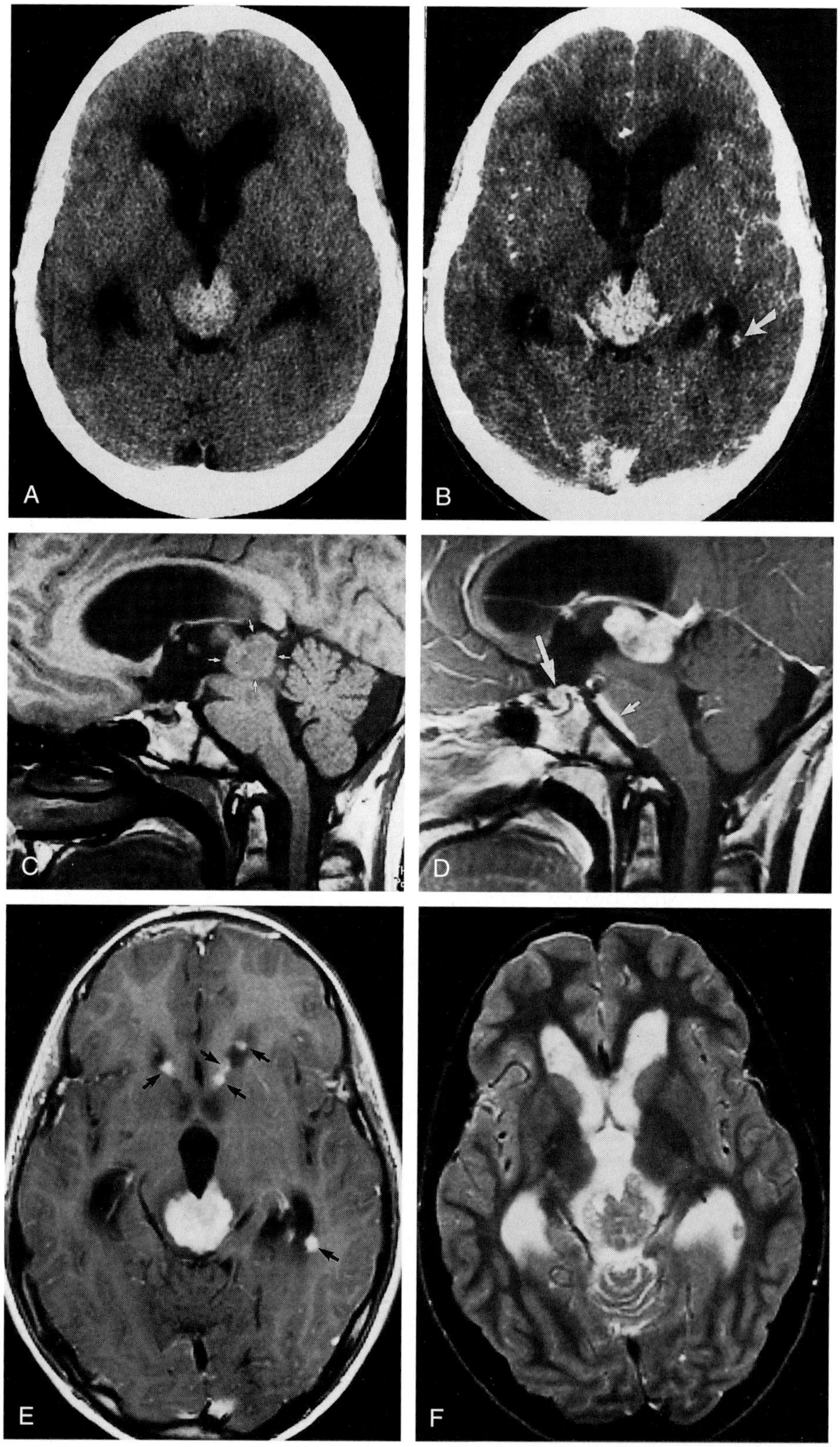

Figure 4–67. Germinoma. CT **(A)** before and **(B)** after contrast shows a uniformly hyperdense and enhancing mass of the pineal region with hydrocephalus. There is remote ependymal enhancement (arrow) due to CSF tumor spread. **(C)** On sagittal T1-weighted MRI the mass (arrows) is isointense with gray matter and there is severe dilatation of the third ventricle. **(D)** Contrast-enhanced MRI shows homogeneous enhancement of the primary mass with enhancing tumor also seen in the floor of the third ventricle (long arrow) and prepontine cistern (short arrow). **(E)** Axial contrast-enhanced MRI shows more extensive ependymal metastases (arrows) than does CT. **(F)** On T2-weighted MRI the primary mass is slightly hyperintense relative to gray matter.

Teratoma

The teratoma is the second most common germ cell tumor of the pineal region. Most intracranial teratomas occur in the pineal region, followed by the sella and suprasellar region. They usually present in the first two decades and occur almost exclusively in males. Mature teratomas contain cells of all three embryologic cell lines (ectoderm, mesoderm, and endoderm). They usually contain cartilage, bone, hair, and fat and are nearly always partly cystic.

CT Findings. CT shows an extremely heterogeneous mass with cysts, linear or nodular calcification, usually fat, and irregular or no contrast enhancement. The margins are usually sharp. Immature (malignant) teratomas tend to be large with cystic and necrotic areas and are less likely to contain visible fat.

MRI Findings. Benign teratomas are heterogeneous with areas of hyperintensity and hypointensity on T1-weighted images. They are heterogeneously hyperintense on T2-weighted images. Ringlike enhancement may be observed after intravenous contrast. Malignant teratomas tend to be large (>4 cm), heterogeneous, hypointense on T1-weighted images, and hyperintense on T2-weighted images. Malignant teratomas visibly invade adjacent structures, especially the tectum and tegmentum.

Differential Diagnosis

See Tables 4–18 and 4–19.

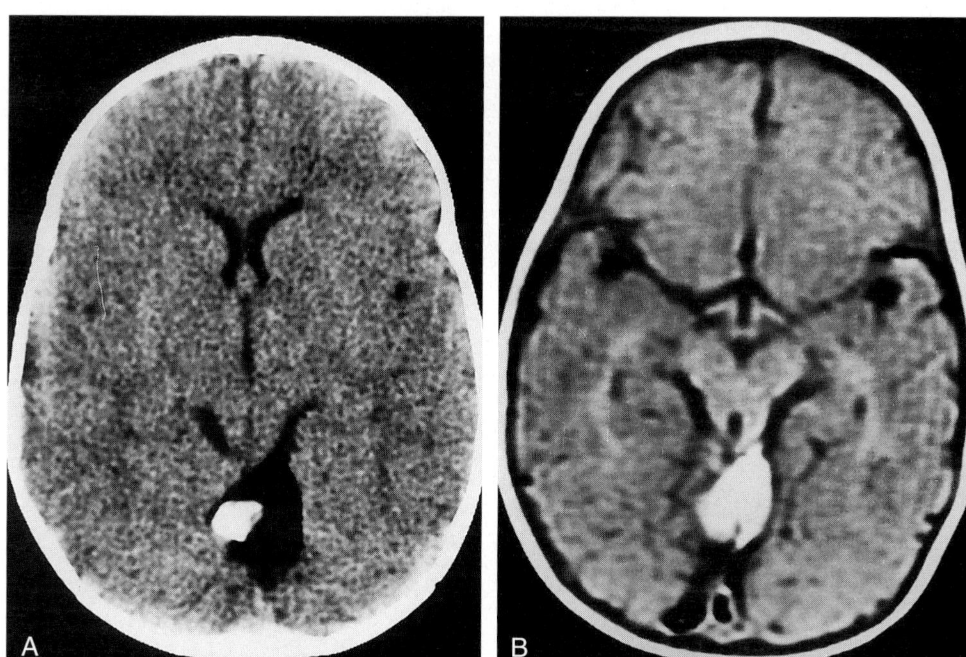

Figure 4–68. Teratoma. **(A)** CT shows a posterior midline mass composed mostly of fat with a solitary large dense calcification. **(B)** Axial T1-weighted MRI shows a hyperintense fatty mass of the pineal region.

Pineocytoma

Pineocytomas are true benign neoplasms of pineal parenchymal cells but constitute only a small percentage of tumors in this region. They usually occur in adults with no sex predilection. These tumors are slow growing, and patients may survive for decades. Dissemination throughout the CSF may occur.

CT Findings. CT usually shows a well-circumscribed isodense to hyperdense mass with homogeneous enhancement. Calcifications are present in slightly less than half of cases.

MRI Findings. Pineocytomas are usually heterogeneous on T1-weighted images and heterogeneously hyperintense on T2-weighted images. The margins are usually well defined. Homogeneous enhancement occurs after intravenous contrast. As with most pineal region tumors, CSF spread is common.

Differential Diagnosis

See Tables 4–18 and 4–19.

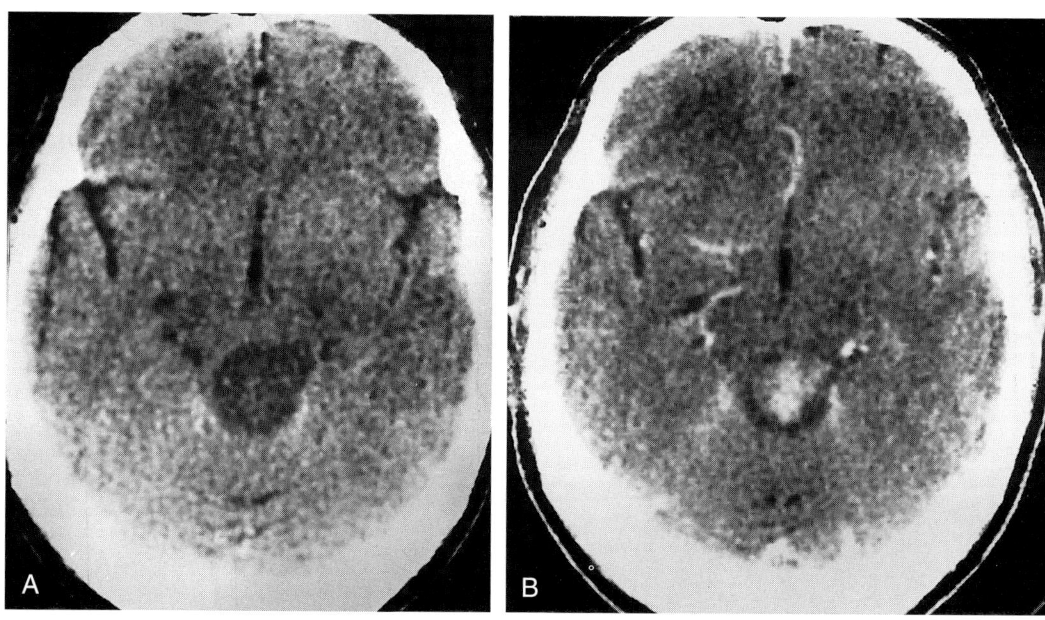

Figure 4–69. Pineocytoma. CT **(A)** before and **(B)** after contrast shows a hypodense mass of the pineal region with solid enhancement.

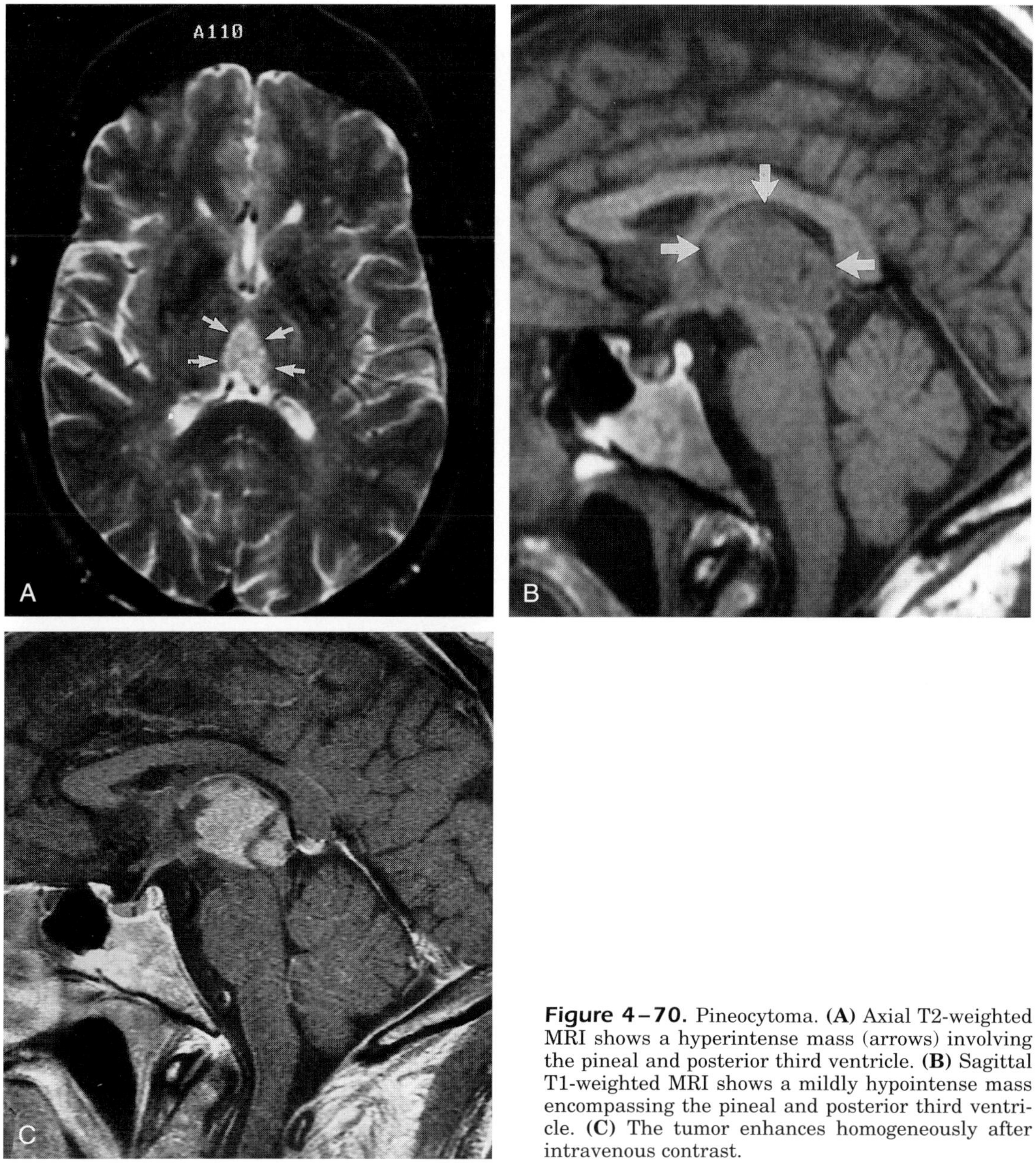

Figure 4–70. Pineocytoma. **(A)** Axial T2-weighted MRI shows a hyperintense mass (arrows) involving the pineal and posterior third ventricle. **(B)** Sagittal T1-weighted MRI shows a mildly hypointense mass encompassing the pineal and posterior third ventricle. **(C)** The tumor enhances homogeneously after intravenous contrast.

Pineoblastoma

Pineoblastomas represent a malignant transformation of pineal parenchymal cells into a tumor that is indistinguishable from, and sometimes categorized as, a primitive neuroectodermal tumor. Its peak incidence is in the first decade of life. There is a high incidence of subarachnoid seeding and infiltration of brain. Occasionally areas of differentiation into retinoblastoma are encountered. The so-called trilateral retinoblastoma consists of bilateral retinoblastomas and a pineoblastoma. Few patients survive more than 2 years.

CT Findings. CT typically shows a hyperdense, heterogeneously enhancing mass with cystic or necrotic areas. Calcifications are sometimes seen. Leptomeningeal tumor spread is common.

MRI Findings. MRI reveals a large lobulated mass isointense to hypointense on T1-weighted images and isointense to slightly hyperintense on T2-weighted images. Cystic or necrotic areas are common. Hemorrhage may be present. Pineoblastomas tend to be larger (>4 cm) than other pineal tumors. The solid portions show heterogeneous enhancement.

Differential Diagnosis

See Tables 4–18 and 4–19.

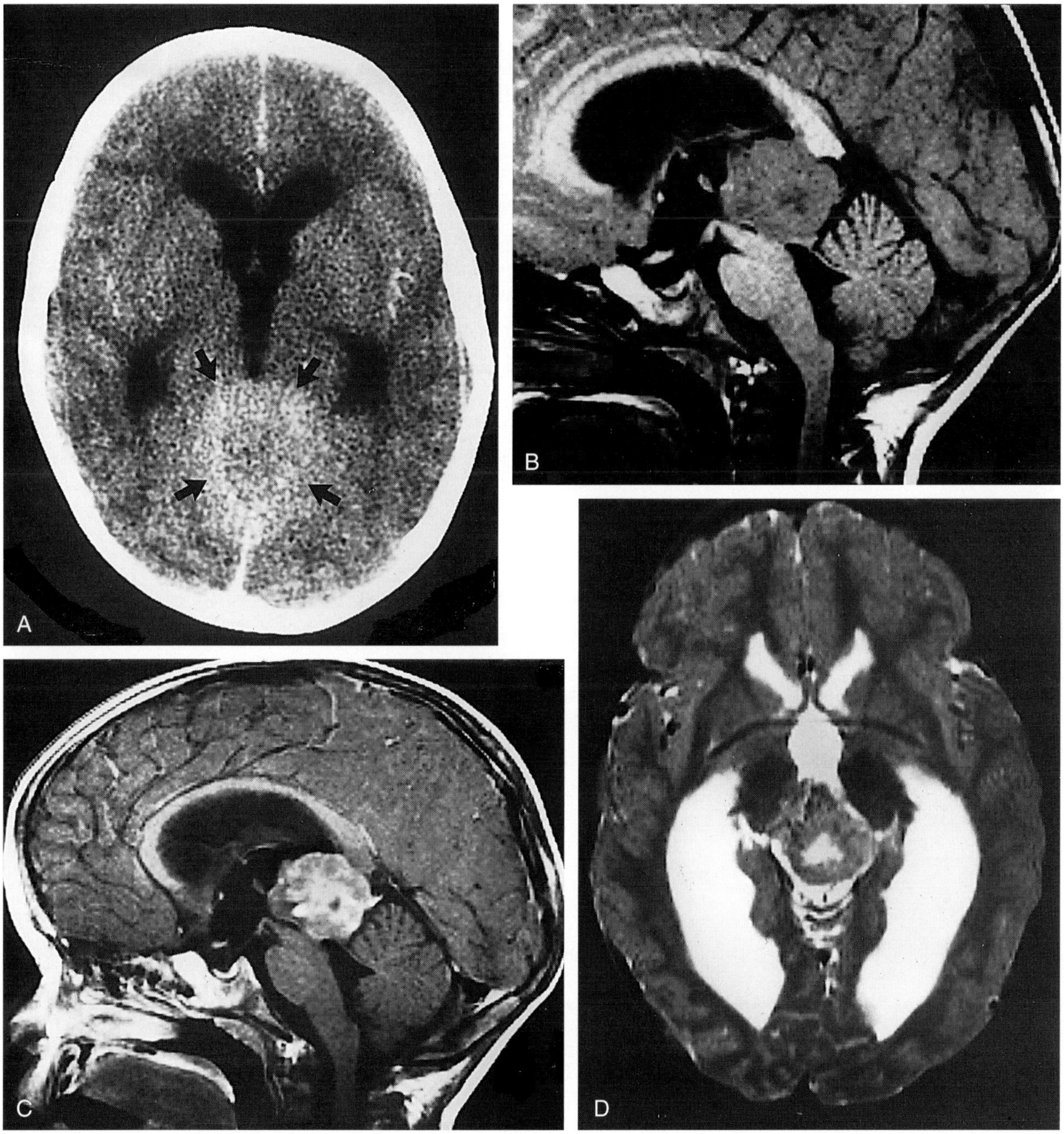

Figure 4–71. Pineoblastoma. **(A)** Contrast-enhanced CT shows a uniformly enhancing mass (arrows) filling the superior cerebellar cistern. Hydrocephalus is present. **(B)** On sagittal T1-weighted MRI the mass is isointense with gray matter and arises from the pineal region. **(C)** Solid enhancement is seen after intravenous contrast. **(D)** On axial T2-weighted MRI the mass is heterogeneously hyperintense relative to brain.

Pineal Cyst

Pineal cysts are a common incidental finding on MRI. They are rarely symptomatic and if typical in appearance do not require treatment or follow-up.

CT Findings. Pineal cysts are seldom recognized on CT because their fluid content is usually isodense with CSF of the quadrigeminal cistern. Their detection may be enhanced with thin slices, improving visualization of the thin wall of the cyst.

MRI Findings. Pineal cysts are frequently recognized on MRI with a reported incidence of 1.5–4.3%. The cyst has a smooth thin wall (<2 mm) and is usually less than 10 mm but may be up to 15 mm in diameter. Larger cysts may produce mass effect upon the tectum and displace the vein of Galen. The cyst contents are homogeneously isointense to slightly hyperintense relative to CSF on T1-weighted images and hyperintense relative to CSF on proton-density and T2-weighted images. Thin rim enhancement may be seen after intravenous contrast, although with a long postinjection delay the cyst contents may enhance as well.

Differential Diagnosis

With a straightforward MRI appearance as described above, the appearance is virtually pathognomonic. Pineal cysts may be distinguished from neoplasms by the absence of symptoms and their smooth sharp margins, internal homogeneity, and typical signal characteristics.

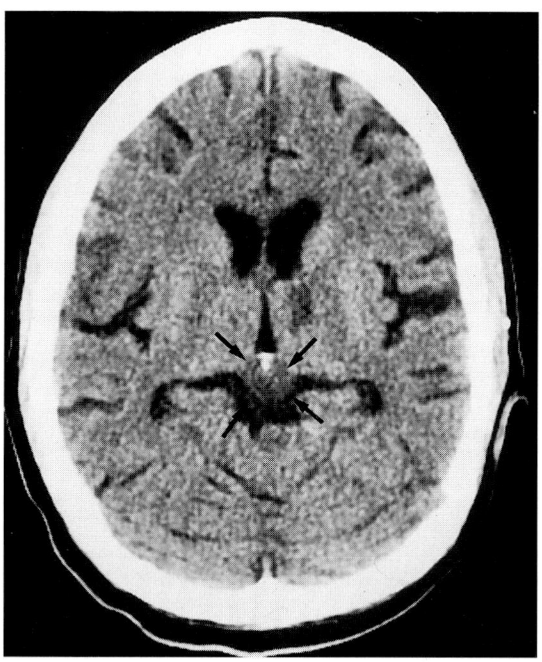

Figure 4–72. Pineal cyst. CT without contrast shows a pineal cyst (arrows) slightly higher in attenuation than adjacent CSF.

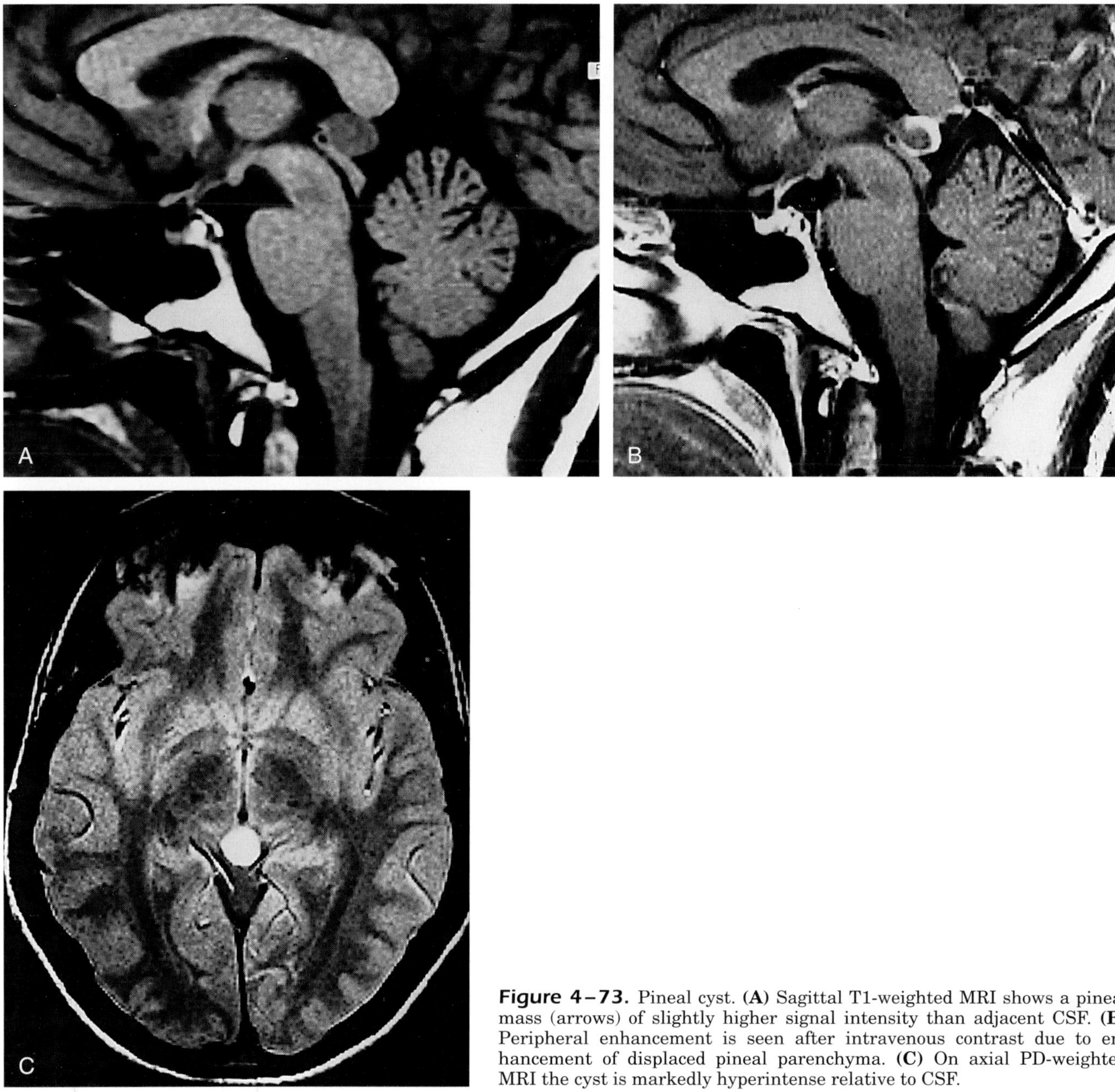

Figure 4–73. Pineal cyst. **(A)** Sagittal T1-weighted MRI shows a pineal mass (arrows) of slightly higher signal intensity than adjacent CSF. **(B)** Peripheral enhancement is seen after intravenous contrast due to enhancement of displaced pineal parenchyma. **(C)** On axial PD-weighted MRI the cyst is markedly hyperintense relative to CSF.

Effects of Treatment

Postoperative Changes

Imaging findings in the postoperative patient may be related to normal postoperative changes, postoperative complications, and tumor recurrence. The ability to distinguish normal postoperative events, especially regarding contrast enhancement, from tumor recurrence is fundamental to the follow-up evaluation of tumor patients. Certain points should be kept in mind:

1. Intravenous contrast may not show residual tumor if the tumor did not enhance preoperatively.
2. Tumors that at first did not enhance may progress to more malignant forms that do enhance.
3. Malignant gliomas almost always recur at some time.

CT Findings. The immediate postoperative CT may normally show subdural and epidural fluid collections, blood-soaked Gelfoam, air, edema, and cavities at the site of resection. No significant contrast enhancement should be seen in the first few days after surgery. Enhancement of postoperative tissue reaction may appear in weeks and persist for months.

MRI Findings. The acute postoperative MRI following a tumor resection will typically show scalp swelling; air, blood, or CSF collections at the craniotomy site; and edema or hemorrhage of the adjacent parenchyma. Postoperative enhancement of brain and meninges unrelated to tumor has been documented as soon as 18 hours after surgery for intraaxial tumors and will develop in two thirds by 6 months. Postoperative parenchymal enhancement will usually disappear by 1 year, whereas meningeal enhancement (arachnoid or dura), although subsiding somewhat, may persist for decades. The parenchymal enhancement usually is seen along the margins of the encephalotomy site. Thick nodular enhancement, increasing area of enhancement, or enhancement beyond 1 year should suggest tumor recurrence.

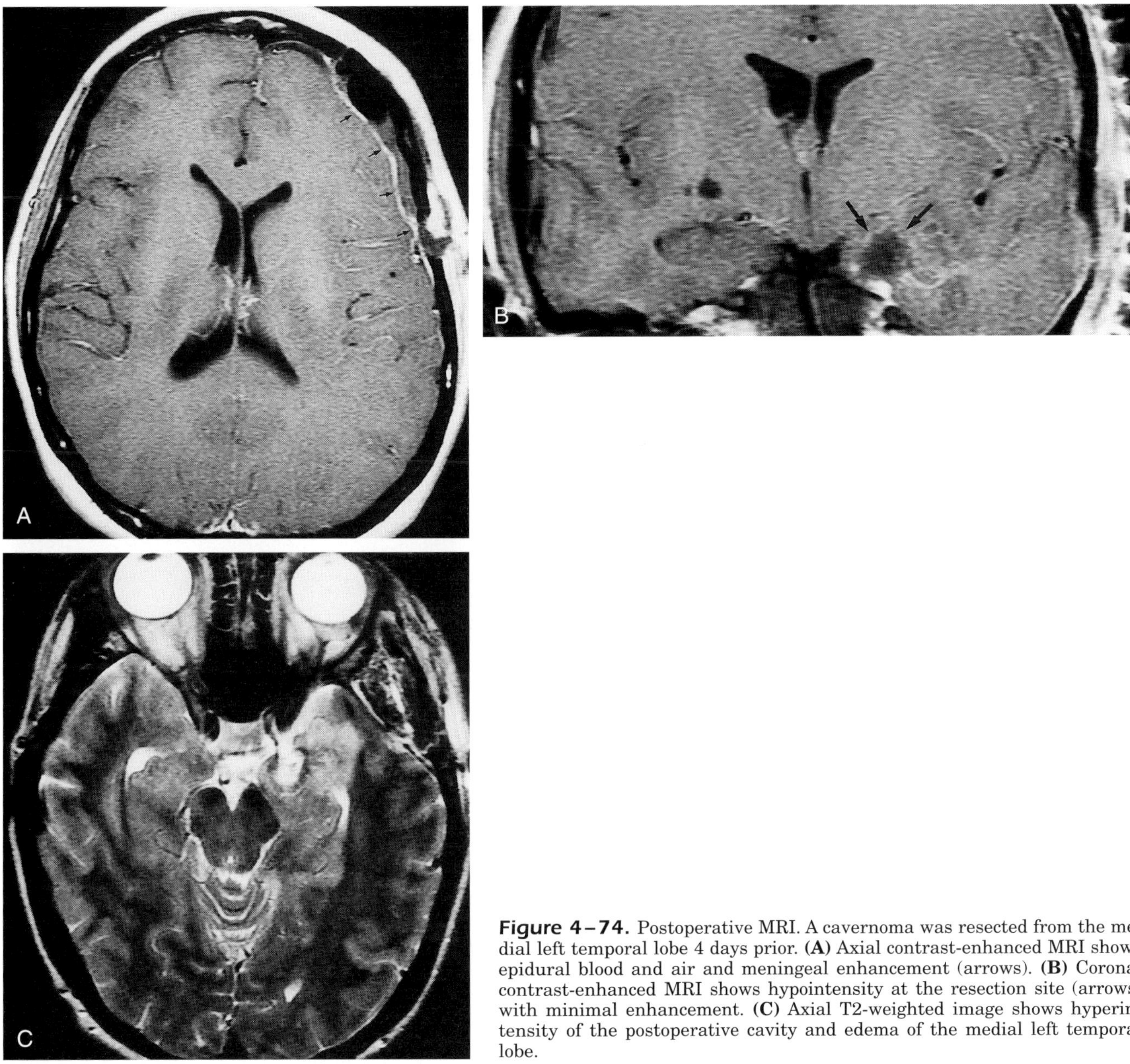

Figure 4–74. Postoperative MRI. A cavernoma was resected from the medial left temporal lobe 4 days prior. **(A)** Axial contrast-enhanced MRI shows epidural blood and air and meningeal enhancement (arrows). **(B)** Coronal contrast-enhanced MRI shows hypointensity at the resection site (arrows) with minimal enhancement. **(C)** Axial T2-weighted image shows hyperintensity of the postoperative cavity and edema of the medial left temporal lobe.

Radiation Injury

Complications of cranial radiation are usually divided into early and late radiation injuries. The injuries of greatest clinical significance are usually delayed several months to 10 or more years after treatment. These injuries include radiation necrosis, diffuse white matter injury, radiation vasculitis, and necrotizing leukoencephalopathy. Tables 4–20 and 4–21 list the CNS sequelae of oncologic therapy and cerebral complications of antineoplastic therapy.

TABLE 4–20 | CNS Sequelae of Oncologic Therapy

Atrophy
Chemical meningitis
Radiation injuries
Necrosis
Diffuse white matter injury
Vasculitis
Necrotizing leukoencephalopathy
Mineralizing microangiopathy
Cerebellar sclerosis
Spinal cord dysfunction
Secondary neoplasms

TABLE 4–21 | Cerebral Complications of Antineoplastic Therapy

Condition	Clinical Findings	Imaging Findings
Atrophy	Very common, results from radiation or chemotherapy, and most likely asymptomatic	Enlargement of ventricles, cortical fissures, and sulci
Necrotizing leukoencephalopathy	Neurologic deterioration beginning 2 to 12 months after treatment	White matter edema, enhancement, and calcifications
Mineralizing microangiopathy	Occurs mostly in children following combined cranial radiation and chemotherapy given during the first decade of life	Extensive calcification of the basal ganglia and thalami on CT and may also involve subcortical white matter, caudate nuclei, and dentate nuclei
Radiation necrosis	Symptoms of mass lesion presenting 3 months to 2 years after treatment	White matter edema, enhancing mass, and usually very close to tumor site
Diffuse radiation injury	Most often asymptomatic, presenting months to years after treatment	Bilateral symmetric white matter hypodensity on CT and hyperintensity on T2 MRI
Tumor induction	Complication of cranial irradiation in childhood with latency of 5 to 30 years and incidence of 3–5%	Meningiomas and nerve sheath tumors show greatest increase in incidence

Radiation Necrosis

Radiation necrosis presents as a new or enlarging mass lesion following cranial irradiation. About 70% of cases occur in the first 2 years following treatment. It is characterized pathologically by demyelination and coagulative necrosis of the white matter and fibrinoid necrosis of small arteries and arterioles. Radiation necrosis typically occurs at or near the original tumor bed.

CT Findings. CT shows localized vasogenic edema in the white matter with irregular ring enhancement following intravenous contrast. The enhancing mass typically is at or near the original tumor bed.

MRI Findings. MRI findings parallel those on CT with vasogenic edema and an enhancing mass. Diffuse white matter injury may be present concurrently.

Differential Diagnosis

Differentiating radiation necrosis from recurrent tumor is a historic diagnostic dilemma. No anatomically based imaging findings allow a confident distinction to be made, although the treatment is radically influenced by the diagnosis. Physiologic investigation by positron-emission tomography (PET) or MRI spectroscopy shows promise, with each showing decreased metabolic activity in radiation necrosis and increased activity in tumor.

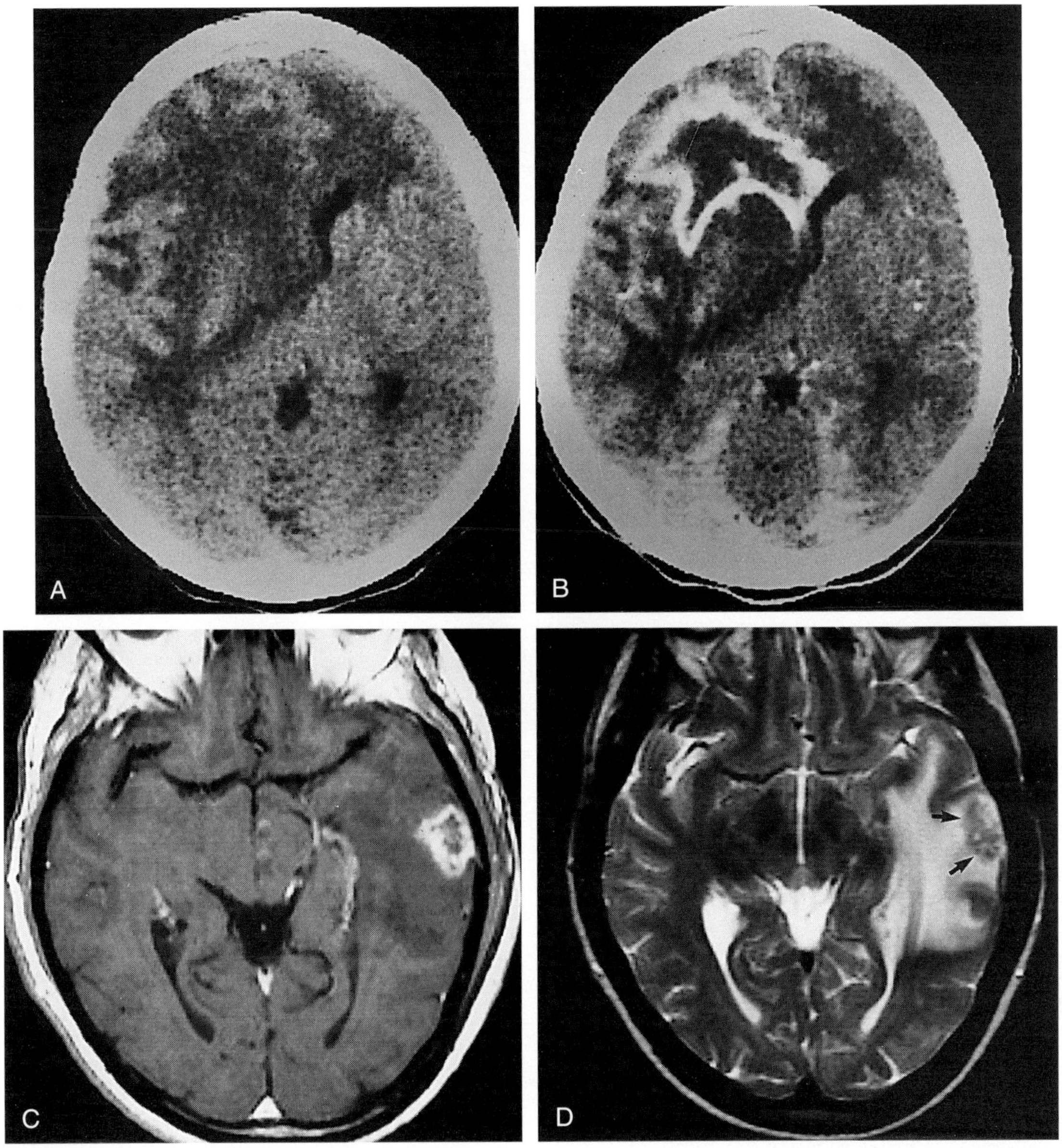

Figure 4–75. Radiation necrosis. **(A)** Unenhanced CT shows massive vasogenic edema of both frontal lobes extending into the lentiform nuclei and temporal lobe on the right. **(B)** After intravenous contrast a large irregular necrotic cavity is demarcated by intense peripheral enhancement. **(C)** Patient received localized radiotherapy for superficial scalp malignancy. Contrast-enhanced MRI shows a superficial, irregular ring–enhancing mass of the left temporal lobe with surrounding edema. **(D)** T2-weighted scan shows marked vasogenic edema. The arrow of necrosis (arrows) is slightly hyperintense relative to brain.

Diffuse White Matter Injury

Diffuse white matter injury is an extremely common finding after cranial irradiation, eventually becoming manifest on MRI in over one third of all radiated patients. Most are asymptomatic; those with more severe injury tend to manifest mild to severe cognitive deficits. The abnormal white matter signal on MRI relates to increased tissue water probably accompanying demyelination.

CT Findings. The primary finding on CT is the presence of symmetric low attenuation in the periventricular white matter. Atrophy may be present. Because CT is less sensitive than MRI in this condition, an abnormal CT indicates more severe involvement and is more likely to correlate with the presence of cognitive deficits.

MRI Findings. MRI reveals periventricular hyperintensity on proton-density and T2-weighted scans. The hyperintensity is usually bilaterally symmetric but may range in extent from small foci adjacent to the frontal horns and trigones to diffuse disease spanning the white matter from the cortex to the ependyma of the lateral ventricles.

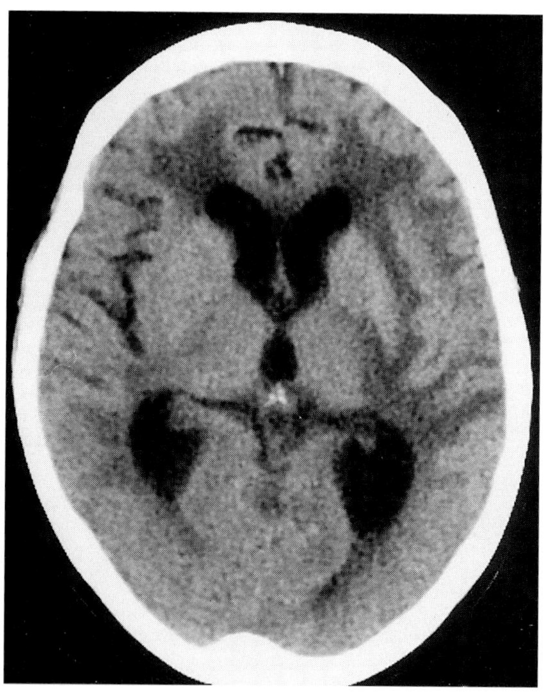

Figure 4–76. Diffuse white matter injury. Unenhanced CT shows diminished attenuation in the frontal white matter bilaterally, left external and internal capsules, and left temporal white matter.

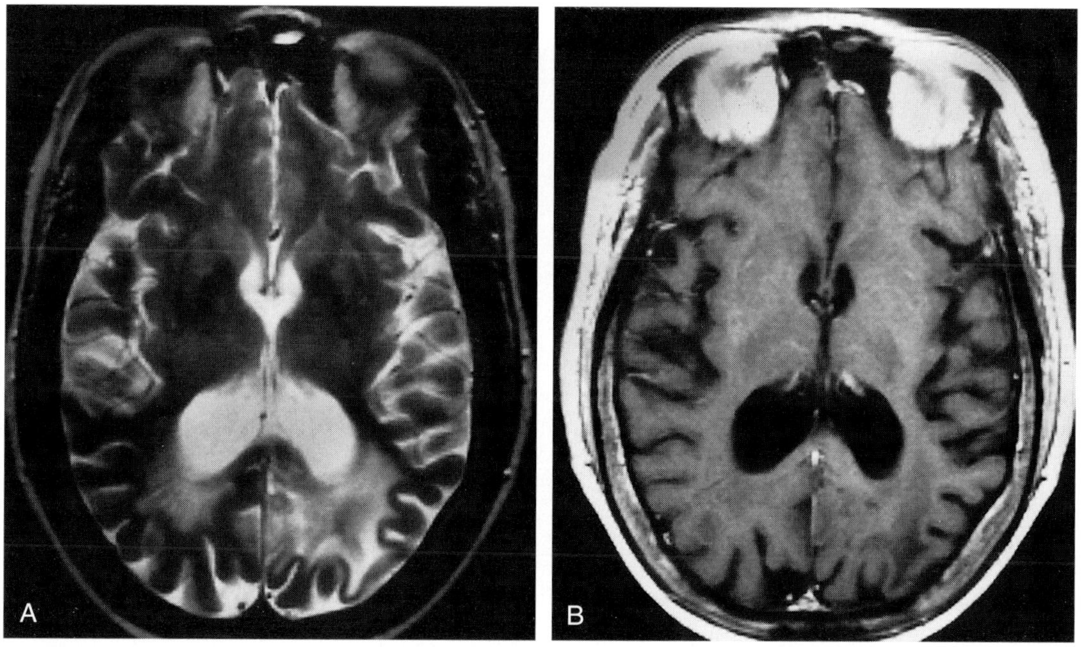

Figure 4–77. Diffuse white matter injury. **(A)** Axial T2-weighted MRI shows hyperintensity in the peritrigonal white matter bilaterally, which developed subsequent to radiotherapy. There was an added component of vasogenic edema on the left associated with a small enhancing focus. **(B)** Axial contrast-enhanced MRI shows absence of enhancement within the white matter. Diminished signal is only apparent on the left where there was an additional component of vasogenic edema.

Radiation Vasculitis

Although radiation usually affects only medium and small arteries, progressive disease of larger cerebral arteries occasionally develops. Pathologically this resembles an accelerated form of atherosclerosis, and ischemic complications may ensue. Symptoms usually do not develop until many years after treatment.

CT Findings. CT may show calcifications in the parenchyma related to the affected vessels or dystrophic calcification of ischemic tissue. Secondary effects of ischemia (atrophy, demyelination, and infarction) are the major CT findings.

Angiographic Findings. Angiography reveals irregular narrowing, either focal or diffuse, of the major cerebral arteries.

Necrotizing Leukoencephalopathy

Necrotizing leukoencephalopathy is a rare complication of oncologic therapy that may follow cranial irradiation, systemic or intrathecal methotrexate, or any combination thereof. Other chemotherapeutic agents have also been implicated. Its onset is characterized clinically by progressive irritability, seizures, and neurologic deficits progressing to coma or death. Histology reveals white matter coagulation necrosis, axonal edema with fragmentation, and reactive gliosis leading to parenchymal atrophy and calcifications.

CT Findings. CT may show periventricular low attenuation or mild edema with occasional contrast enhancement. The process may occur focally around a ventriculostomy catheter. In later stages, CT shows parenchymal atrophy and calcifications.

MRI Findings. T2-weighted images show white matter hyperintensity that tends to be asymmetrical between hemispheres. Marked enhancement may occur after intravenous contrast.

Differential Diagnosis
Recurrent tumor
Radiation necrosis

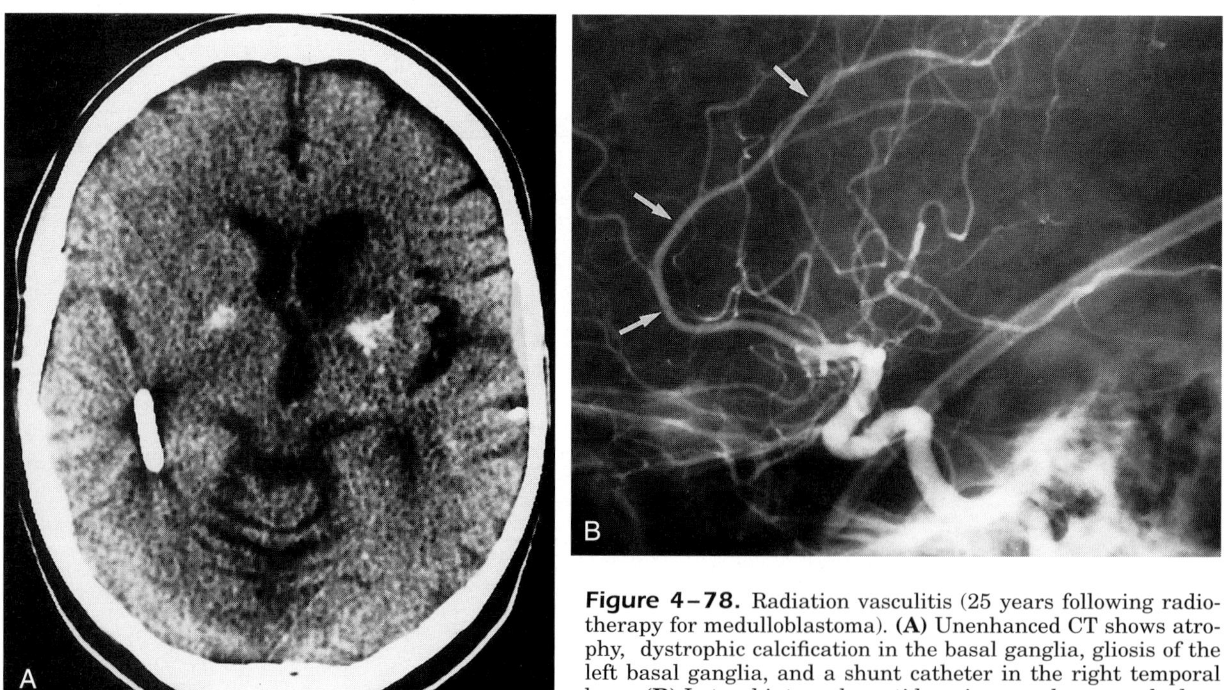

Figure 4–78. Radiation vasculitis (25 years following radiotherapy for medulloblastoma). **(A)** Unenhanced CT shows atrophy, dystrophic calcification in the basal ganglia, gliosis of the left basal ganglia, and a shunt catheter in the right temporal horn. **(B)** Lateral internal carotid angiogram shows marked attenuation and irregularity of the middle cerebral branches. Compare to caliber of normal anterior cerebral artery (arrows).

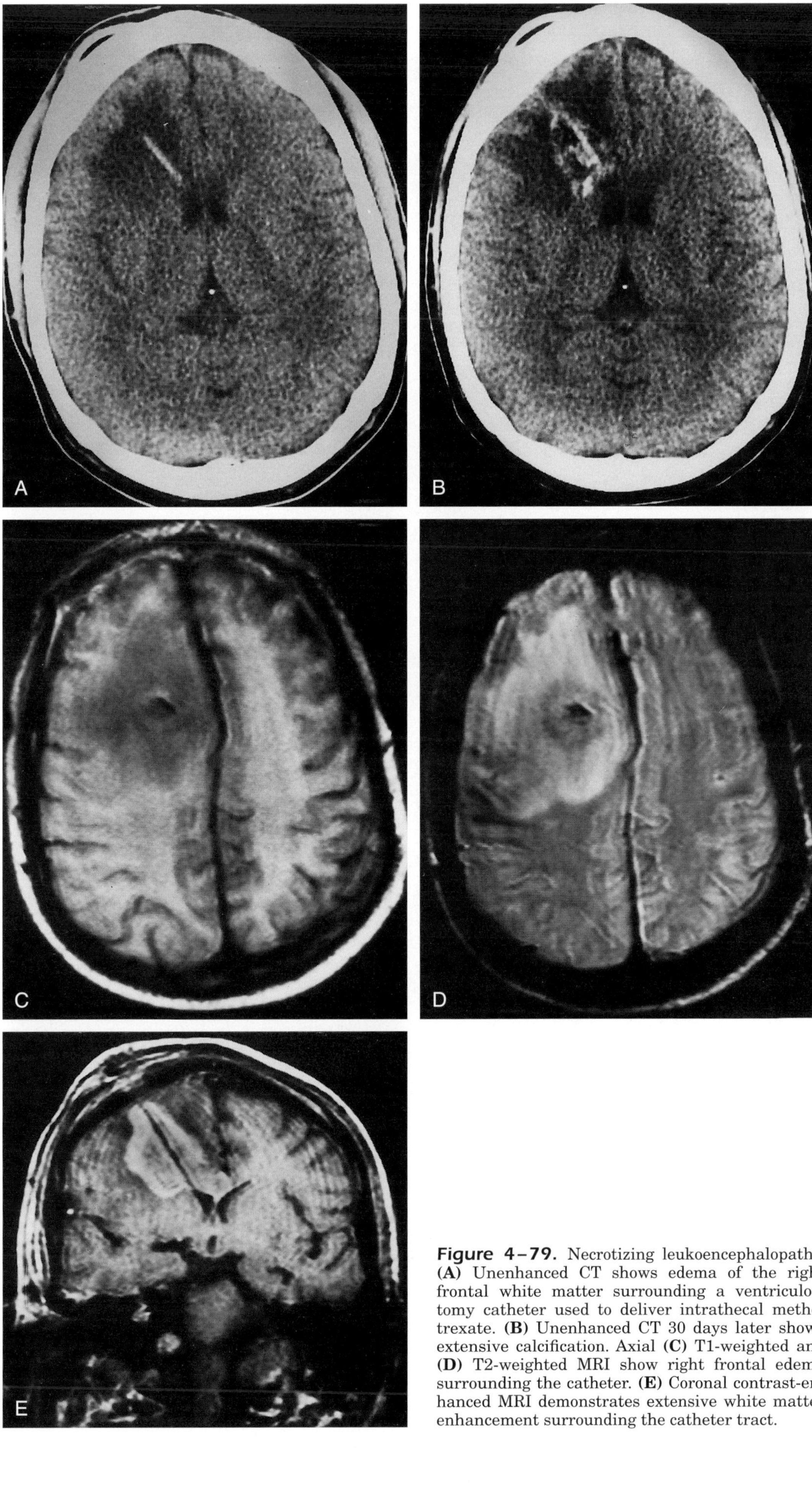

Figure 4–79. Necrotizing leukoencephalopathy. **(A)** Unenhanced CT shows edema of the right frontal white matter surrounding a ventriculostomy catheter used to deliver intrathecal methotrexate. **(B)** Unenhanced CT 30 days later shows extensive calcification. Axial **(C)** T1-weighted and **(D)** T2-weighted MRI show right frontal edema surrounding the catheter. **(E)** Coronal contrast-enhanced MRI demonstrates extensive white matter enhancement surrounding the catheter tract.

RECOMMENDED READINGS

Meningioma

Aoki,S, Sasaki,Y, Machida,T, Tanioka,H. Contrast-Enhanced MR Images in Patients with Meningioma: Importance of Enhancement of the Dura Adjacent to the Tumor. *AJNR* 11:935–938,1990.

Elster,AD, Challa,VR, Gilbert,TH, Richardson,DN, Contento,JC. Meningiomas: MR and Histopathologic Features. *Radiology* 170:857–862, 1989.

Rosenbaum,AE, Rosenbloom,SB. Meningiomas Revisited. *Semin Roentgenol* 19:8–26, 1984.

Terstegge,K, Schorner,W, Henkes,H, et al. Hyperostosis in Meningiomas: MR Findings in Patients with Recurrent Meningioma of the Sphenoid Wings. *AJNR* 15:555–560, 1994.

Zee,CS, Chin,T, Segall,HD, Destian,S, Ahmadi,J. Magnetic Resonance Imaging of Meningiomas. *Semin Ultrasound CT MR* 13:154–169, 1992.

Arachnoid Cysts

Kolawole,TM, Patel,PJ, Mahdi,AH. Arachnoid Cysts: Computed Tomography Findings. *J Comput Assist Tomogr* 11:156–159, 1987.

Robertson,SJ, Wolpert,SM, Runge,VM. MR Imaging of Middle Cranial Fossa Arachnoid Cysts: Temporal Lobe Agenesis Syndrome Revisited. *AJNR* 10:1007–1010, 1989.

Wiener,SN, Pearlstein,AE, Eiber,A. MR Imaging of Intracranial Arachnoid Cysts. *J Comput Assist Tomogr* 11:236–241, 1987.

Dermoid

Smith,AS, Benson,JE, Blaser,SI, Mizushima,A, Tarr,RW, Bellon,EM. Diagnosis of Ruptured Intracranial Dermoid Cysts: Value of MR over CT. *AJNR* 12:175–180, 1991. *AJR* 156:807–812, 1991.

Wilms,G, Casselman,J, Demaerel,P, Plets,C, De Haene,I, Baert,AL. CT and MRI of Ruptured Intracranial Dermoids. *Neuroradiology* 33:149–151, 1991.

Epidermoid

Steffey,DJ, De Filipp,GJ, Spera,T, Gabrielsen,TO. MR Imaging of Primary Epidermoid Tumors. *J Comput Assist Tomogr* 12:428–440, 1988.

Tampieri,D, Melanson,D, Romeo,E. MR Imaging of Epidermoid Cysts. *AJNR* 10:351–356, 1989.

Schwannoma

Stack,JP, Ramsden,RT, Antoun,NM, Lye,RH, Isherwood,I, Jenkins, JPR. Magnetic Resonance Imaging of Acoustic Neuromas: The Role of Gadolinium-DTPA. *Br J Radiol* 61: 800–805, 1988.

Wu,EH, Tang,Y, Zhang,Y, Bai,R. CT in Diagnosis of Acoustic Neuromas. *AJNR* 7:645–650, 1986.

Pituitary Adenoma

Colombo,N, Loli,P, Vignati,F, Scialfa,G. MR of Corticotropin-Secreting Pituitary Microadenomas. 15:1591–1595, 1994.

Sakamoto,Y, Takahashi,M, Korogi,Y, Bussaka,H, Ushio,Y. Normal and Abnormal Pituitary Glands: Gadopentetate Dimeglumine-enhanced MR Imaging. *Radiology* 178:441–445, 1991.

Schwartzberg,DG. Imaging of Pituitary Gland Tumors. *Semin Ultrasound CT MR* 13:207–223, 1992.

Stadnik,T, Stevenaert,A, Beckers,A, Luypaert,R, Buisseret, Osteaux,M. Pituitary Microadenomas: Diagnosis with Two- and Three-dimensional MR Imaging at 1.5T before and after Injection of Gadolinium. *Radiology* 176:419–428, 1990.

Sumida,M, Uozumi,T, Mudada,K, et al. Rathke Cleft Cysts: Correlation of Enhanced MR and Surgical Findings. *AJNR* 15:525–532, 1994.

Teramoto,A, Hirakawa,K, Sanno,N, Osamura,Y. Incidental Pituitary Lesions in 1,000 Unselected Autopsy Specimens. *Radiology* 193:161–164, 1994.

Craniopharyngioma

Freeman,MP, Kessler,RM, Allen,JH, Price,AC. Craniopharyngioma: CT and MR Imaging in Nine Cases. *J Comput Assist Tomogr* 11:810–814, 1987.

Pusey,E, Korman,KE, Flannigan,BD, Tsuruda,J, Bradley,WG. MR of Craniopharyngiomas: Tumor Delineation and Characterization. *AJNR* 8:439–444, 1987.

Chordoma

Meyer,JE, Oot,RF, Lindfors,KK. CT Appearance of Clival Chordomas. *J Comput Assist Tomogr* 10:34–38, 1986.

Meyers,SP, Hirsch,WL, Curtin,HD, Barnes,L, Sekhar,LN, Sen,C. Chordomas of the Skull Base: MR Features. *AJNR* 13:1627–1636, 1992.

Sze,G, Uichanco III,LS, Brant-Zawadski,MN, et al. Chordomas: MR Imaging. *Radiology* 166:187–191, 1988.

Weber,AL, Liebsch,NJ, Sanchez,R, Sweriduk,ST. Chordomas of the Skull Base: Radiologic and Clinical Evaluation. *Neuroimaging Clin North Am* 4:515–527, 1994.

Meningeal Metastasis

Lee,YY, Glass,JP, Geoffray,A, Wallace,S. Cranial Computed Tomographic Abnormalities in Leptomeningeal Metastasis. *AJNR* 5:559–563, 1984. *AJR* 143:1035–1039, 1984.

Lee,YY, Tien,RD, Bruner,JM, DePena,CA, Van Tassel,P. Loculated Intracranial Leptomeningeal Metastases: CT and MR Characteristics. *AJNR* 10:1171–1179, 1989, *AJR* 154: 351–359, 1990.

Sze,G, Soletsky,S, Bronen,R, Krol,G. MR Imaging of the Cranial Meninges with Emphasis on Contrast Enhancement and Meningeal Carcinomatosis. *AJNR* 10:965–975, 1989. *AJR* 153:1039–1049, 1989.

Glioblastoma Multiforme

Castillo,M, Scatliff,JH, Bouldin,TW, Suzuki,K. Radiologic-Pathologic Correlation: Intracranial Astrocytoma. *AJNR* 13: 1609–1616, 1992.

Dean,BL, Drayer,BP, Bird,CR, et al. Gliomas: Classification with MR Imaging. *Radiology* 174:411–415, 1990.

Leeds,NE, Elkin,CM, Zimmerman,RD. Gliomas of the Brain. *Semin Roentgenol* 19:27–43, 1984.

Anaplastic Astrocytoma

Krol,G, Muraki,A, Kearney,A. MR Characteristics of Anaplastic Astrocytomas. Presented at the American Society of Neuroradiology, Washington D.C., 1991.

Fibrillary Astrocytoma

Dean,BL, Drayer,BP, Bird,CR, et al. Gliomas: Classification with MR Imaging. *Radiology* 174:411–415, 1990.

Leeds,NE, Elkin,CM, Zimmerman,RD. Gliomas of the Brain. *Semin Roentgenol* 19:27–43, 1984.

Oligodendroglioma

Lee,YY, Van Tassel,P. Intracranial Oligodendrogliomas: Imaging Findings in 35 Untreated Cases. *AJR* 152:361–369,1989. *AJNR* 10:119–127,1989.

Ganglioglioma

Castillo,M, Davis,PC, Takei,Y, Hoffman,JC. Intracranial Ganglioglioma: MR, CT, and Clinical Findings in 18 Patients. *AJNR* 11:109–114, 1990, *AJR* 154:607–612, 1990.

Dorne,HL, O'Gorman,AM, Melanson,D. Computed Tomography of Intracranial Gangliogliomas. *AJNR* 7:281–285,1986.

Tampieri,D, Moumdjian,R, Melanson,D, Ethier,R. Intracerebral Gangliogliomas in Patients with Partial Complex Seizures: CT and MR Imaging Findings. *AJNR* 12:749–755, 1991. *AJR* 157:843–849, 1991.

Lymphoma

Jack,CR, O'Neill,BP, Banks,PM, Reese,DF. Central Nervous System Lymphoma: Histologic Types and CT Appearance. *Radiology* 167:211–215.

Schwaighofer,BW, Hesselink,JR, Press,GA, Wolf,RL, Healy,ME, Berthoty,DP. Primary Intracranial CNS Lymphoma: MR Manifestations. *AJNR* 10:725–729, 1989.

Hemangioblastoma

Lee,SR, Sanches,J, Mark,AS, Dillon,WP, Norman,D, Newton, TH. Posterior Fossa Hemangioblastomas: MR Imaging. *Radiology* 171:463–468, 1989.

Seeger,JF, Burke,DP, Knake,JE, Gabrielsen,TO. Computed Tomographic and Angiographic Evaluation of Hemangioblastomas. *Radiology* 138:65–73, 1981.

Juvenile Pilocytic Astrocytoma

Lee,YY, Van Tassel,P, Bruner,JM, Moser,RP, Share,JC. Juvenile Pilocytic Astrocytomas: CT and MR Characteristics. *AJR* 152:1263–1270, 1989. *AJNR* 10:363–370, 1989.

Medulloblastoma

Lee,YY, Glass,JP, van Eys,J, Wallace,S. Medulloblastoma in Infants and Children: Computed Tomographic Follow-up after Treatment. *Radiology* 154:677–682, 1985.

Meyers,SP, Kemp,SS, Tarr,RW. MR Imaging Features of Medulloblastomas. *AJR* 158:859–865, 1992.

Rollins,N, Mendelsohn,D, Mulne,A, et al. Recurrent Medulloblastoma: Frequency of Tumor Enhancement on Gd-DTPA MR Imaging. *AJNR* 11:583–587, 1990. *AJR* 155:153–157, 1990.

Sandhu,A, Kendall,B. Computed Tomography in Management of Medulloblastomas. *Neuroradiology* 29:444–452, 1987.

Supratentorial Primitive Neuroectodermal Tumor

Altman,N, Fitz,CR, Chuang,S, Harwood-Nash,D, Cotter,C, Armstrong,D. Radiological Characteristics of Primitive Neuroectodermal Tumors in Children. *AJNR* 6:15–18, 1985.

Figueroa,RE, El Gammal,T, Brooks,BS, Holgate,R, Miller,W. MR Findings on Primitive Neuroectodermal Tumors. *J Comput Assist Tomogr* 13:773–778, 1989.

Robles,HA, Smirniotopoulis,JG, Figueroa,RE. Understanding the Radiology of Intracranial Primitive Neuroectodermal Tumors From a Pathological Perspective: A Review. *Semin Ultrasound CT MR* 13:170–181, 1992.

Hamartoma

Boyko,OB, Curnes,JT, Oakes,WJ, Burger,PC. Hamartomas of the Tuber Cinereum: CT, MR, and Pathologic Findings. *AJNR* 12:309–314, 1991. *AJR* 156:1053–1058, 1991.

Burton,EM, Ball,WS, Crone,K, Dolan,LM. Hamartoma of the Tuber Cinereum: A Comparison of MR and CT Findings in Four Cases. *AJNR* 10:497–501, 1989.

Parenchymal Brain Metastasis

Bentson,JR, Steckel,RJ, Kagan,AR. Diagnostic Imaging in Clinical Cancer Management: Brain Metastases. *Invest Radiol* 23:335–341, 1988.

Carrier,DA, Mawad,ME, Kirkpatrick,JB, Schmid,MF. Metastatic Adenocarcinoma to the Brain: MR with Pathologic Correlation. *AJNR* 15:155–159, 1994.

Potts,DG, Abbott,GF, von Sneidern,JV. National Cancer Institute Study: Evaluation of Computed Tomography in the Diagnosis of Intracranial Neoplasms. III. Metastatic Tumors. *Radiology* 136:657–664, 1980.

Sze,G, Milano,E, Johnson,C, Heier,L. Detection of Brain Metastases: Comparison of Contrast-Enhanced MR with Unenhanced MR and Enhanced CT. *AJNR* 11:785–791, 1990.

Metastatic Melanoma

Atlas,SW, Grossman,RI, Gomori,JM, et al. MR Imaging of Intracranial Metastatic Melanoma. *J Comput Assist Tomogr* 11:577–582, 1987.

Ginaldi,S, Wallace,S, Shalen,P, Luna,M, Handel,S. Cranial Computed Tomography of Malignant Melanoma. *AJR* 136:145–149,1981.

Ependymoma

Armington,WG, Osborne,AG, Cubberly,DA, et al. Supratentorial Ependymoma: CT Appearance. *Radiology* 157:367–372, 1985.

Spoto,GP, Press,GA, Hesselink,JR, Solomon,M. Intracranial Ependymoma and Subependymoma: MR Manifestations. *AJNR* 11:83–91, 1990. *AJR* 154:837–845, 1990.

Swartz,JD, Zimmerman,RA, Bilaniuk,LT. Computed Tomography of Intracranial Ependymomas. *Radiology* 143:97–101, 1982.

Choroid Plexus Papilloma

Coates,TL, Minshaw,DB Jr, Peckman,N, et al. Pediatric Choroid Plexus Neoplasms: MR, CT, and Pathologic Correlation. *Radiology* 173:81–88, 1989.

Jelinek,J, Smirniotopoulos,JG, Parisis,JE, Kanzer,M. Lateral Ventricular Neoplasms of the Brain: Differential Diagnosis Based on Clinical, CT, and MR Findings. *AJNR* 11:567–574, 1990. *AJR* 155:365–372, 1990.

Colloid Cyst

Ganti,SR, Antunes,JL, Louis,KM, Hilal,SK. Computed Tomography in the Diagnosis of Colloid Cysts of the Third Ventricle. *Radiology* 138:385–391, 1981.

Maeder,PP, Holtas,SL, Basibuyuk,LN, Salford,LG, Tapper,UAS, Brun,A. Colloid Cysts of the Third Ventricle: Correlation of MR and CT Findings with Histology and Chemical Analysis. *AJNR* 11:575–581, 1990. *AJR* 155:135–141, 1990.

Wilms,G, Marchal,G, Van Hecke,P, et al. Colloid Cysts of the Third Ventricle: MR Findings. *J Comput Assist Tomogr* 14:527–531, 1990.

Ependymal (Neuroepithelial) Cyst

Czervionke,LF, Daniels,DL, Meyer,GA, Pojunas,KW, Williams, AL, Haughton,VM. Neuroepithelial Cysts of the Lateral Ventricles: MR Appearance. *AJNR* 8:609–613, 1987.

New,PFJ, Davis,KR. Intraventricular Noncolloid Neuroepithelial Cysts. *AJNR* 2:569–576, 1981.

Sherman,JL, Camponovo,E, Citrin,CM. MR Imaging of CSF-like Choroidal Fissure and Parenchymal Cysts of the Brain. *AJNR* 11:939, 1990. *AJR* 155:1069–1075, 1990.

Germinoma

Ganti,SR, Hilal,SK, Stein,BM, Silver,AJ, Mawad,M, Sane,P. CT of Pineal Region Tumors. *AJNR* 7:97–104, 1986.

Higano,S, Takahashi,S, Ishii,K, et al. Germinoma Originating in the Basal Ganglia and Thalamus: MR and CT Evaluation. *AJNR* 15:1435–1441, 1994.

Moon,WK, Chang,KH, Kim,IO, et al. Germinomas of the Basal Ganglia and Thalamus: MR Findings and a Comparison Between MR and CT. *AJR* 162:1413–1417, 1994.

Soejima,T, Takeshita,I, Yamamoto,H, Tsukamoto,Y, Fukui,M, Matsuoka,S. Computed Tomography of Germinomas in

Basal Ganglia and Thalamus. *Neuroradiology* 29:366–370, 1987.

Tien,RD, Barkovich,AJ, Edwards,MSB. MR Imaging of Pineal Tumors. *AJNR* 11:557–565, 1990. *AJR* 155:143–151 , 1990.

Teratoma

Muller-Forell,W, Schroth,G, Egan,PJ. MR Imaging in Tumors of the Pineal Region. *Neuroradiology* 30:224–231, 1988.

Tien,RD, Barkovich,AJ, Edwards,MSB. MR Imaging of Pineal Tumors. *AJNR* 11:557–565, 1990. *AJR* 155:143–151, 1990.

Zee,CS, Segall,H, Apuzzo,M, et al. MR Imaging of Pineal Region Neoplasms. *J Comput Assist Tomogr* 15:56–63, 1991.

Pineocytoma

Chang,T, Teng,MMH, Guo,WY, Sheng,WC. CT of Pineal Tumors and Intracranial Germ Cell Tumors. *AJNR* 10:1039–1044, 1989. *AJR* 153:1269–1274, 1989.

Ganti,SR, Hilal,SK, Stein,BM, Silver,AJ, Mawad,M, Sane,P. CT of Pineal Region Tumors. *AJNR* 7:97–104, 1986.

Zee,CS, Segall,H, Apuzzo,M, et al. MR Imaging of Pineal Region Neoplasms. *J Comput Assist Tomogr* 15:56–63, 1991.

Pineoblastoma

Ganti,SR, Hilal,SK, Stein,BM, Silver,AJ, Mawad,M, and Sane,P. CT of Pineal Region Tumors. *AJNR* 7:97–104, 1986.

Robles,HA, Smirniotopoulis,JG, Figueroa,RE. Understanding the Radiology of Intracranial Primitive Neuroectodermal Tumors From a Pathological Perspective: A Review. Semin Ultrasound CT MR 13:170–181, 1992.

Tien,RD, Barkovich,AJ, Edwards,MSB. MR Imaging of Pineal Tumors. *AJNR* 11:557–565, 1990. *AJR* 155:143–151, 1990.

Pineal Cyst

Fleege,MA, Miller,GM, Fletcher,GP, et al. Benign Glial Cysts of the Pineal Gland: Unusual Imaging Characteristics with Histologic Correlation. *AJNR* 15:161–166, 1994.

Lee,DH, Norman,D, Newton,TH. MR Imaging of Pineal Cysts *J Comput Assist Tomogr* 11:586–590, 1987.

Mamourian,AC Towfighi,J. Pineal Cysts: MR Imaging. *AJNR* 7:1081–1086, 1986.

Mamourian,AC, Yarnell,T. Enhancement of Pineal Cysts on MR Images. *AJNR* 12:773–774, 1991.

Postoperative Changes

Burke,JW, Podrasky,AE, Bradley,WG. Meninges: Benign Postoperative Enhancement on MR Images. *Radiology* 174: 99–102, 1990.

Elster,AD, DiPersio,DA. Cranial Postoperative Site: Assessment with Contrast-enhanced MR Imaging. *Radiology* 174:93–98, 1990.

Radiation Injury

Atlas,SW, Grossman,RI, Packer,RJ, et al. Magnetic Resonance Imaging Diagnosis of Disseminated Necrotizing Leukoencephalopathy. *J Comput Tomogr* 11:39–43, 1987.

Brant-Zawadski,M, Anderson,M, DeArmond,SJ, Conley,FK, Jahnke,RW. Radiation-Induced Large Intracranial Vessel Occlusive Vasculopathy. *AJR* 134:51–55, 1980.

Shalen,PR, Ostrow,PT, Glass,PJ. Enhancement of the White Matter Following Prophylactic Therapy of the Central Nervous System for Leukemia. Radiology 140:409–412, 1981.

Valk,PE, Dillon,WP. Radiation Injury of the Brain. *AJNR* 12:45–62, 1991, *AJR* 156:689–706, 1991.

CHAPTER
FIVE

Degenerative Brain Disease

Degenerative diseases of the CNS occur throughout all decades of life. The specific diagnosis relies on clinical presentation, laboratory results, and imaging findings. In many cases, only biopsy (or autopsy) can finally establish the correct diagnosis. With most of the disorders discussed in this chapter, a specific diagnosis cannot be made from the imaging findings alone. The most common finding, atrophy, is routinely observed in healthy elderly individuals and is so nonspecific as to be almost useless. Furthermore, the imaging findings described herein are in most instances drawn from retrospective reviews, and the predictive value of the various findings for a given disease is in most instances uncertain.

In patients presenting either with dementia or progressive neurologic deficit, the first priority of imaging is to exclude a potentially reversible cause such as tumor, hydrocephalus, or chronic subdural hematoma. In the detection of normal pressure hydrocephalus and ischemic leukoencephalopathy, imaging provides a primary diagnostic role. Multiple sclerosis and mesial temporal sclerosis are diagnosed by a combination of history, imaging, and laboratory data.

The major primary degenerative diseases of the elderly are characterized by progressive intellectual decline or progressive motor deficits and are represented by Alzheimer's disease (the leading cause of dementia in the elderly) or Parkinson's disease. The present state of imaging does not enable a specific diagnosis of such conditions, although methods of functional imaging and spectroscopy may offer potential. The two major degenerative disorders are imitated by a number of other less common entities that may be difficult to diagnose prospectively. It is likely that as research continues our ability to diagnose degenerating disease of the CNS will improve. Practically speaking, accurate diagnosis will be required only when effective treatments become available.

Dementing Diseases

Alzheimer's Disease

Alzheimer's disease is the leading cause of dementia in the elderly and accounts for 50–60% of such cases. Its incidence increases rapidly after age 65 with an average prevalence among the elderly of 6%. The earliest symptom is a mild personality change, progressing to aphasia, memory loss, and severe intellectual impairment. Neuropathology reveals atrophy of the temporal, parietal, and frontal gray matter with severe hippocampal atrophy. Neurofibrillary tangles and senile plaques are the prominent histologic findings.

CT Findings. The most common CT finding is atrophy, especially of the angular gyrus, medial temporal lobe (limbic structures), and inferior and middle temporal gyri. This pattern of atrophy results in disproportionate enlargement of the Sylvian fissures, suprasellar cistern, temporal horns of the lateral ventricles, and the third ventricle. Generally, however, CT exhibits poor sensitivity and specificity, and the findings are most evident late in the disease course.

MRI Findings. As with CT, MRI may show atrophy of the angular gyrus, amygdala, hippocampus, and inferior and middle temporal gyri along with dilatation of the adjacent ventricles and fissures. Hyperintensity of involved structures, especially the hippocampus, may be observed on T2-weighted images. Cortical hypointensity on T2-weighted images, especially in the parietal region, may be present and has been attributed to iron accumulation. A smooth, thin halo of hyperintensity surrounding the lateral ventricles has been described as a common finding but is nonspecific. Patchy white matter hyperintensities, especially periventricular, are common but probably unrelated to the Alzheimer's disease process. MRI appears to be more sensitive and specific than CT early in the disease course.

PET and SPECT Findings. Using a variety of tracers, these methods show diminished cerebral blood flow and hypometabolism in affected areas of the brain, especially the parietal cortex. PET in particular may be more sensitive than MRI in the early stages of Alzheimer's disease.

Differential Diagnosis

The major challenge is to distinguish Alzheimer's disease from simple atrophy and ischemic leukoencephalopathy. Deep white matter involvement is not a significant component of Alzheimer's disease. Since both Alzheimer's disease and ischemic leukoencephalopathy are common disorders, however, many patients present with *both* conditions. See Table 5–1.

TABLE 5–1 Primary Dementing Diseases of Adults

Disorder	Clinical Manifestations	Primary Areas Affected	CT Findings	MRI Findings
Alzheimer's disease	Progressive memory loss, confusion, and disorientation	Hippocampus and gray matter of frontal and temporal lobes	Atrophy of anteromedial temporal lobes and global atrophy	Temporal lobe atrophy, hippocampal atrophy and hyperintensity, and cortical hypointensity on T2-weighted images (especially parietal)
Pick's disease	Loss of concentration and memory	Frontal and temporal lobes and caudate nucleus	Localized or asymmetric atrophy of frontal and temporal lobes	Atrophy of inferior frontal lobes, anterior temporal lobes, and caudate nucleus
Huntington's chorea	Hyperkinesia, intellectual deterioration, and autosomal dominant with complete penetrance	Caudate nucleus and putamen	Atrophy of caudate nucleus	Atrophy of caudate and putamen +/− hyperintensity on T2-weighted images
Ischemic leukoencephalopathy	Dementia and pseudobulbar palsy, often hypertensive	Periventricular white matter, basal ganglia, and central pons	Low attenuation of deep white matter and enlargement of ventricles and sulci	Irregular hyperintensity of deep white matter and central pons on T2-weighted images, ventricular enlargement, and atrophy
Wernicke's encephalopathy	Confusion and ataxia in a chronic alcoholic	Mamillary bodies, dorsomedial nucleus of thalamus, and brainstem nuclei	Generalized cerebral and cerebellar atrophy	Atrophy of superior vermis and mamillary bodies and hyperintensity of periaqueductal gray and medial thalamus on T2-weighted images
Creutzfeldt-Jakob disease	Rapidly progressive dementia and myoclonic seizures	Gray matter, especially frontal and temporal lobes	Initially normal with rapidly progressive atrophy	Atrophy and hyperintensity of affected gray matter on T2-weighted images
Normal pressure hydrocephalus	Classic triad of dementia, ataxia, and incontinence	Ventricular system, perhaps periventricular white matter (?)	Enlargement of ventricles out of proportion to sulcal enlargement	Hydrocephalus and exaggerated flow void in aqueduct

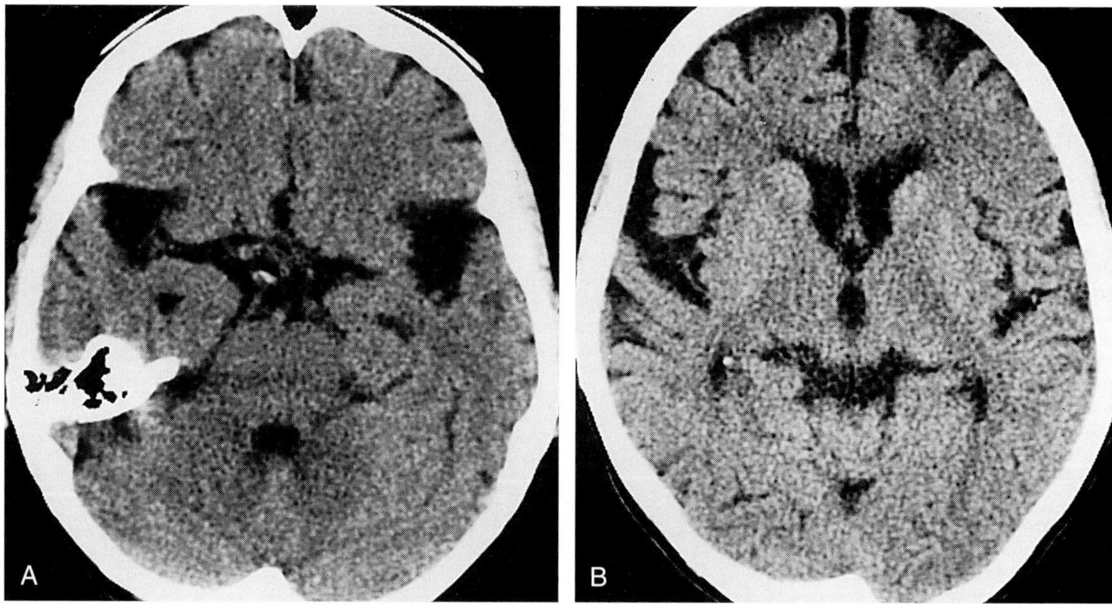

Figure 5–1. Alzheimer's disease (72-year-old female). **(A)** CT through middle fossae shows mild temporal horn enlargement and marked widening of the Sylvian fissures. **(B)** Higher section shows bifrontal and right temporal lobe atrophy.

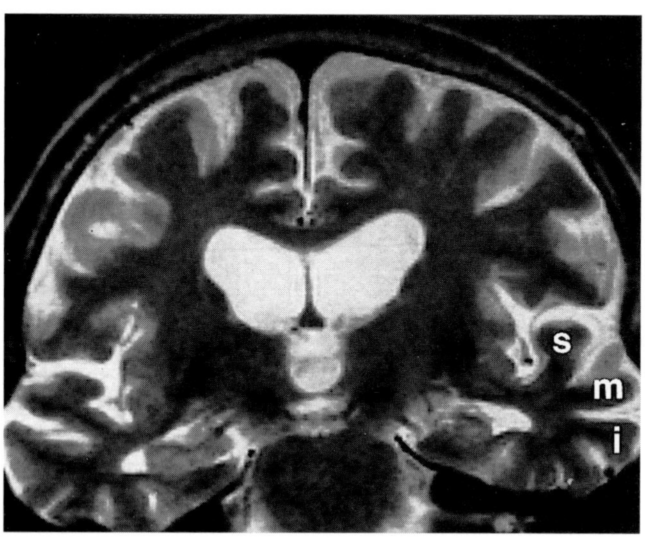

Figure 5–2. Alzheimer's disease (62-year-old male). Coronal MRI shows generalized atrophy with small gyri, large sulci, and marked enlargement of third and lateral ventricles. Temporal lobe atrophy is prominent. s=superior temporal gyrus, m=middle temporal gyrus, i=inferior temporal gyrus.

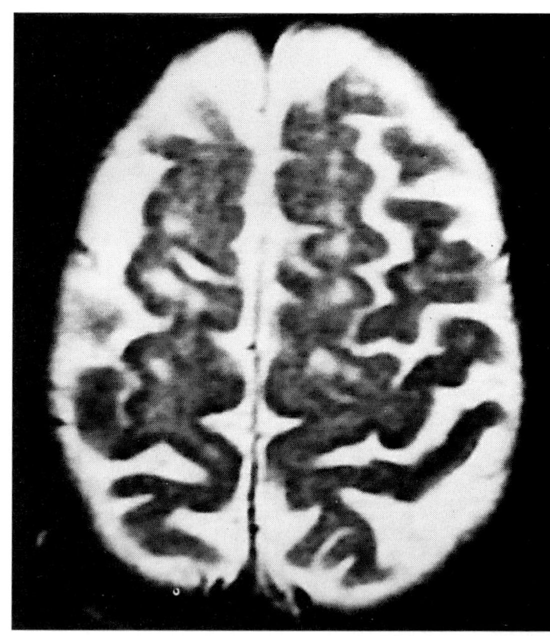

Figure 5–3. Alzheimer's disease (74-year-old male). T2-weighted MRI shows gyral hypointensity in the parietal convexity.

Figure 5–4. Alzheimer's disease. Tc-99m HMPAO SPECT scan of **(A)** a normal 27-year-old male and **(B)** a 66-year-old female with probable Alzheimer's disease by National Institute of Neurologic Disorders and Stroke (NINDS) criteria show marked reduction of tracer uptake in the posterior temporal and parietal regions, which is worse on the left. (Courtesy of Dr. James M. Mountz and Dr. Georg Deutsch, Birmingham, AL.)

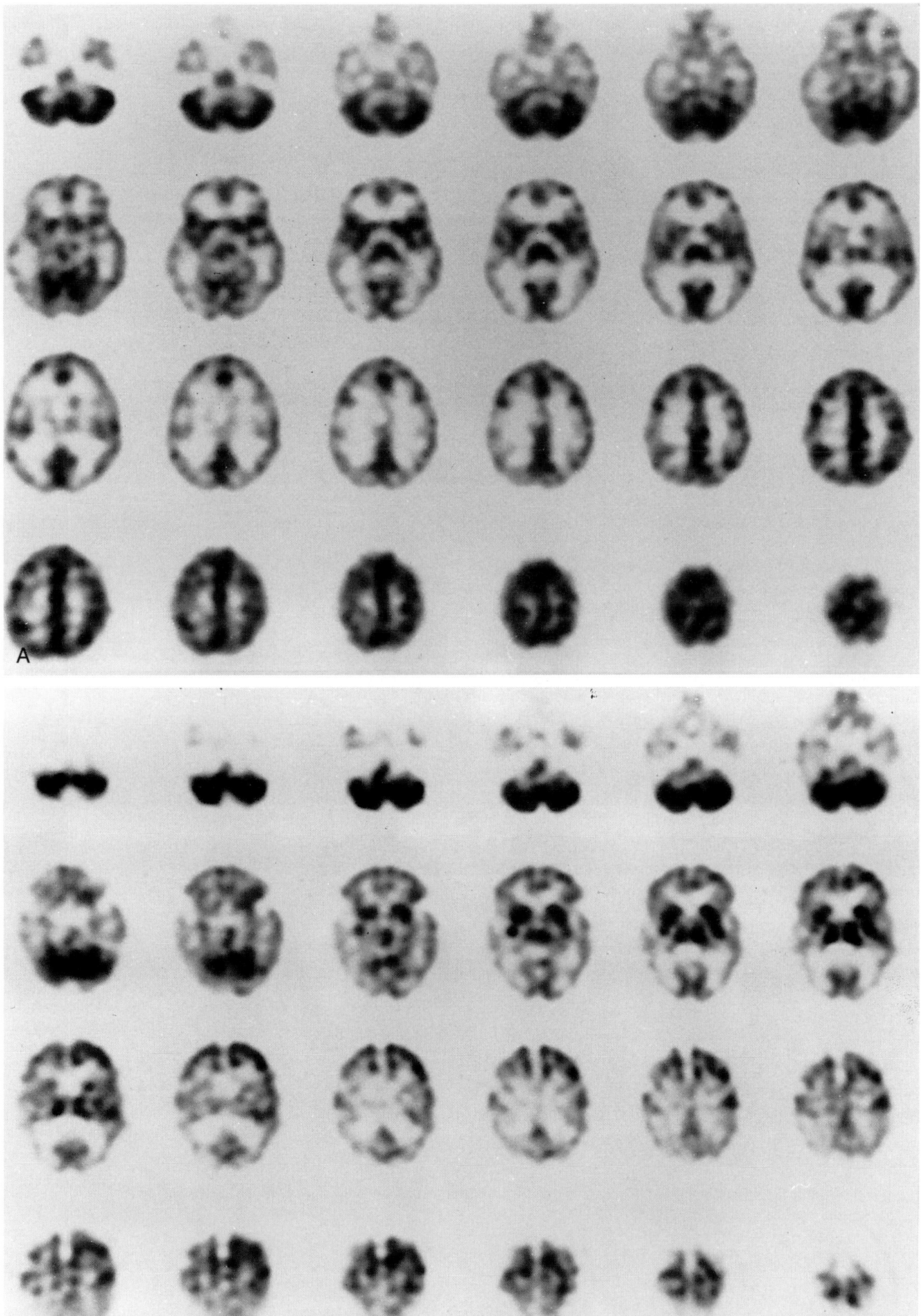

Figure 5–4. *See legend on opposite page*

Huntington's Disease

Synonym: Huntington's chorea.

Huntington's disease is an inherited autosomal dominant condition characterized by progressive neuronal loss and gliosis in the putamen and caudate nucleus. Affected patients present during the third through fifth decades with choreiform involuntary movements, progressing to dementia and death within 15 years of onset. A subset of patients paradoxically presents with rigidity and bradykinesia, the rigid form of Huntington's.

CT Findings. CT scans may be normal or show mild to severe atrophy especially of the caudate nucleus. This results in flattening of the inferior and lateral walls of the frontal horn.

MRI Findings. Atrophy of the caudate nucleus and putamen is again the primary imaging abnormality. T2-weighted images may show hypointensity of the caudate and putamen due to increased iron. Hyperintensity of these nuclei on T2-weighted images has also been described, particularly in the rigid variant of Huntington's disease.

Differential Diagnosis

See Table 5—1.

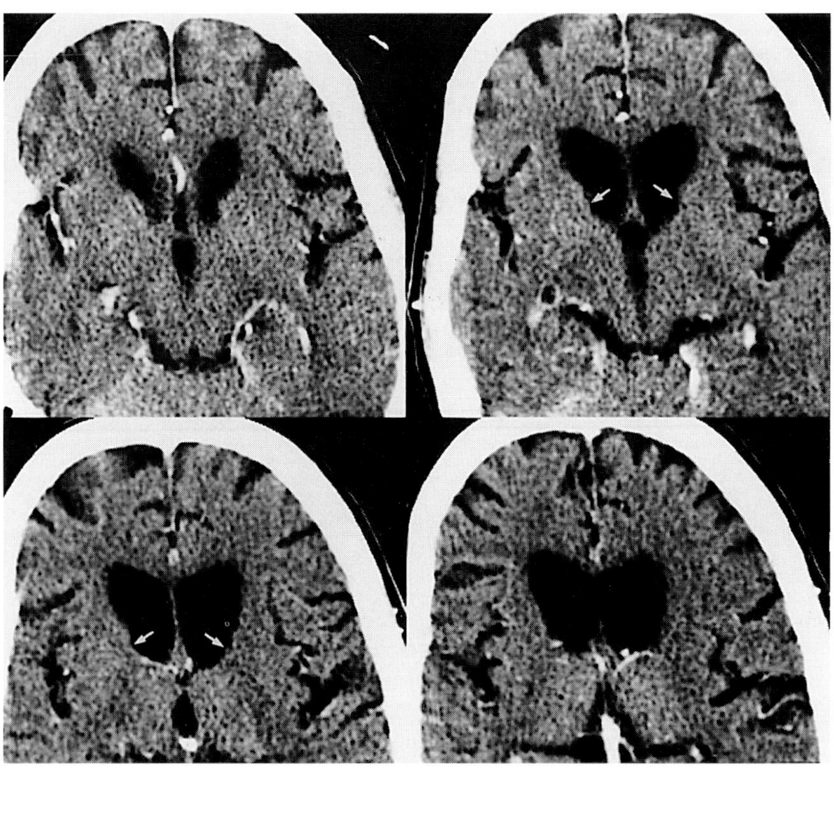

Figure 5–5. Huntington's disease (34-year-old female). Axial CT sections show enlargement of the frontal horns with flattening of the caudate heads (arrows). Generalized atrophy is also present.

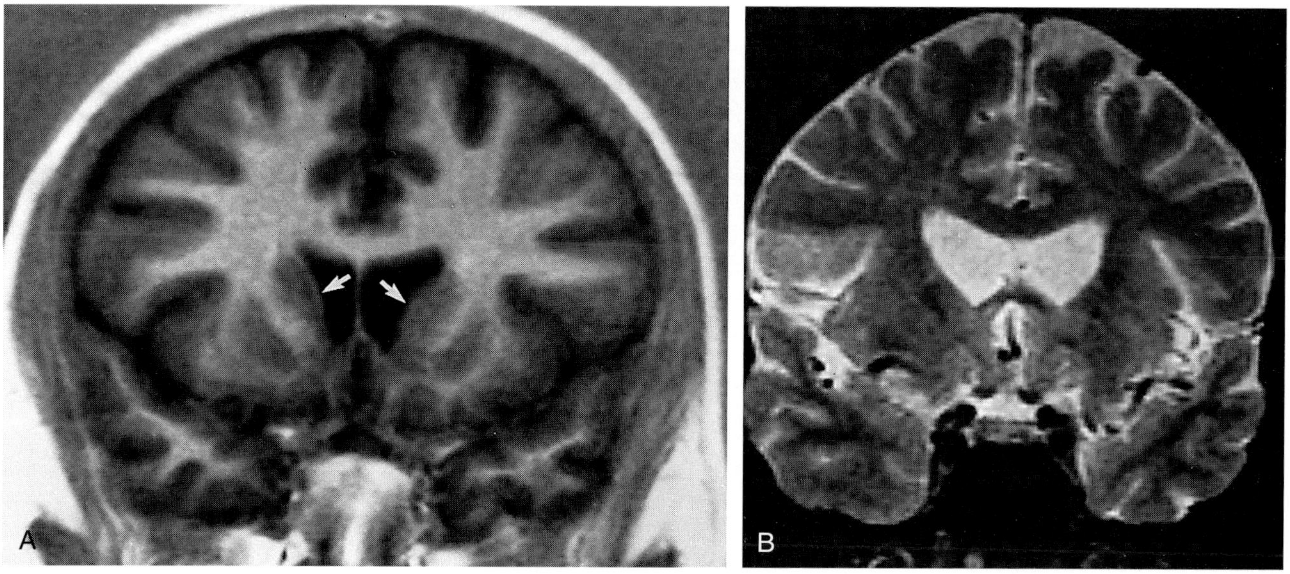

Figure 5–6. Huntington's disease **(A)** Coronal inversion-recovery MRI shows the normal caudate nuclei (arrows) creating a convex impression on the frontal horns. **(B)** T2-weighted MRI in a 44-year-old male with chorea of 3 years' duration shows severe bilateral caudate atrophy. The inferolateral frontal horns are convex rather than concave.

Ischemic Leukoencephalopathy

Synonyms: Binswanger's disease, microangiopathy, subcortical arteriosclerotic leukoencephalopathy, multi-infarct dementia.

The following terms refer strictly to the imaging finding of abnormal or altered white matter without regard to the presence or absence of dementia: leukoaraiosis, white matter lucency (CT), periventricular hyperintensity (MRI), and unidentified bright objects (UBO's), a term whose use is to be discouraged.

Vascular dementia may result from multiple large vessel infarcts, critically located small infarcts, or chronic hypoperfusion of small penetrating and medullary arteries. Histology in the latter reveals atrophy, demyelination, and hyalinoid thickening of small arterial and arteriolar walls. The diagnosis is usually confirmed by MRI, although the majority of patients with deep white matter hyperintensities show no signs of dementia.

CT Findings. CT shows low attenuation of the periventricular white matter, especially adjacent to the ventricular trigones and in the centrum semiovale. Atrophy of the white matter is usually present, resulting in a corresponding enlargement of the third and lateral ventricles. The white matter lesions do not enhance with contrast.

MRI Findings. T2-weighted images show varying-sized areas of hyperintensity, either patchy or confluent, in the periventricular white matter. They occur with greatest frequency in the centrum semiovale, basal ganglia, and central pons. Discreet lacunar infarctions are commonly present in the basal ganglia. The better perfused subcortical U fibers and corpus callosum are rarely involved. The lesions do not enhance with contrast and are typically subtle or inapparent on T1-weighted images. Generalized atrophy is usually present, resulting in ventricular dilatation (hydrocephalus ex vacuo).

TABLE 5–2 Differential Diagnosis of Periventricular White Matter Hyperintensities

Differential Diagnosis
Vascular/Ischemic
Normal aging
Multiple infarcts
Microangiopathy/chronic ischemic change
Systemic lupus erythematosus
Radiation vasculitis
Inflammatory
Sarcoidosis
Sjögren's syndrome
Behçet's disease
Progressive multifocal leukoencephalopathy
AIDS
Encephalitis
Lyme disease
Demyelinating/dysmyelinating
Multiple sclerosis
Acute disseminated encephalomyelitis
Leukodystrophies
Vitamin B12 deficiency
Tumors
Glioma
Lymphoma
Lymphomatoid granulomatosis
Subependymal tumor
Trauma
Diffuse axonal injury
Other
Hydrocephalus
Pseudotumor cerebri

Differential Diagnosis

The greatest difficulty is distinguishing ischemic leukoencephalopathy with atrophy from normal pressure hydrocephalus (NPH). The findings that aid in distinguishing hydrocephalus from atrophy are reviewed in Chapter 1. See Table 5–2.

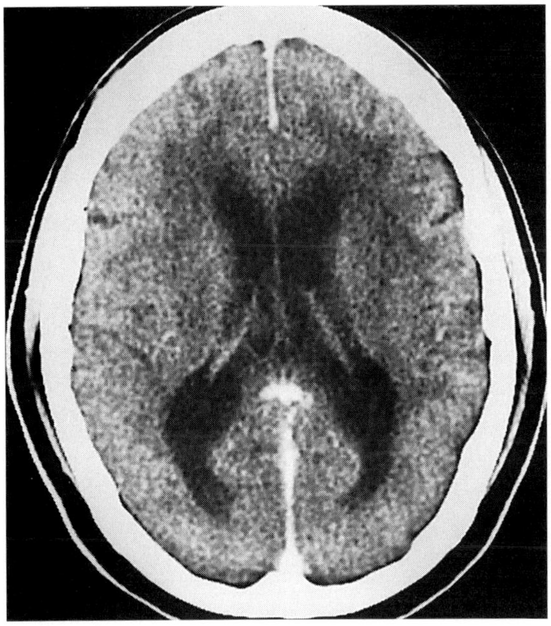

Figure 5–7. Ischemic leukoencephalopathy. CT shows bilateral low attenuation in the periventricular and subcortical white matter. The lateral ventricles are mildly enlarged.

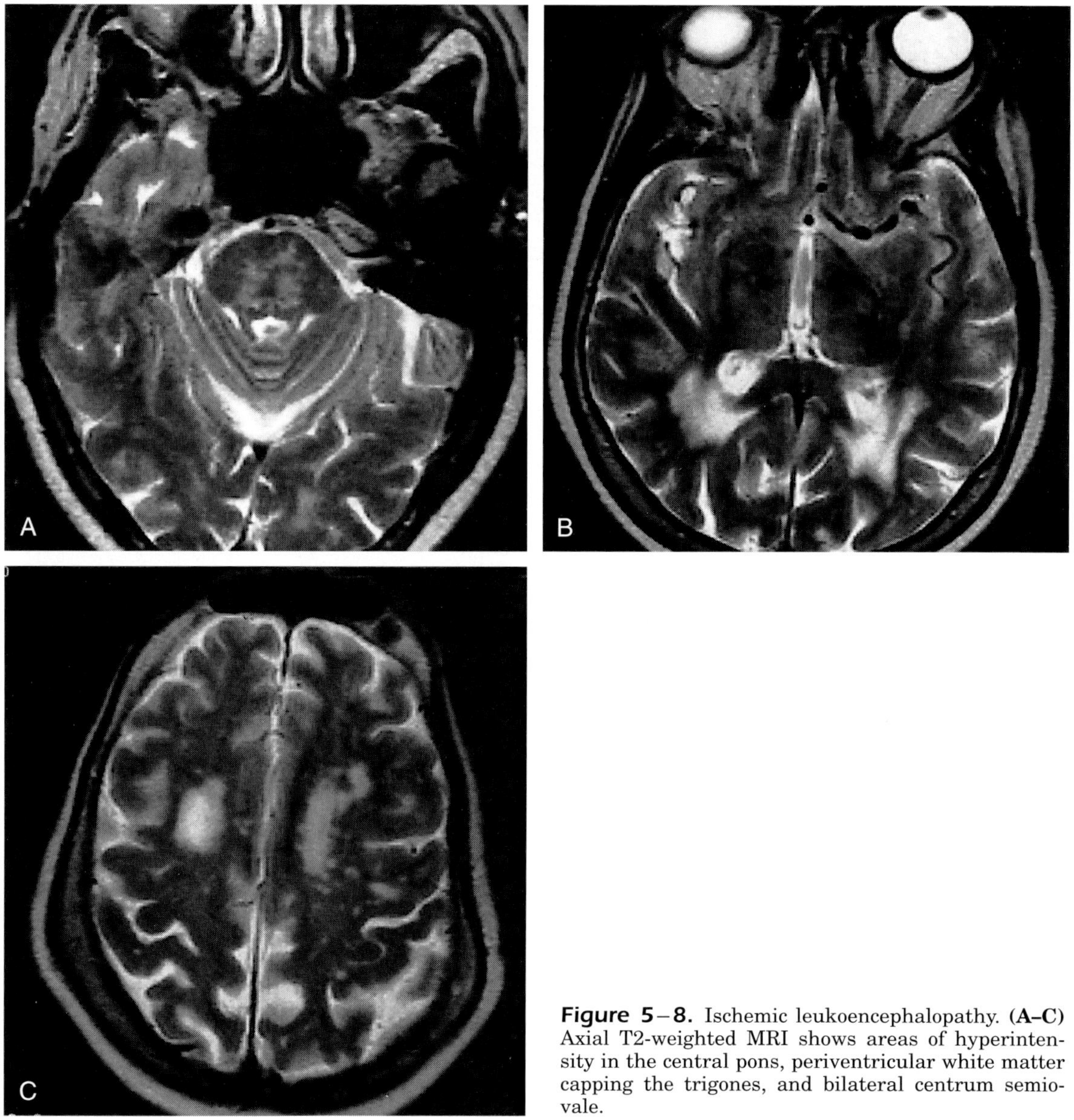

Figure 5–8. Ischemic leukoencephalopathy. **(A–C)** Axial T2-weighted MRI shows areas of hyperintensity in the central pons, periventricular white matter capping the trigones, and bilateral centrum semiovale.

Normal Pressure Hydrocephalus

Among the degenerative conditions of the elderly brain, perhaps none is more mysterious or controversial than the NPH. It has been recognized for some time that some elderly patients who present with enlarged ventricles along with a symptom complex of ataxia, dementia, and incontinence manifest symptomatic improvement after ventricular shunting. It is equally clear that many others do not improve. The major controversies center on questions of etiology and patient selection for a shunting procedure, and in regard to the latter, neuroimaging may play a useful role.

CT Findings. CT shows dilatation of the third, fourth, and lateral ventricles with low attenuation of the periventricular white matter. The ventricular enlargement should be disproportionately greater than that of cortical sulci. Dilatation of the temporal horns in the absence of gross temporal lobe atrophy (normal sylvian fissures) is an especially helpful finding.

MRI Findings. MR shows evidence of ventricular dilatation disproportionate to the degree of sulcal enlargement. The most specific signs include upward bowing of the corpus callosum, inferior displacement of the fornix, enlargement of the temporal horns without temporal lobe atrophy, and flattening of cortical gyri against the inner table. (The CSF spaces overlying the gyri are enlarged with simple atrophy). Another, albeit controversial, sign of NPH is the presence of exaggerated signal void in the aqueduct, posterior third ventricle, and fourth ventricle due to CSF flow.

Differential Diagnosis

The major difficulty lies in differentiating NPH from ischemic leukoencephalopathy and deep atrophy. See preceding section and Hydrocephalus, Chapter 1.

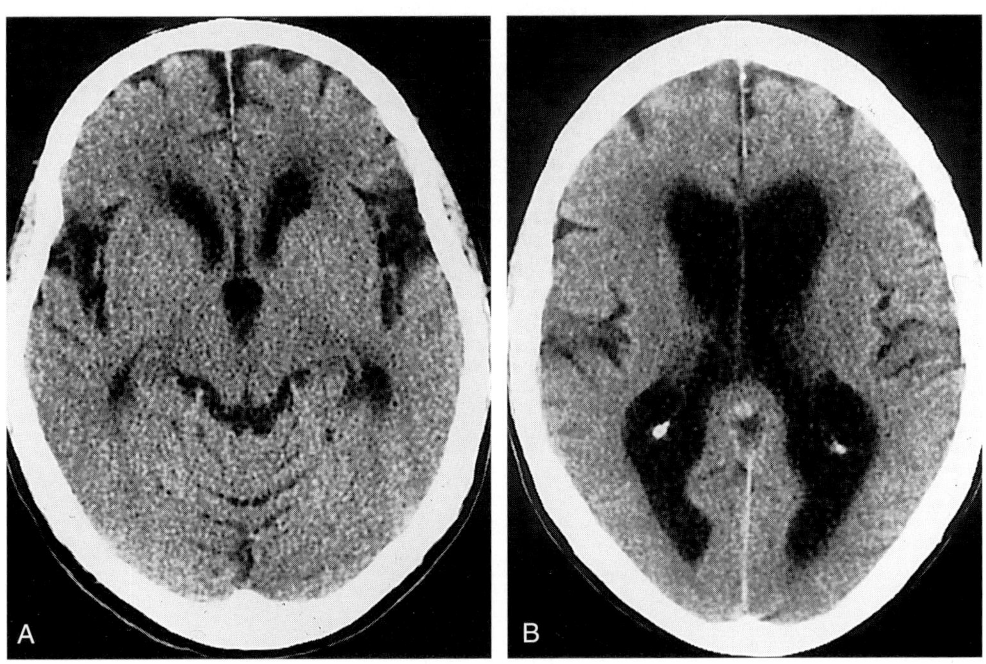

Figure 5–9. Normal pressure hydrocephalus. **(A,B)** CT shows marked enlargement of the third and lateral ventricles. The sylvian fissures are enlarged, but the cortical sulci remain small. On postshunting CT (not shown) there was marked reduction in size of both the ventricles and sylvian fissures.

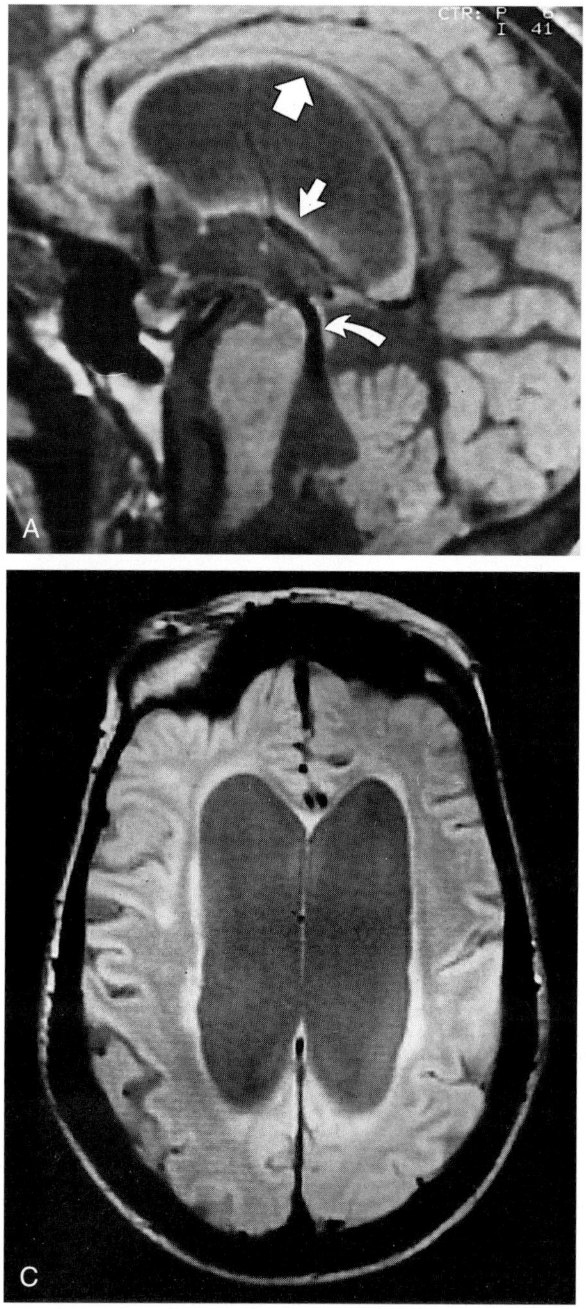

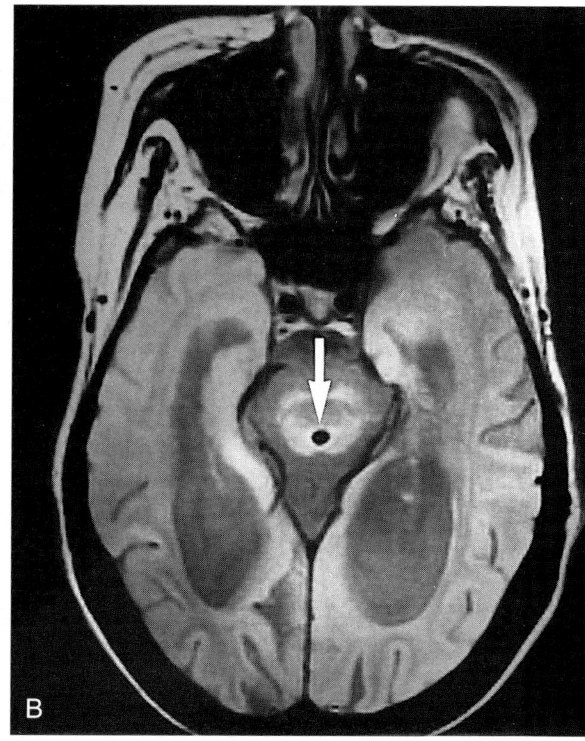

Figure 5–10. Normal pressure hydrocephalus. **(A)** Sagittal T1-weighted MRI shows marked upward bowing of the corpus callosum (large arrow) and depression of the fornix (small arrow). There is prominent flow void in the aqueduct (curved arrow) and enlargement of both third and lateral ventricles. **(B,C)** Axial PD-weighted MRI shows prominent flow void in the aqueduct (arrow), marked ventricular enlargement, and relatively small sulci. (Courtesy of Dr. Taher El Gammal; **(A)** reprinted with permission from *AJR* 149:807–813, 1987.)

Wilson's Disease

Synonym: Hepatolenticular degeneration.

Wilson's disease results from an inherited autosomal recessive defect of ceruloplasmin synthesis that causes abnormal accumulations of copper, especially in liver and brain. This in turn leads to atrophy, gliosis, edema, and sometimes necrosis of the involved regions. Affected patients present with rigidity, tremor, gait impairment, decreased coordination, and dysarthria. The diagnosis is confirmed by low serum ceruloplasmin and copper levels and by increased urinary copper excretion.

CT Findings. CT may show ventricular enlargement, cortical atrophy, and diminished attenuation in the basal ganglia.

MRI Findings. In symptomatic cases, T2-weighted images show bilateral and symmetrical hyperintensity in the caudate nuclei, lentiform nuclei, thalami, subcortical white matter, or pons. Hypointensity has also been observed in the caudate nucleus and putamen, tentatively attributed to iron deposition. The signal abnormalities often resolve with treatment. Contrast enhancement has not been noted.

Differential Diagnosis

Similar patterns of signal abnormality may be encountered in central pontine myelinolysis, Huntington's disease, and carbon monoxide poisoning, to name a few. The diagnosis is readily confirmed by laborabory findings.

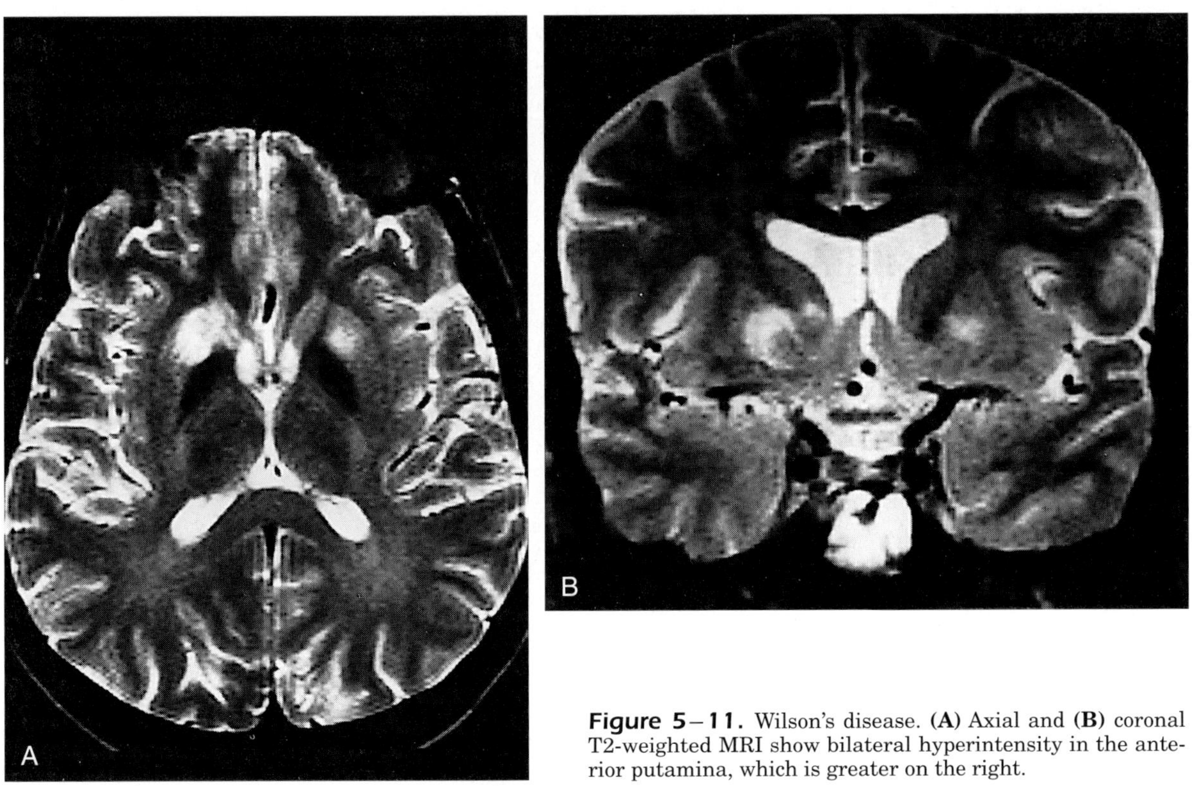

Figure 5–11. Wilson's disease. **(A)** Axial and **(B)** coronal T2-weighted MRI show bilateral hyperintensity in the anterior putamina, which is greater on the right.

Degenerative Motor Diseases

Parkinson's Disease

Parkinson's disease is a common degenerative disease of the elderly, affecting approximately 1% of those over age 50. The patients present after age 45 with symptoms of pill-rolling hand tremor, rigidity, bradykinesia, ataxia, and autonomic dysfunction. The primary pathologic lesion is neuronal degeneration in the substantia nigra and locus ceruleus, with the appearance of intracytoplasmic inclusions (Lewy bodies) in the remaining neurons.

CT Findings. CT usually shows atrophy, with enlargement of both the ventricular system and cortical sulci. No distinctive features have been identified to distinguish Parkinson's disease from other causes of atrophy.

MRI Findings. Nonspecific MRI changes include generalized cerebral atrophy and focal hyperintensities in the globus pallidus or substantia nigra. There is a statistically significant decrease in the thickness of the pars compacta of the substantia nigra, the relatively hyperintense band seen on T2-weighted images of normal subjects between the hypointense red nucleus and the hypointense pars reticulata of the substantia nigra. However, this finding is of limited use since there is considerable overlap in width between parkinsonian and normal populations. Currently, MRI is useful primarily in the exclusion of other disease processes.

In a subset of patients, the so-called Parkinson's plus syndrome, abnormal hypointensity in the putamen (due to increased iron), is a common finding. The Parkinson's plus syndrome encompasses a number of diseases, including striatonigral degeneration, Shy-Drager syndrome, olivopontocerebellar atrophy, and progressive supranuclear palsy.

Differential Diagnosis

See Table 5–3. It is difficult to make the diagnosis with certainty from imaging findings alone.

TABLE 5–3 **Degenerative Diseases of the Brain Presenting with Sensorimotor Deficits**

Disorder	Clinical Manifestations	Primary Areas Affected	CT Findings	MRI Findings
Parkinson's disease	Bradykinesia Rigidity Resting tremor	Pars compacta of the substantia nigra	Normal or generalized atrophy	Atrophy Thinning of pars compacta
Shy-Drager syndrome	Bradykinesia Tremor Orthostatic hypotention Autonomic nervous system failure	Substantia nigra Pons Cerebellum	Hemispheric, brainstem, and cerebellar atrophy	Marked hypointensity in putamen and pars compacta on T_2-weighted images
Progressive supranuclear palsy	Supranuclear ophthalmoplegia Dementia Rigidity	Substantia nigra Pons Periaqueductal gray matter	Midbrain atrophy	Hyperintensity of periaqueductal gray matter on T_2-weighted images Atrophy of midbrain, especially superior colliculi
Striatonigral degeneration	Extremity weakness and spasticity Positive family history Autosomal dominant transmission	Substantia nigra Putamen	Atrophy	Atrophy
Olivopontocerebellar atrophy	Progressive ataxia Dysarthria Cranial nerve deficits	Pons Cerebellum Cerebellar peduncles	Progressive atrophy of brainstem and cerebellum	Atrophy of inferior pons and cerebellum with mild hyperintensity on T_2-weighted images

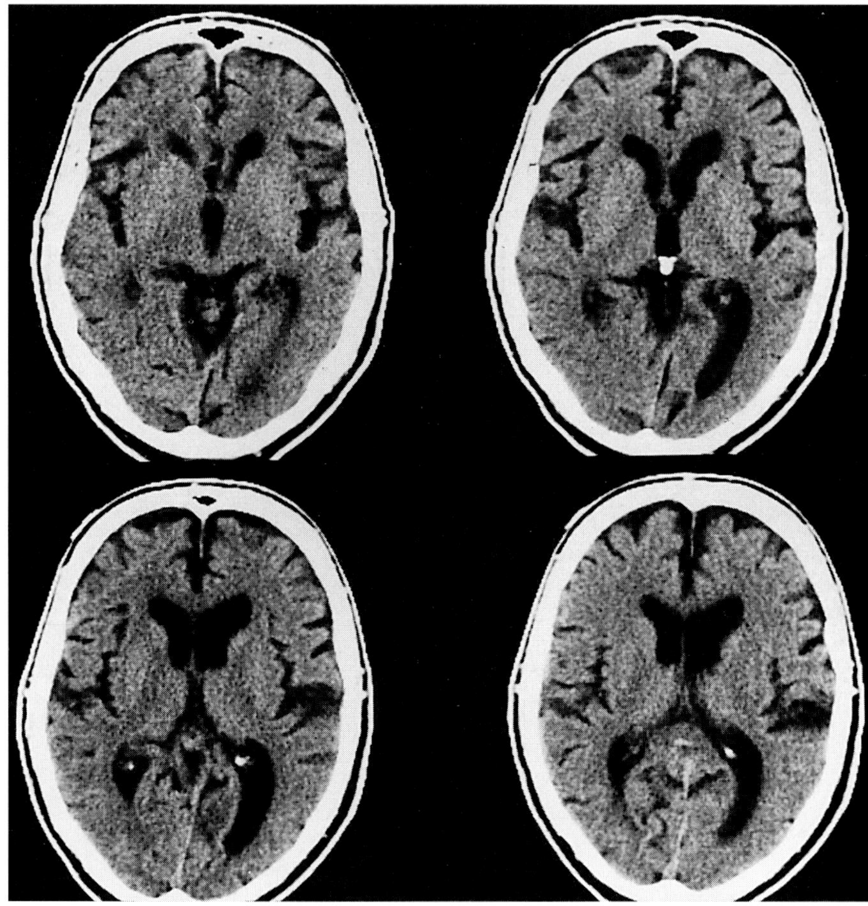

Figure 5–12. Parkinson's disease (72-year-old male). Sequential CT sections show a nonspecific pattern of generalized cortical atrophy.

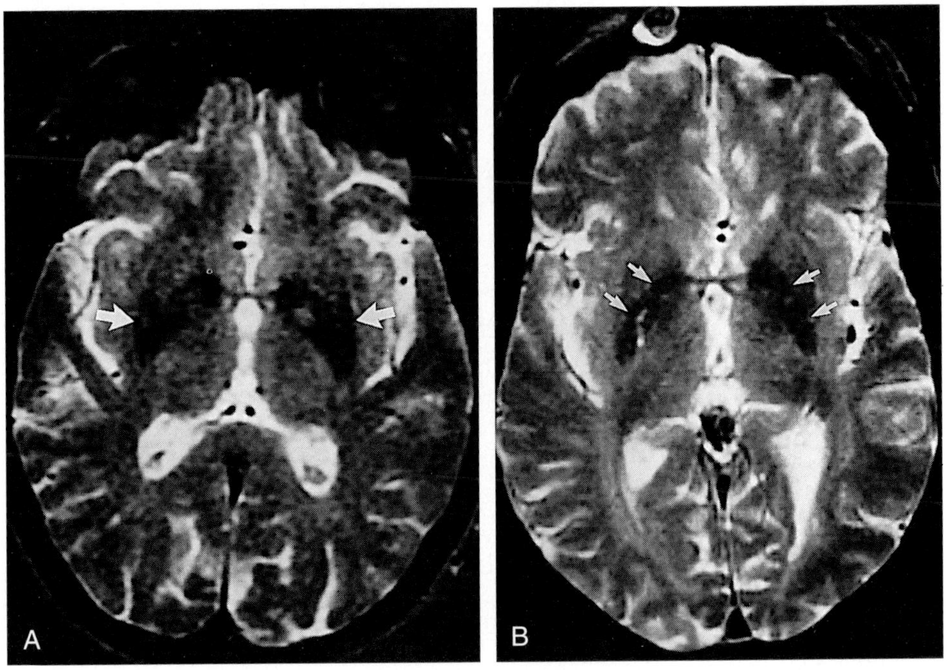

Figure 5–13. Suspected Shy-Drager syndrome in a 57-year-old female with severe orthostatic hypotension. **(A)** Axial T2-weighted MRI shows hypointensity (arrows) in the putamen bilaterally obscuring its interface with the normally hypointense globus pallidus. **(B)** In an age-matched control the interface between the globus pallidus and putamen is readily visible (arrows).

Olivopontocerebellar Atrophy

Olivopontocerebellar atrophy encompasses a spectrum of degenerative disorders in which the common denominator is progressive atrophy of the pons, middle cerebellar peduncles, and cerebellar hemispheres. It occurs both in sporadic and familial forms. Patients present with ataxia, progressing to bulbar palsies and mental deterioration. Some cases also manifest extrapyramidal and autonomic dysfunction, meriting the designation of multisystem atrophy. These disorders selectively involve the transverse fibers of the pons, middle cerebellar peduncles, and Purkinje cells of the cerebellum, but spare the pyramidal tracts and tegmentum. Degeneration of the inferior olives occurs secondary to the cerebellar degeneration.

CT Findings. CT shows moderate to severe atrophy of the brainstem and cerebellum with an enlarged fourth ventricle and enlarged hemispheric and vermian sulci. Cerebral hemispheric atrophy is usually also present.

MRI Findings. Sagittal T1-weighted images show flattening of the anteroinferior pons, while coronal images show atrophy of the middle cerebellar peduncles causing a pointed appearance of the lateral pons. Atrophy of the brainstem and cerebellum exceeds the severity of cerebral atrophy. T2-weighted images show mild diffuse hyperintensity of the cerebellum compared to the occipital or temporal lobes. Focal hyperintensity is seen in the middle cerebellar peduncles, the transverse pontine fibers, and the pontine raphe. The latter abnormalities result in relative hypointensity and increased conspicuity of the normal, unaffected pyramidal tracts.

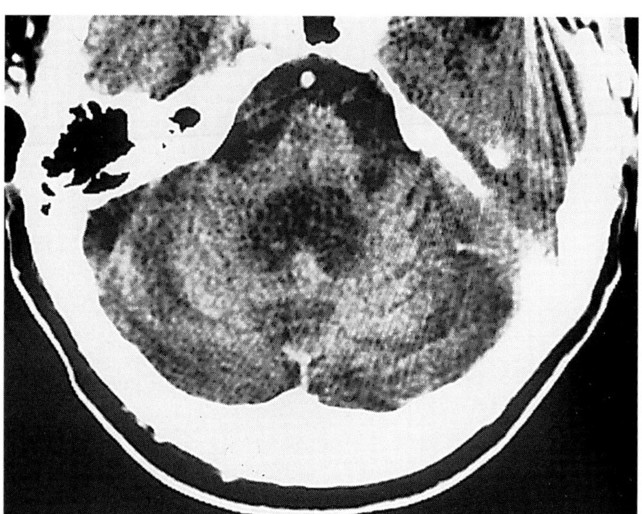

Figure 5–14. Olivopontocerebellar atrophy. CT shows severe atrophy of the pons, middle cerebellar peduncles, and cerebellar hemispheres.

TABLE 5–4 Causes of Cerebellar Atrophy
Dilantin therapy
Alcohol abuse
Olivopontocerebellar atrophy
Ataxia telangiectasia
Multiple sclerosis
Subacute cerebellar degeneration (paraneoplastic phenomenon)

Differential Diagnosis

See Tables 5–3 and 5–4.

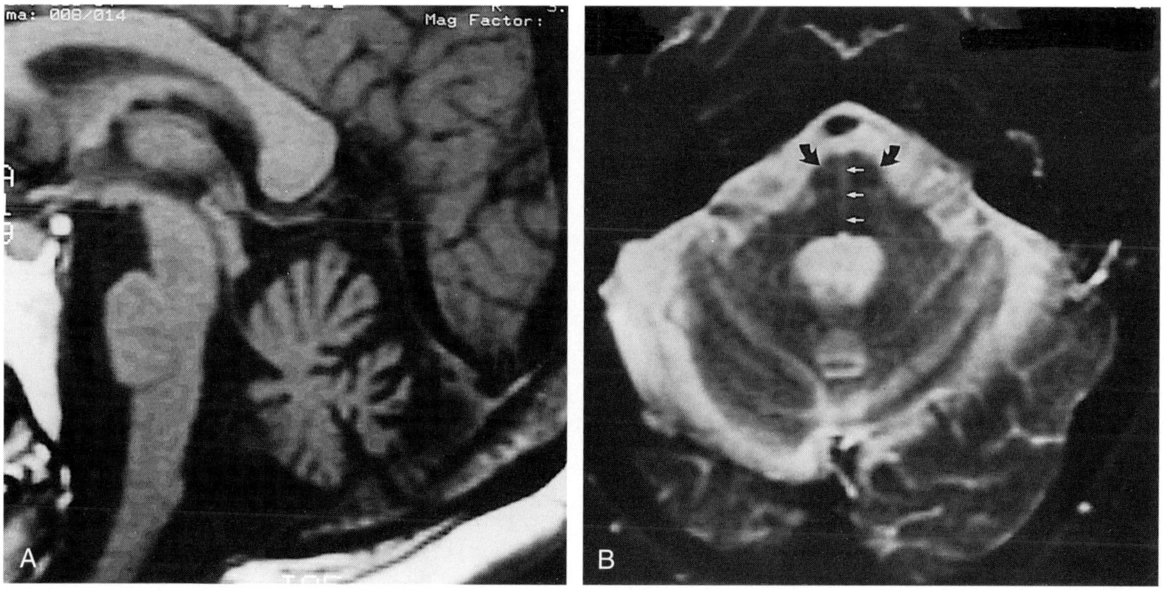

Figure 5–15. Olivopontocerebellar atrophy. **(A)** Sagittal MRI shows atrophy of the vermis and flattening of the ventral pons. **(B)** Axial T2-weighted MRI shows hyperintensity in the pontine raphe (small arrows) and transverse pontine fibers with increased conspicuity of the hypointense pyramidal tracts (curved arrows). There is atrophy of the pons, middle cerebellar peduncles, and cerebellum.

Multiple Sclerosis

Multiple sclerosis (MS) is a disorder characterized by inflammatory plaques of demyelination in the brain and spinal cord. It is a common condition, and the lifetime risk of developing the disease is about 1 in 1,000. Progressive disability is the hallmark of the disease, with a mean survival of 35 to 40 years. MS is a disease of young adults, with 95% of cases diagnosed between ages 18 and 50. Presenting symptoms run the gamut of neurologic disability, including motor or sensory deficits, pain, optic neuritis (see Chapter 10), and cognitive or personality alterations. The diagnosis rests on a combination of clinical examination, history, imaging, CSF studies, and evoked potentials.

The most common form (70% of cases), is characterized by a pattern of relapse and remission with a progressive cumulative disability. A chronic progressive form occurs in about 20% of patients. Acute, fulminant disease leading to death within months (the Marburg form) occurs in a small percentage. Treatment generally has relied on corticosteroids during periods of clinical relapse. Recently beta-interferon has been demonstrated to slow the progression of disease.

CT Findings. The basic CT abnormality is the presence of multiple areas of low attenuation in the white matter, usually periventricular, without mass effect. Contrast enhancement in a patchy, uniform, or ringlike pattern is often present in active disease. High-dose delayed postcontrast scanning has been shown to increase the sensitivity. Long-standing disease results in atrophy. All this aside, the initial CT is normal in most patients. Because of its higher sensitivity, MRI is the modality of choice when MS is suspected clinically.

MRI Findings. On MRI, one typically sees multiple areas of hyperintensity within the deep white matter in a periventricular distribution, which are most apparent on PD-weighted images and usually less than 2.5 cm in diameter. The nonspecificity of white matter hyperintensity has been discussed in Chapter 1, Edema. Features that are particularly characteristic of MS plaques include (1) smooth margins; (2) ovoid configuration with the longer axis perpendicular to the ventricular surface; (3) lumpy, bumpy pattern of hyperintensity; (4) involvement of the corpus callosum, especially at its interface with the septum pellucidum; (5) involvement of cerebellar peduncles; (6) prominent hypointensity on T1-weighted images; and (7) involvement of subcortical U fibers. These features serve primarily to distinguish MS from ischemic and aging-related white matter changes, which are widely prevalent.

Mass effect is very rare but can occur in acute disease. Hypointensity in the putamen and thalamus may be present on T2-weighted images, putatively ascribed to abnormal iron accumulation. Both infratentorial white matter and spinal cord lesions are common. Isolated spinal cord disease may exist in a small percentage of patients.

MS is usually chronic and progressive, and MRI is more sensitive than clinical examination in the detection of new lesions. New or active lesions tend to enhance with contrast; enhancement is usually uniform but may be ringlike. Enhancement usually lasts 4 to 8 weeks but has been shown to persist up to 5 months. Most acute plaques show some reduction in size over time, and many plaques, especially the smaller ones, may completely disappear.

Differential Diagnosis

Hyperintense foci in the white matter on T2-weighted MRI may be the most nonspecific finding in neuroimaging (see Table 5–2). Sarcoidosis, Lyme disease, and vasculitis may especially be confused with MS. One must rely upon clinical history, laboratory findings, and the MRI features as described to make a confident diagnosis of MS.

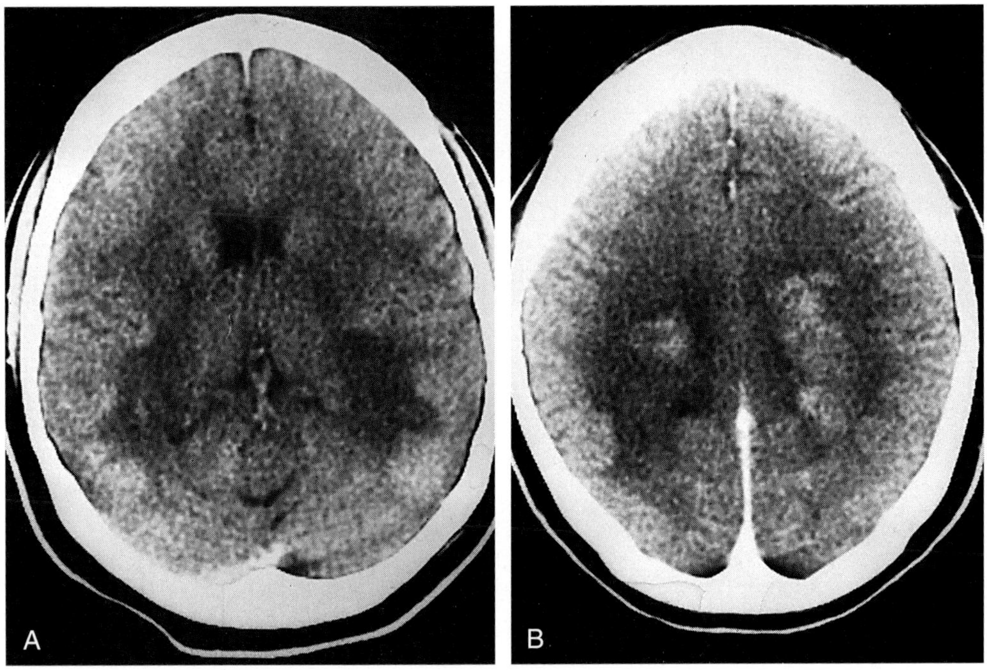

Figure 5–16. Multiple sclerosis (acute). **(A,B)** Contrast-enhanced CT shows extensive low attenuation in the white matter with patchy enhancement, which is greater on the left.

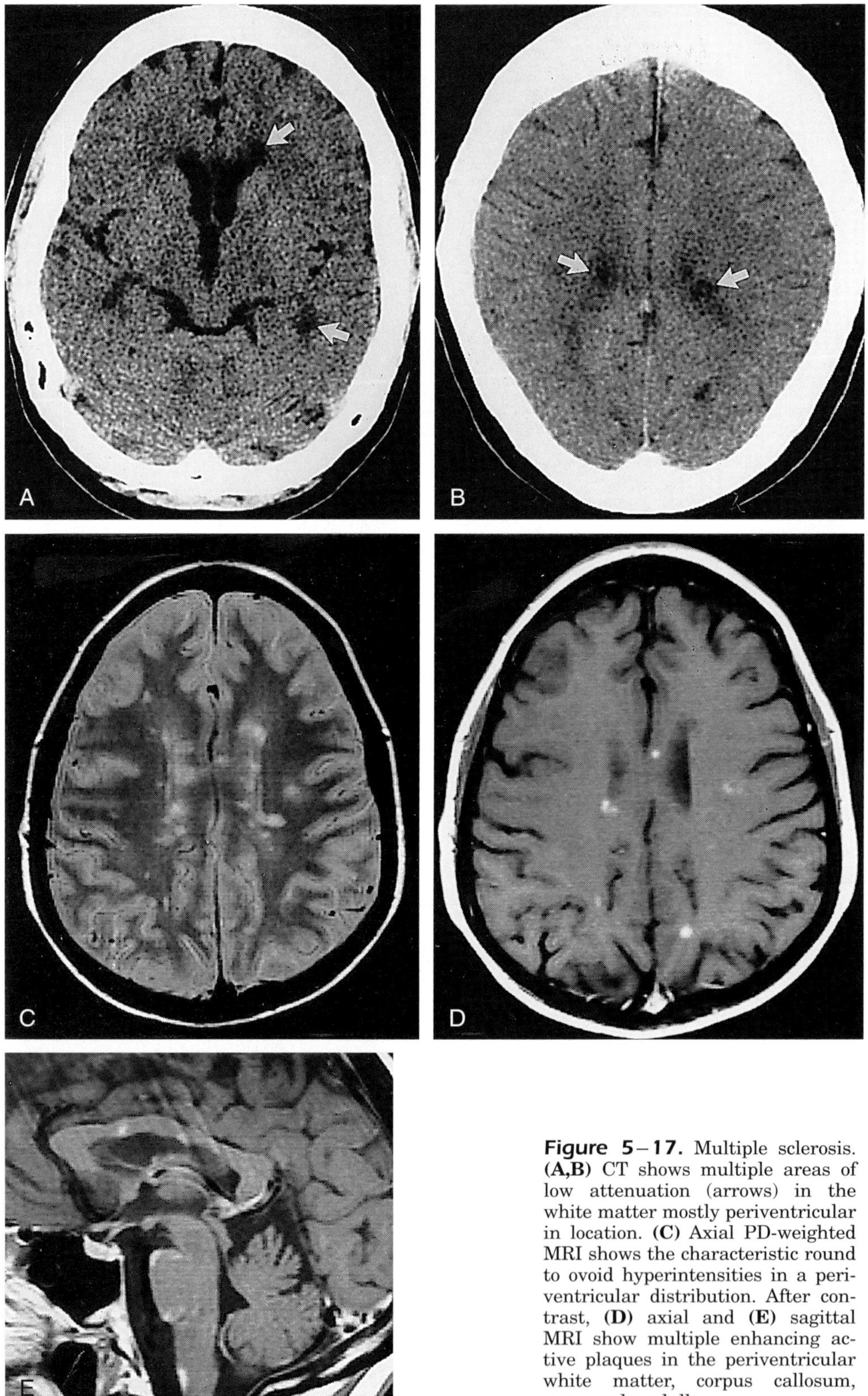

Figure 5–17. Multiple sclerosis. **(A,B)** CT shows multiple areas of low attenuation (arrows) in the white matter mostly periventricular in location. **(C)** Axial PD-weighted MRI shows the characteristic round to ovoid hyperintensities in a periventricular distribution. After contrast, **(D)** axial and **(E)** sagittal MRI show multiple enhancing active plaques in the periventricular white matter, corpus callosum, pons, and medulla.

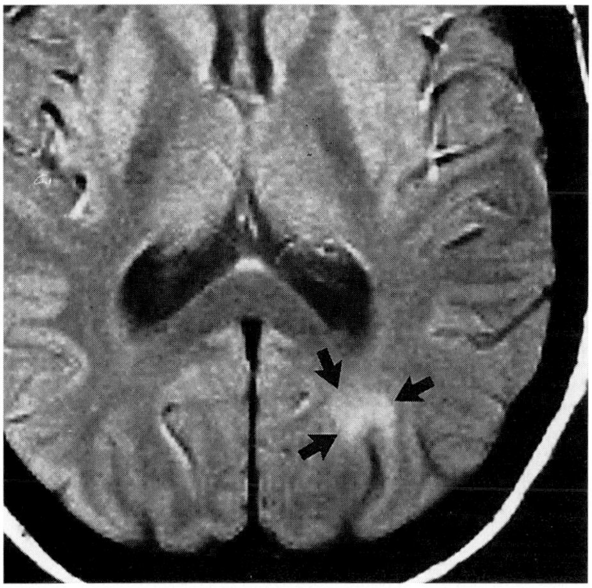

Figure 5–18. Multiple sclerosis. PD-weighted MRI shows a subcortical plaque in the left occipital lobe. The plaque involves subcortical U fibers and is confluent with the gray matter. Ischemic disease tends to spare the subcortical U fibers and remain distinct from the gray matter. (See also Figure 1–39.)

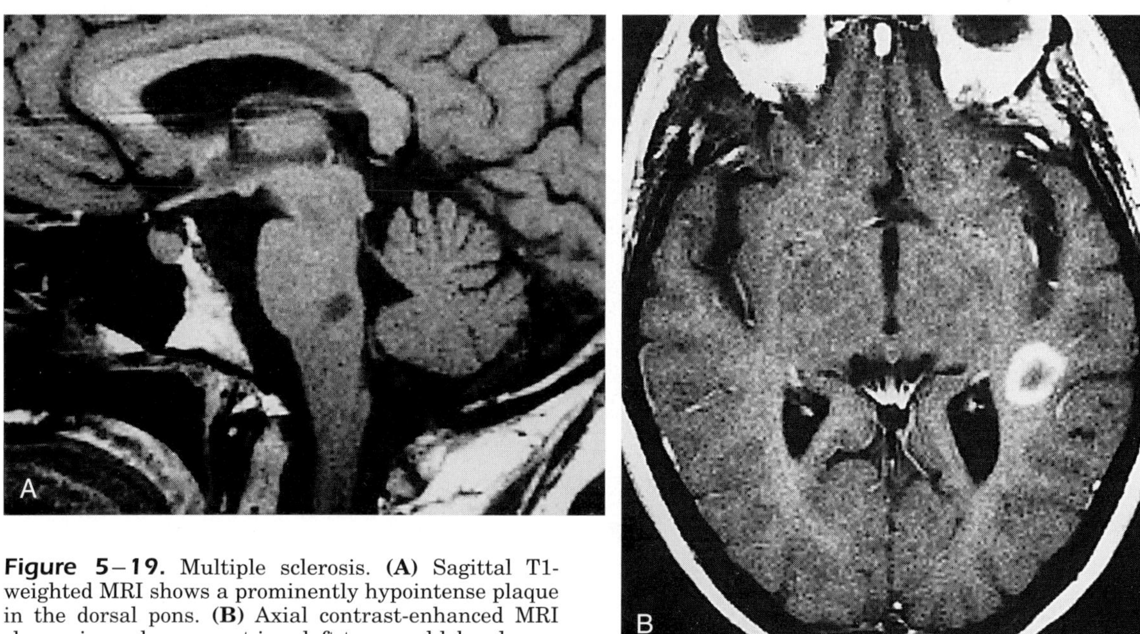

Figure 5–19. Multiple sclerosis. **(A)** Sagittal T1-weighted MRI shows a prominently hypointense plaque in the dorsal pons. **(B)** Axial contrast-enhanced MRI shows ring enhancement in a left temporal lobe plaque.

Epileptic Disease

Mesial Temporal Sclerosis

Synonym: Hippocampal sclerosis.

The pyramidal layer of the hippocampus is highly vulnerable to anoxia or hypoglycemia. Repeated episodes of anoxia, such as those that might occur with a chronic seizure disorder, can lead to hippocampal atrophy and gliosis, a condition known as mesial temporal sclerosis. Mesial temporal sclerosis is the underlying cause in 50–70% of cases of intractable epilepsy. Anterior temporal lobe resection may be curative in 70–90% of such cases. MRI is important in both the preoperative localization of the seizure focus and the exclusion of other disorders.

CT Findings. CT is highly insensitive for mesial temporal sclerosis and therefore of limited value. The abnormality most often identified is asymmetric enlargement of the temporal horn. This finding is a common normal variant and therefore quite nonspecific. Diminished attenuation in the medial temporal lobe is occasionally seen.

MRI Findings. Visual inspection of coronal MRI most often reveals atrophy of the hippocampal formation, seen best on heavily T1-weighted images. This is manifested by a reduction in the cross-sectional area of the hippocampus compared with the opposite side and enlargement of the temporal horn (which may be a normal variant) and choroidal fissure. Hyperintensity of the hippocampus is present on T2-weighted images in 70% or more of cases depending on the scanning technique. Quantitative methods, such as T2 measurement and volumetric analysis, may allow enhanced diagnostic confidence in subtle cases. Intravenous contrast is useful only for excluding tumors or other mass lesions.

TABLE 5–5 | Principal Causes of Intractable Epilepsy

Injuries
Mesial temporal sclerosis
Infarct
Trauma
Infection
Congenital
Heterotopic gray matter
Focal cortical dysplasia
Hamartoma
Vascular malformation
Neoplastic
Astrocytoma
Ganglioglioma

Differential Diagnosis

Other potential causes of signal abnormality in the medial temporal lobe include gliosis unrelated to seizures, glioma (especially ganglioglioma), hamartoma, and choroidal fissure cyst. In a patient with intractable seizures localized to the temporal lobe, surgery will still be required for each of these conditions except a cyst. Cysts can be readily diagnosed by reference to T1-weighted images. See Table 5–5.

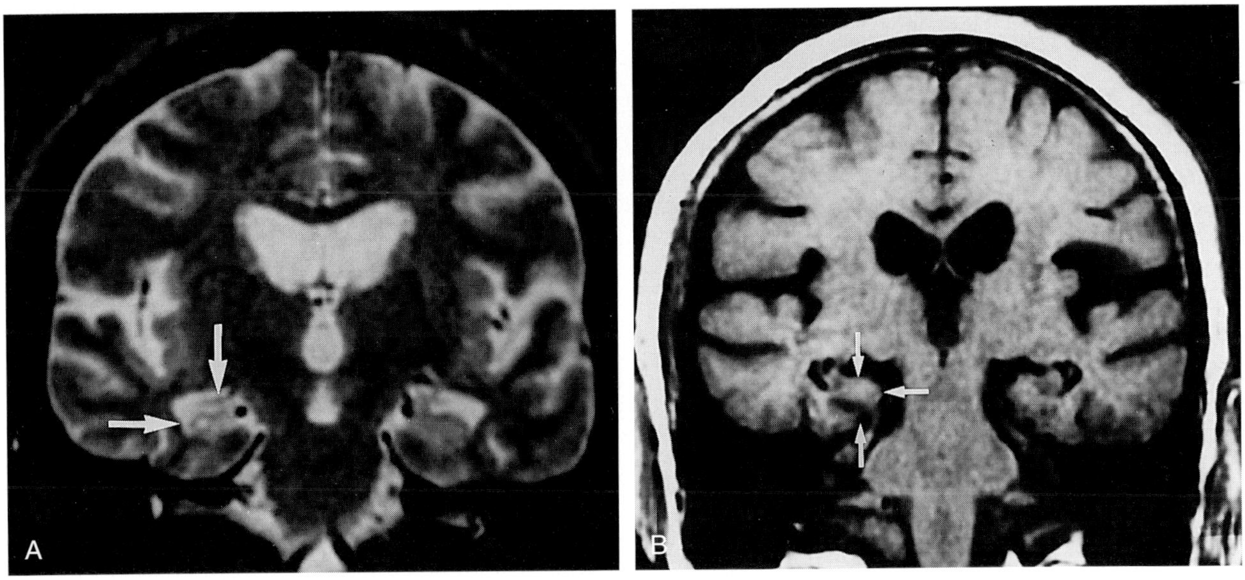

Figure 5–20. Mesial temporal sclerosis. **(A)** Coronal T2-weighted MRI shows hyperintensity in the right hippocampus (arrows) compared with the normal left side. **(B)** Coronal T1-weighted MRI shows diminished cross-sectional area (arrows) of the right parahippocampal gyrus with loss of gray and white matter.

RECOMMENDED READINGS

General

Davis,PC, Mirra,SS, Alazraki,N. The Brain in Older Persons With and Without Dementia: Findings on MR, PET, and SPECT Images. *AJR* 162:1267–1278, 1994.

Drayer,BP. Degenerative Disorders of the Central Nervous System: An Integrated Approach to the Differential Diagnosis. *Neuroimaging Clin North Am* 5:135–154, 1995.

LeMay,M. CT Changes in Dementing Diseases: A Review. *AJNR* 7:841–853, 1986. *AJR* 147:963–975, 1986.

Tien,RD, Felsberg,GJ, Ferris,NJ, Osumi,AK. The Dementias: Correlation of Clinical Features, Pathophysiology, and Neuroradiology. *AJR* 161:245–255, 1993.

Alzheimer's Disease

Bonte,FJ, Tintner,R, Weiner,MF, Bigio,EH, White,CL. Brain Blood Flow in the Dementias: SPECT with Histopathologic Correlation. *Radiology* 186:361–365, 1993.

de Leon,MJ, Golomb,J, George,AE, et al. The Radiologic Prediction of Alzheimer Disease: The Atrophic Hippocampal Formation. *AJNR* 14:897–906, 1993.

Fazekas,F, Chawluk,JB, Alavi,A, Hurtig,HI, Zimmerman,RA. MR Signal Abnormalities at 1.5T in Alzheimer's Dementia and Normal Aging. *AJR* 149:351–356, 1987.

Kido,DK, Caine,ED, LeMay,M, Ekholm,S, Booth,H, Panzer,R. Temporal Lobe Atrophy in Patients with Alzheimer Disease: A CT Study. *AJNR* 10:551–555, 1989.

Ohnishi,T, Hoshi,H, Nagamachi,S, et al. Regional Cerebral Blood Flow Study with ^{123}I-IMP in Patients with Degenerative Dementia. *AJNR* 12:513–520, 1991.

Tanna,NK, Kohn,MI, Horwich,DN, et al. Analysis of Brain and Cerebrospinal Fluid Volumes with MR Imaging: Impact on PET Data Correction for Atrophy. Part II. Aging and Alzheimer Dementia. *Radiology* 178:123–130, 1991.

Wisniewski,HM, Wegiel,J. The Neuropathology of Alzheimer's Disease. *Neuroimaging Clin North Am* 5:45–58, 1995.

Huntington's Disease

Rutledge,JN, Hilal,SK, Silver,AJ, Defendini,R, Fahn,S. Study of Movement Disorders and Brain Iron by MR. *AJNR* 8:397–411, 1987. *AJR* 149:365–379, 1987

Savoiardo,M, Strada,L, Oliva,D, Girotti,F, D'Incerti,L. Abnormal MRI Signal in the Rigid Form of Huntington's Disease. J Neurol Neurosurg Psychiatry 54:888–891, 1991.

Ischemic Leukoencephalopathy

Bowern,BC, Barker,WW, Loewenstein,DA, Sheldon,J, Duara,R. MR Signal Abnormalities in Memory Disorder and Dementia. *AJNR* 11:283–290, 1990, *AJR* 154:1285–1292, 1990.

Heier,L. White Matter Disease in the Elderly. *Neuroimaging Clin N Am.* 2:441–461, 1992.

Salomon,A, Yeates,AE, Burger,PC, Heinz,ER. Subcortical Arteriosclerotic Encephalopathy: Brain Stem Findings with MR Imaging. *Radiology* 165:625–629, 1987.

Normal Pressure Hydrocephalus

Bradley,WG, Whittemore,AR, Kortman,KE, et al. Marked Cerebrospinal Fluid Void: Indicator of Successful Shunt in Patients with Suspected Normal-Pressure Hydrocephalus. *Radiology* 178:459–466, 1991.

Bradley,WG, Whittemore,AR, Watanabe,AS, et al. Association of Deep White Matter Infarction with Chronic Communicating Hydrocephalus: Implications Regarding the Possible Origin of Normal-Pressure Hydrocephalus. *AJNR* 12:31–39, 1991

George,AE, Holodny,A, Golomb,J, de Leon,MJ. The Differential Diagnosis of Alzheimer's Disease: Cerebral Atrophy Versus Normal Pressure Hydrocephalus. *Neuroimaging Clin North Am* 5:19–32, 1995.

Román,GC. White Matter Lesions and Normal-Pressure Hydrocephalus: Binswanger Disease or Hakim Syndrome? *AJNR* 12:40–41, 1991.

Wikkelso,C, Andersson,H, Blomstrand,C, Matousek,M, Svendsen,P. Computed Tomography of the Brain in the Diagnosis of and Prognosis in Normal Pressure Hydrocephalus. *Neuroradiology* 31:160–165, 1989.

Wilson's Disease

Nazer,H, Brismar,J, Al-Kawi,MZ, Guasekaran,TS, Jorulf,HK. Magnetic Resonance Imaging of the Brain in Wilson's Disease. *Neuroradiology* 35:130–133, 1993.

Thuomas,K, Aquilonius,SM, Bergström,K, Westermark,K. Magnetic Resonance Imaging of the Brain in Wilson's Disease. *Neuroradiology* 35:134–141, 1993.

Parkinson's Disease

Braffman,BH, Grossman,RI, Goldberg,HI, et al. MR Imaging of Parkinson Disease with Spin-Echo and Gradient-Echo Sequences. *AJNR* 9:1093–1099, 1988. *AJR* 152:159–165, 1989.

Rutledge,JN, Hilal,SK, Silver,AJ, Defendini,R, Fahn,S. Study of Movement Disorders and Brain Iron by MR. *AJNR* 8:397–411, 1987. *AJR* 149:365–379, 1987.

Olivopontocerebellar Atrophy

Savoiardo,M, Bracchi,M, Passerini,A, Visciani,A, Di Donato,S, Cocchini,F. Computed Tomography of Olivopontocerebellar Degeneration. *AJNR* 4:509–512, 1983.

Savoiardo,M, Strada,L, Girotti,F, et al. Olivopontocerebellar Atrophy: MR Diagnosis and Relationship to Multisystem Atrophy. Radiology 174:693–696, 1990.

Multiple Sclerosis

Barkhof,F, Scheltens,P, Frequin,STF, et al. Relapsing-Remitting Multiple Sclerosis: Sequential Enhanced MR Imaging vs Clinical Findings in Determining Disease Activity. *AJR* 159:1041–1047, 1992.

Farlow,MR, Bonnin,JM. Clinical and Neuropathologic Features of Multiple Sclerosis. *Neuroimaging Clin N Am.* 3:213–228, 1993.

Grossman,RI, Lenkinski,RE, Ramer,KN, Gonzalez-Scarano,F, Cohen,JA. MR Proton Spectroscopy in Multiple Sclerosis. *AJNR* 13:1535–1543, 1992.

Nesbit,GM, Forbes,GS, Scheithauer,BW, Okazaki,H, Rodriguez,M. Multiple Sclerosis: Histopathologic and MR and/or CT Correlation in 37 Cases at Biopsy and Three Cases at Autopsy. *Radiology* 180:467–474, 1991.

Simon,JH. Neuroimaging of Multiple Sclerosis. *Neuroimaging Clin N Am.* 3:229–246, 1993.

Wallace,CJ, Seland,TP, Fong,TC. Multiple Sclerosis: The Impact of MR Imaging. *AJR* 158:849–857, 1992.

Mesial Temporal Sclerosis

Bronen,RA. Epilepsy: The Role of MR Imaging. *AJR* 159: 1165–1174, 1992.

Bronen,RA, Cheung,G, Charles,JT, et al. Imaging Findings in Hippocampal Sclerosis: Correlation with Pathology. *AJNR* 12:933–940, 1991.

Jack,CR. Epilepsy: Surgery and Imaging. *Radiology* 189:635–646, 1993.

Jack,CR, Sharbrough,FW, Twomey,CK, et al. Temporal Lobe Seizures: Lateralization with MR Volume Measurements of the Hippocampal Formation. *Radiology* 175:423–429, 1990.

Jackson,GD, Berkovic,SF, Duncan,JS, Connelly,A. Optimizing the Diagnosis of Hippocampal Sclerosis Using MR Imaging. *AJNR* 14:753–762, 1993.

Heinz,R, Ferris,N, Lee,EK, et al. MR and Positron Emission Tomography in the Diagnosis of Surgically Correctable Temporal Lobe Epilepsy. *AJNR* 15:1341–1348, 1994.

Meiners,LC, van Gils,A, Jansen,GH, et al. Temporal Lobe Epilepsy: The Various MR Appearances of Histologically Proven Mesial Temporal Sclerosis. *AJNR* 15:1547–1555, 1994.

Tien,RD, Felsberg,GJ, de Castro,CC, et al. Complex Partial Seizures and Mesial Temporal Sclerosis: Evaluation with Fast Spin-Echo MR Imaging. *Radiology* 189:835–842, 1993.

CHAPTER SIX

Head Trauma

Depressed Skull Fracture

Leptomeningeal Cyst

Subarachnoid Hemorrhage

Acute Epidural Hematoma

Acute Subdural Hematoma

Chronic Subdural Hematoma

Subdural Hygroma

Cerebral Contusions

Intracerebral Hematoma

Diffuse Axonal Injury

Post-traumatic Cerebral Edema

Battered Child Syndrome

Head injury is one of the most common indications for the performance of cranial CT, which in most instances remains the imaging procedure of choice. However, there are some conditions, such as diffuse axonal injury and child abuse, for which MRI may be required to make the diagnosis.

The pathologic changes associated with head trauma constitute a fairly short list of common injuries (Table 6–1). The most important injuries are described herein. Some entities, such as scalp injuries and linear skull fractures, are of less clinical significance and are not discussed. Secondary cerebral infarction and traumatic vascular injuries are discussed in Chapter 7. Temporal bone fractures are covered in Chapter 9.

TABLE 6–1 | Imaging Findings in Head Trauma

Cranial Injuries
Subgaleal hematoma
Laceration
Linear skull fracture
Depressed skull fracture
Skull base fractures
Leptomeningeal cyst
Intracranial Extracerebral Injuries
Acute epidural hematoma
Acute subdural hematoma
Chronic subdural hematoma
Subdural hygroma
Primary Cerebral Injuries
Contusion
Hematoma
Diffuse axonal injury
Secondary Cerebral Injuries
Edema
Infarct
Herniation
Hemorrhage
Secondary Findings
Pneumocephalus
Subarachnoid hemorrhage
Hydrocephalus
CSF leak

Depressed Skull Fracture

Most skull fractures are self-healing events requiring no specific medical intervention. Although skull fractures are not inconsequential—the incidence of intracranial hemorrhage is much higher when a skull fracture is present—the diagnosis of intracranial injury takes precedence. Hence CT has replaced skull radiography in the evaluation of head injury, even though some linear fractures may remain undiagnosed. More complex fractures, however, may require surgical treatment.

CT Findings. A depressed skull fracture is a fracture with inward displacement of the inner table or bone fragments. Depressions greater than 5 mm are usually treated surgically. Underlying contusions (coup injuries) are present in about one half of cases. Contrecoup contusions occur in about one third. Overlying scalp swelling or hematoma is nearly universally present.

MRI Findings. MRI is of little use in the diagnosis of skull fractures but may be of use in the detection of associated cerebral injuries.

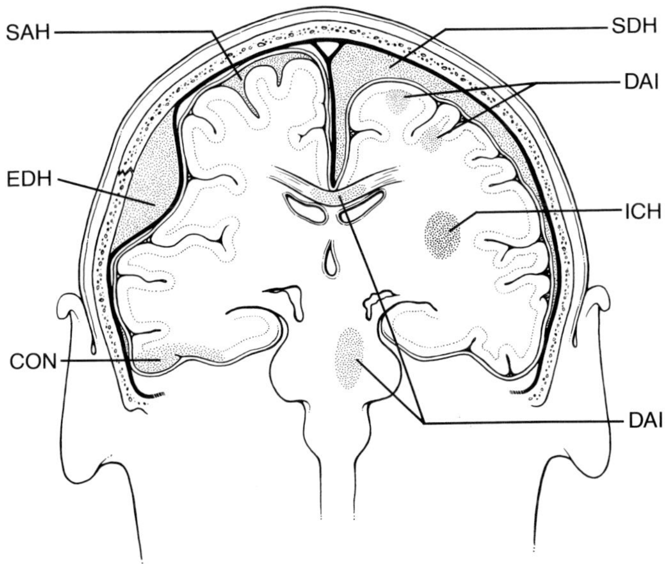

Figure 6–1. Summary of the major types of intracranial injury and their anatomic bases. CON = contusion, DAI = diffuse axonal injury, EDH = epidural hematoma, ICH = intracerebral hematoma, SAH = subarachnoid hemorrhage, SDH = subdural hematoma. Heavy black line represents dura.

CON: Contusions connote a focal brain injury at a point of bony impact. Superficial gray matter is most involved with relative sparing of white matter and deeper gray matter.

DAI: Axonal disruption is present most commonly in the corpus callosum, subcortical white matter, and brainstem (Adams' triad). Hemorrhage may be present, and mass effect tends to be minimal.

EDH: Hemorrhage between the inner table and the dura displaces the dura away from the skull. A skull fracture is present in over 90%. The displaced dura usually can be visualized on MRI.

ICH: Intracerebral hemorrhage results from rupture of intracerebral blood vessels with hemorrhage into deep white matter and possibly ventricles.

SAH: Hemorrhage into the subarachnoid space extends into the depths of cortical sulci and rarely is sufficient to produce mass effect.

SDH: Subdural hemorrhage displaces the arachnoid from the dura forming a localized mass. Subdural hematoma cannot cross the falx or tentorium. The arachnoid prevents blood from entering the sulci, which are flattened and compressed.

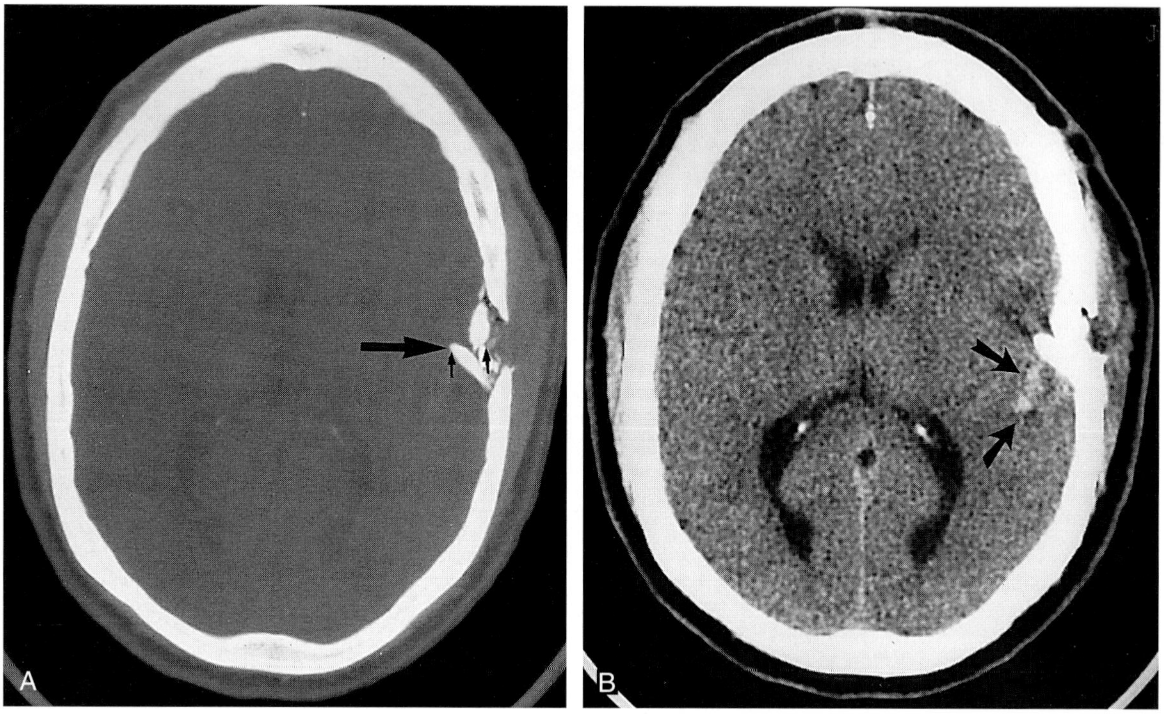

Figure 6–2. Depressed skull fracture. **(A)** Bone window shows the depressed fragment (large arrow) and allows measurement of the depth of depression (small arrows), which is 12 mm. **(B)** Soft tissue window shows hemorrhagic cortical contusion (arrows) beneath the depressed fragment.

Leptomeningeal Cyst

Synonyms: Pseudomeningocele, growing skull fracture.

Dural and arachnoidal lacerations at the site of a skull fracture may result in an arachnoid cyst or a pseudomeningocele, which in turn may cause progressive, erosive enlargement of the skull defect. The leptomeningeal cyst occurs almost exclusively in infants and young children who typically present months to years after the causative injury. It is one of the few disorders for which skull radiography is still of value as an easy and inexpensive means for following a child at risk of developing a growing fracture.

CT Findings. CT shows an elliptical skull defect with indistinct margins developing at the site of a previous fracture. There is usually greater erosion of the inner table than the outer. There may be herniation of brain or a collection of CSF protruding through the defect. Low attenuation of the subjacent parenchyma may be seen owing to gliosis or encephalomalacia.

MRI Findings. Because of the absence of beam-hardening artifacts, MRI may more effectively display the relationship of CSF, meninges, and cranial defects. There may also be signal abnormality (decreased on T1, increased on T2) and atrophy of the subjacent brain parenchyma due to gliosis or encephalomalacia.

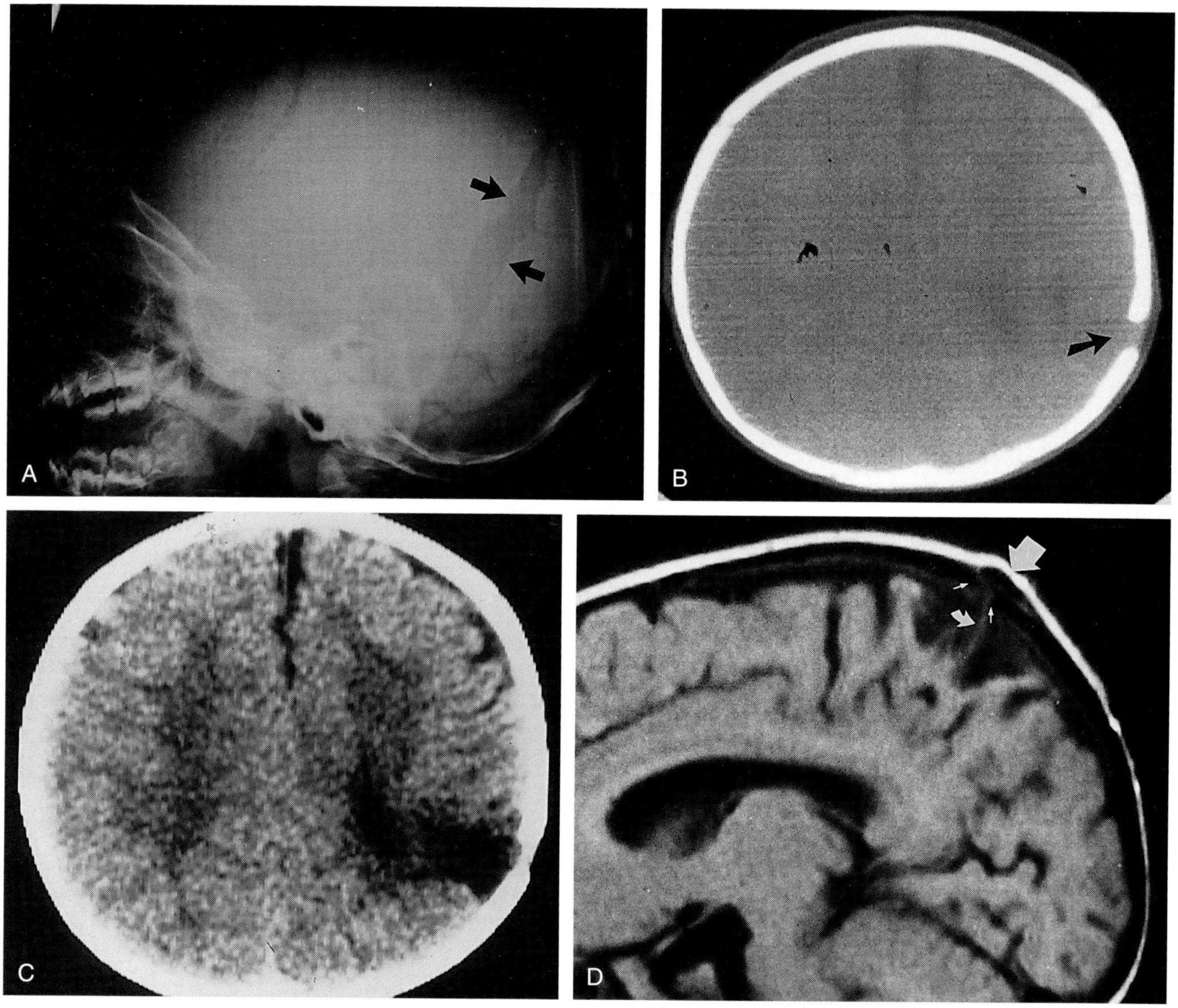

Figure 6–3. Leptomeningeal cyst. **(A)** Skull film reveals wide linear defect (arrows) at site of previous fracture. **(B)** Bone window shows a well-marginated and complete cortical defect (arrow). **(C)** Soft tissue window of **B** shows gliosis of underlying parenchyma. **(D)** Sagittal T1-weighted MRI shows the calvarial defect with herniation of meninges and CSF (large arrow), arachnoid adhesions (small curved arrow), and underlying cortical atrophy.

Subarachnoid Hemorrhage

Post-traumatic subarachnoid hemorrhage (SAH) usually arises from hemorrhagic contusion with bleeding into the subarachnoid space. SAH after blunt trauma is usually mild and almost never life threatening. Occasional morbidity may result from acute or delayed hydrocephalus.

CT Findings. CT shows increased attenuation in the cortical fissures and sulci or the basal cisterns. SAH due to trauma is seen more often in the cortical sulci near the brain surface than in the basal cisterns as with aneurysmal rupture. Increased density may be observed in the anterior and superior interhemispheric fissure with a zigzag configuration due to blood extending into adjacent sulci. SAH in the posterior interhemispheric fissure is unusual, and blood here is more likely to be subdural.

MRI Findings. MRI is less sensitive than CT for the detection of SAH. (See Hemorrhage, Chapter 1.)

Differential Diagnosis

Mildly increased attenuation must be distinguished from normal or calcified dura (falx and tentorium). Intrathecal contrast causes a similar appearance to SAH but is usually more diffuse than traumatic SAH. Occasionally it may be unclear whether SAH is traumatic or aneurysmal in origin. Traumatic SAH is less likely to be present in the basal cisterns or to be associated with vasospasm or infarcts.

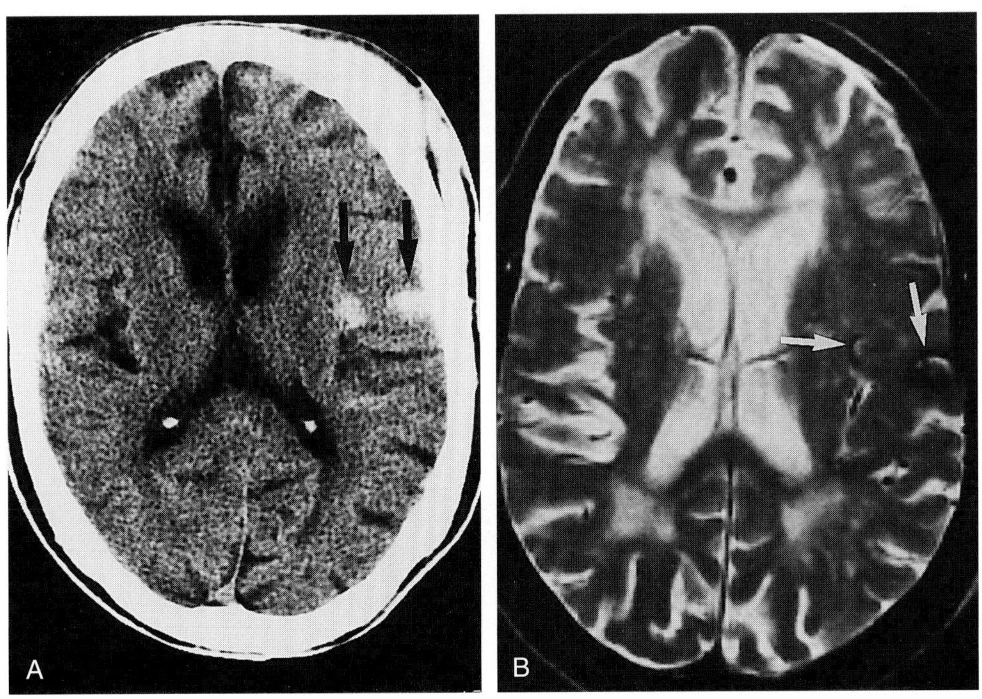

Figure 6–4. Subarachnoid hemorrhage. **(A)** CT shows hemorrhage in the left sylvian fissure (arrows). **(B)** T2-weighted MRI 4 months later shows localized superficial siderosis (arrows) at sites corresponding to hemorrhage seen in **A**.

Acute Epidural Hematoma

Epidural hemorrhage usually arises from laceration of a meningeal artery (most commonly the middle meningeal) with the rapid formation of hematoma stripping the dura from the inner table of the skull. A few cases of epidural hematoma (EDH) result from rupture of a major venous sinus. Over 90% of EDHs are associated with an overlying skull fracture. Affected patients may initially remain quite lucid but progressively deteriorate as the hematoma enlarges. The prognosis is usually excellent if the hematoma is evacuated before serious secondary injuries ensue. Certain small nonexpanding EDHs can be managed nonoperatively with careful CT follow-up.

CT Findings. CT demonstrates a high attenuation, biconvex mass adjacent to the inner table of the skull. Epidural hemorrhage tends not to cross cranial sutures, where the dura is tightly adherent. A lower attenuation swirl may be present within the clot, reflecting active bleeding mixed with serum from clotted blood. Skull fractures adjacent to the hematoma are present in over 90% of cases. Because they lie outside the dura, epidural hematomas may cross the falx or displace dural venous sinuses from the inner table.

MRI Findings. MRI may show the displaced dura as a linear hypointensity separating the hematoma from the subjacent brain. The signal characteristics of the clot are complex and time dependent. (See Hemorrhage, Chapter 1.)

Differential Diagnosis

In the setting of acute trauma, the appearance of CT and MRI is virtually pathognomonic. Acute EDHs may be mimicked by chronic subdural hematomas, meningiomas, or meningeal or calvarial metastases.

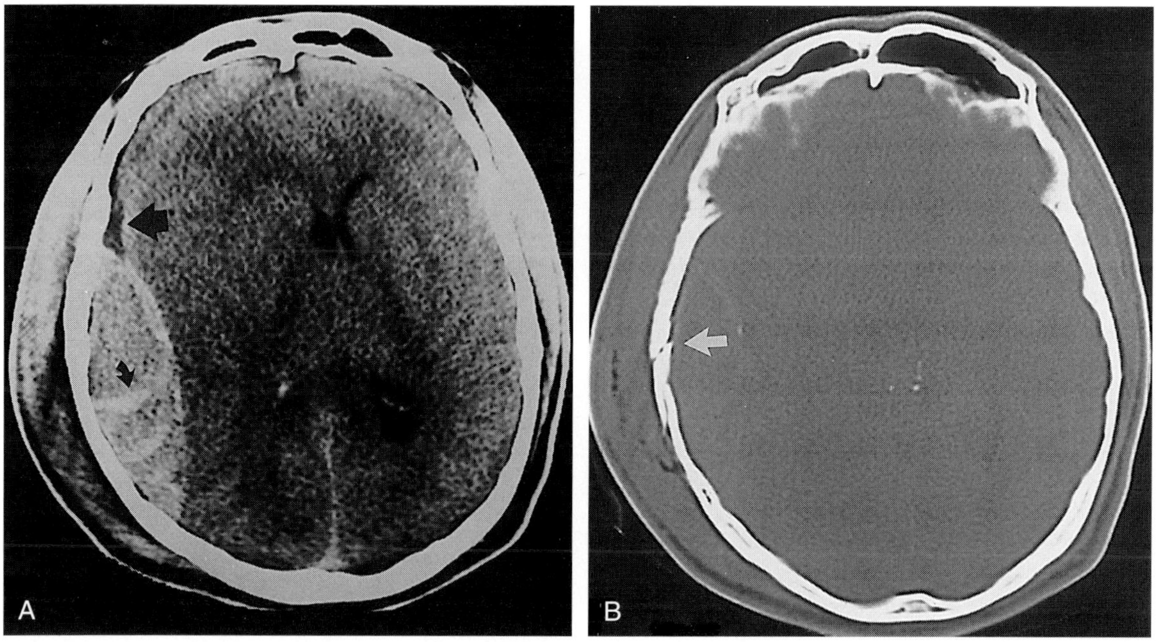

Figure 6–5. Epidural hematoma. **(A)** CT shows convex clot limited anteriorly at site of coronal suture and posteriorly near the lambdoid suture. Alternating areas of higher and lower density (small curved arrow) represent a mixture of clotted and unclotted blood. Note enlargement of the subarachnoid space anteriorly (large arrow), a general feature of extraaxial masses. **(B)** Fracture (arrow) corresponds to the location of epidural hematoma in **A**.

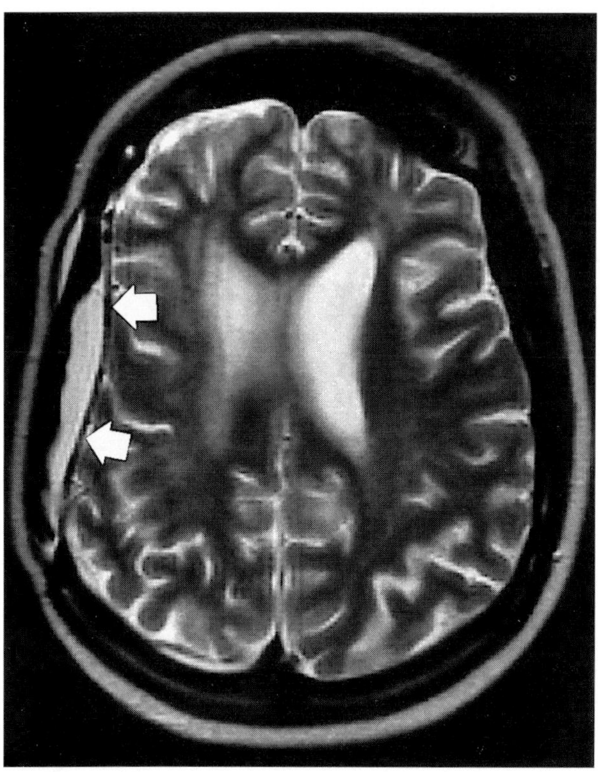

Figure 6–6. Chronic postoperative epidural hematoma. On T2-weighted MRI the displaced dura (arrows) is seen as a thick hypointense line.

Acute Subdural Hematoma

Subdural hemorrhage most often results from ruptured cerebral veins passing through the subdural space to the major venous sinuses. Since the bleeding is venous, expansion ordinarily develops more slowly than that with epidural hemorrhage. Underlying cerebral injuries are more frequent with SDH than EDH. Swelling of the underlying hemisphere is common, so that the mass effect is greater than expected based on the size of the clot alone. Occasionally spontaneous subdural hematomas (SDHs) may result from a ruptured aneurysm or an ateriovenous malformation. Small hematomas are sometimes managed conservatively with careful follow-up imaging.

CT Findings. CT typically shows a crescentic band of high attenuation (with a concave medial aspect) following the inner table of the skull. The attenuation of the clot may be lower than expected due to unclotted blood, low hematocrit value, or admixture with CSF. Associated contusions are present in 50%. The degree of mass effect and shift is typically greater than that expected from the hematoma alone.

After several days to weeks, the hematoma becomes isodense with the underlying brain. It may be identified through the presence of mass effect or the aid of intravenous contrast. Contrast-enhanced CT may show an enhancing membrane or displaced cortical veins.

Interhemispheric Subdural Hematoma. CT shows a band of increased attenuation along the falx and remote from the sagittal sinus. The hematoma manifests a flat medial and convex lateral border usually along the posterior falx and often extending over the tentorium. Anteriorly it does not contact the rostrum of the corpus callosum, whereas subarachnoid blood can and does. Anterior interhemispheric SDH is thought not to occur in the absence of a posterior interhemispheric SDH. Blood in the anterior interhemispheric fissure is more likely to be subarachnoid.

MRI Findings. Even in the acute stage, MRI has demonstrated superior sensitivity to CT in the detection of acute SDH. However, the additional hematomas detected by MRI tend to be clinically insignificant. CT is still generally preferred because of the medical considerations and technical requirements of imaging victims of acute trauma. One important exception is in the evaluation of suspected child abuse, where the detection of any hematoma is significant. In such cases, MRI should be performed. Associated intracerebral injuries are visualized in nearly all patients with SDH.

TABLE 6–2 Differential Diagnosis of Thickened Hyperdense Falx

- Subdural hematoma
- Normal falx (cerebral edema or atrophy)
- Calcified or ossified falx
- Meningioma
- Subarachnoid hemorrhage
- Pachymeningitis
- Dural carcinomatosis

Differential Diagnosis

In the setting of documented acute trauma, the appearance is virtually pathognomonic. See Tables 6–2 and 6–3.

TABLE 6–3 Differential Diagnosis of Acute Post-Traumatic Extraaxial Fluid Collection

	Epidural Hematoma	Acute Subdural Hematoma	Subdural Hygroma
Inner margin	Convex	Concave	Concave
Sutures	Usually does not cross	Crosses easily	Crosses easily
Falx/tentorium	Crosses easily	Cannot cross	Cannot cross
Skull fractures	Nearly 100%	Randomly associated	Randomly associated
Contents	Blood	Blood	CSF
Mass effect	Proportionate	Disproportionately large	Proportionate
Blood serum level	Absent	Sometimes present	Absent
Swirl sign	Sometimes present	Unclotted blood may yield similar appearance	Absent

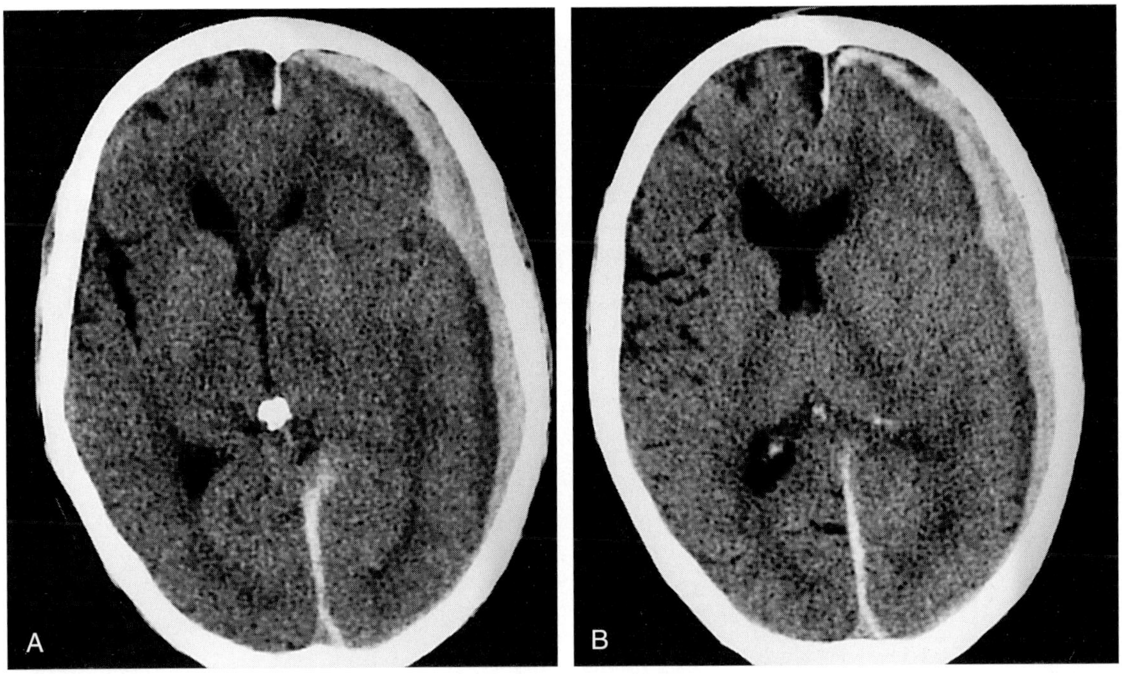

Figure 6–7. Acute subdural hematoma. **(A,B)** Axial CT shows acute left subdural hematoma that crosses the coronal suture and has concave inner margin. Subdural blood is also present in the posterior interhemispheric fissure.

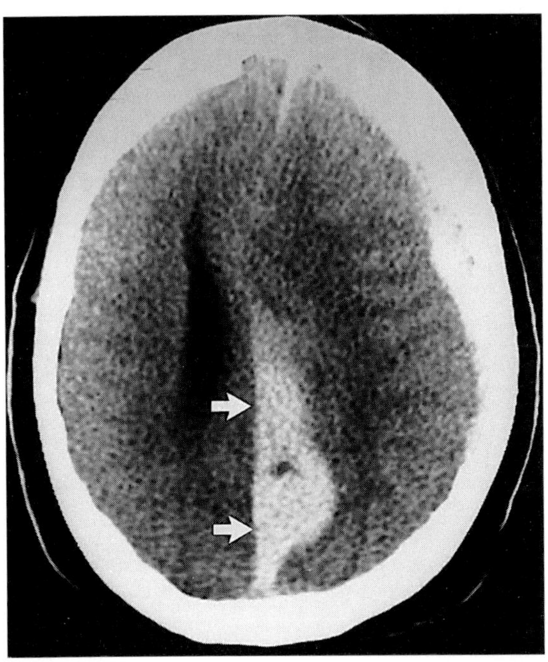

Figure 6–8. Interhemispheric subdural hematoma. Note the flat medial (arrows) and convex lateral borders. There is also a left frontal subdural hematoma.

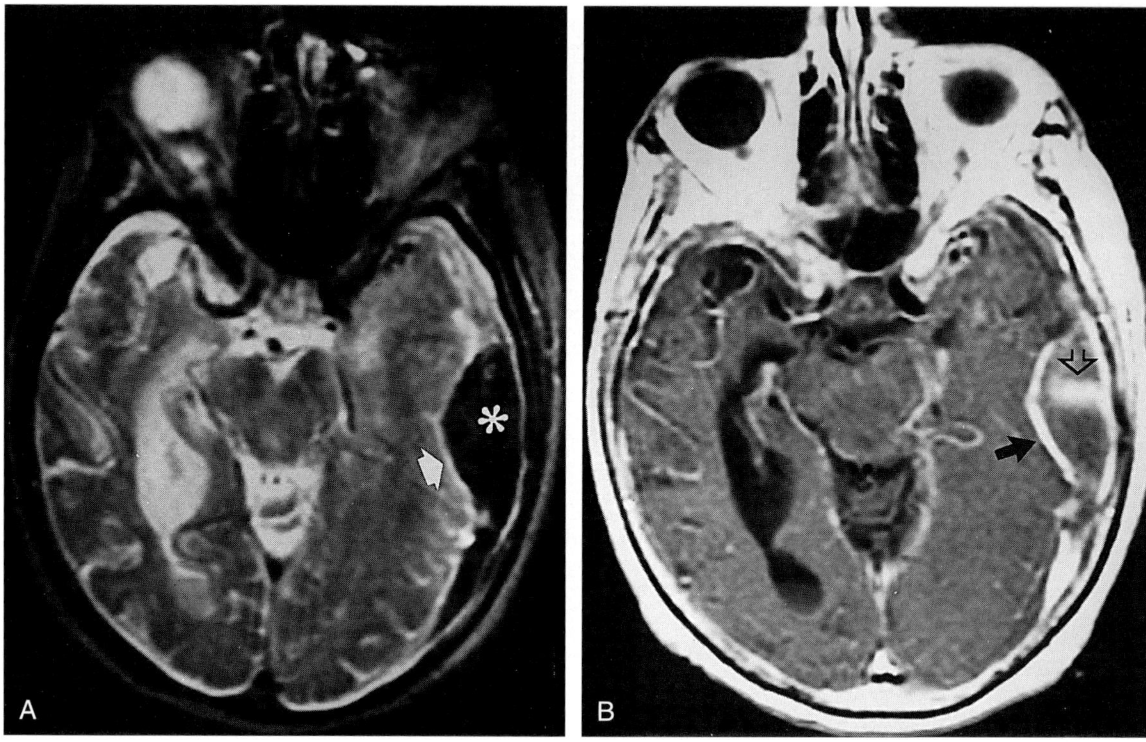

Figure 6–9. Acute subdural hematoma. **(A)** T2-weighted MRI shows hypointensity owing to intracellular hemoglobin derivatives within an acute left subdural hematoma (asterisk). There is a thin rim of hyperintensity reflecting CSF in the subarachnoid space (arrow). **(B)** Contrast-enhanced T1-weighted MRI shows enhancement of the medial border (solid arrow). Note central hyperintensity due to the release of free extracellar methemoglobin (open arrow).

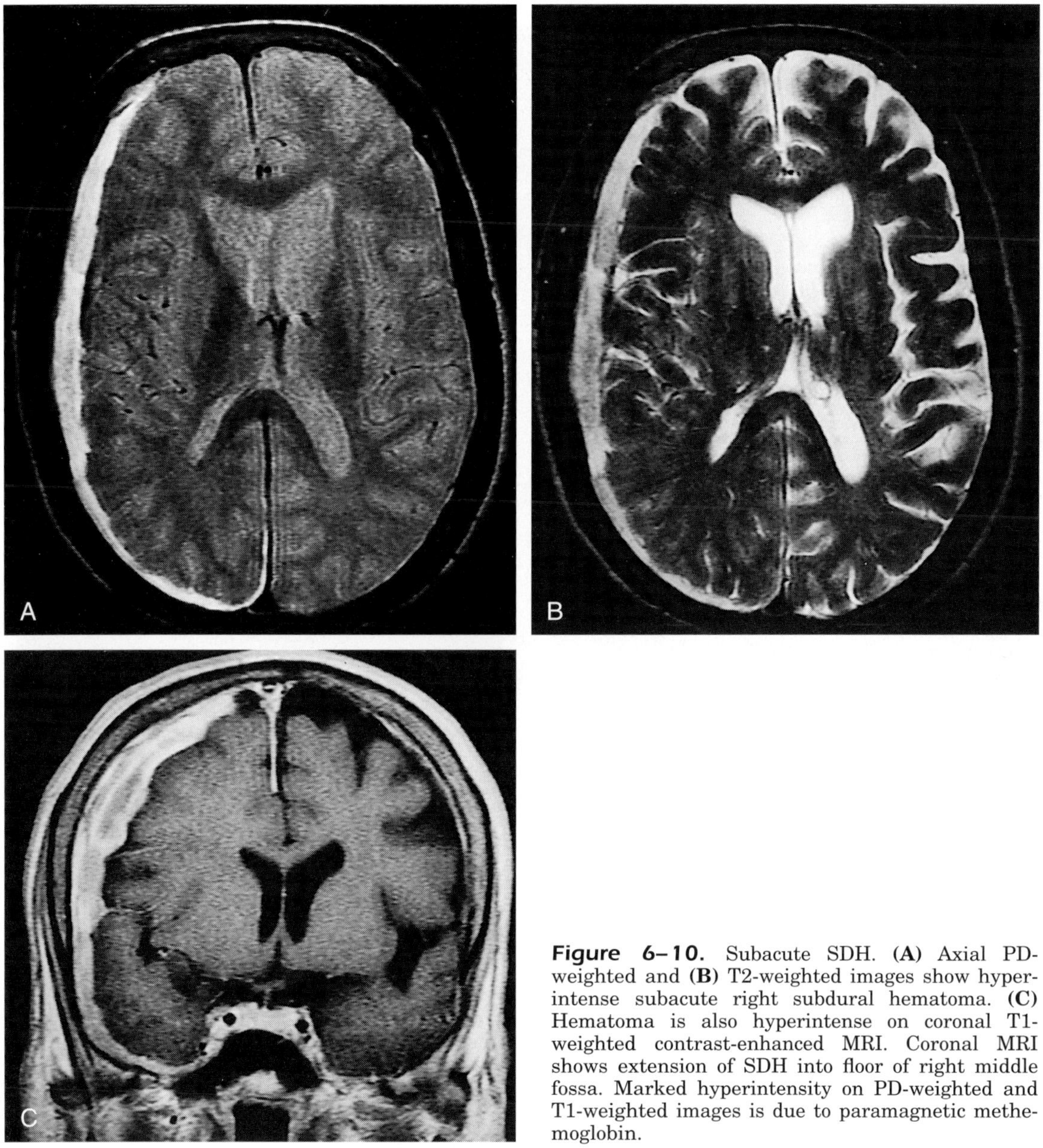

Figure 6–10. Subacute SDH. **(A)** Axial PD-weighted and **(B)** T2-weighted images show hyperintense subacute right subdural hematoma. **(C)** Hematoma is also hyperintense on coronal T1-weighted contrast-enhanced MRI. Coronal MRI shows extension of SDH into floor of right middle fossa. Marked hyperintensity on PD-weighted and T1-weighted images is due to paramagnetic methemoglobin.

Chronic Subdural Hematoma

Elderly patients are subject to the development of chronic subdural hematomas, often following relatively trivial injuries. A richly vascular membrane may form around the hematoma, leading to recurrent hemorrhage in 10–30% of patients. Chronic subdural hematomas are often bilateral and owing to the presence of atrophy can become quite large before provoking symptoms.

CT Findings. On CT a chronic subdural hematoma usually appears as a crescentic band of low attenuation closely applied to the inner table. The hematoma may be isodense, hyperdense, or of mixed attenuation as a result of rebleeding and may occasionally be biconvex due to adhesions. The ipsilateral sulci are usually effaced, and contrast injection demonstrates enhanced cortical veins interposed between the displaced cortical surface and the subdural collection. An enhancing membrane may be seen on the arachnoid side of the hematoma along a variable distance. The hematoma may enhance diffusely on contrast-enhanced CT delayed 3 to 6 hours after injection.

MRI Findings. On MRI, a chronic hematoma that has not rebled is isointense or slightly hypointense relative to gray matter on T1-weighted images and hyperintense on T2-weighted images. Displacement of cortical veins away from the inner table is seen. If rebleeding has occurred, blood in different stages of evolution is visible. (See Hemorrhage, Chapter 1.)

Differential Diagnosis	
Subdural hygroma	More closely identical to CSF on CT and T1-weighted MRI
Acute subdural hematoma	May be hypodense on CT in the presence of low hematocrit
Epidural hematoma	Both EDH and chronic SDH may be biconvex (see Table 6–2) MRI can help by demonstrating the older age of the chronic hematoma and offering direct visualization of the displaced dura

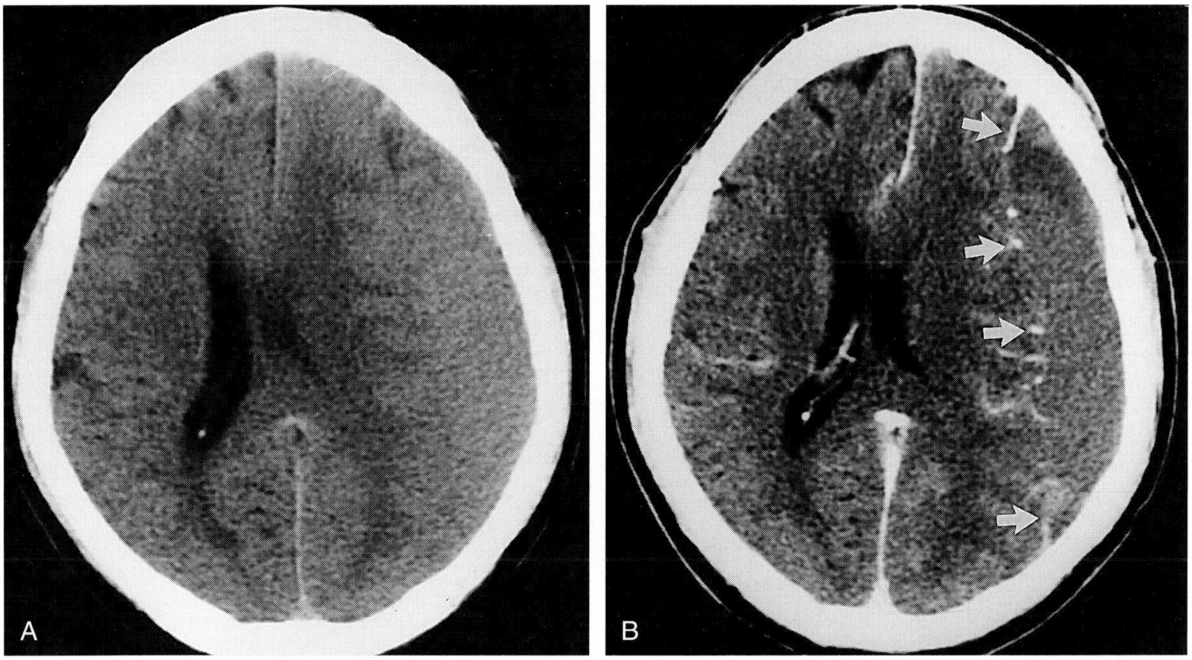

Figure 6–11. Chronic subdural hematoma. **(A)** CT shows left hemisphere mass isodense with gray matter with compression of left lateral ventricle and left to right shift. Most anterior portion is slightly hypodense due to layering of blood components. **(B)** Following intravenous contrast, there is clear delineation of hematoma from cortex by enhancing membrane and displaced cortical veins (arrows).

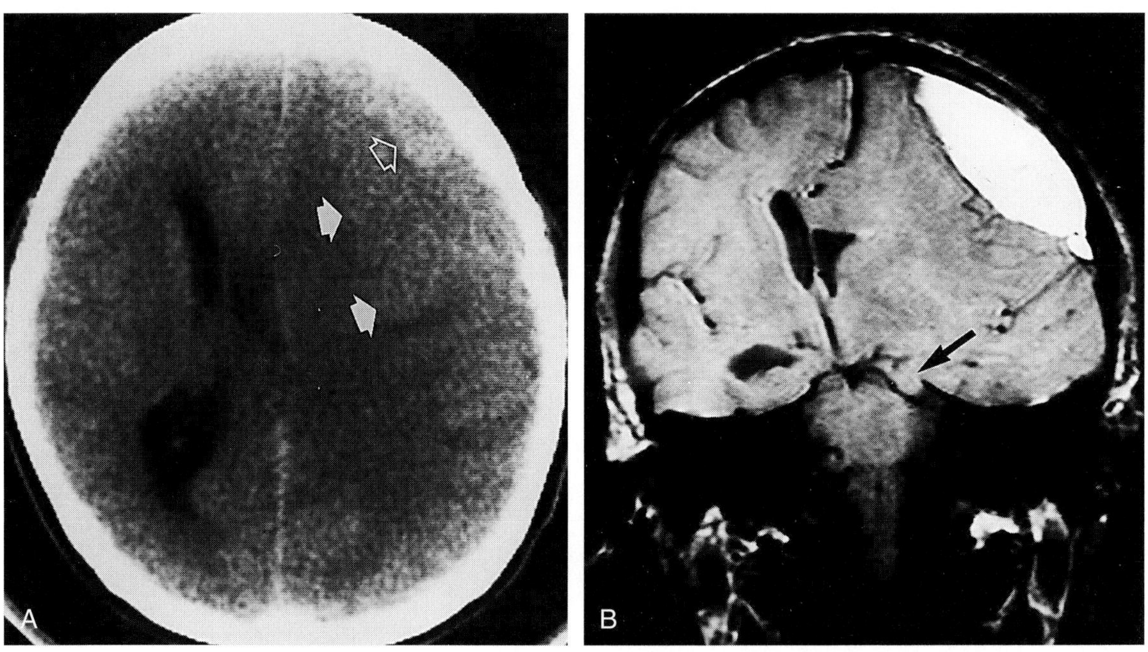

Figure 6–12. Chronic isodense subdural hematoma. **(A)** CT shows left to right shift with subfalcine herniation. There is slightly dense clot anteriorly (open arrow). Note inward displacement of gray-white junction referred to as white matter buckling (solid arrows). **(B)** Coronal T1-weighted MRI shows to much better advantage the large clot, which is hyperintense due to methemoglobin. Uncal (transtentorial) herniation is indicated by arrow.

Subdural Hygroma

A tear in the arachnoid without vascular injury may result in leakage and accumulation of CSF in an enlarging subdural space. This phenomenon is referred to as a subdural hygroma. Such hygromas are usually small and self-limited.

CT Findings. CT shows an extracerebral fluid collection isodense with CSF. Hygromas are crescentic following the inner table and concave with respect to the cerebral cortex. The sulci may be flattened, and cortical veins seen on contrast-enhanced scans are displaced away from the inner table.

MRI Findings. MRI reveals an extracerebral fluid collection isointense to CSF on all pulse sequences. Displaced cortical veins from the inner table may be seen by their signal void or flow-related enhancement.

Differential Diagnosis	
Chronic subdural hematoma	Shows evidence of blood products, especially on MRI
Atrophy	No inward displacement of cortical vessels Sulci are enlarged, not compressed

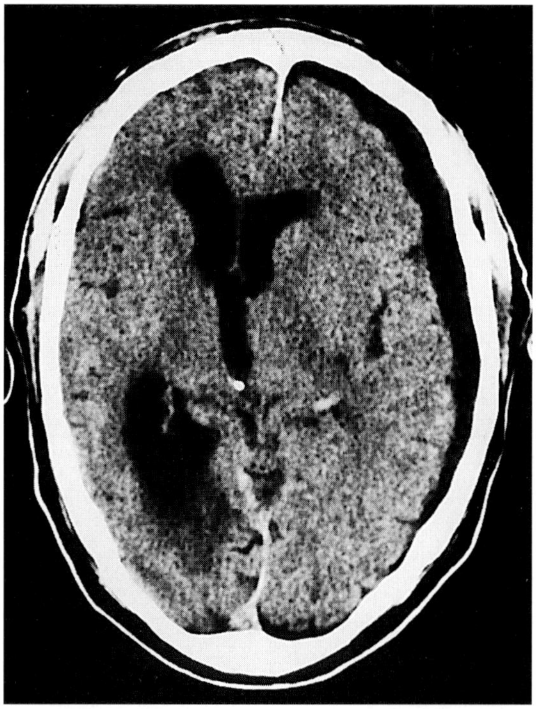

Figure 6–13. Subdural hygroma. Contrast-enhanced CT shows large left-sided fluid collection isodense with CSF and compressing brain, crossing suture lines, and limited anteriorly by the falx. Note the absence of enhancing membrane.

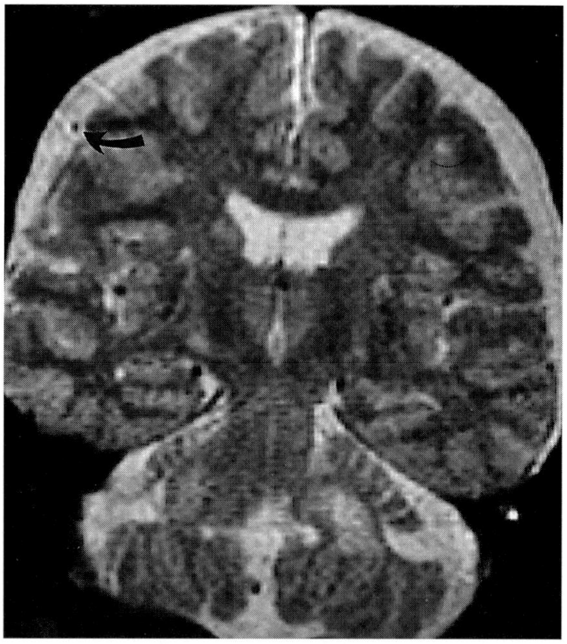

Figure 6–14. Bilateral subdural hygromas. Coronal T2-weighted MRI shows bilateral subdural hygromas. They are distinguished from atrophy by the flattened gyri, compression of the sulci, and displacement of the cortical veins (arrow).

Cerebral Contusions

Contusions are a focal injury of the brain surface due to direct impact with the calvarium. They are usually associated with superficial cortical hemorrhage. Contusions are most common at sites of bony protuberances of the skull base and therefore are seen in the frontal poles, orbital surface of the frontal lobes, temporal poles, and inferior surface of the temporal lobes and adjoining the anterior sylvian fissure near the lesser sphenoid wing. Progression of hemorrage often occurs during the first 24 to 48 hours (see Intracerebral Hematoma).

CT Findings. Hemorrhagic contusions are perhaps the most frequent intracranial CT abnormality in victims of head trauma. Such contusions appear as cortical foci of high attenuation interspersed with areas of low attenuation representing necrosis or edema. Hemorrhagic contusions are multiple in approximately 30% and are commonly associated with extracerebral hematomas or skull fractures. Occurring at points of bony impact, contusions are observed at the apex of gyri with progressively less involvement of deeper structures. The temporal lobes are the most common site, followed by the frontal lobes. Nonhemorrhagic contusions are hypodense and often difficult to visualize. Scans performed 24 to 48 hours after injury commonly show previously undetected contusions, more extensive hemorrhage, and increased edema.

MRI Findings. MRI is much more sensitive than CT in the detection of contusions after the first 24 hours. Nonhemorrhagic contusions are hypointense on T1-weighted images and hyperintense on T2-weighted images. Hemorrhagic contusions exhibit varied signal characteristics as a function of age (see Hemorrhage, Chapter 1). Contusions affect the gyral surfaces, and larger ones may involve several adjacent gyri. With MRI, multiple lesions are seen in the vast majority of cases.

Differential Diagnosis

Infarct	Usually appears in a characteristic vascular distribution
Chronic injury with gliosis	Local atrophy is seen rather than mass effect

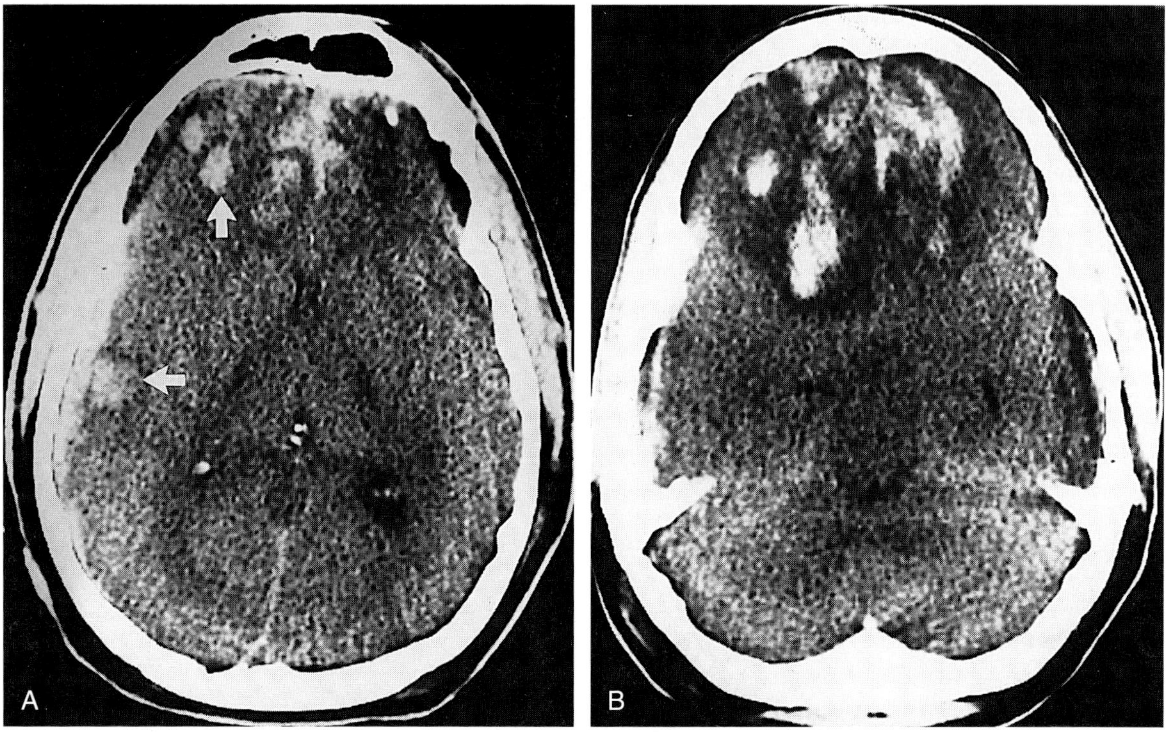

Figure 6–15. Cerebral contusions and hematoma. **(A)** CT scan shows acute right subdural hematoma, subarachnoid hemorrhage in anterior interhemispheric fissure, and multiple subfrontal and temporal hemorrhage contusions (arrows). **(B)** CT 1 day later shows formation of delayed intracerebral hematoma in the right frontal lobe.

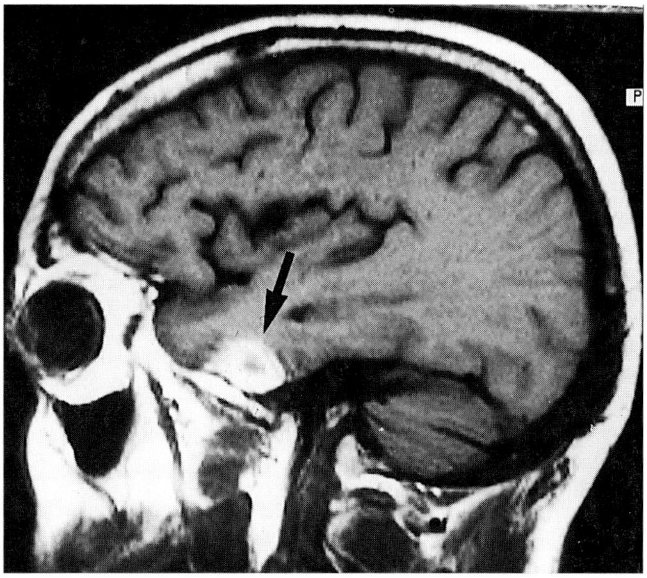

Figure 6–16. Subacute contusion. Sagittal T1-weighted MRI shows hyperintense clot (arrow) in the inferior temporal lobe, one of the classic sites of contusion.

Intracerebral Hematoma

Intracerebral hemorrhage results from the rupture of intracerebral blood vessels caused by either blunt or penetrating trauma. Intracerebral hematomas (ICHs) tend to be larger than contusions and involve the white matter or basal ganglia. Delayed ICH occurs hours to days after injury, affecting up to 8% of those with severe closed head injury.

CT Findings. CT shows a large high attenuation intraaxial mass usually in the frontal or temporal lobes or the basal ganglia. Surrounding low attenuation due to edema develops rapidly. Hematomas are bilateral in 20% of cases and extend into the ventricles in about 30% of cases. Intracerebral hematomas are frequently associated with epidural or subdural hematomas.

MRI Findings. The distribution of lesions is the same as that described for CT. The signal characteristics are complex and time dependent. (See Hemorrhage, Chapter 1.)

Differential Diagnosis

The appearance of a cerebral hematoma is usually specific. The list of possible etiologies, however, is quite lengthy. (See Hemorrhage, Chapter 1.)

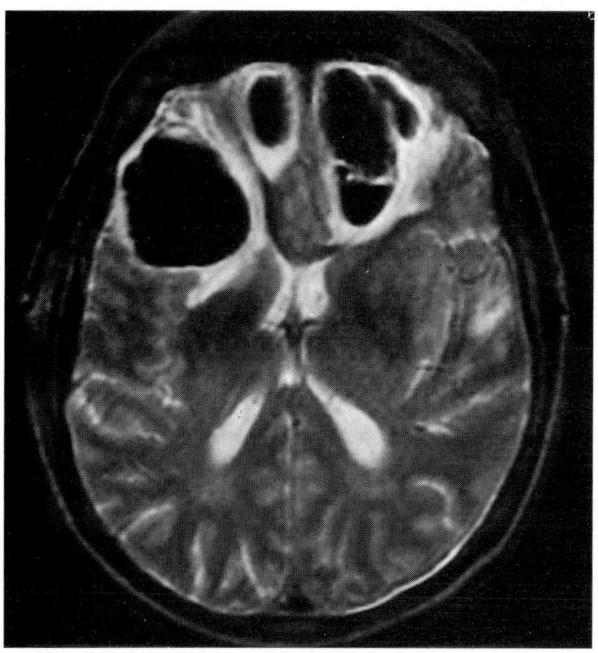

Figure 6–17. Acute intracerebral hematoma. Axial T2-weighted MRI shows large hypointense hematomas in both frontal lobes with surrounding edema.

Diffuse Axonal Injury

Synonym: White matter shear injury.

Severe rotational accelerative/decelerative forces upon the brain may result in widespread disruption of axons often with hemorrhage. This injury is most often identified in the corpus callosum, hemispheric white matter, and dorsolateral quadrants of the rostral brainstem. The combination of all three is called Adams' triad. The lesions are most common and numerous in the corticomedullary junction of the frontotemporal regions. Affected patients are usually immediately comatose but may slowly improve over days to weeks. Diffuse axonal injury (DAI) is the most common cause of post-traumatic coma in the absence of intracranial hematoma. It portends the worst prognosis of any primary cerebral injury.

CT Findings. CT is relatively insensitive for the diagnosis of DAI. Abnormalities are present in 20–50%. The lesions may appear as low attenuation foci in the hemispheric white matter, brainstem, and corpus callosum. Hemorrhage may be present and facilitates the CT diagnosis. The degree of hemorrhage may range from petechial hemorrhages in the subcortical white matter to large hematomas in the corpus callosum or deep white matter.

MRI Findings. The lesions of DAI appear as multiple small ovoid foci of hyperintensity on T2-weighted images with central hypointensity if hemorrhagic. They are hypointense on T1-weighted images. About 50% of lesions appear in the subcortical white matter of the hemispheres. Additional lesions may be present in the corpus callosum, superior cerebellar peduncles, and dorsolateral quadrants of the midbrain and upper pons.

Differential Diagnosis	
Infarction	Lesions occur in a vascular distribution
Demyelinating disease	Absence of major head trauma
Primary hemorrhage	May be impossible to distinguish from hemorrhagic DAI

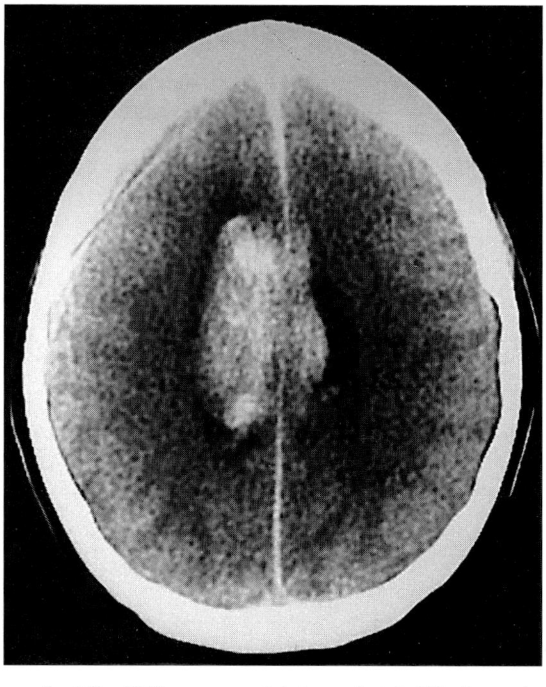

Figure 6–18. Diffuse axonal injury. Axial CT shows hemorrhage in the corpus callosum.

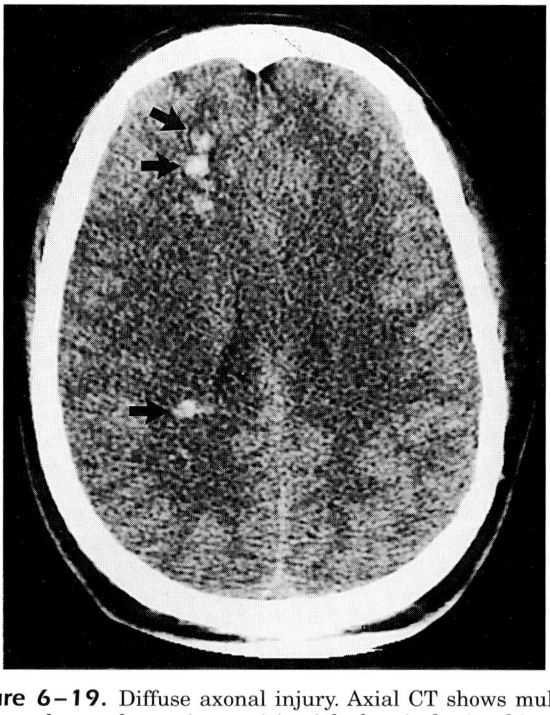

Figure 6–19. Diffuse axonal injury. Axial CT shows multiple punctate hemorrhages (arrows) in right hemispheric white matter tracts.

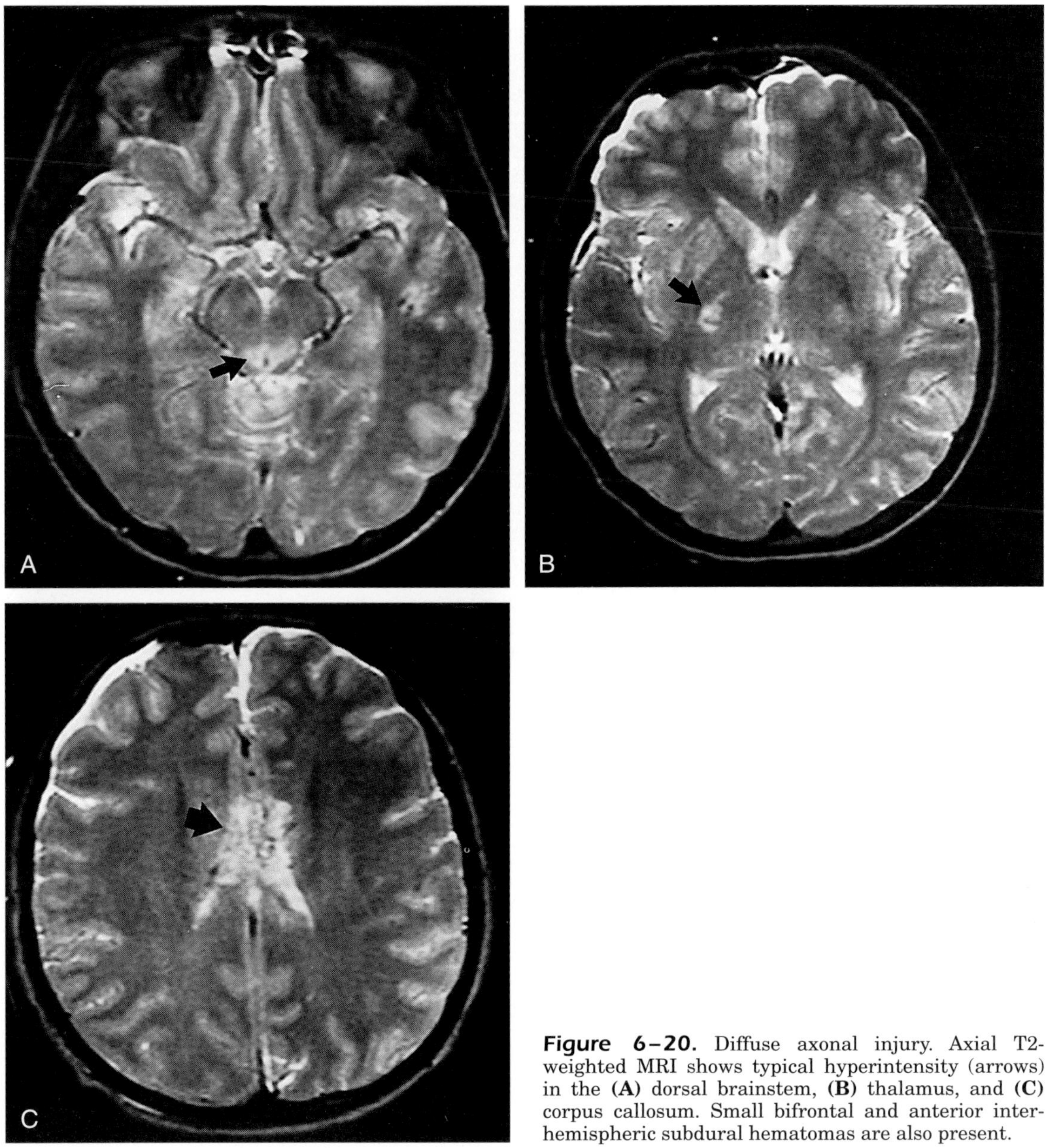

Figure 6–20. Diffuse axonal injury. Axial T2-weighted MRI shows typical hyperintensity (arrows) in the **(A)** dorsal brainstem, **(B)** thalamus, and **(C)** corpus callosum. Small bifrontal and anterior interhemispheric subdural hematomas are also present.

Post-traumatic Cerebral Edema

Post-traumatic cerebral swelling occurs via a variety of mechanisms, including primary neuronal injuries and secondary ischemia and infarction, or as a distinct clinical syndrome unrelated to other injuries. In the latter case, blunt head injury sometimes results in acute diffuse swelling of both cerebral hemispheres. This phenomenon occurs mostly in children and adolescents and may follow severe or relatively minor injuries. Post-traumatic cerebral edema is probably a misnomer when applied to this syndrome, as most studies indicate increased cerebral blood volume as the cause of brain swelling and increased pressure. If severe, however, intracranial pressure may exceed arterial perfusion pressure leading to secondary anoxic injury. Cytotoxic and vasogenic edemas then ensue with typical imaging findings of edema (see Chapter 1).

CT Findings. CT shows diminution or effacement of the ventricles and cortical sulci and compression of the basal cisterns. There is no decrease in parenchymal attenuation, as would be expected in true edema. Follow-up examinations showing return of the CSF spaces to their expected size are helpful in confirming the diagnosis, albeit retrospectively.

MRI Findings. As with CT, the brain is enlarged with sulcal, cisternal, and ventricular effacement. Studies have documented the absence of alteration in parenchymal signal intensity, specifically the absence of hyperintensity on T2-weighted images, which would be expected with true edema.

Differential Diagnosis

Pseudotumor cerebri	History of headaches not related to trauma
Isodense subarachnoid hemorrhage	Causes obliteration of cisterns Ventricles remain normal in size

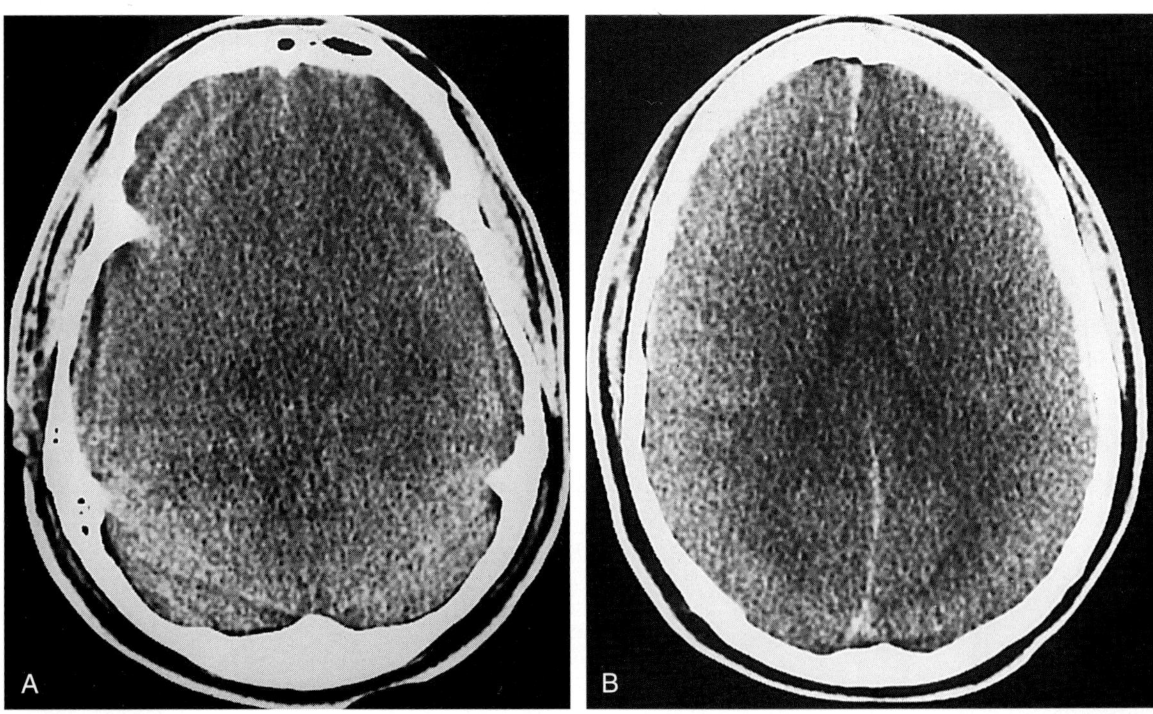

Figure 6–21. Post-traumatic cerebral edema. Axial CT shows **(A)** complete obliteration of the basal cisterns and **(B)** marked compression of the ventricles without hematoma or shift.

Battered Child Syndrome

Synonyms: Child abuse, nonaccidental trauma.

Battered child syndrome refers to a spectrum of injuries resulting from direct physical abuse usually from an adult caregiver and usually occurring over a period of time. Most injured children are less than 2 years old, and head injury is the leading cause of morbidity and mortality. Head injuries occur in about half of all cases and may result from either blows to the head or severe shaking. Cutaneous injuries (bruises, lacerations) are present in 90% of cases. Other common findings are ocular hemorrhages and long bone fractures often of varying ages and in different stages of healing.

CT Findings. All the injuries described in this chapter may be seen in the battered child. The most common injury is acute subdural hematoma, especially interhemispheric or posterior fossa. Other common findings include skull fractures, subarachnoid hemorrhages, cerebral edemas, infarcts, and parenchymal hematomas. Subdural hematomas of varying ages are a strong indication of abuse. Infarctions may develop in the cortex or basal ganglia. The reversal sign is present when the gray matter becomes distinctly lower in attenuation than the brainstem, thalami, cerebellum, and white matter. It is believed to represent extensive cortical ischemic necrosis, and the prognosis is extremely poor. CT in the chronic stage may show focal or generalized atrophy and encephalomalacia.

MRI Findings. MRI is more sensitive than CT in the demonstration of subdural hematoma, contusion, and white matter shearing injury but less sensitive for the detection of subarachnoid hemorrhage. Since the detection of any subdural hematoma is significant, MRI is the preferred modality. A strong case can be made for performing both CT and MRI in the evaluation of these patients.

Differential Diagnosis

It is essential to exclude other etiologies for intracerebral hemorrhage, including accidental injuries and bleeding disorders.

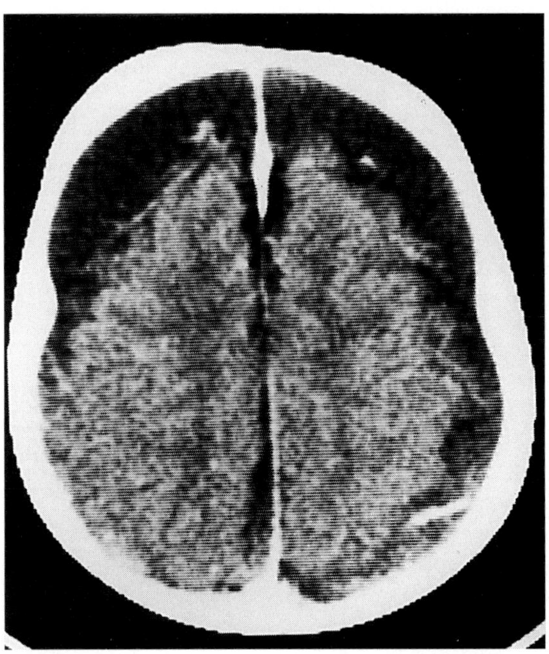

Figure 6–22. Battered child syndrome. Axial contrast-enhanced CT shows bilateral chronic subdural hematomas. Note inward displacement of enhancing cortical veins.

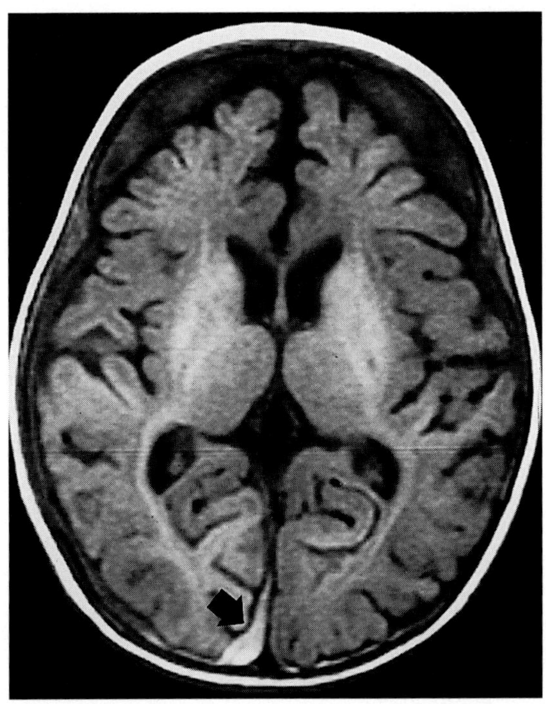

Figure 6–23. Battered child syndrome. Axial T1-weighted MRI shows bilateral chronic subdural hematomas. Note more recent SDH in the posterior interhemispheric fissure (arrow). (Courtesy of Dr. Pamela Van Tassel, Charleston, SC.)

RECOMMENDED READINGS

Depressed Skull Fracture

Hackney,DB. Skull Radiography in the Evaluation of Acute Head Trauma: A Survey of Current Practice. *Radiology* 181:711–714, 1991.

Healy,JF, Crudale,AS. Computed Tomographic Evaluation of Depressed Skull Fractures and Associated Intracranial Injury. *Comput Radiol* 6:323–330, 1982.

Leptomeningeal Cyst

Barkovich,AJ. Metabolic and Destructive Brain Disorders. In *Contemporary Neuroimaging: Volume I. Pediatric Neuroimaging.* New York: Raven Press, 1990, pp 35–76.

Eames,FA, Waldman,JB. CT of Posttraumatic Intradiploic Pseudomeningocele of the Skull Base: A Case Report. *AJNR* 12:985–987, 1991.

Numerow,LM, Krcek,JP, Wallace,CJ, Tranmer,BI, Auer,RN, Fong,TC. Growing Skull Fracture Simulating a Rounded Lytic Calvarial Lesion. *AJNR* 12:783–784, 1991.

Subarachnoid Hemorrhage

Cornelius,RS, Gaskill,MF, Lukin,RR. Traumatic Intracranial Hemorrhage. *Neuroimaging Clin N Am.* 1:433–441, 1991.

Cornell,SH, Chiu,LC, Christie,JH. Diagnosis of Extracerebral Fluid Collections by Computed Tomography. *AJR* 131: 107–110, 1978

Zimmerman,RD, Yurberg,E, Russell,EJ, Leeds,NE. Falx and Interhemispheric Fissure on Axial CT: II. Recognition and Differentiation of Interhemispheric Subarachnoid and Subdural Hemorrhage. *AJNR* 3:635–642, 1982.

Acute Epidural Hematoma

Gentry,LR, Godersky,JC, Thompson,B, Dunn,VD. Prospective Comparative Study of Intermediate-Field MR and CT in the Evaluation of Closed Head Trauma. *AJNR* 9:91–100, 1988.

Mathis,JM, Sowers,JJ, Zelenik,ME. Pathognomonic CT Findings of Posterior Fossa Epidural Hematomas. *Comput Radiol* 8:395–401, 1984.

Zimmerman,RA, Bilaniuk,LT. Computed Tomographic Staging of Traumatic Epidural Bleeding. *Radiology* 144:809–812, 1982.

Zimmerman,RA, Bilaniuk,LT, Gennarelli,T, Bruce,D, Dolinskas,C, Uzzell,B. Cranial Computed Tomography in Diagnosis and Management of Acute Head Trauma. *AJR* 131: 27–34, 1978.

Acute Subdural Hematoma

Fobben,ES, Grossman,RI, Atlas,SW, et al. MR Characteristics of Subdural Hematomas and Hygromas at 1.5 T. *AJR* 153: 589–595, 1989.

Hadley,DM, Teasdale,GM, Jenkins,A, et al. Magnetic Resonance Imaging in Acute Head Injury. *Clin Radiol* 39:131–139, 1988.

Osborn,AG, Anderson,RE, Wing,SD. The False Falx Sign. *Radiology* 134:421–425, 1980.

Zimmerman,RA, Bilaniuk,LT, Gennarelli,T, Bruce,D, Dolinskas, C, Uzzell,B. Cranial Computed Tomography in Diagnosis and Management of Acute Head Trauma. *AJR* 131: 27–34, 1978.

Chronic Subdural Hematoma

Cornell,SH, Chiu,LC, Christie,JH. Diagnosis of Extracerebral Fluid Collections by Computed Tomography. *AJR* 131: 107–110, 1978.

Fobben,ES, Grossman,RI, Atlas,SW, et al. MR Characteristics of Subdural Hematomas and Hygromas at 1.5 T. *AJR* 153: 589–595, 1989.

Karasawa,H, Tomita,S, Suzuki,S. Chronic Subdural Hematomas: Time-Density Curve and Iodine Concentration in Enhanced CT. *Neuroradiology* 29:36–39, 1987.

Subdural Hygroma

Cornell,SH, Chiu,LC, Christie,JH. Diagnosis of Extracerebral Fluid Collections by Computed Tomography. *AJR* 131: 107–110, 1978.

Fobben,ES, Grossman,RI, Atlas,SW, et al. MR Characteristics of Subdural Hematomas and Hygromas at 1.5 T. *AJR* 153: 589–595, 1989.

Cerebral Contusions

Hadley,DM, Teasdale,GM, Jenkins,A, et al. Magnetic Resonance Imaging in Acute Head Injury. *Clin Radiol* 39:131–139, 1988.

Hesselink,JR, Dowd,CF, Healy,ME, et al. MR Imaging of Brain Contusions: A Comparative Study with CT. *AJR* 150: 1133–1142, 1988.

Orrison,WW, Gentry,LR, Stimac,GK, Tarrel,RM, Espinosa,MC, Cobb,LC. Blinded Comparison of Cranial CT and MR in Closed Head Injury Evaluation. *AJNR* 14:351–356, 1994.

Zimmerman,RA, Bilaniuk,LT, Gennarelli,T, Bruce,D, Dolinskas, C, Uzzell,B. Cranial Computed Tomography in Diagnosis and Management of Acute Head Trauma. *AJR* 131:27–34, 1978.

Intracerebral Hematoma

Adams,JH. Pathology of Nonmissile Head Injury. *Neuroimaging Clin North Am* 1:397–410, 1991.

Hadley,DM, Teasdale,GM, Jenkins,A, et al. Magnetic Resonance Imaging in Acute Head Injury. *Clin Radiol* 39:131–139, 1988.

Zimmerman,RA, Bilaniuk,LT, Gennarelli,T, Bruce,D, Dolinskas, C, Uzzell,B. Cranial Computed Tomography in Diagnosis and Management of Acute Head Trauma. *AJR* 131:27–34, 1978.

Diffuse Axonal Injury

Gentry,LR. Primary Neuronal Injuries. *Neuroimaging Clin North Am* 1:411–431, 1991.

Gentry,LR, Godersky,JC, Thompson,B. MR Imaging of Head Trauma: Review of the Distribution and Radiopathologic Features of Traumatic Lesions. *AJNR* 9:101–110, 1988. *AJR* 150:663–672, 1988.

Gentry,LR, Godersky,JC, Thompson,B. Traumatic Brain Stem Injury: MR Imaging. *Radiology* 171:177–187, 1989.

Mittl,RL, Grossman,RI, Hiehle,JF, et al. Prevalence of MR Evidence of Diffuse Axonal Injury in Patients with Mild Head Injury and Normal Head CT Findings. *AJNR* 15:1583–1598, 1994.

Zimmerman,RA, Bilaniuk,LT, Gennarelli,T. Computed Tomography of Shearing Injuries of the Cerebral White Matter. *Radiology* 127:393–396, 1978.

Post-traumatic Cerebral Edema

Bruce,D, Alavi,A, Bilaniuk,L, Dolinskas,C, Obrist,W, Uzzell,B. Diffuse Cerebral Swelling Following Head Injuries in Children: The Syndrome of "Malignant Brain Edema." *J Neurosurg* 54:170–178, 1981.

Grossman,R, Atlas,S, Hackney,D, et al. MR Imaging Observations in Head Injury and Their Importance in Understanding the Pathophysiology of Head Trauma. *Radiology* 169(P):309, 1988.

Battered Child Syndrome

Cohen,RA, Kaufman,RA, Myers,PA, Towbin,RB. Cranial Computed Tomography in the Abused Child with Head Injury. *AJR* 146:97–102, 1986.

Harwood-Nash,DC. Abuse to the Pediatric Central Nervous System. *AJNR* 13:569–575, 1992.

Radkowski,MA, Merten,DF, Leonidas,JC. The Abused Child: Criteria for the Radiologic Diagnosis. *Radiographics* 3: 262–297, 1983.

Sato,Y, Smith,WL. Head Injury in Child Abuse. *Neuroimaging Clin N Am* 1:475–492, 1991.

Sato,Y, Yuh,W, Smith,W, Alexander,R, Kao,S, Ellerbroek,C. Head Injury in Child Abuse: Evaluation with MR Imaging. *Radiology* 173:653–657, 1989.

CHAPTER SEVEN

Vascular Diseases

With stroke the third leading cause of death in the United States, cerebrovascular diseases are among the most common disorders in the usual practice of neuroradiology. Stroke is a catchall term that applies to any acute neurologic syndrome of vascular etiology. The disorders described in this chapter span a wide range of pathologic categories. They are unique in that invasive angiography still performs a vital service in their diagnosis, follow-up, and, in some cases, treatment.

Congenital/Pediatric

Persistent Fetal Anastomoses

Trigeminal Artery. The trigeminal artery is the most common persistent fetal anastomosis between the internal carotid and vertebrobasilar systems. This artery arises from the internal carotid at the bend between precavernous and cavernous segments and passes posteromedially to fill the basilar artery between the superior cerebellar and anterior inferior cerebellar arteries. The posterior communicating artery is usually absent or hypoplastic. The basilar artery below the trigeminal artery is usually hypoplastic. Trigeminal arteries are associated with an increased incidence of aneurysms and arteriovenous malformations (AVMs).

Hypoglossal Artery. The hypoglossal artery is the second most common fetal carotid-vertebral anastomosis. This artery arises from the cervical internal carotid around C1, ascends through the hypoglossal canal (usually enlarged), and joins the basilar artery just at or above its origin from the vertebral artery. The vertebral arteries are usually hypoplastic.

Proatlantal Intersegmental Artery. The type 1 proatlantal artery arises from the internal carotid at C2 and anastomoses with the vertebral artery at the atlanto-occipital junction. The type 2 proatlantal artery arises from the external carotid artery and anastomoses with the vertebral artery at the C1-C2 interspace.

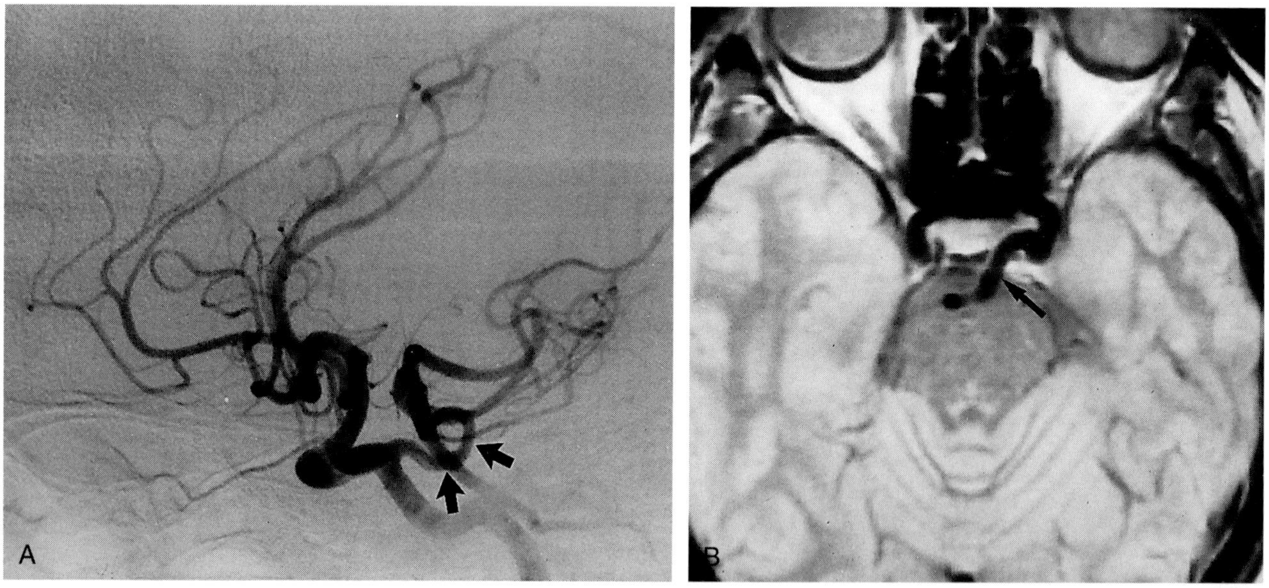

Figure 7–1. Trigeminal artery. **(A)** Lateral internal carotid angiogram shows a persistent trigeminal artery (arrows) connecting the precavernous internal carotid artery to the basilar artery. **(B)** Axial PD-weighted MRI of a different case shows a persistent trigeminal artery (arrow) connecting the left internal carotid and basilar arteries. (Figure **B** reprinted with permission from El Gammal, T, Brooks, BS. Conventional MR Neuroangiography. *AJR* 156:1075–1080, 1991.)

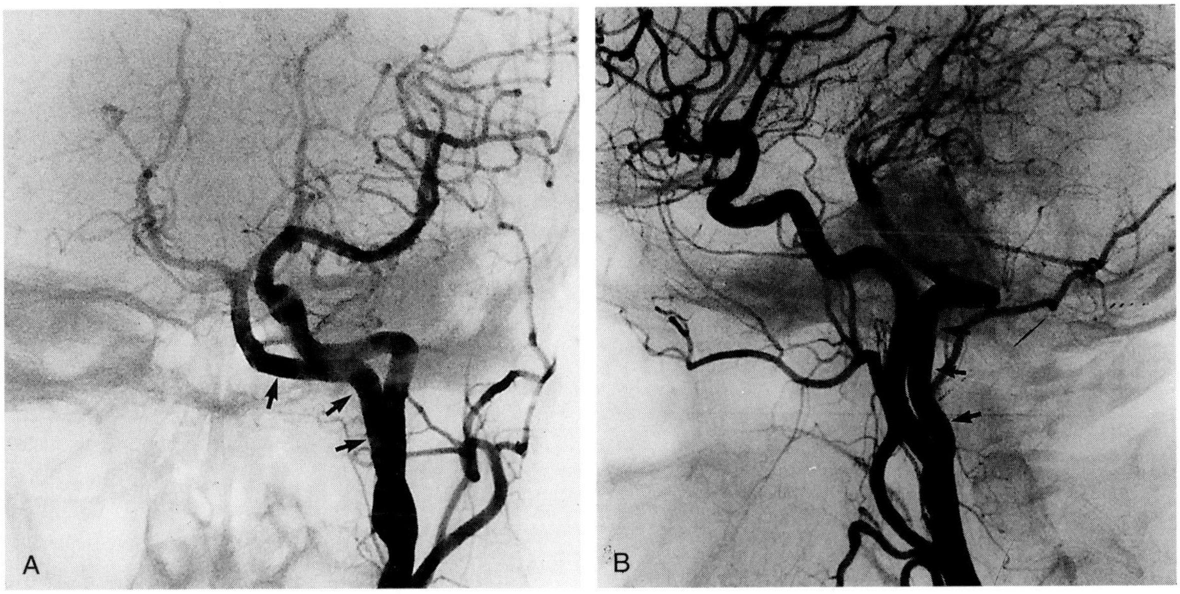

Figure 7–2. Hypoglossal artery. **(A)** AP and **(B)** lateral common carotid angiograms show a persistent hypoglossal artery (arrows) connecting the internal carotid at C1 to the basilar artery.

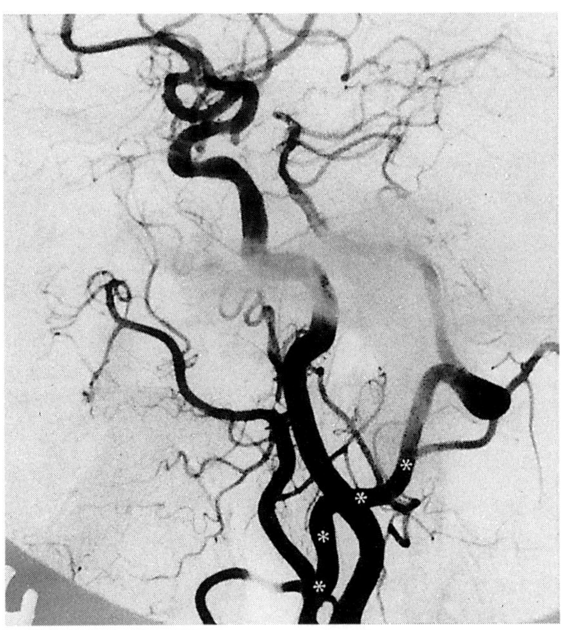

Figure 7–3. Type 2 proatlantal intersegmental artery. The vertebral artery is supplied by a direct connection (asterisks) from the external carotid artery.

Vein of Galen Malformation

Synonyms: Vein of Galen aneurysm, vein of Galen ectasia.

The vein of Galen malformation is an uncommon congenital vascular malformation characterized by a midline arteriovenous shunt and posterior deep venous drainage. Recognized types include (1) a single or multiple direct arteriovenous fistulas to a dilated draining vein, (2) a thalamic AVM draining into the midline venous varix, and (3) a combination of an arteriovenous fistula and AVM. The reference to the vein of Galen is an anatomic misnomer, as the enlarged draining vein is usually not the vein of Galen but a persistent fetal median vein of the prosencephalon. The classic clinical presentation is an infant with hydrocephalus and high output congestive heart failure, although less severe cases may present in childhood or later.

Sonographic, CT, and MRI Findings. The essential finding is the presence of a large vascular mass in the pineal region (vein of Galen aneurysm). Its vascular nature is established on ultrasound by the use of Doppler, on CT by intense contrast enhancement, and on MRI by the striking flow void. This dilated vein may produce mass effect upon the posterior third ventricle. Enlarged feeding arteries and enlarged draining deep venous sinuses may be seen on CT or MRI. An AVM nidus is seen in the thalamus in about 50% of cases. Hydrocephalus is present in about 70%. Parenchymal calcifications are infrequently encountered. Subarachnoid or intracerebral hemorrhage occasionally occurs in older age groups.

Angiographic Findings. Angiography reveals marked dilatation of the feeding arteries and draining veins with rapid arteriovenous shunting. The shunting tends to be more rapid and severe with fistulas than with AVMs. Focal severe aneurysmal dilatation of the draining veins is usually present and is sometimes present in feeding arteries. With direct fistulas, the dominant arterial supply is usually from posterior choroidal arteries. AVMs are usually supplied by enlarged thalamoperforators. Anomalies of venous drainage are common and include focal stenoses of the draining veins, absence of the straight sinus, and persistence of the fetal venous channels, especially the falcine sinus.

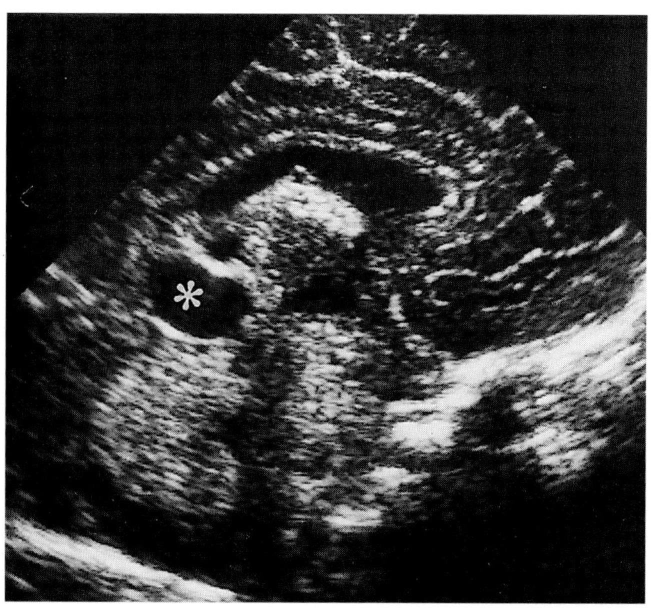

Figure 7–4. Vein of Galen malformation. Sagittal sonogram shows an anechoic mass (asterisk) posterior to the thalamus and third ventricle. Doppler analysis showed rapid flow.

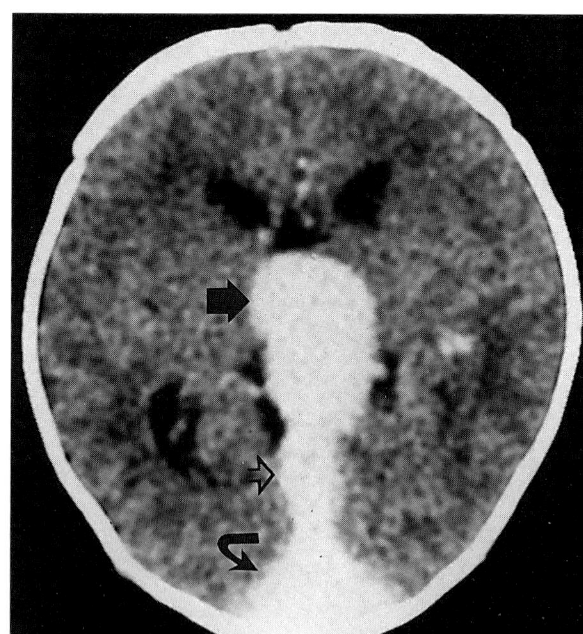

Figure 7–5. Vein of Galen malformation. Axial contrast-enhanced CT shows intense enhancement of a massive midline varix (large arrow) draining via a falcine sinus (open arrow) to the torcular (curved arrow).

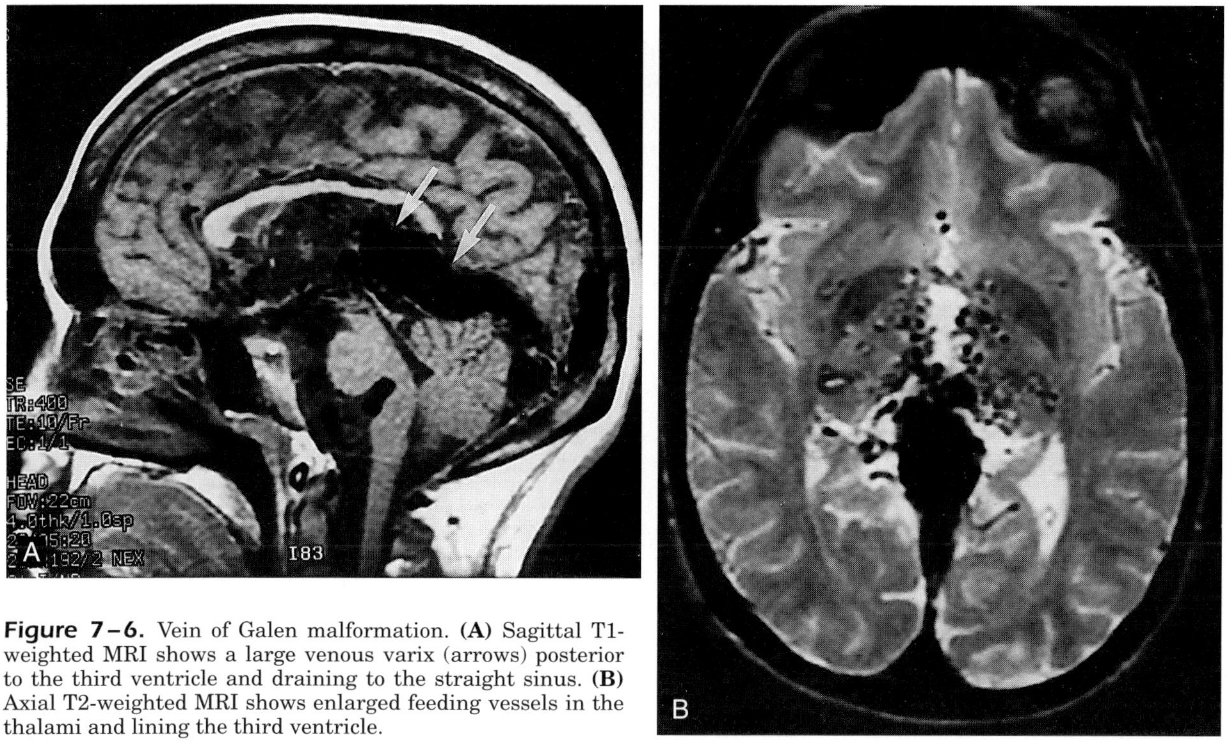

Figure 7–6. Vein of Galen malformation. **(A)** Sagittal T1-weighted MRI shows a large venous varix (arrows) posterior to the third ventricle and draining to the straight sinus. **(B)** Axial T2-weighted MRI shows enlarged feeding vessels in the thalami and lining the third ventricle.

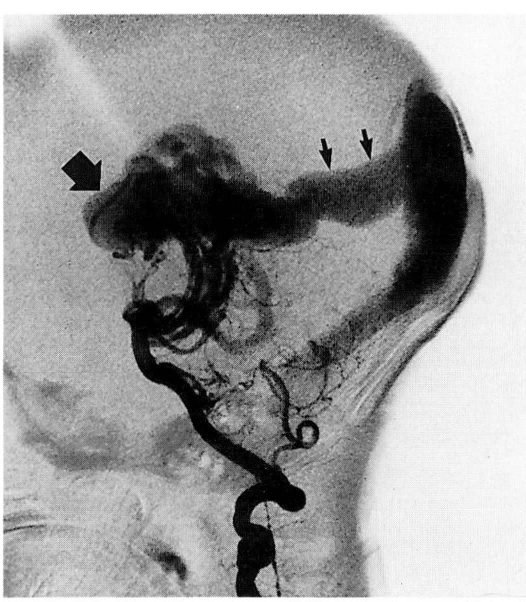

Figure 7–7. Vein of Galen malformation. Lateral vertebral angiogram shows enlarged choroidal arteries feeding a fistula to the median vein of the prosencephalon (large arrow). Drainage occurs via a falcine sinus (small arrows) to the enlarged sagittal sinus. The straight sinus is absent.

Neonatal Intracerebral Hemorrhage

Spontaneous germinal matrix hemorrhage is a common event among premature infants and the leading cause of neurologic morbidity and mortality. This type of hemorrhage occurs in up to 50% of infants of 28 weeks or less of gestation, declines rapidly with increasing gestational age, and is extremely rare among term infants. The survival rate ranges from excellent with a grade 1 hemorrhage (Table 7–1) to 90% mortality with grade 4, along with a similarly wide spectrum of neurologic sequelae.

The germinal matrix in the premature infant is still quite prominent and contains a rich network of fragile vessels. Independent risk factors that have been associated with hemorrhage include hypoxia, hyaline membrane disease, pneumothorax, patent ductus arteriosus, and acidosis. Other forms of primary intracranial hemorrhage are summarized in Table 7–2.

Sonographic Findings. Acute clot is highly echogenic. In grade 1 hemorrhage, increased echogenicity is present in the region of the caudate head or caudothalamic groove. Intraventricular clot (grade 2) forms an echogenic mass that must be distinguished from the normal choroid plexus. The distinction of the normal choroid plexus, choroid plexus hemorrhage, and intraventricular hemorrhage can be quite difficult because of the wide range of appearances of the normal choroid plexus, which may appear quite bulky (Table 7–3). In grade 3 hemorrhage, hydrocephalus is present with the ventricles distended by either CSF or blood. In grade 4, blood extends into the frontoparietal white matter or basal ganglia.

Regardless of location, the clot eventually decreases in echogenicity beginning centrally, leading to an anechoic mass with an echogenic rim. All of the clot resorbs within 1 to 2 months in grades 1 and 2. Late findings of intraventricular hemorrhage may include subependymal gliosis (echogenic ventricular lining) and hydrocephalus. Intraparenchymal hemorrhage will usually result in porencephalic cysts, ventricular dilatation, and/or atrophy.

CT Findings. All of the findings described for sonography also apply to CT. Because of its ease of use, ultrasound is always the screening procedure of choice. CT is superior in distinguishing an intraventricular clot from the choroid plexus and is much more sensitive in the detection of subarachnoid and subdural hemorrhage.

TABLE 7–1 Classification of Neonatal Germinal Matrix Hemorrhage

Grade	Criteria
Grade 1	Hemorrhage limited to germinal matrix or choroid plexus
Grade 2	Hemorrhage into lateral ventricle
Grade 3	Ventricular hemorrhage and ventricular dilatation or hydrocephalus
Grade 4	Germinal matrix and intraventricular hemorrhage with intraparenchymal hemorrhage, especially into periventricular white matter

TABLE 7–2 Other Types of Primary Hemorrhage in the Neonate

Type	Comments
Choroid plexus hemorrhage	Usually term infants Good prognosis
Cerebellar hemorrhage	From germinal matrix of fourth ventricle Grim prognosis
Hemorrhagic periventricular leukomalacia	May account for a high proportion of parenchymal hemorrhage in premature infants Hard to distinguish from nonhemorrhagic PVL with ultrasound alone
Subarachnoid hemorrhage	Lumbar puncture most sensitive diagnostic procedure, followed by CT Clinical significance uncertain Excellent prognosis
Subdural hematoma	Usually related to birth trauma CT is diagnostic procedure of choice

TABLE 7–3 Choroid Plexus Versus Intraventricular Clot

Choroid Plexus	Intraventricular Clot
May extend short distance into occipital horns	May be seen in posterior occipital horns
Stationary	May change with position
Clear CSF	May see blood-CSF level
Smooth crescent shape	Bulky and irregular
Isodense to brain on CT	Bright on CT

Differential Diagnosis

See Tables 7–1 to 7–3.

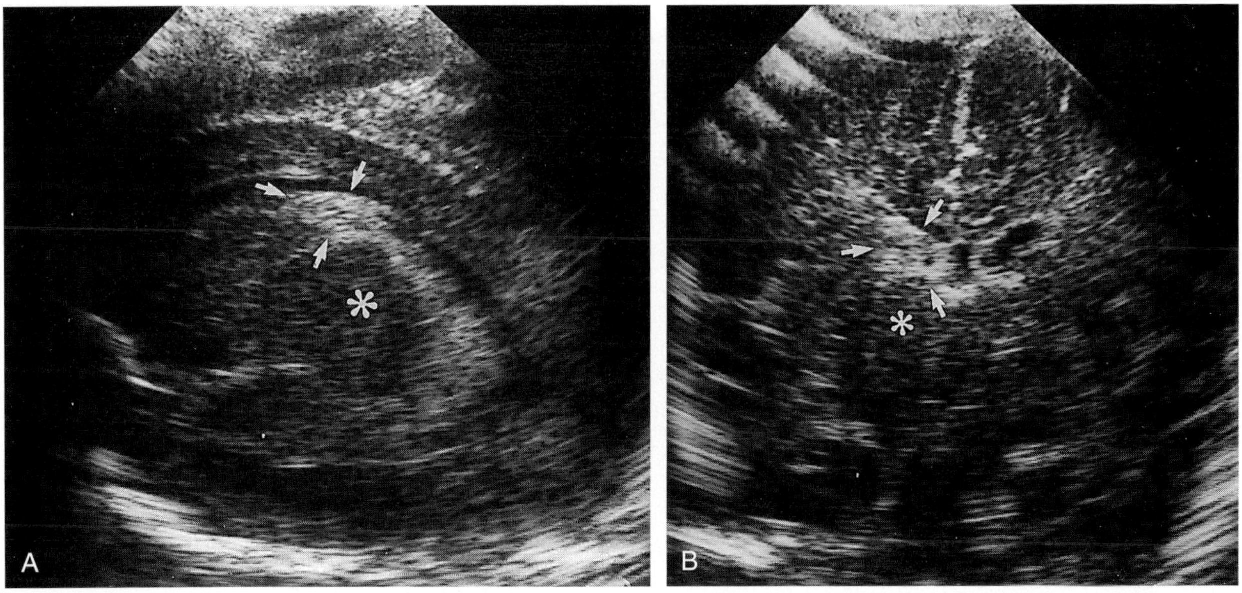

Figure 7–8. Grade 1 ICH. **(A)** Parasagittal and **(B)** coronal sonograms show an area of increased echogenicity (arrows) in the caudothalamic groove. Asterisk indicates the thalamus.

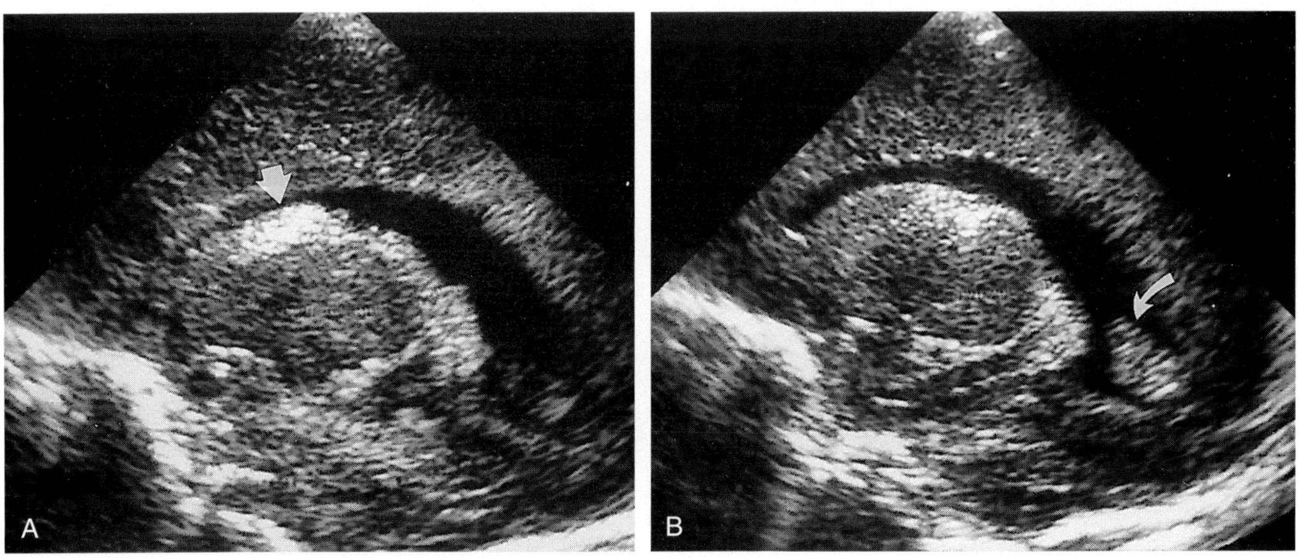

Figure 7–9. Grade 2 ICH. Parasagittal sonograms show **(A)** a hematoma (arrow) in the caudate head and **(B)** intraventricular clot (curved arrow) in the occipital horn of the lateral ventricle.

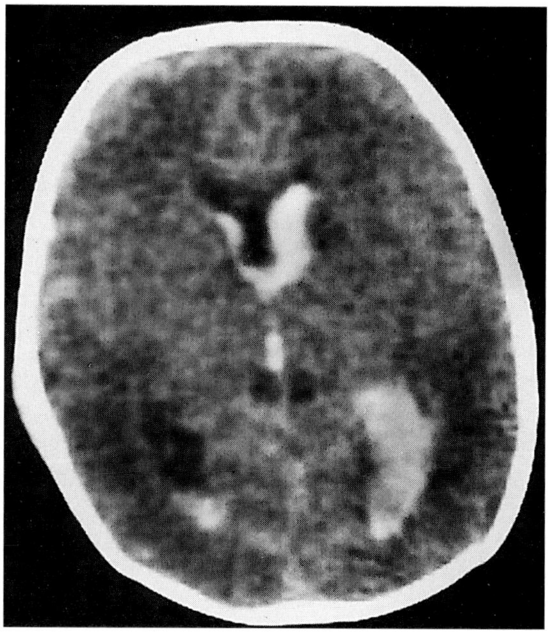

Figure 7–10. Grade 2 ICH. Axial CT shows blood in the third ventricle and both lateral ventricles without dilatation.

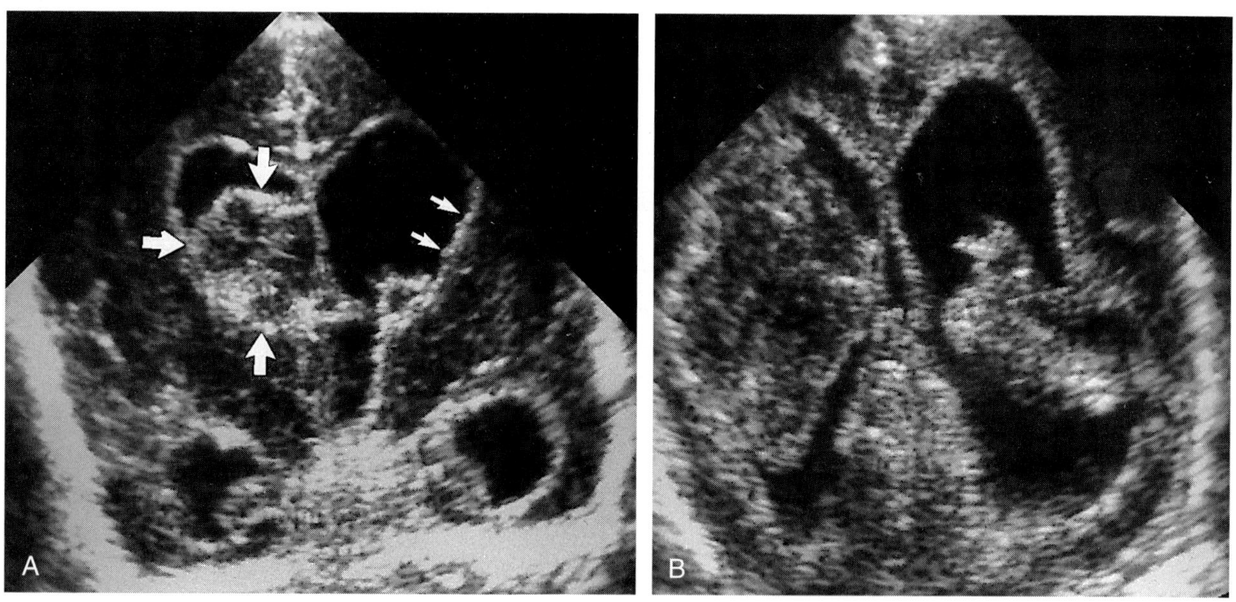

Figure 7–11. Grade 3 ICH (subacute). **(A)** Coronal sonogram shows a large hematoma (large arrows) of the caudate extending in the lateral ventricle with marked hydrocephalus. Increased echogenicity of the ependyma (small arrows) represents gliosis. **(B)** Semi-axial sonogram through lateral ventricles shows large bilateral intraventricular clots.

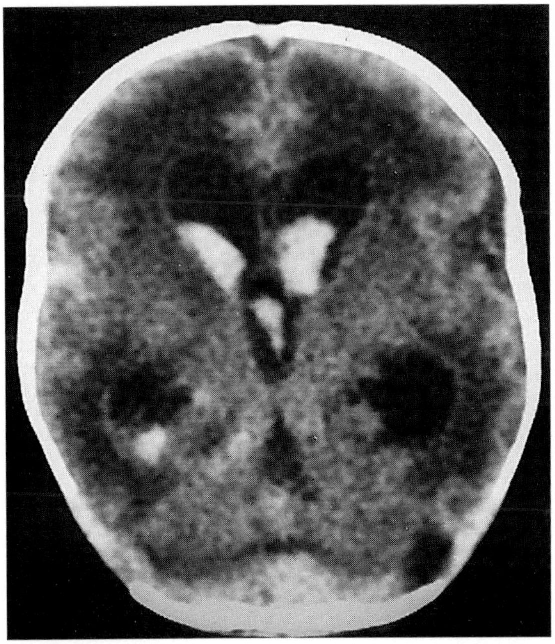

Figure 7–12. Grade 3 ICH. Axial CT shows clot in the third ventricle and both lateral ventricles with hydrocephalus.

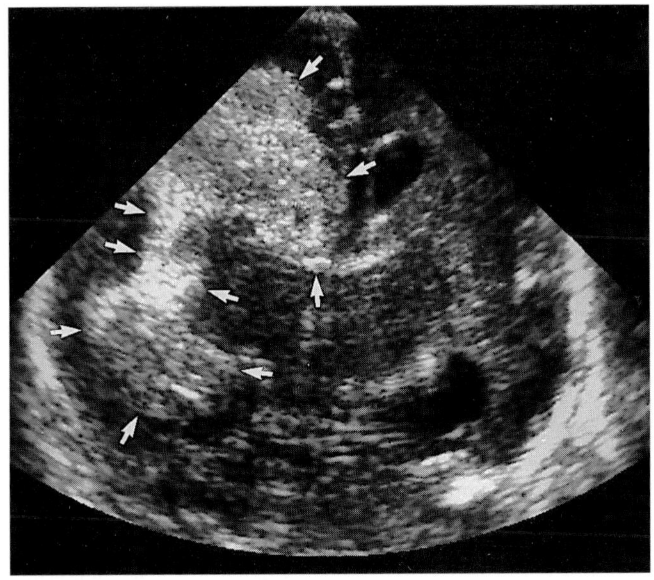

Figure 7–13. Grade 4 ICH. Coronal sonogram shows a large hematoma (arrows) extending into the frontal white matter, lateral basal ganglia, and temporal lobe.

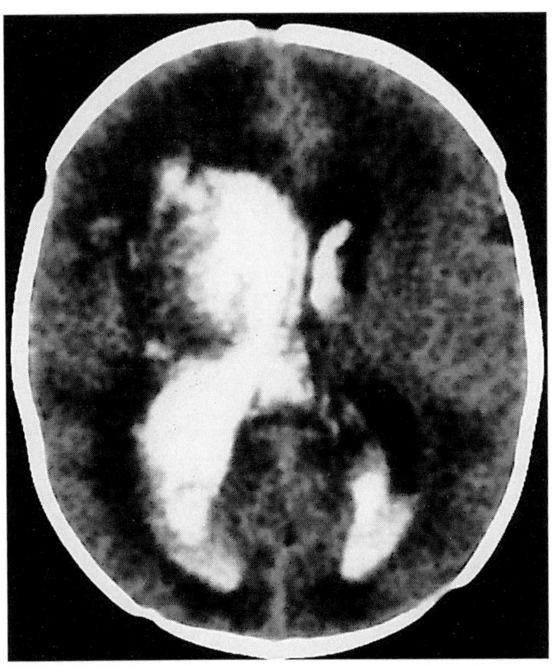

Figure 7–14. Grade 4 ICH. Axial CT shows massive intraventricular hemorrhage with extension into the periventricular white matter of the right hemisphere.

Periventricular Leukomalacia

Periventricular leukomalacia (PVL) is a complication of hypoxia in the premature infant and is characterized by ischemic necrosis of the cerebral white matter. It most commonly affects the white matter adjacent to the trigones of the lateral ventricles followed by the frontal white matter near the foramen of Monro. This condition results in both high mortality and significant neurologic morbidity, particularly spastic diplegia and intellectual deficits. The various forms of anoxic injury to the newborn brain are summarized in Table 7–4.

Sonographic Findings

Up to Two Weeks. Sonography reveals increased echogenicity of the white matter at the angles of lateral ventricles, especially adjacent to the trigones and frontal horns. This must be distinguished from a mild hyperechogenicity found in the peritrigonal white matter, which is normal. Bilateral involvement is usual. Superimposed white matter hemorrhage is common pathologically and on CT, but hemorrhagic and nonhemorrhagic PVL cannot be accurately distinguished by ultrasound.

More Than Two Weeks. The echogenicity of the involved areas begins to diminish. Cysts begin to develop in the white matter and range in diameter from microscopic to 1 cm. The cysts may later coalesce into larger cysts or become incorporated into the lateral ventricle, forming a pseudoventricle or ventriculomegaly. Smaller cysts typically disappear after a few months.

CT Findings. The white matter of premature infants contains little myelin and is normally of very low attenuation, approaching that of water. Since the early lesions of PVL are characterized by necrosis and edema, CT manifests diminished white matter attenuation that may be quite difficult to distinguish from the normal appearance. Hemorrhage, however, is much more readily apparent on CT than ultrasound. Following the onset of gross cavitation, cysts are more easily recognized in the white matter. In late stages, the dominant CT finding is atrophy with enlargement of the ventricles and sulci.

MRI Findings. In the early stages of PVL, MRI reveals focal, sharply defined areas of hypointensity in the white matter on T1-weighted images. Atrophy, ventricular dilatation, and delayed myelination (corrected for gestational age) are also commonly present.

In late PVL, MRI reveals thinning and abnormal hyperintensity of the white matter on T2-weighted images with focal dilatation of the adjacent lateral ventricle most pronounced in the vicinity of the trigones. This appearance typically persists into adulthood.

Differential Diagnosis

Nonhemorrhagic PVL must be distinguished from thromboembolic cerebral infarction, whereas hemorrhagic PVL may resemble other forms of primary hemorrhage in the neonate. (See Table 7–4.)

TABLE 7–4 | Hypoxic-Ischemic Encephalopathy in the Neonate

Pathology	Sonography	Comments
Major vessel infarcts	Focally increased parenchymal echogenicity Late cyst formation	Middle cerebral artery distribution most common
Periventricular hemorrhagic infarction	Same as grade 4 intraventricular hemorrhage	Spastic hemiparesis
Global ischemia (multicystic encephalomalacia)	Diffusely increased parenchymal echogenicity Late cyst formation	History of severe anoxia Term infants
White matter ischemia (PVL)	Increased echogenicity of periventricular white matter Late cyst formation	Prematurity Spastic diplegia

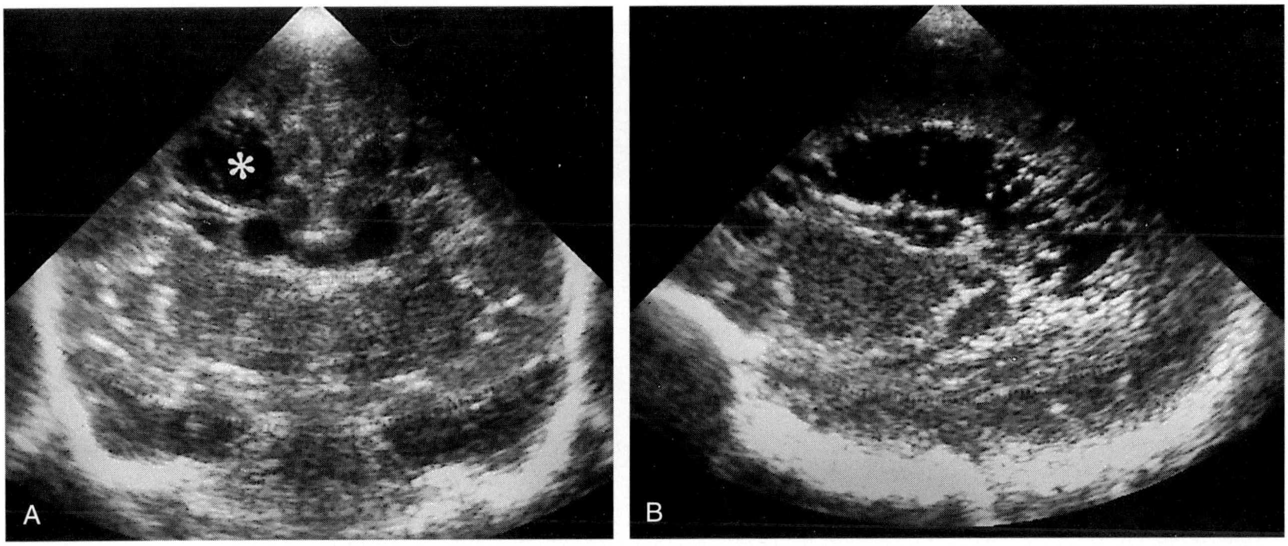

Figure 7–15. Periventricular leukomalacia. **(A)** Coronal sonogram shows a large anechoic region (asterisk) in the periventricular white matter. **(B)** Parasagittal sonogram lateral to lateral ventricle shows extensive multicystic changes in frontal and parietal white matter. The cysts were in continuity with dilated lateral ventricles.

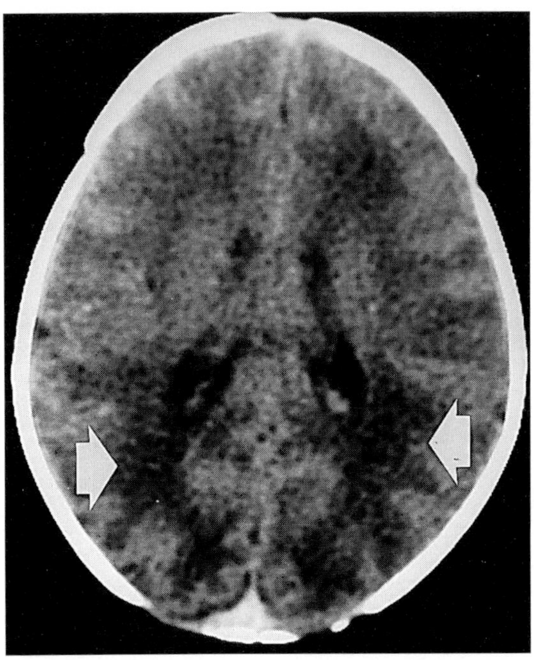

Figure 7–16. Periventricular leukomalacia. CT shows markedly diminished attenuation of the parietal white matter bilaterally (arrows) relative to the frontal white matter. The hypodense regions were hyperechoic on sonography. (Estimated gestational age is 34 weeks.)

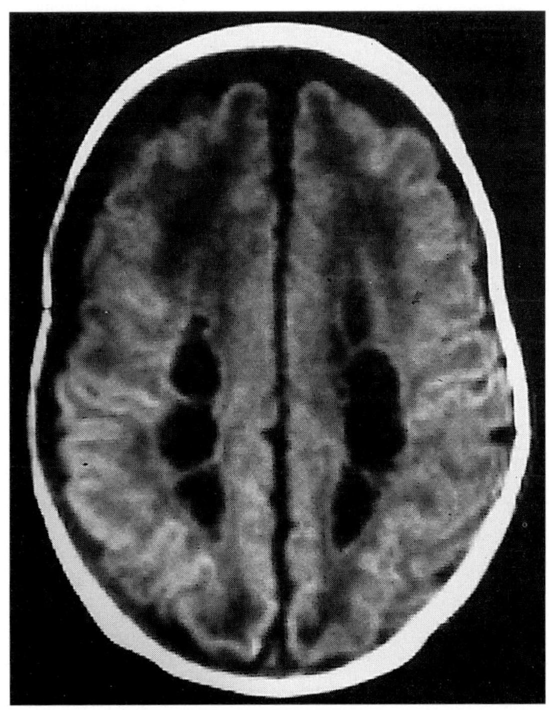

Figure 7–17. Periventricular leukomalacia. Axial T1-weighted MRI shows cystic changes of the parietal white matter bilaterally. (Courtesy of Dr. Yoginder Vaid, Birmingham, AL.)

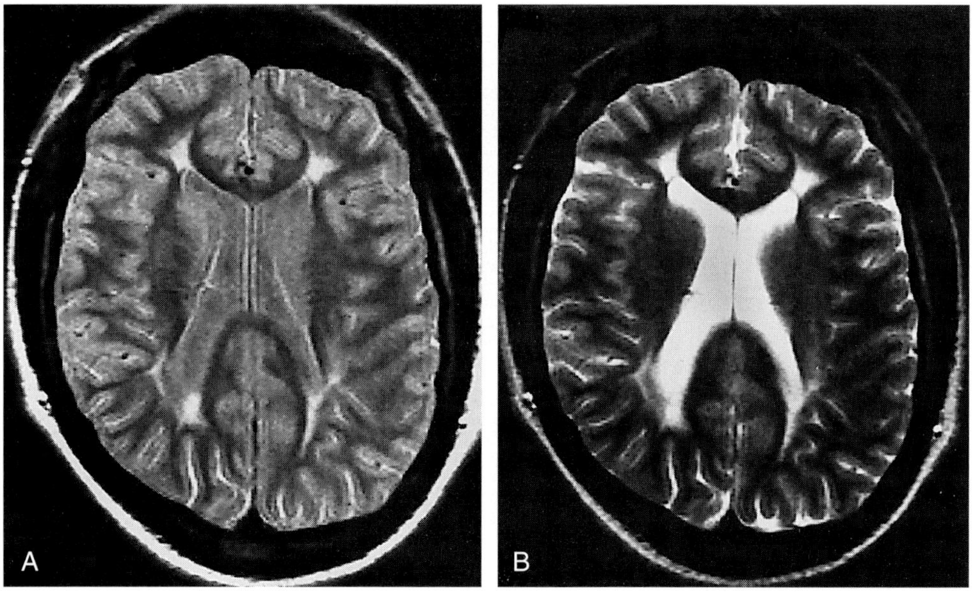

Figure 7–18. Late periventricular leukomalacia. **(A)** Axial PD-weighted and **(B)** T2-weighted MRI in an adult show abnormal white matter hyperintensity confined to the white matter adjacent to the frontal horns and trigones of the lateral ventricles.

Vascular Malformations

Arteriovenous Malformation

An AVM is a vascular anomaly characterized by a network of abnormal thick-walled vessels with direct connections to feeding arteries and draining veins bypassing an intervening capillary bed. As a result, there is arteriovenous shunting with rapid flow and enlargement of both afferent and efferent vessels (Table 7–5).

AVMs usually present in early adulthood, with 64% diagnosed in persons less than 40 years old. AVMs are most common in the cerebral hemispheres but may occur anywhere. Patients may present with seizures, ischemic symptoms, or hemorrhages. Spontaneous hemorrhage may be either subarachnoid or parenchymal and ranges in severity from minor to massive and fatal.

CT Findings. CT shows a mass of mixed attenuation, often with globular calcifications. Surrounding gliosis or atrophy is common. Secondary hemorrhage may be present and intraventricular, parenchymal, or subarachnoid, in order of decreasing frequency. Following intravenous contrast, there is homogeneous central enhancement with irregular margins (the individual vessels within the nidus cannot be resolved, as with MRI) as well as enhancement of enlarged feeding arteries and draining veins. Thrombosed AVMs appear as a hyperdense mass with little or no contrast enhancement. They are usually peripheral and often lobulated in contour.

MRI Findings. Findings directly related to the AVM include enlarged cerebral arteries feeding the AVM, a cluster of signal voids representing the nidus, and enlarged draining veins. Secondary findings may consist of gliosis or encephalomalacia from prior hemorrhage or ischemia and areas of hypointensity caused by hemosiderin from old hemorrhage.

Angiographic Findings. The angiographic findings in unthrombosed AVMs are diagnostic. The essential finding is a cluster (nidus) of enlarged terminal arteries with arteriovenous shunting. Usually there is gross enlargement of both feeding arteries and draining veins. Ancillary findings may include aneurysms of the feeder arteries, aneurysms within the nidus, venous strictures, and venous varices.

The following angiographic findings are associated with an increased risk of hemorrhage:

- Deep or periventricular location
- Intranidal aneurysm
- Central venous drainage

Differential Diagnosis

See Table 7–5.

TABLE 7–5 | Classification of Intracranial Vascular Malformations

	Relative Frequency*	Pathology	Clinical
Venous angioma	65%	Anomalous venous drainage	Usually silent and rarely causes seizures or hemorrhage
Cavernous hemangioma	10%	Enlarged cavernous postcapillary spaces without intervening brain substance	Occasionally hemorrhage
Arteriovenous malformation	25%	Arteriovenous shunting without intervening capillaries	Often hemorrhage or causes ischemic steal phenomena and seizures
Capillary telangiectasia	?	Enlarged capillary spaces with intervening brain tissue	Rarely produces symptoms

*Estimates of prevalence are derived from the literature and should reflect the relative frequency with which these entities are encountered in an unselected population of MRI patients.

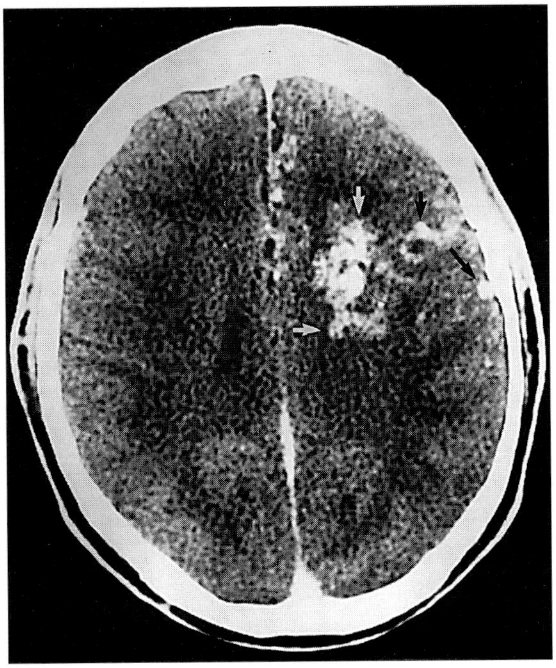

Figure 7–19. Arteriovenous malformation. Axial contrast-enhanced CT shows enhancement of irregular and curvilinear structures (short arrows) in the left frontal lobe with an enlarged cortical vein (long arrow).

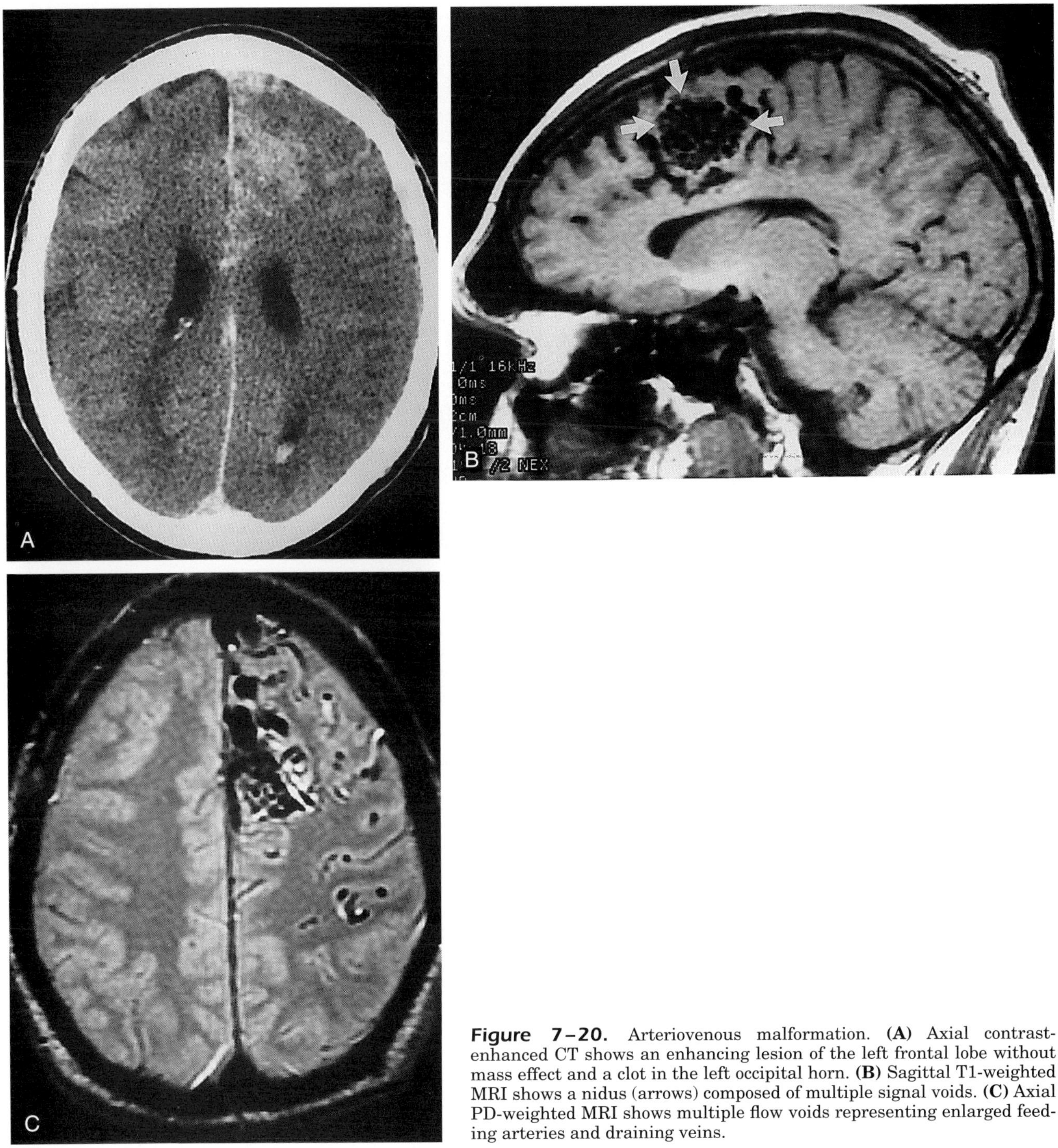

Figure 7–20. Arteriovenous malformation. **(A)** Axial contrast-enhanced CT shows an enhancing lesion of the left frontal lobe without mass effect and a clot in the left occipital horn. **(B)** Sagittal T1-weighted MRI shows a nidus (arrows) composed of multiple signal voids. **(C)** Axial PD-weighted MRI shows multiple flow voids representing enlarged feeding arteries and draining veins.

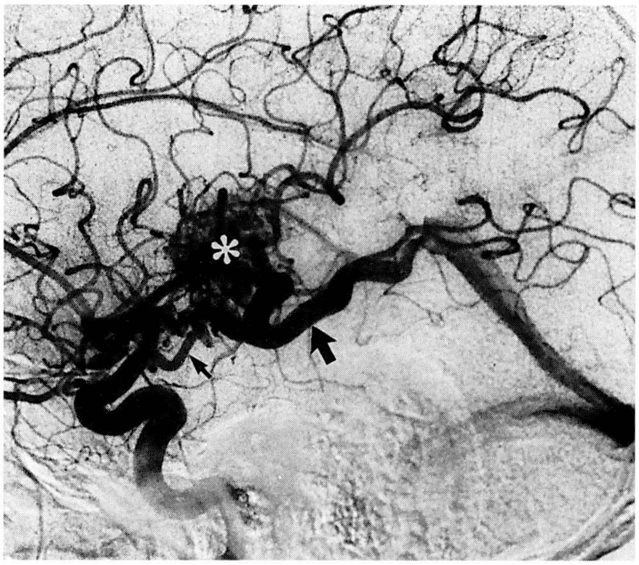

Figure 7–21. Arteriovenous malformation. Lateral internal carotid angiogram shows the three essentials of an AVM: enlarged feeding arteries (small arrow), nidus (asterisk), and early venous drainage (large arrow). The nidus is in the thalamus, supplied by thalamoperforators and draining via the basal vein of Rosenthal to the straight sinus.

Cavernous Hemangioma

Synonyms: Cavernoma, occult vascular malformation.

The cavernous hemangioma contains a compact network of dilated vascular spaces resembling veins with little or no intervening neural parenchyma. There is no arteriovenous shunting and very slow flow. It is seldom demonstrated angiographically, hence the term occult vascular malformation. An accumulation of hemosiderin-laden macrophages in the periphery is usually present and has been attributed to diapedesis of red blood cells. Acute hemorrhage is infrequent but may be catastrophic if the malformation is in a critical area such as the brainstem.

A seizure disorder is the most common clinical manifestation, although many are asymptomatic and discovered incidentally on MRI. Multiple lesions are common, occurring in up to one third of patients.

CT Findings. CT shows a small hyperdense mass with mild contrast enhancement. Calcifications are common. Cavernomas are usually supratentorial and often multiple. Hemorrhage is infrequent.

MRI Findings. MRI shows a well-demarcated mass with central mottled hyperintensity on both T1- and T2-weighted images. A prominent hypointense rim due to hemosiderin is seen on T2-weighted images. Mild central enhancement is usually observed after intravenous contrast.

Angiographic Findings. Angiography is usually normal. With larger lesions, secondary signs of mass effect may be observed. Visible staining of the malformation is quite rare.

Differential Diagnosis

Cavernomas may be mimicked by hemorrhagic tumors (especially metastases), thrombosed AVMs, and subacute or chronic primary hemorrhage. The primary differential consideration in the usual case would be other vascular malformations. However, the point is academic since the clinical course and treatment are similar for true cavernomas and angiographically occult AVMs.

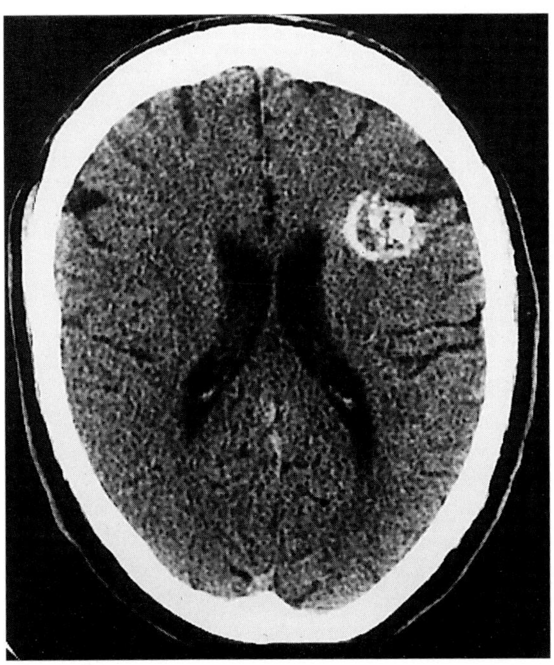

Figure 7–22. Cavernous hemangioma. Axial unenhanced CT shows a small mass in the left frontal lobe with central speckled calcifications and partial rim calcification.

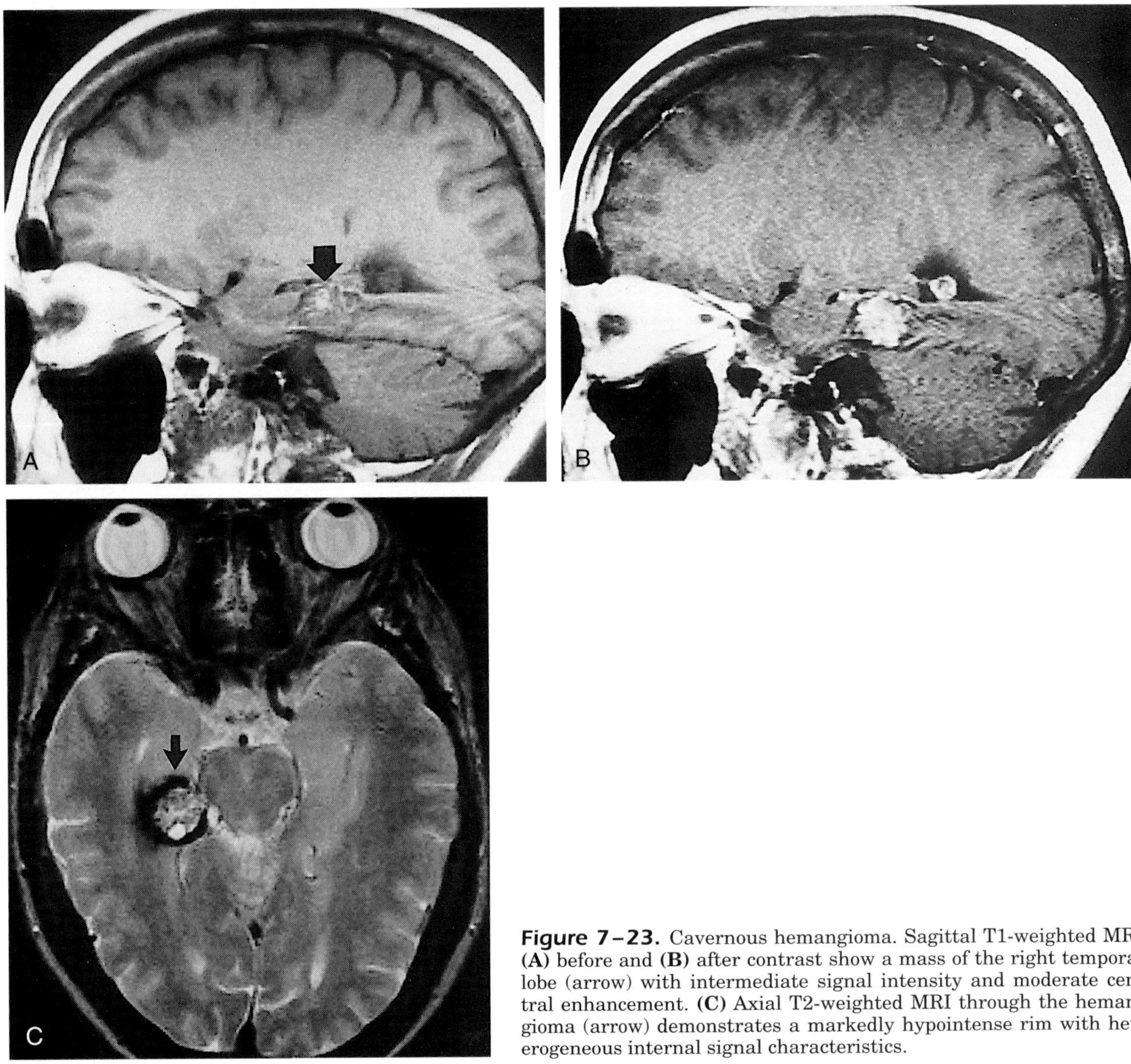

Figure 7–23. Cavernous hemangioma. Sagittal T1-weighted MRI **(A)** before and **(B)** after contrast show a mass of the right temporal lobe (arrow) with intermediate signal intensity and moderate central enhancement. **(C)** Axial T2-weighted MRI through the hemangioma (arrow) demonstrates a markedly hypointense rim with heterogeneous internal signal characteristics.

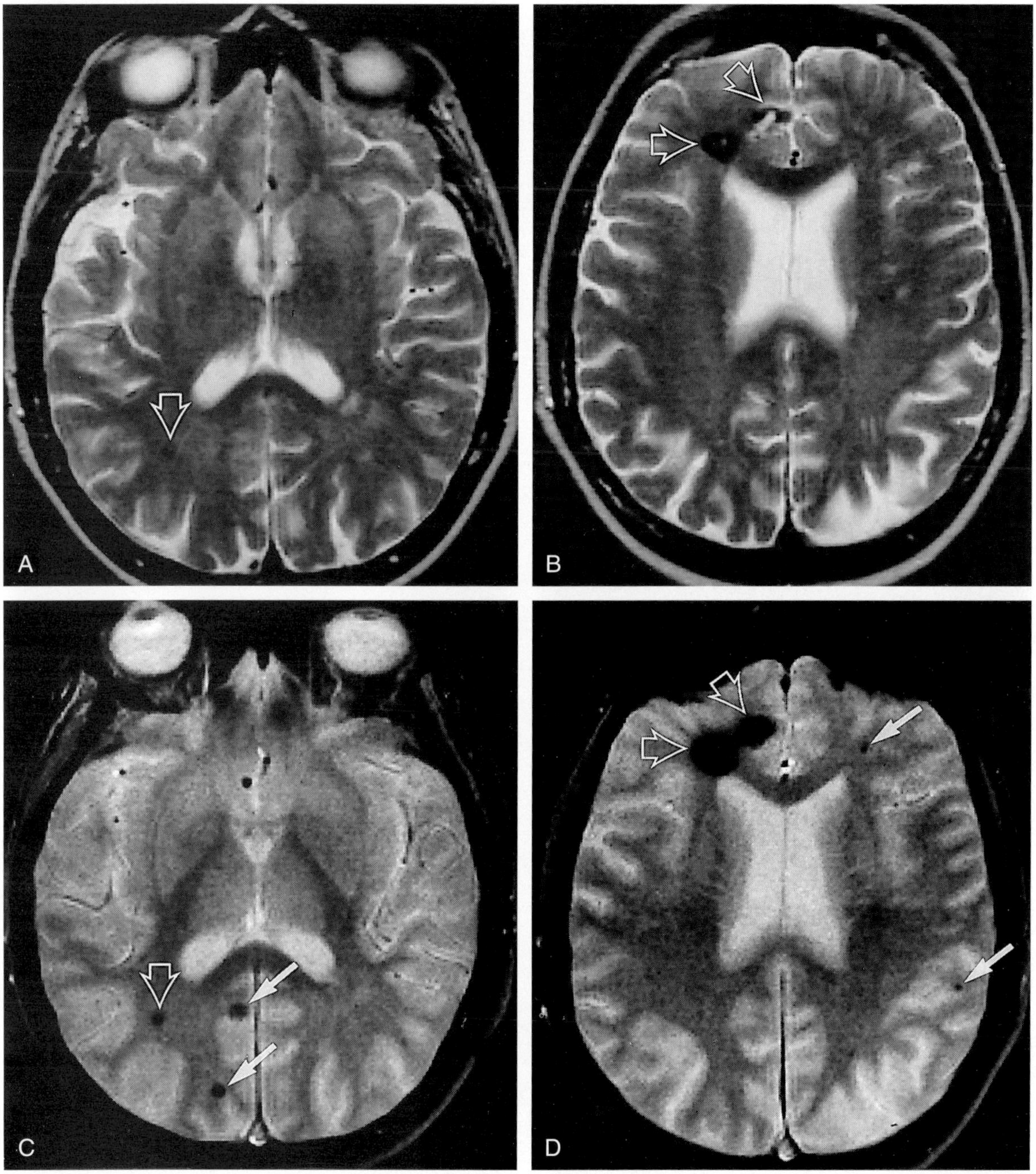

Figure 7–24. Multiple cavernomas. **(A,B)** Axial fast spin echo (FSE) and **(C,D)** gradient echo (GE) technique show multiple cavernomas (open arrows). Because GE techniques are more sensitive to magnetic susceptibility effects, more lesions appear on the GE sequence (solid arrows), and those seen on the FSE scan appear larger (blossoming effect).

Venous Angioma

A venous angioma is a malformation composed of a loose network of medullary veins with intervening neural tissue, which converges into a single large draining vein. Arteriovenous shunting is not present. Venous angiomas are common incidental findings on MRI. Hemorrhage is very rare.

CT Findings. Contrast-enhanced CT shows an enhancing tubular structure leading toward the pial surface. The tubular structure may be round or linear depending on the plane of section. Most venous angiomas are supratentorial. Mild enhancement may also be seen related to the converging venous network (tuft).

MRI Findings. Unenhanced MRI typically shows a curvilinear hypointense structure coursing through the brain substance toward the pial surface. Depending on the pulse sequence, flow velocity, size, and section plane, the actual signal intensity of the draining vein may be quite variable. After intravenous contrast, there is nearly consistent demonstration of an umbrella-shaped tuft of medullary veins supplying a single enlarged enhancing vein that usually drains toward the pial surface. Associated hemorrhage is rarely noted but may occur. Most venous angiomas cannot be seen on MR angiography.

Angiographic Findings. The essential angiographic findings consist of the following:

1. Converging dilated medullary veins that may fill during the early, middle, or late venous phase.
2. A single large draining vein coursing through the brain parenchyma toward a dural sinus, superficial cortical vein, or occasionally subependymal ventricular vein.
3. Diminished or absent normal venous drainage in the region of the abnormality.

Differential Diagnosis

The angiographic appearance is pathognomonic, and the enhanced CT and MRI nearly so.

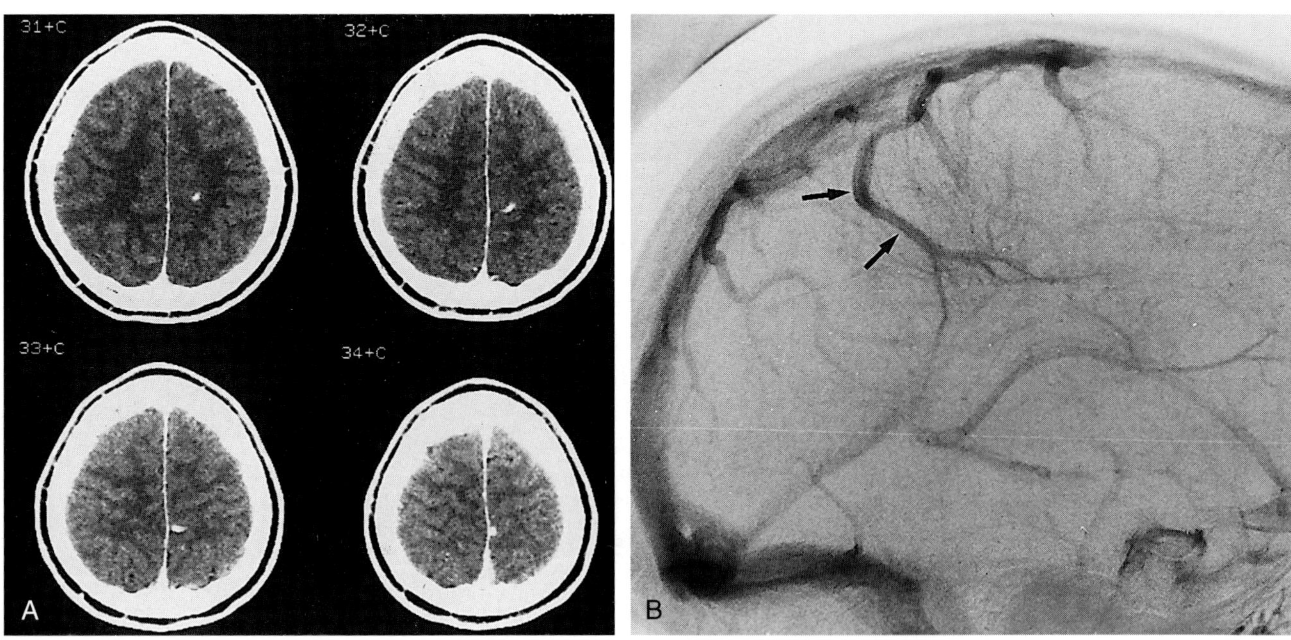

Figure 7–25. Venous angioma. **(A)** Axial contrast-enhanced CT through serial ascending levels shows a linear enhancing structure in the left parietal lobe coursing to the sagittal sinus. **(B)** Late venous phase of internal carotid angiogram shows a venous angioma draining (arrows) to the sagittal sinus.

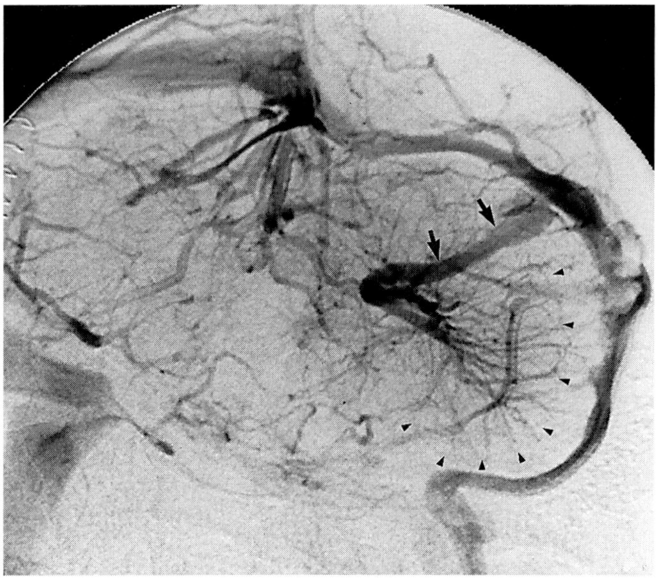

Figure 7–26. Venous angioma. AP projection of vertebral angiogram (venous phase) shows a large left cerebellar venous angioma composed of a radiating tuft (arrowheads) and a large central draining vein (arrows) that empties into the left transverse sinus.

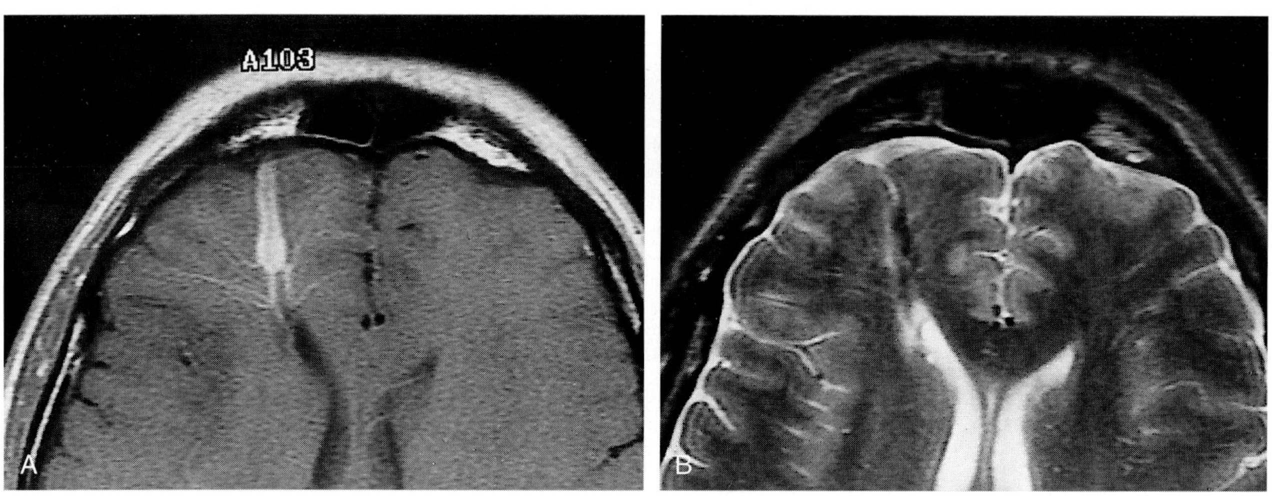

Figure 7–27. Venous angioma. **(A)** Axial contrast-enhanced T1-weighted MRI shows a tuft of converging enhanced medullary veins with large vein draining anteriorly toward the pial surface. **(B)** On T2-weighted MRI the draining vein exhibits mixed signal due to the slow flow.

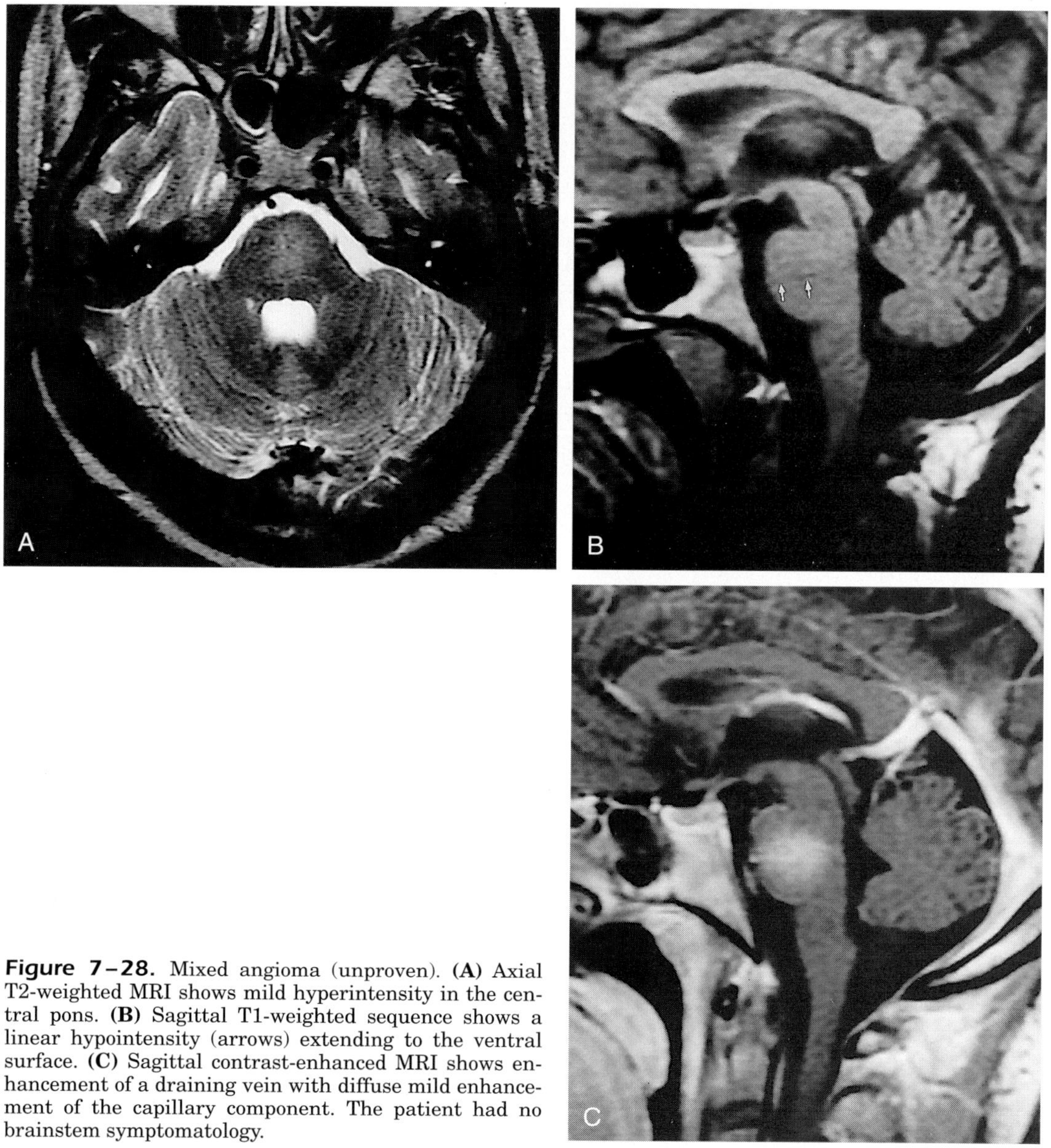

Figure 7–28. Mixed angioma (unproven). **(A)** Axial T2-weighted MRI shows mild hyperintensity in the central pons. **(B)** Sagittal T1-weighted sequence shows a linear hypointensity (arrows) extending to the ventral surface. **(C)** Sagittal contrast-enhanced MRI shows enhancement of a draining vein with diffuse mild enhancement of the capillary component. The patient had no brainstem symptomatology.

Dural Arteriovenous Fistula

Synonym: Low flow carotid cavernous fistula.

Dural arteriovenous fistulas (DAVFs) are composed of abnormal connections between dural arteries and venous sinuses, with arteriovenous shunting an essential component. They comprise about 10–15% of intracranial AVMs. DAVFs are found in middle-aged and older adults who present with various symptoms, including headaches, pulsatile tinnitus, diplopia, or proptosis. Intracranial venous hypertension may develop, leading to infarction or hemorrhage. The cavernous sinus is most commonly affected.

CT Findings. CT is often insensitive for the detection of dural fistulas. One may see enlargement of the cortical veins or enlargement of the affected dural sinus. Secondary findings may include focal cortical atrophy or hemorrhage. Cavernous sinus fistulas may produce enlarged ophthalmic veins and extraocular muscles and proptosis.

MRI Findings. MRI may show enlargement of the meningeal and external carotid branches supplying the fistula, with enlargement of the affected dural sinus. Varying degrees of stenosis or occlusion of the affected dural sinuses are encountered. Since the normal cavernous sinus does not exhibit a flow void on MRI, an intracavernous flow void separate from the internal carotid artery should suggest the diagnosis of DAVF. MR angiography may demonstrate the enlarged arterial feeders and fistula site.

Angiographic Findings. Angiography reveals shunting of blood from small dural branches of the internal and external carotid arteries to a major dural sinus. The cavernous, transverse, and sigmoid sinuses are affected in descending order. Cavernous sinus fistulas may be supplied by the inferolateral trunk and meningohypophyseal trunk of the internal carotid and by the ascending pharyngeal, middle meningeal, accessory meningeal, and foramen rotundum branches of the external carotid. A variety of venous drainage patterns are seen. Anterior drainage to the ophthalmic veins causes ocular symptoms, and cortical venous drainage may cause cerebral complications. Venous drainage may also occur via the petrosal sinuses, intercavernous sinuses to the opposite cavernous sinus, or pterygoid plexus.

Differential Diagnosis

Angiography is diagnostic.

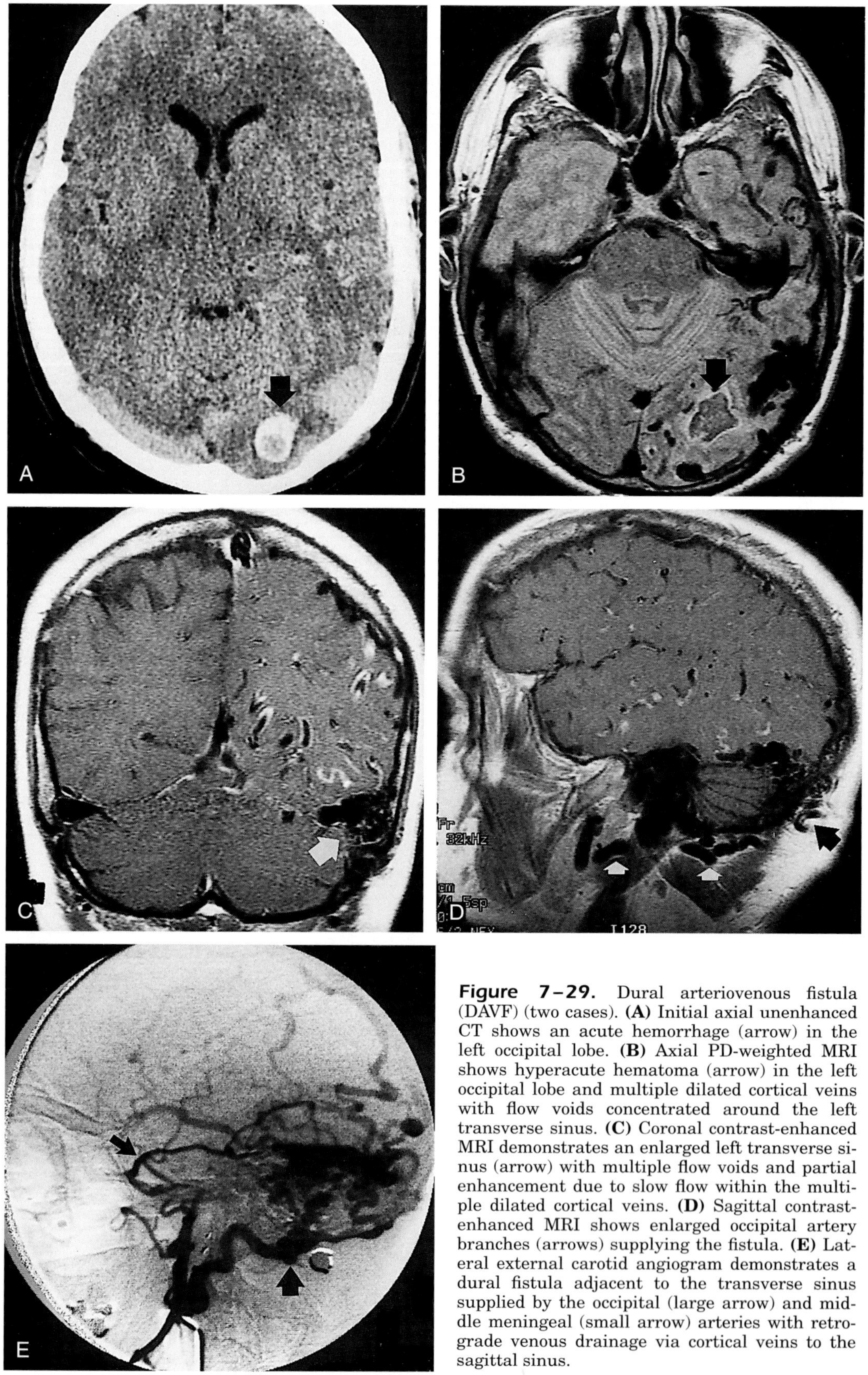

Figure 7–29. Dural arteriovenous fistula (DAVF) (two cases). **(A)** Initial axial unenhanced CT shows an acute hemorrhage (arrow) in the left occipital lobe. **(B)** Axial PD-weighted MRI shows hyperacute hematoma (arrow) in the left occipital lobe and multiple dilated cortical veins with flow voids concentrated around the left transverse sinus. **(C)** Coronal contrast-enhanced MRI demonstrates an enlarged left transverse sinus (arrow) with multiple flow voids and partial enhancement due to slow flow within the multiple dilated cortical veins. **(D)** Sagittal contrast-enhanced MRI shows enlarged occipital artery branches (arrows) supplying the fistula. **(E)** Lateral external carotid angiogram demonstrates a dural fistula adjacent to the transverse sinus supplied by the occipital (large arrow) and middle meningeal (small arrow) arteries with retrograde venous drainage via cortical veins to the sagittal sinus.

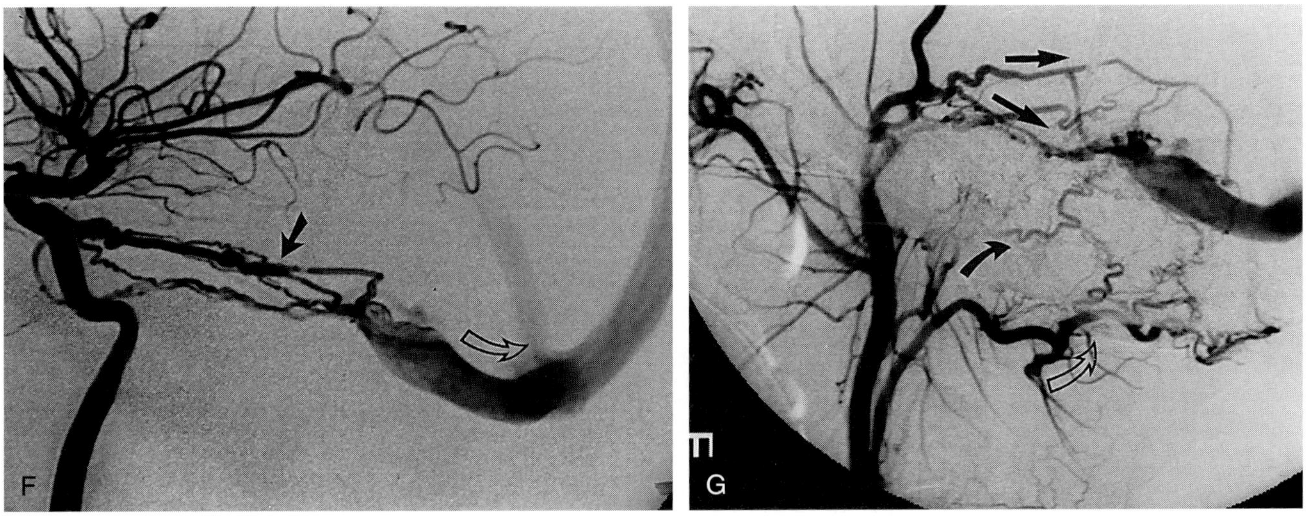

Figure 7–29. **(F)** Left internal carotid angiogram shows an arteriovenous shunt of the left transverse sinus. The fistula is supplied by the tentorial artery (solid arrow) and multiple meningeal branches. Venous drainage (open arrow) is retrograde to the sagittal sinus and opposite transverse sinus. The distal transverse sinus is occluded. **(G)** Left external carotid angiogram shows the supply to the fistula by branches of the middle meningeal (straight solid arrows), posterior auricular (curved solid arrow), and occipital (open arrow) arteries.

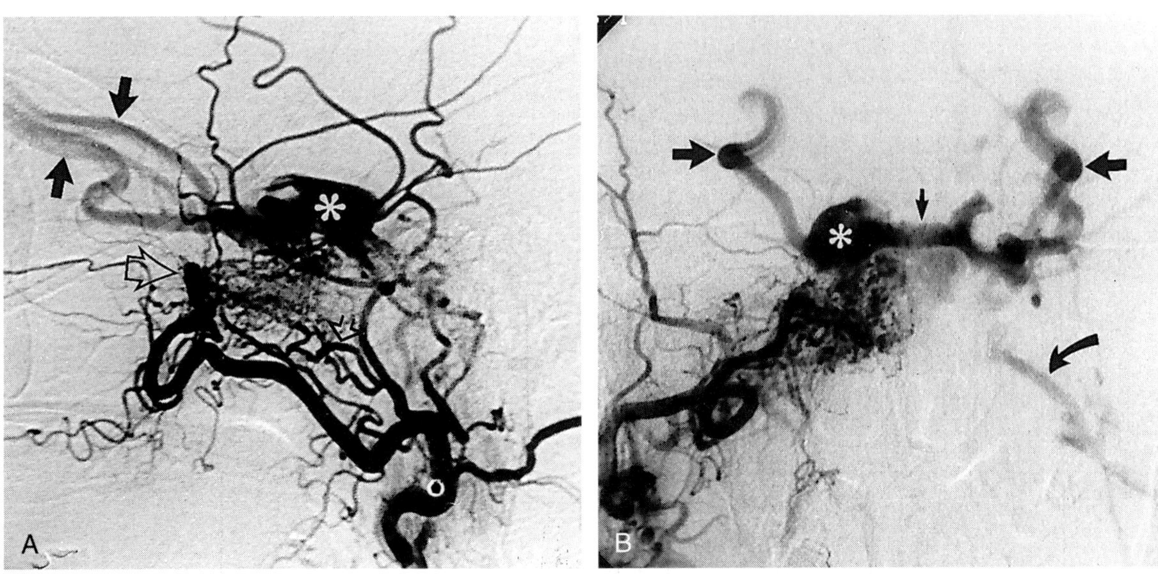

Figure 7–30. Cavernous DAVF. **(A)** Lateral and **(B)** AP external carotid angiograms show a dural fistula of the right cavernous sinus. The fistula is supplied by multiple small dural branches of the internal maxillary (large open arrow) and accessory meningeal (small open arrow) arteries. The cavernous sinus (asterisk) drains via the superior ophthalmic vein (large solid arrow) and intercavernous vein (small solid arrow) to the left cavernous sinus. Curved arrow indicates inferior petrosal vein.

Aneurysms

Aneurysms

Congenital berry aneurysms are a common cerebrovascular lesion, occurring in up to 2% of the general population. They are the leading cause of spontaneous subarachnoid hemorrhage. Pathologically there is thinning or absence of the arterial media with dilatation of the lumen, usually at a bifurcation and almost always in the proximal circle of Willis. The probability of rupture strongly correlates with the size of the aneurysm, with rupture very uncommon in those less than 5 mm in diameter. Ninety percent of aneurysmal ruptures occur in persons between 30 and 70 years of age.

Mycotic aneurysms are usually associated with endocarditis and occur in peripheral intracranial vessels. They may cause primary intracerebral hematoma. The term is a misnomer, as these are actually pseudoaneurysms and almost never a result of fungal infection.

CT Findings. Aneurysms appear on CT as a round mass isodense or mildly hyperdense relative to the brain. Rapid dynamic scanning shows contrast enhancement equal in degree to the arteries of the circle of Willis. There may be a characteristic peripheral curvilinear calcification of the aneurysm wall and mural filling defects (which do not enhance) indicating thrombus.

TABLE 7–6 | Correlation of Aneurysm Location with Location of SAH on CT

Aneurysm Site	Location of Hemorrhage on CT
Middle cerebral artery	Frontal operculum Unilateral sylvian fissure Basal cisterns
Posterior communicating artery	Basal cisterns
Anterior communicating artery	Gyrus rectus Third ventricle Septum pellucidum Basal cisterns
Pericallosal artery	Corpus callosum Anterior interhemispheric fissure
Basilar tip	Posterior third ventricle Basal cisterns
Posterior inferior cerebellar artery	Fourth ventricle Posterior fossa cisterns

MRI Findings. MRI reveals a mass in which signal characteristics are flow dependent. The internal signal is a function of flow direction and velocity, turbulence, contrast administration, and scanning techniques. The lumen may appear homogeneous or heterogeneous and ranges from a complete absence of signal (flow void) to very bright.

Giant aneurysms are somewhat arbitrarily and inconsistently defined as those exceeding 1.5 to 2.5 cm in real outer diameter. The cavernous carotid is the most common location (43%). Mass effect is often seen with giant aneurysms, and intraluminal thrombus is more common. Thrombus results in concentric layers of blood clot of different ages and signal intensities, with the most recent clot located centrally.

MR angiography can be used to diagnose aneurysms, but the clinical role of this technique has yet to be established.

Angiographic Findings. Angiography reveals the classic and pathognomonic outpouching of a vessel lumen that is round to oval in shape and fills with contrast. Most aneurysms occur at points of bifurcation or origins of major branches. Berry aneurysms are most common in the circle of Willis and multiple in 20–25%. Mycotic aneurysms tend to occur in peripheral intracranial branches.

When more than one aneurysm is found in a patient with subarachnoid hemorrhage, it is of paramount importance to ascertain which of the aneurysms ruptured. The following features strongly implicate a particular aneurysm as the source of hemorrhage:

- Vasospasm adjacent to the aneurysm
- Nipple sign, a small outpouching of contrast beyond the aneurysm's outer contour
- Origin from the anterior communicating artery
- Larger size
- Correspondence to site of hemorrhage on CT (Table 7–6)

Distribution of berry aneurysms:

40% Internal carotid/posterior communicating artery
30% Anterior communicating artery/anterior cerebral artery
20% Middle cerebral artery
10% Vertebrobasilar (most are basilar tip)

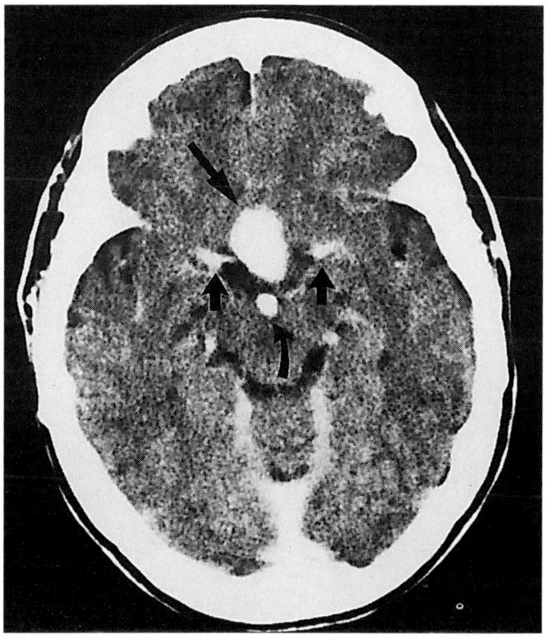

Figure 7–31. Aneurysm. Axial dynamic contrast-enhanced CT shows a mass (long arrow) in the suprasellar cistern that enhances to the same degree as the basilar (curved arrow) and internal carotid (short arrow) arteries.

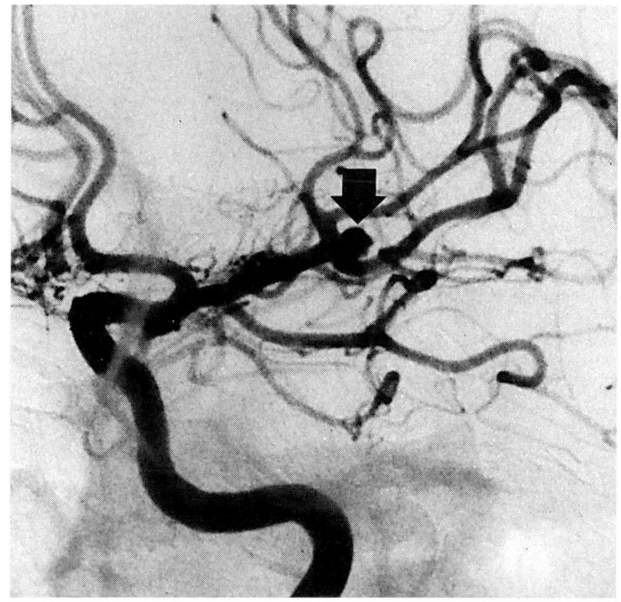

Figure 7–32. Middle cerebral aneurysm. Oblique internal carotid angiogram shows an aneurysm (arrow) of the middle cerebral trifurcation.

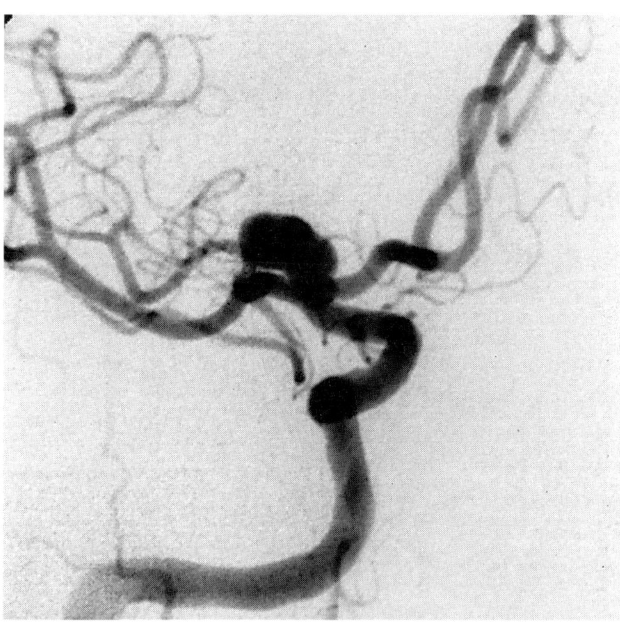

Figure 7–33. Internal carotid aneurysm. Anteroposterior oblique view of right common carotid angiogram shows a bilobulated aneurysm of the internal carotid bifurcation.

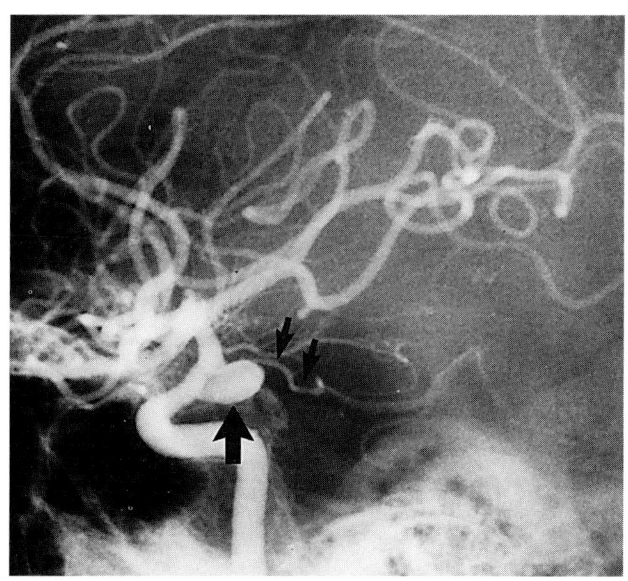

Figure 7–34. Posterior communicating aneurysm. Lateral internal carotid angiogram shows an aneurysm (large arrow) at the origin of the posterior communicating artery (small arrows).

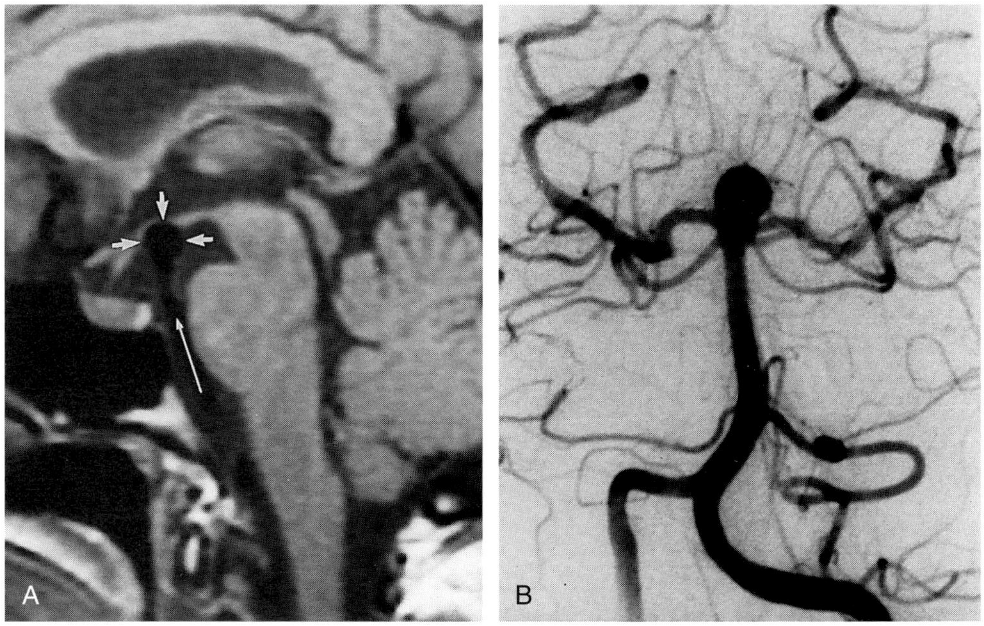

Figure 7–35. Basilar tip aneurysm. **(A)** Sagittal T1-weighted MRI shows an aneurysm (short arrows) at the tip of the basilar artery (long arrow). The aneurysm presses upon the hypothalamus just anterior to the mammillary bodies. **(B)** Left vertebral angiogram (AP projection) shows a typical basilar tip aneurysm.

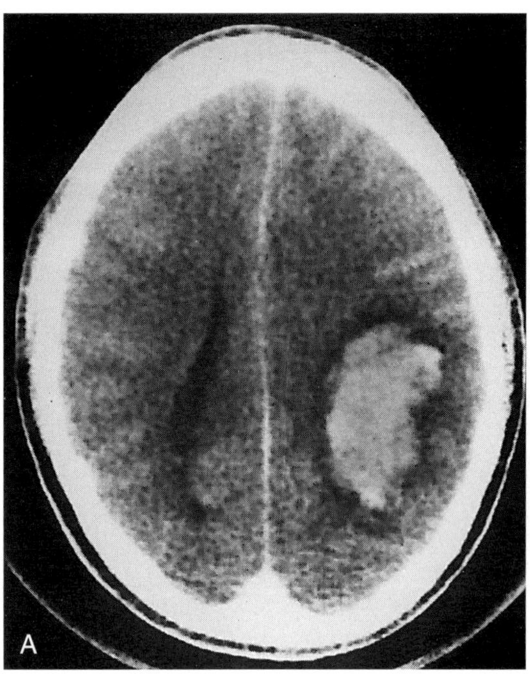

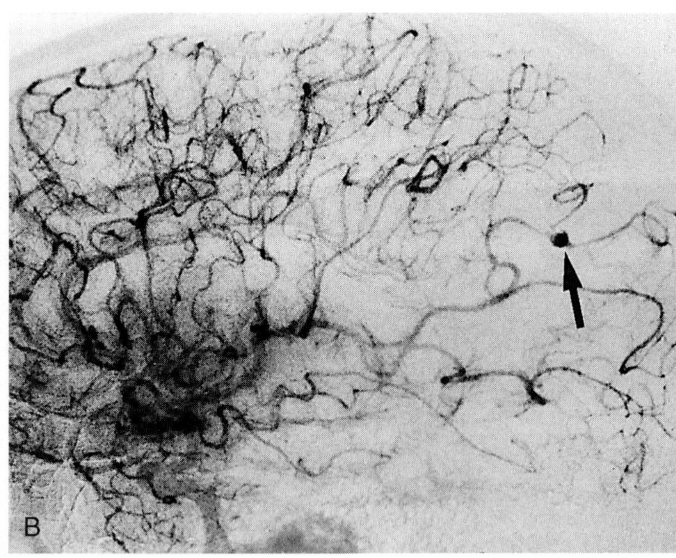

Figure 7–36. Mycotic aneurysm. **(A)** Axial unenhanced CT shows acute hemorrhage in the left parietal white matter. **(B)** Lateral internal carotid angiogram shows a pseudoaneurysm (arrow) arising from a small distal branch of the angular artery.

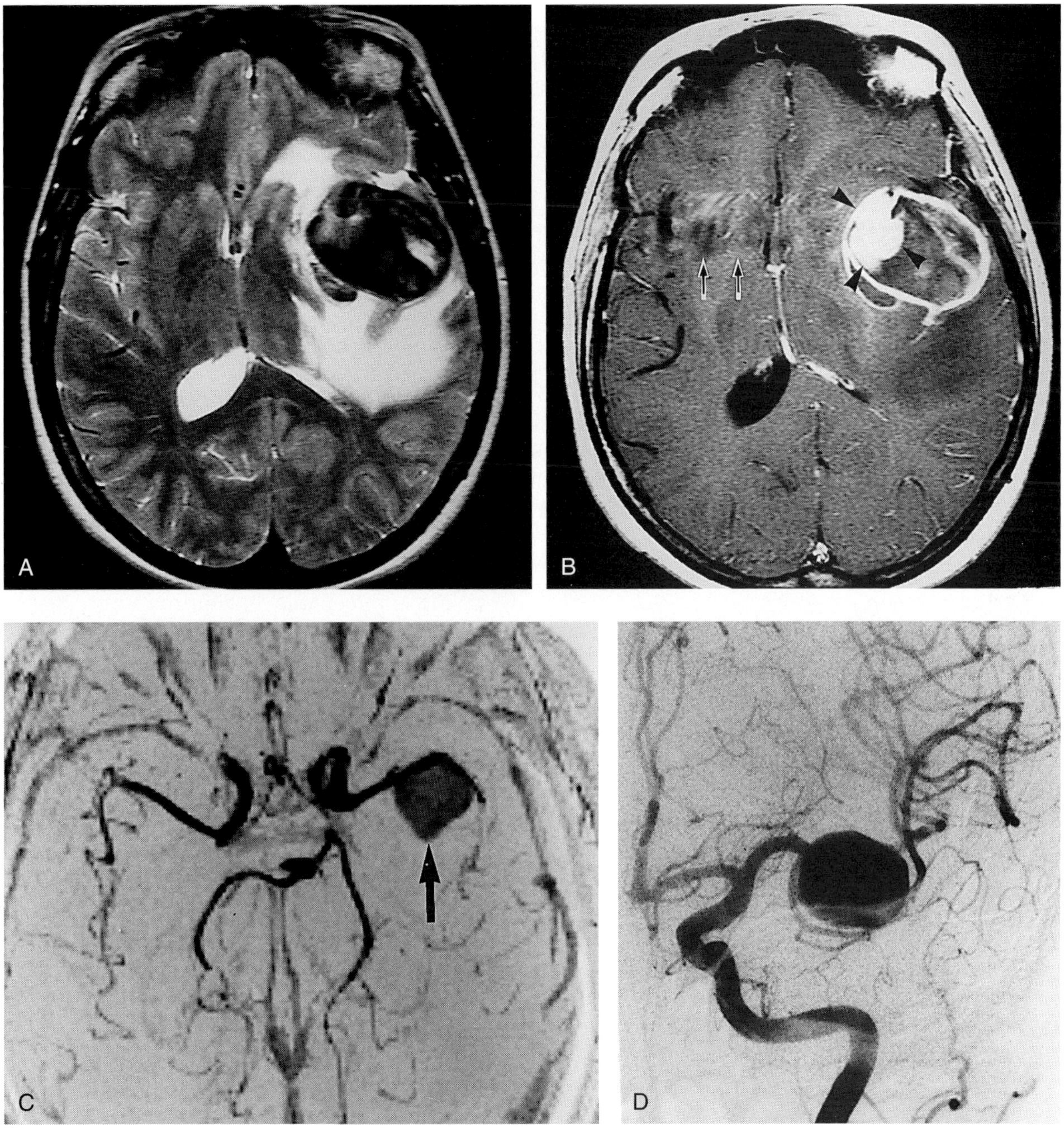

Figure 7–37. Giant aneurysm. **(A)** Axial T2-weighted MRI shows a 3.8- by 4.4-cm mass in the left middle fossa. The mass is mostly hypointense reflecting acute thrombus. There is marked vasogenic edema of the surrounding brain. **(B)** Axial contrast-enhanced MRI shows marked ring enhancement of the aneurysm wall and intense enhancement of the lumen (arrowheads). The luminal thrombus does not enhance. Note the artifact (arrows) along the phase-encoding direction indicating flow within the enhanced lumen. **(C)** MR angiography (3D time-of-flight, axial projection) shows an aneurysm (arrow) of the left middle cerebral artery. **(D)** AP left internal carotid angiogram shows a large aneurysm arising from the middle cerebral artery trifurcation. Observe how angiography underrepresents the size of the aneurysm because of its inability to depict mural thrombus.

Subarachnoid Hemorrhage

Primary (nontraumatic) subarachnoid hemorrhage (SAH) occurs with an annual incidence of 10 to 20 per 100,000 population in the United States, with a 30-day mortality rate of 30–40%. It accounts for approximately 6% of all strokes. Hence, SAH represents a major cause of neurologic morbidity and mortality. A ruptured berry aneurysm is the most common cause. Patients usually present with severe headache, meningismus, or altered mental status. The morbidity related to SAH is ongoing with important delayed complications, including rebleeding (especially in the first 2 weeks), hydrocephalus, and infarctions.

CT Findings. CT scans may show the following:

1. Blood in cisterns, ventricles, and other subarachnoid spaces: The sensitivity of CT for SAH is quite good (70 to >90%). However, a normal CT does not rule out the diagnosis of acute subarachnoid hemorrhage. Blood in the CSF clears rapidly and may become undetectable within days of onset.
2. Hydrocephalus: Hydrocephalus may be noncommunicating, owing to clots in the ventricular system, or communicating, owing to blood impairing CSF resorption by the arachnoid villi.
3. Infarcts: Infarcts may develop secondary to severe vasospasm, usually in an anterior or a middle cerebral artery distribution.
4. Source of hemorrhage: An aneurysm or AVM may be directly identified.

Idiopathic SAH (no history of trauma, negative angiogram) tends to be most prominent in the prepontine and interpeduncular cisterns of the posterior fossa. Traumatic SAH is discussed in Chapter 2. Neonatal SAH is usually secondary to birth trauma and tends to appear in the posterior interhemispheric fissure and superior cerebellar and quadrigeminal cisterns.

MRI Findings. MRI plays almost no role in the evaluation of acute subarachnoid hemorrhage. Although some investigators claim good sensitivity for SAH, MRI is probably less sensitive than CT, and the findings are often very subtle. Subacute SAH may demonstrate hyperintensity in the cisterns on T1-weighted images owing to methemoglobin within localized clots. Chronic SAH may result in accumulation of hemosiderin-laden macrophages in the leptomeninges and subpial tissue, producing the so-called superficial siderosis. This phenomenon manifests itself as superficial cortical hypointensity on T2-weighted images.

Angiographic Findings. Angiography may reveal the following:

1. Vasospasm: SAH may induce severe narrowing of the cerebral vasculature, usually most severe in the vicinity of the aneurysm. It is seldom present at onset and reaches a peak incidence at 7 to 10 days post-ictus.
2. Mass effect due to midline shift, herniation, or hematoma may be seen.
3. Etiology of hemorrhage: The principal purpose of angiography in subarachnoid hemorrhage is to determine the source of bleeding. The various etiologies of SAH are listed in Table 7–7.

TABLE 7–7 Etiology of Primary Subarachnoid Hemorrhage

Berry aneurysm	up to 85%
Arteriovenous malformation	10%
Idiopathic (some estimates as high as 15%)	5%
Vasculitis	<1%
Mycotic aneurysm	<1%
Moyamoya disease	<1%

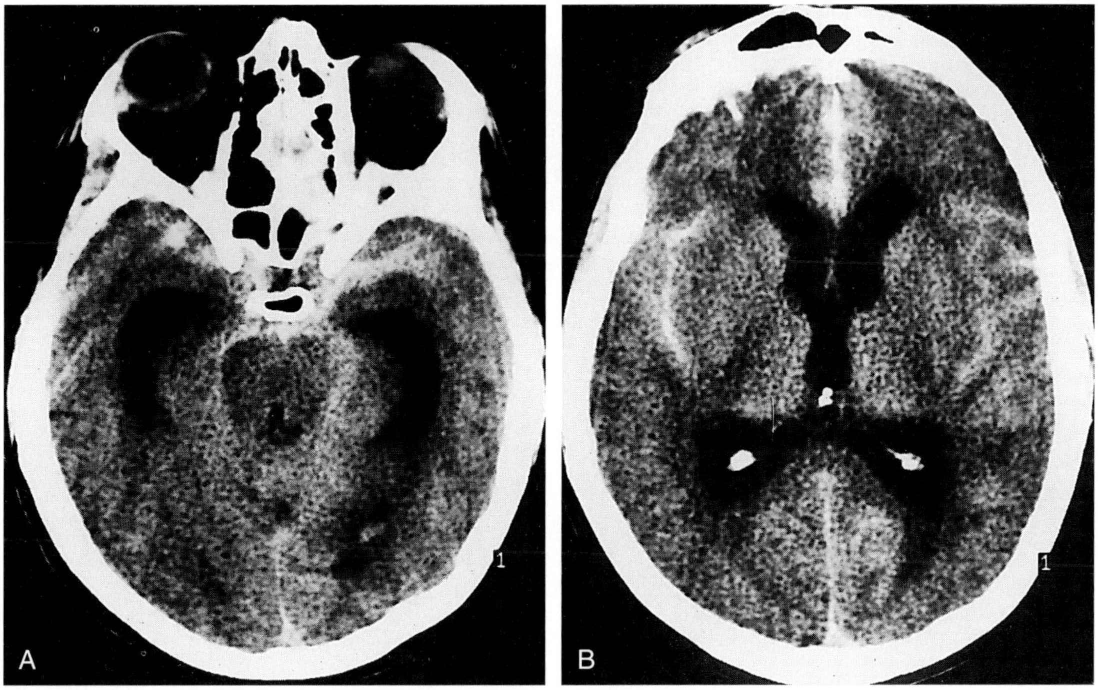

Figure 7–38. Subarachnoid hemorrhage (anterior communicating aneurysm rupture). Axial unenhanced CT through **(A)** level of sella and **(B)** foramen of Monro show high attenuation of acute blood in the prepontine and ambient cisterns, sylvian fissures, and anterior interhemispheric fissure.

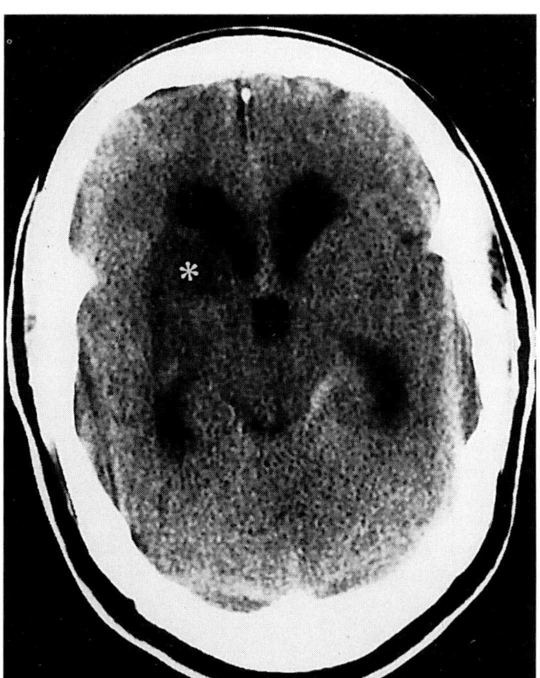

Figure 7–39. Subarachnoid hemorrhage (vasospasm and infarction). Axial unenhanced CT shows low attenuation in the right lentiform nuclei (asterisk), an early sign of middle cerebral infarction.

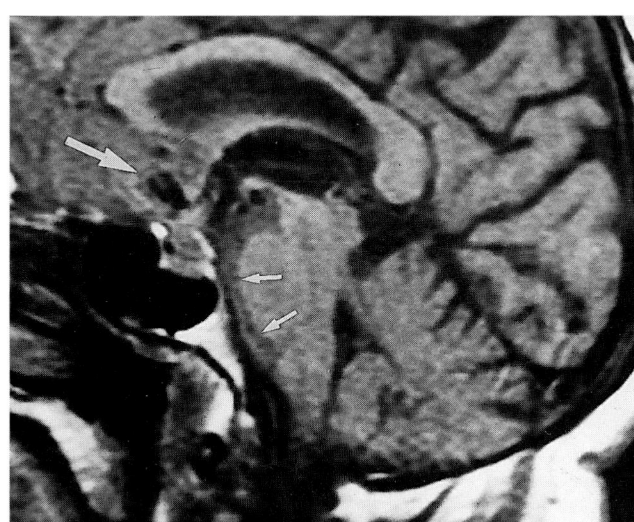

Figure 7–40. Subarachnoid hemorrhage. Sagittal T1-weighted MRI shows increased signal in the prepontine cistern (small arrows) due to massive SAH from a ruptured anterior communicating artery aneurysm (long arrow).

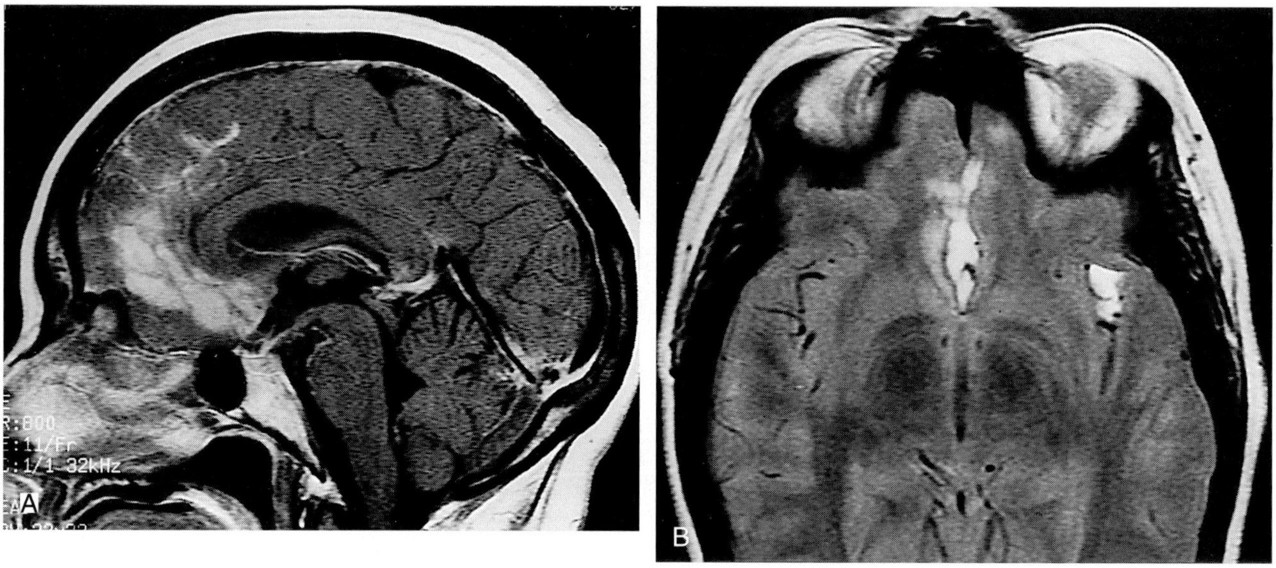

Figure 7–41. Subarachnoid hemorrhage. **(A)** Sagittal T1-weighted MRI (contrast enhanced) shows marked hyperintensity in the anterior interhemispheric fissure representing subacute subarachnoid hemorrhage from a ruptured anterior communicating artery aneurysm. **(B)** Axial PD-weighted MRI shows hyperintense clot in the anterior interhemispheric fissure and left sylvian fissure.

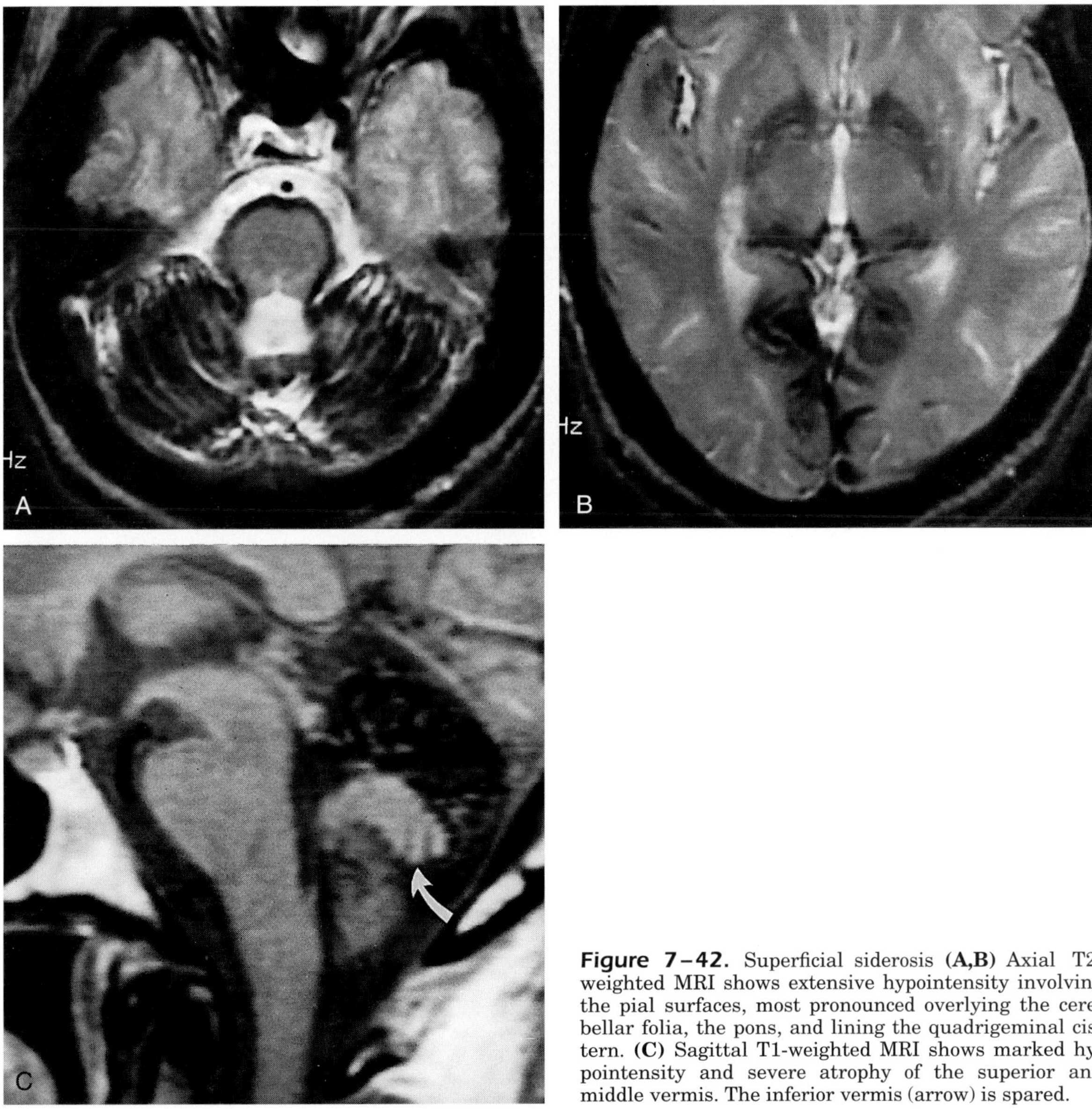

Figure 7–42. Superficial siderosis **(A,B)** Axial T2-weighted MRI shows extensive hypointensity involving the pial surfaces, most pronounced overlying the cerebellar folia, the pons, and lining the quadrigeminal cistern. **(C)** Sagittal T1-weighted MRI shows marked hypointensity and severe atrophy of the superior and middle vermis. The inferior vermis (arrow) is spared.

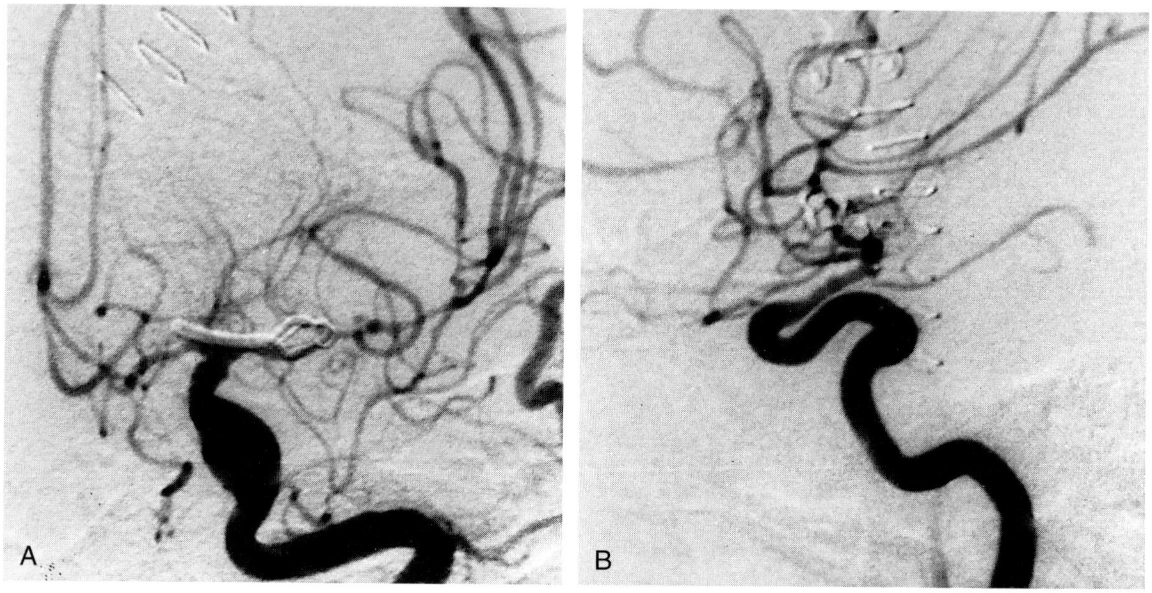

Figure 7–43. Subarachnoid hemorrhage—vasospasm. **(A)** AP and lateral **(B)** internal carotid angiograms show marked spasm of the supraclinoid ICA and the A1 and M1 segments of the anterior and middle cerebral arteries after clipping of a ruptured internal carotid bifurcation aneurysm.

Thromboembolic

Atherosclerosis

Synonym: Arteriosclerosis.

Atherosclerosis is the cause of over 90% of thrombotic cerebral infarctions in developed countries. The most common site of cerebral vascular involvement is in the first 3 cm of the proximal internal carotid artery, followed by the cavernous internal carotid. Diffuse involvement of peripheral intracranial vasculature may sometimes occur.

A stenosis of 75% or greater is necessary to cause a significant decrease in cerebral blood flow under normotensive conditions. However, less severe stenosis may lead to infarction by the release of emboli or acute thrombosis. Current therapeutic strategies begin with the identification of affected patients through screening methods such as ultrasound, leading to medical management with antiplatelet agents or surgical treatment with endarterectomy. These treatments can decrease the probability of subsequent cerebral infarction.

Sonographic Findings. The combination of cross-sectional sonographic imaging with Doppler velocity analysis is an effective screening test for disease of the carotid bifurcation. Real-time imaging shows echogenic plaque encroaching on the anechoic vascular lumen. Stenosis of the internal carotid causes increased flow velocity, and there is good correlation between velocity and degree of stenosis (Table 7–8). Numerous pitfalls exist, the greatest being sonography's total dependence on the skill of the operator.

Other Doppler criteria are useful but generally less sensitive than internal carotid flow analysis. These include the following:

1. Internal carotid/common carotid flow ratio: normal is less than 1.5.
2. Common carotid mean flow: normal is greater than 25 cm/sec.
3. Common carotid diastolic flow: normal is greater than 9 cm/sec.
4. Left/right common carotid flow ratio: normal range is 0.7 to 1.3.

TABLE 7–8 Correlation of Velocity with Stenosis Using Duplex Sonography

Velocity (Peak Systolic)	Percent Area Stenosis
<1.0 m/sec	0–30
1.0–1.19 m/sec	31–49
1.20–2.5 m/sec	50–90
>2.5 m/sec	91–99
Variable, distorted	>95

CT Findings. Dynamic high resolution CT with bolus administration of intravenous contrast can yield information comparable to MRI and angiography but is not widely employed.

MRI Findings. MR angiography is a rapidly evolving technique whose role is yet to be determined. Although MR angiography can image the carotid bifurcation with an accuracy approaching that of invasive angiography, it is limited in area of coverage and spatial resolution for smaller vessel disease and is subject to various artifacts.

Angiographic Findings. The angiographic hallmark of atherosclerosis is arterial narrowing around the bifurcation of the common carotid artery (CCA). Stenosis is found in the proximal internal carotid artery (ICA) (nearly always in the first 3 cm), the origin of the external carotid artery (ECA), or the terminal artery CCA in decreasing frequency. Less commonly, atherosclerosis may occur anywhere within the cervical or intracranial cerebral vasculature. There may be stenoses or occlusions of the common carotid arteries, vertebral arteries, subclavian arteries, or innominate artery anywhere along their course. Stenosis may be reported as diameter stenosis or area stenosis. Diameter stenosis is derived from the ratio of the minimum diameter at the point of stenosis to the diameter of the distal normal vessel based on a single projection. Area stenosis is more accurate and derived from the product of the diameter stenosis measured in two orthogonal projections.

A subclavian steal is the phenomenon of antegrade flow up one vertebral artery (usually the right) with retrograde flow down the opposite vertebral artery to reconstitute a proximally occluded subclavian artery.

Ulceration within a plaque appears as a contrast-filled outpouching into the plaque. The diagnosis of ulceration by angiography is somewhat inaccurate (about 50%). An outpouching is most likely an ulcer when the connection with the vessel lumen is more narrow than the base of the ulcer. Intraluminal thrombus may be seen as an intravascular filling defect with or without ulceration.

In advanced disease, there may be complete occlusion of the ICA, usually with collateral reconstitution via ECA anastomoses (see Figures 7–45 through 7–49) or the circle of Willis. A string sign is the angiographic visualization of a small residual lumen with subtotal occlusion of the internal carotid. Delayed films of the neck should routinely be obtained when internal carotid occlusion is suspected.

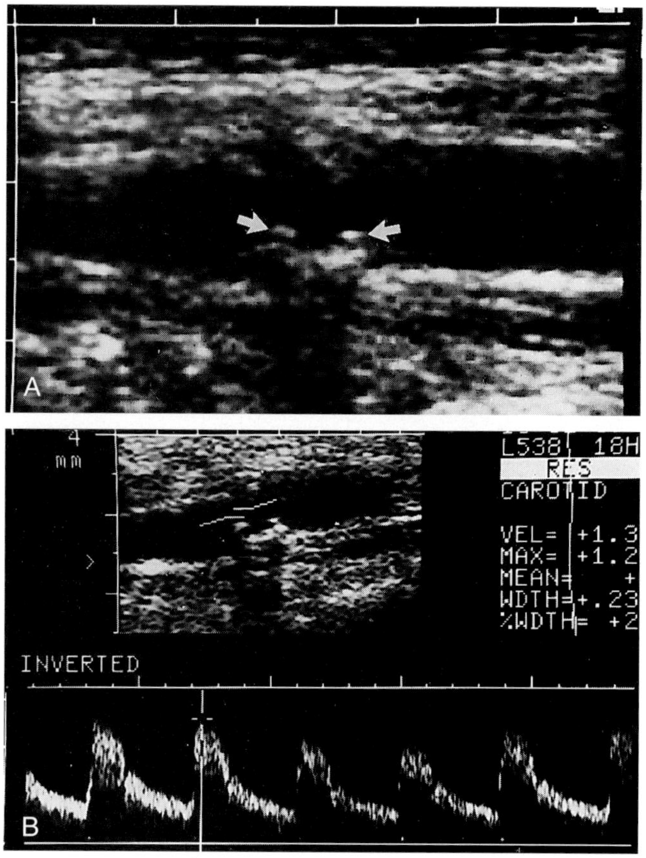

Figure 7–44. Ulcerated plaque with stenosis. **(A)** Sonogram shows a plaque (arrows) of the internal carotid artery with raised sides and a central depression. **(B)** Doppler analysis shows a peak systolic velocity of 1.29 m/sec correlating with a stenosis of 50–90%.

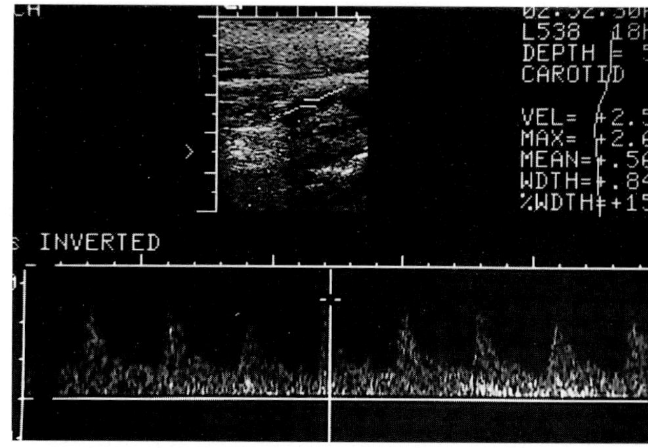

Figure 7–45. High grade stenosis. Doppler analysis of the internal carotid reveals a peak systolic velocity of 2.60 m/sec indicating area stenosis in excess of 90%.

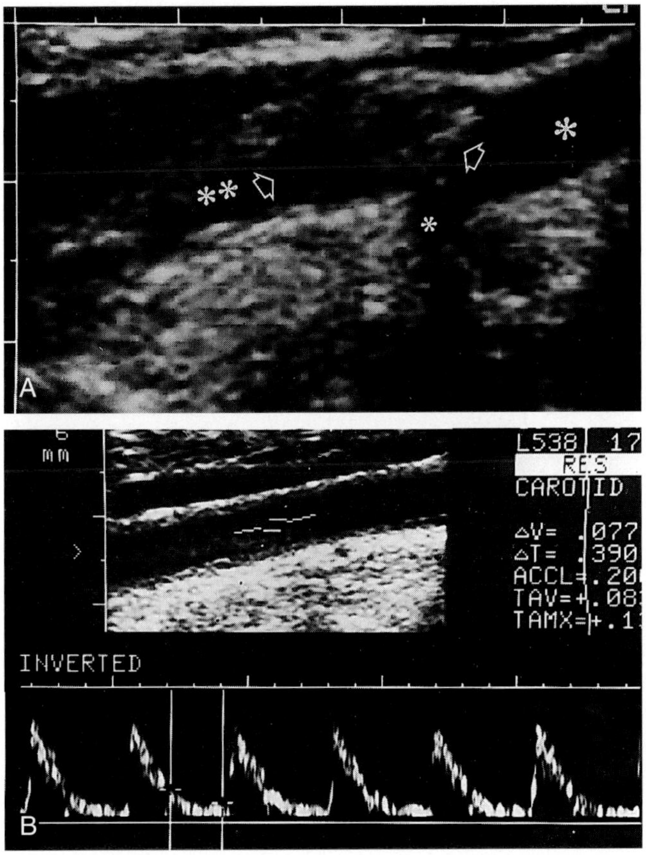

Figure 7–46. Internal carotid occlusion. **(A)** Sonogram shows mildly echogenic plaque (open arrows) filling the carotid bulb with no detectable flow by Doppler. Single asterisk indicates common carotid artery, double asterisk indicates internal carotid artery, and small asterisk indicates trunk of external carotid artery. **(B)** Mean diastolic flow in the common carotid artery is reduced to 0.08 m/sec (8 cm/sec) due to internal carotid occlusion.

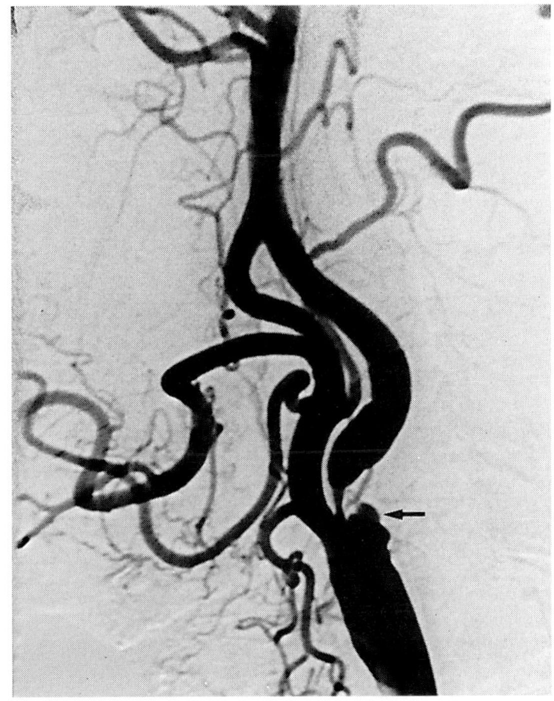

Figure 7–47. Carotid stenosis. Lateral common carotid angiogram shows a severe (>90%) stenosis of the internal carotid origin with an ulcer (arrow).

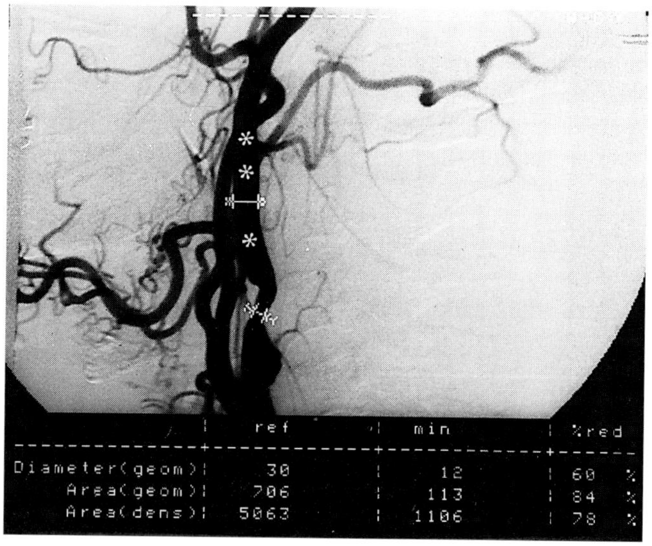

Figure 7–48. Measurement of stenosis. Proprietary software (Siemens Medical Systems) calculates stenosis by operator-placed cursors. Diameters are obtained at point of greatest stenosis and through normal distal internal carotid giving a diameter stenosis of 60%. The same ratio in an orthogonal plane would yield an area stenosis of 84%. Based on the density of contrast opacification, area stenosis is calculated to 78%. Asterisks indicate internal carotid artery.

Major Collateral Pathways of the Cervicocerebral Vasculature

I. Collateral pathways of internal carotid reconstitution (occluded proximal ICA)
   1. ECA → internal maxillary artery → pterygopalatine branches → ethmoidal branches → ophthalmic artery → supraclinoid ICA
   2. ECA → anterior branches of superficial temporal artery → ophthalmic artery → ICA
   3. ECA → middle meningeal artery → lacrimal branches → ophthalmic artery → ICA
   4. ECA → facial artery → angular branch → ophthalmic artery → ICA
   5. ECA → internal maxillary artery → artery of the foramen rotundum → inferolateral trunk → ICA
   6. ECA → internal maxillary artery → vidian artery → petrous ICA
   7. Intracranial reconstitution via anterior or posterior communicating arteries (circle of Willis).
   8. Leptomeningeal collaterals (pial anastomoses)—enlarged cortical anastomoses that allow retrograde reconstitution of proximally occluded cerebral vessels

II. Collateral pathways of internal carotid reconstitution (occluded CCA)
   1. Vertebral artery → muscular branches → occipital artery → ECA → ICA
   2. Contralateral common carotid → ECA → midline facial, internal maxillary, superior thyroid anastomoses → ipsilateral ECA (retrograde flow) → ICA

III. Collateral pathway of vertebral reconstitution ECA → occipital artery → muscular branches → vertebral artery. (This pathway is commonly seen from an occipital artery injection even in the absence of vertebral occlusion.)

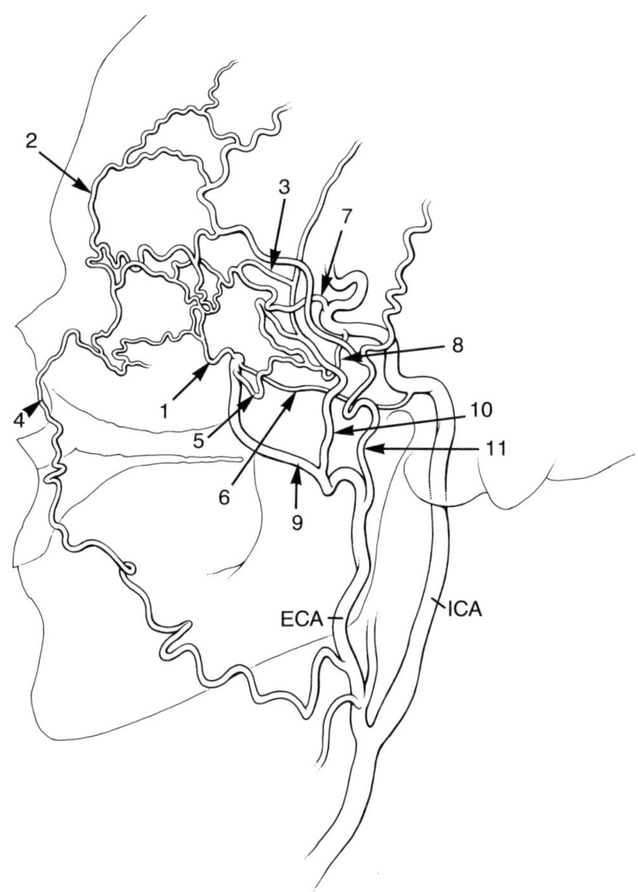

Figure 7–49. Major collateral pathways between external and internal carotid territories. 1 = pterygopalatine (to ethmoidal) artery, 2 = anterior branches of superficial temporal, 3 = recurrent meningeal artery, 4 = facial artery, 5 = artery of the foramen rotundum, 6 = vidian artery, 7 = ophthalmic artery, 8 = inferolateral trunk, 9 = internal maxillary artery, 10 = middle meningeal artery, 11 = superficial temporal artery.

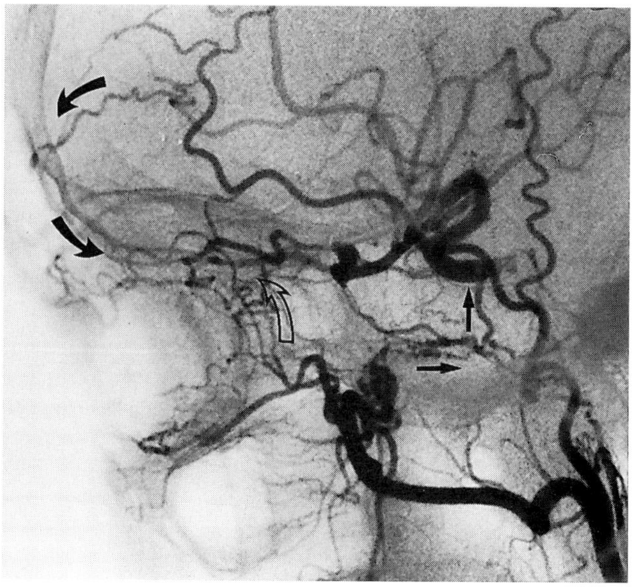

Figure 7–50. Occlusion of internal carotid. Lateral common carotid angiogram shows collateral pathways of internal carotid reconstitution, including superficial temporal to ophthalmic (solid curved arrows), ethmoidal to ophthalmic (open curved arrow), and artery of foramen rotundum to inferolateral trunk (straight arrows).

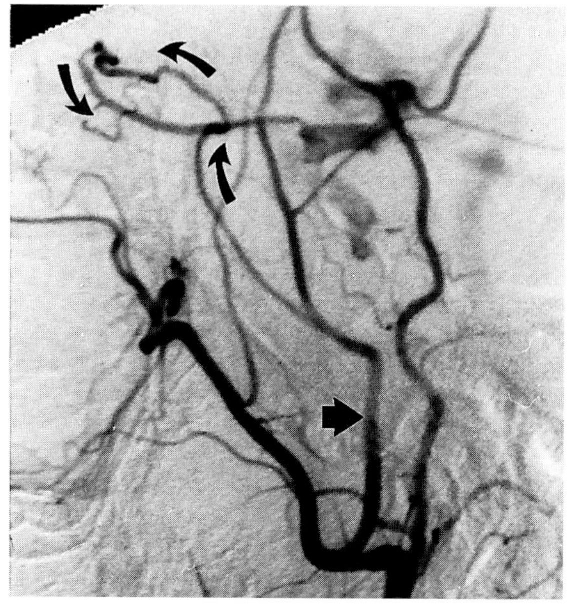

Figure 7–51. Occluded internal carotid. Lateral common carotid angiogram shows internal carotid is reconstituted via the recurrent meningeal artery to the ophthalmic artery (curved arrows). Straight arrow indicates middle meningeal artery.

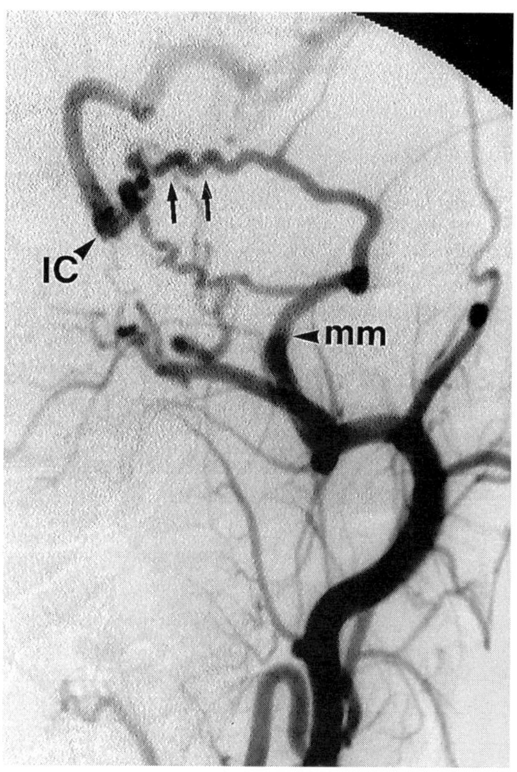

Figure 7–52. Occluded internal carotid. Anteroposterior common carotid angiogram shows the left internal carotid (IC) artery is reconstituted by a direct cavernous anastomosis (arrows) with the middle meningeal artery (mm).

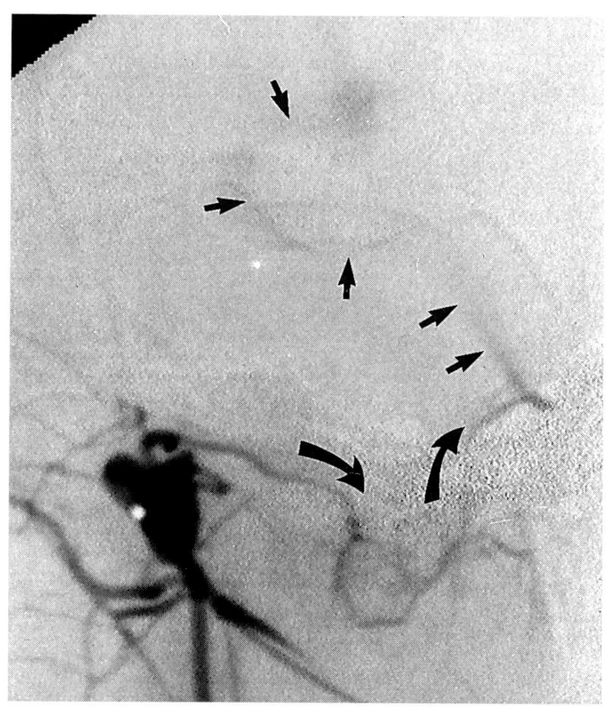

Figure 7–53. Vidian artery. Internal maxillary angiogram shows vidian artery (curved arrows) courses posteriorly to anastomose with the internal carotid (straight arrows) near the foramen lacerum.

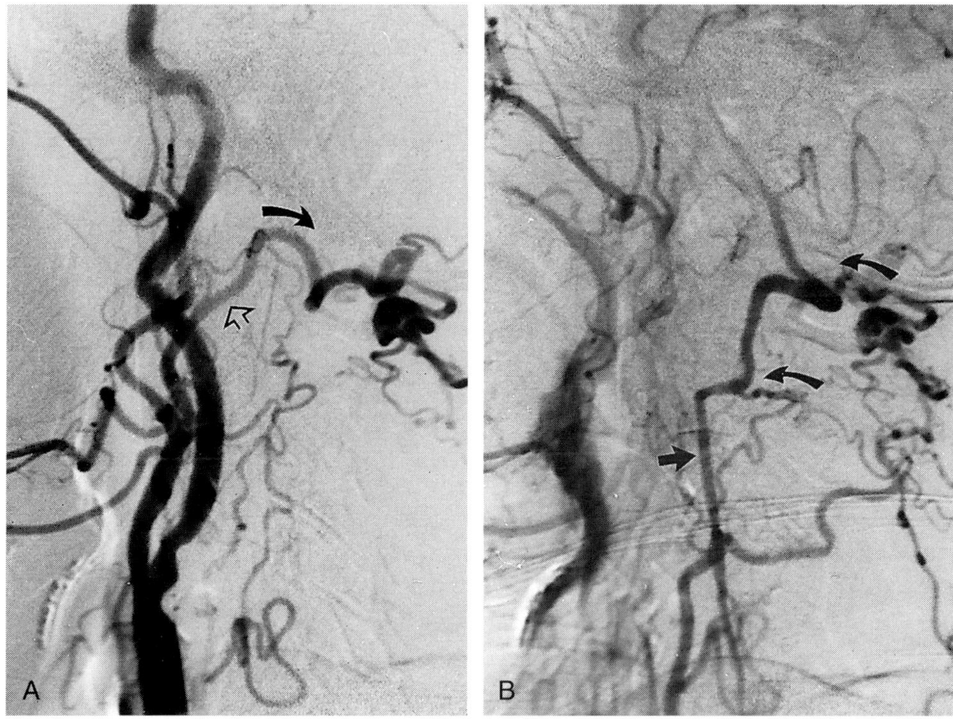

Figure 7–54. Vertebral occlusion. **(A)** Early and **(B)** late arterial images of common carotid injection show the collateral pathway of vertebral reconstitution (curved arrows). Open arrow indicates occipital artery and straight arrow indicates vertebral artery.

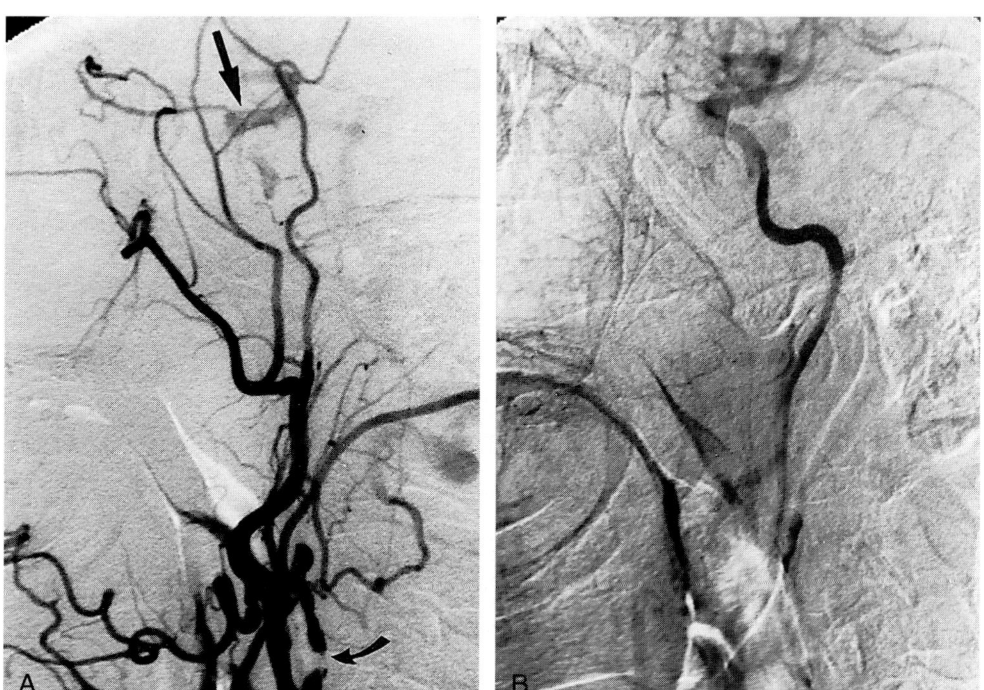

Figure 7–55. String sign. **(A)** Lateral common carotid angiogram shows a severe stenosis (curved arrow) of the internal carotid artery with no distal flow. The intracranial internal carotid (arrow) is reconstituted by collateral flow. **(B)** On delayed film, there is complete filling of the internal carotid artery.

Infarction

Approximately 500,000 cases of stroke occur each year in the United States. Of these, 200,000 die, making stroke the third leading cause of death. Among survivors, 70% are moderately to severely disabled. Although the term stroke may apply to any acute cerebrovascular disorder, including venous thrombosis or aneurysmal rupture, the vast majority are due to acute arterial infarction,

The pathophysiologic events that follow are complex, proceeding from acute edema (both cytotoxic and vasogenic) to coagulative necrosis to liquefaction and absorption to cavitation. Hemorrhagic transformation occurs in up to 30% and is usually associated with embolic occlusion. Because astrocytes are less vulnerable to ischemia than are neurons, glia are preserved in less severe infarcts and at the periphery of larger infarcts.

CT Findings

Acute Infarct (<24 Hours). The following have been described as early CT findings of cerebral infarct:

1. Loss of gray-white differentiation due to decreased attenuation of edematous gray matter
2. Sulcal effacement due to mass effect of edema
3. Insular ribbon sign—diminished attenuation of gray matter in insular cortex and claustrum due to edema, a fairly sensitive sign
4. Obscuration of lentiform nucleus/loss of definition of the internal capsule—nuclei isodense with internal capsule due to edema and diminished attenuation, a fairly sensitive sign
5. Hyperdense middle cerebral artery caused by the high attenuation of intraluminal thromboembolus, insensitive and often inaccurate (positive on the other side)
6. Hemorrhage, rare in first 6 hours

Using current scanners, the reported sensitivity of CT on initial presentation (<24 hours) ranges from 60–90%.

Subacute Infarcts (1 Day to 1 Month). During this period, CT is more than 90% sensitive for acute infarct, with low attenuation representing both cytotoxic and vasogenic edema and presenting in a classic vascular distribution. Mass effect peaks around 3 to 5 days and usually resolves by 21 days. Enhancement, typically gyriform, develops in 3 to 7 days. Hemorrhage into an infarct usually occurs between days 1 and 4. The severity of hemorrhage may range from a mild diffuse petechial hemorrhage (most common) to an isolated massive hematoma with intraventricular extension.

Chronic Infarcts. Smaller infarcts result in gliosis and atrophy, whereas major vessel occlusions usually result in cystic encephalomalacia with areas of brain destruction isodense with CSF. Associated findings may include the following:

- Atrophy with dilatation of adjacent ventricles and sulci
- Wallerian degeneration—denervation atrophy of the ipsilateral cerebral peduncle, basis pontis, and medullary pyramid from an infarction of the motor cortex or internal capsule
- Dystrophic calcification (rare)

MRI Findings

Acute and Subacute Infarcts

- Arterial abnormalities: Increased intraluminal signal, loss of flow void, or arterial enhancement may be seen within minutes of onset of symptoms.
- Morphologic changes: Mild mass effect due to cytotoxic edema with compression of ventricles or sulci may occur as early as 2 hours after onset.
- Signal abnormalities: MRI is slightly more sensitive than CT in the first few hours of an acute infarction. The usual appearance is an area of edema, mostly of gray matter, in a vascular distribution that is hyperintense on proton-density and T2-weighted images. The proton-density images exhibit slightly greater contrast between the infarct and adjacent structures. Hyperintensity begins to appear on T2-weighted images around 8 hours after onset. Hypointensity on T1-weighted sequences may appear in 16 to 24 hours. After 24 hours, signal abnormalities are virtually always present on T2-weighted images.
- Contrast enhancement: Following intravenous contrast, three patterns of abnormal enhancement may be observed. Intravascular enhancement occurs in vessels surrounding the infarcted region. It develops between days 1 and 3 and occurs in 75% or more of cortical infarcts. Meningeal enhancement overlying a cortical infarct also develops in 1 to 3 days and may be seen in about 35% of cortical infarcts. Parenchymal (gyral) enhancement comes in two forms, early intense enhancement and progressive enhancement. Early enhancement develops within the first 3 days, often within 24 hours. The more common progressive enhancement is consistently seen by day 5 and present in nearly 100% after 7 days. It may take from 1 to 6 months to resolve.

Chronic Infarcts (>1 Month). As with CT, the main findings are gliosis, encephalomalacia, wallerian degeneration, and focal atrophy. These findings are not specific and must be distinguished on the basis of history from other forms of brain injury. Enhancement usually disappears in 3 months but may last up to 6 months.

Angiographic Findings. In the acute stages, angiography may reveal small intra-arterial filling defects, branch artery occlusions, major cerebral vessel occlusions, or internal carotid or vertebral artery occlusions. Vessels adjacent to the infarct may fill retrograde via pial collaterals. Later in the course, clot lysis leads to recanalization of the occluded vessels. Reflex vasodilatation may cause a characteristic hypervascularity known as luxury perfusion at the site of infarction.

Differential Diagnosis

See Table 7–9 and Chapter 1, Cytotoxic Edema.

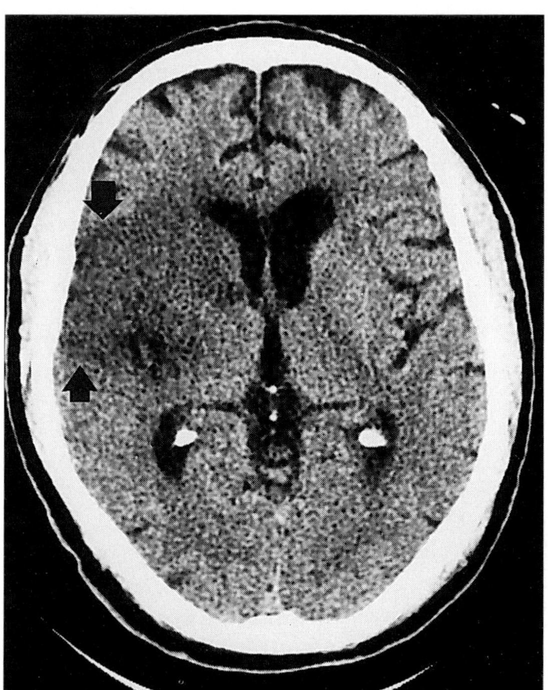

Figure 7–56. Early infarct. Axial unenhanced CT shows loss of the gray-white interface in the region between the arrows. There is also diminished attenuation in the right lentiform nuclei, insular cortex, and caudate head.

TABLE 7–9 | Etiologies of Cerebral Infarction

Hypotensive	Cardiac failure Pulmonary embolism Shock
Embolic	Endocarditis Atrial fibrillation Rheumatic heart disease
Arterial occlusive disease	Moyamoya Dissection Atherosclerosis
Secondary arterial occlusion	Cerebral edema Herniations Tumors
Venous thrombosis	Dehydration Contraceptives Pregnancy
Hematologic	Hyperviscosity states Sickle cell anemia Polycythemia vera
Arteritis	Primary angiitis Lupus erythematosus Polyarteritis nodosa
Infections	Mucormycosis Meningitis (especially tuberculosis)
Drugs	Amphetamines Cocaine Heroin

Text continued on page 339

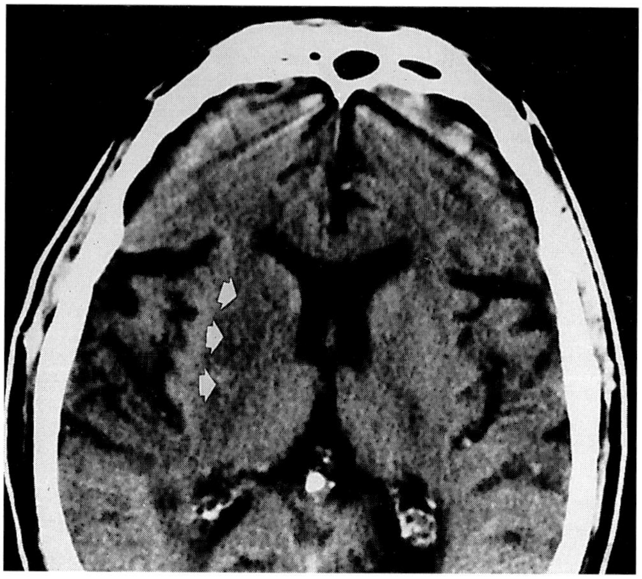

Figure 7–57. Obscuration of lentiform nucleus. Axial unenhanced CT shows diminished attenuation in the right lentiform nucleus (arrows) isodense with the internal capsule.

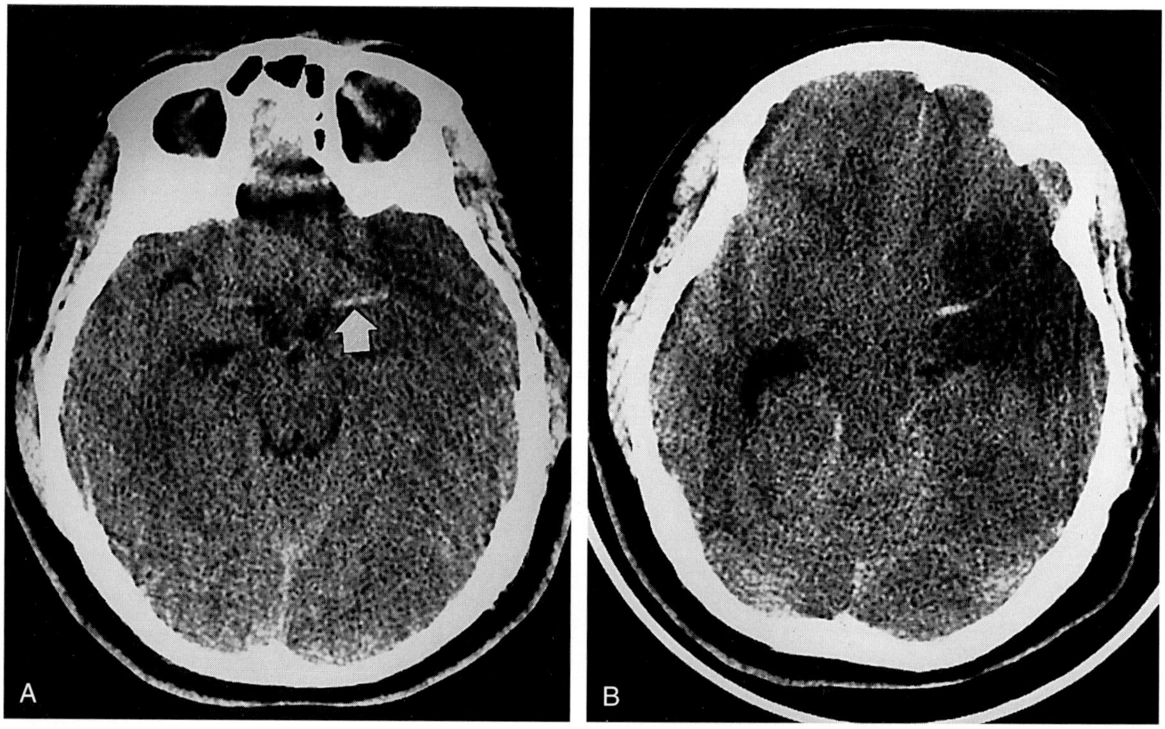

Figure 7–58. Hyperdense middle cerebral artery. **(A)** Axial unenhanced CT on the day of onset shows diminished attenuation in the left temporal lobe. The left middle cerebral artery (arrow) is hyperdense relative to the right. **(B)** On the following day the left MCA remains hyperdense and edema is much more prominent.

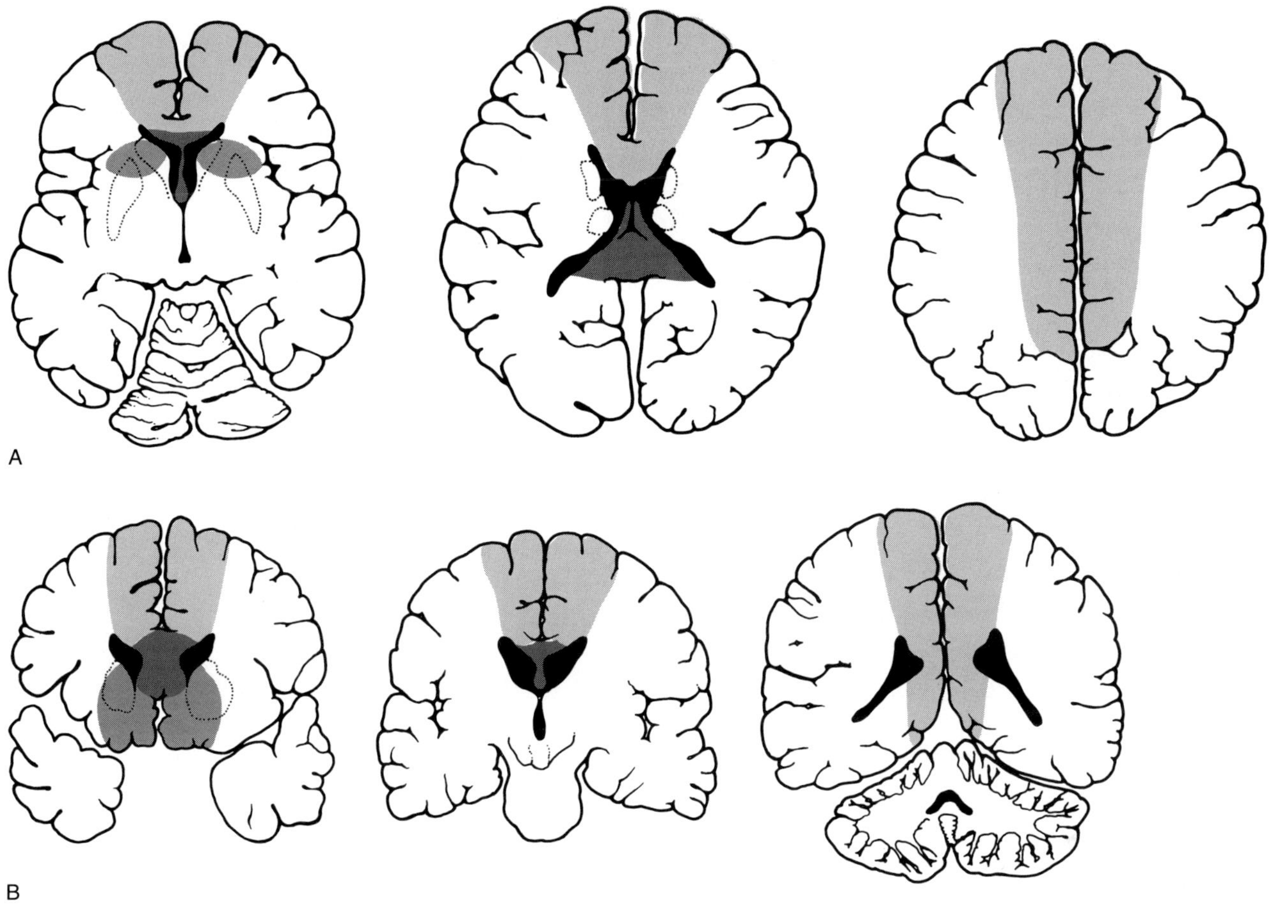

Figure 7–59. Anterior cerebral artery territory. Illustrations of **(A)** axial and **(B)** coronal sections through the brain show the pericallosal (dark shade), medial lenticulostriate (artery of Heubner) (medium shade), and hemispheric (light shade) vascular territories.

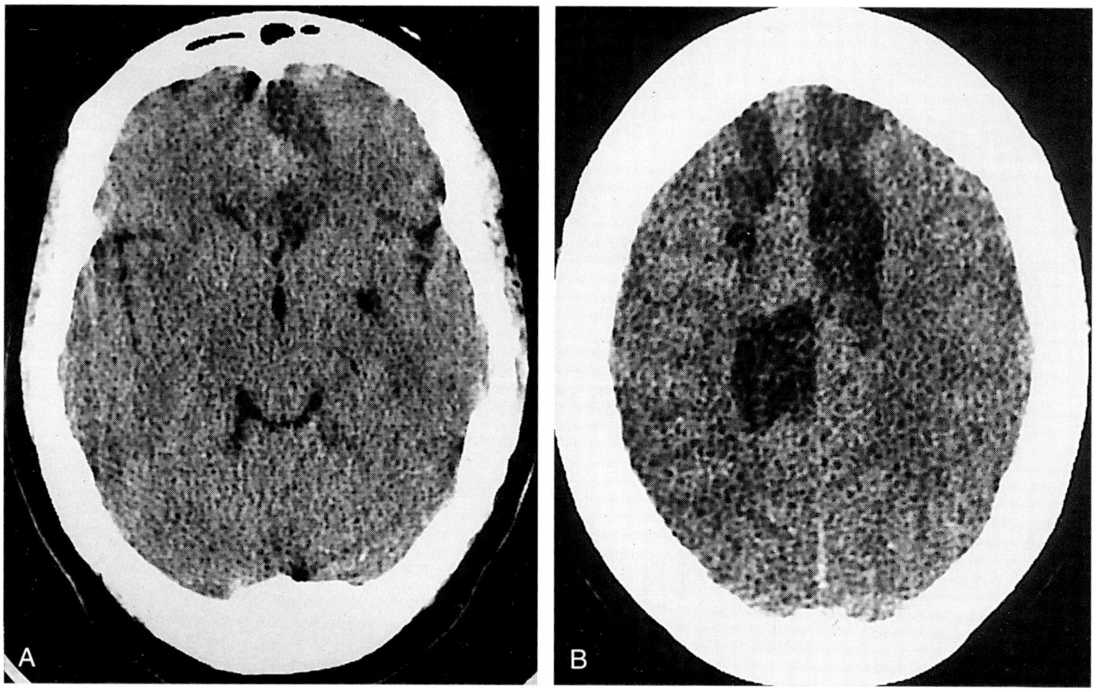

Figure 7–60. Anterior cerebral artery infarcts. Unenhanced scans **(A)** through the level of the third ventricle and **(B)** above the lateral ventricles show patchy low attenuation bilaterally conforming to the territory of the anterior cerebral arteries.

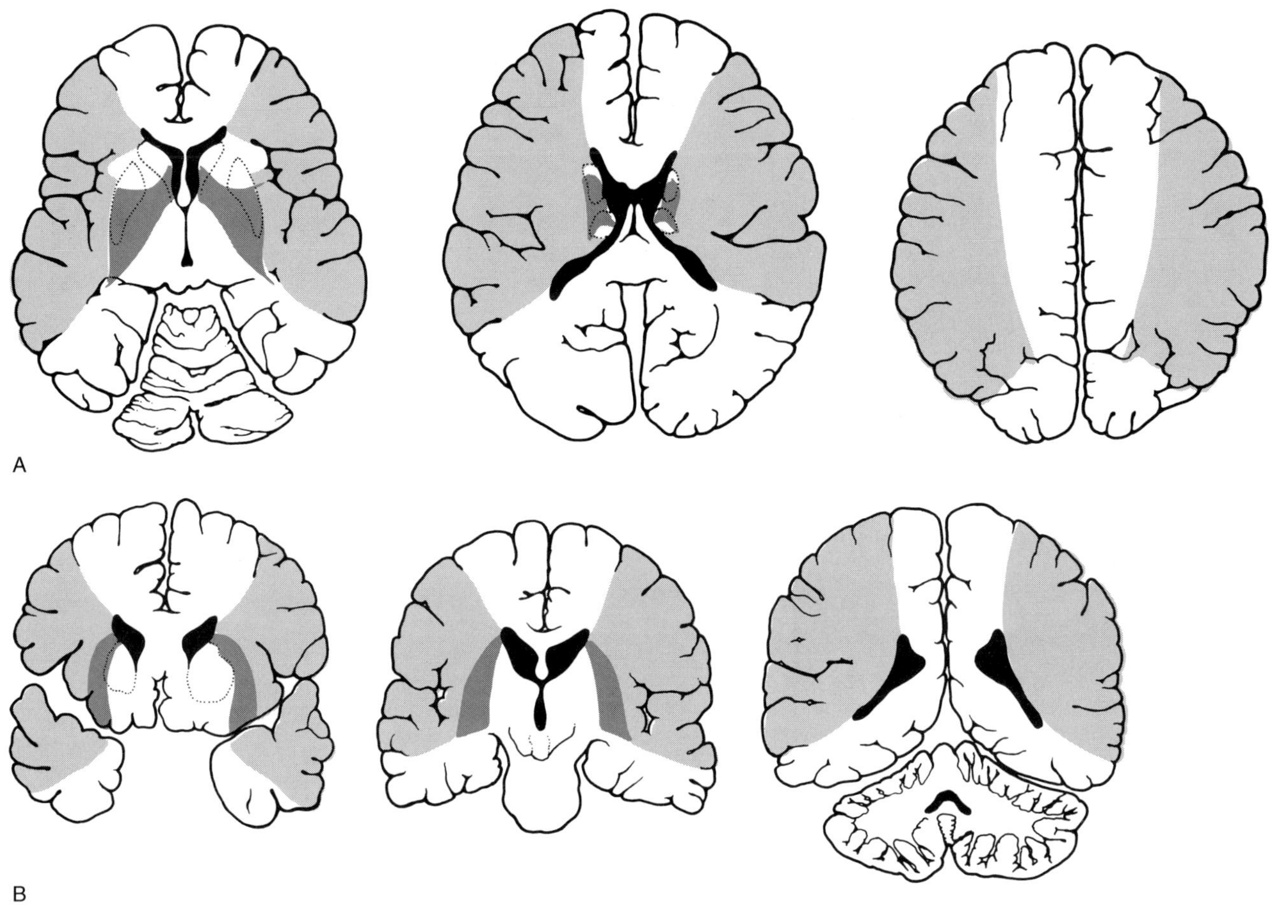

Figure 7–61. Middle cerebral artery territory. Illustrations of **(A)** axial and **(B)** coronal sections through the brain show the lateral lenticulostriate (dark shade) and hemispheric (light shade) vascular territories.

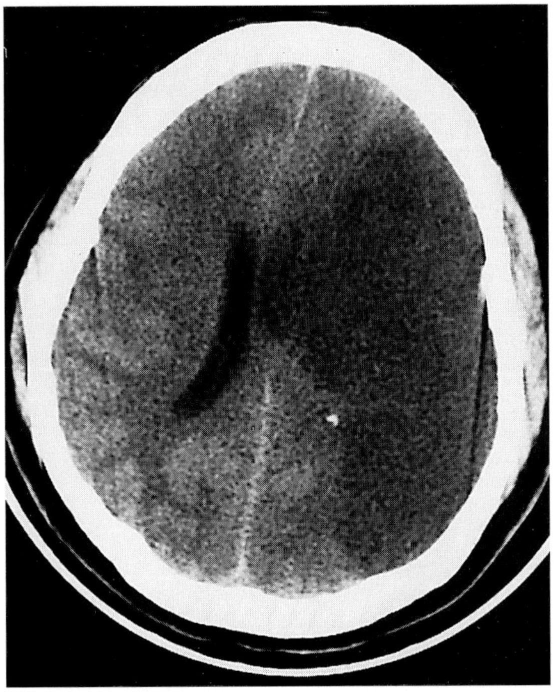

Figure 7–62. Middle cerebral artery infarct. Axial unenhanced CT shows massive edema conforming to the territory of the left middle cerebral artery. The left lateral ventricle is compressed and distorted with left to right shift.

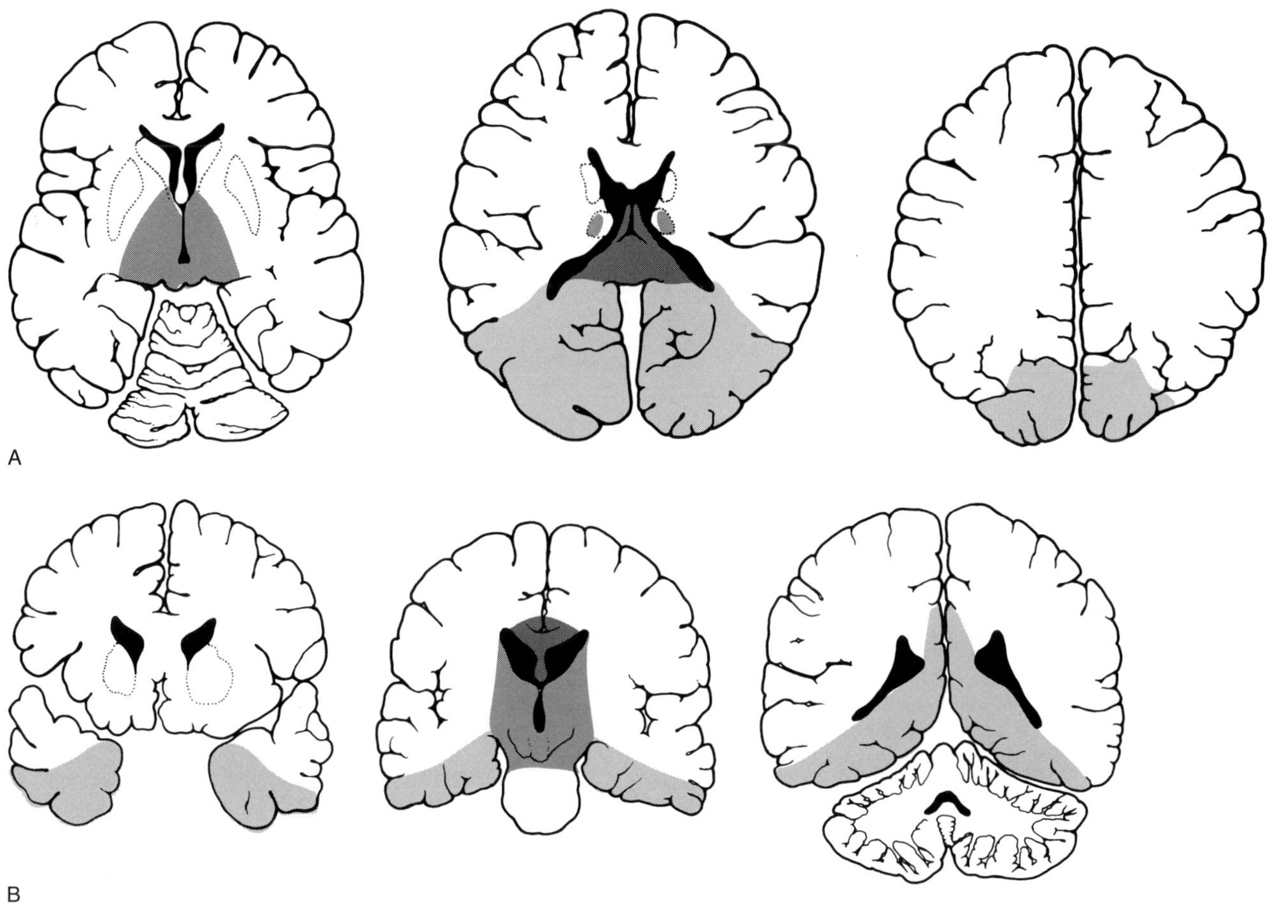

Figure 7–63. Posterior cerebral artery territory. Illustrations of **(A)** axial and **(B)** coronal sections through the brain show the splenial (callosal) (dark shade), thalamic and midbrain perforator (medium shade), and hemispheric (light shade) vascular territories.

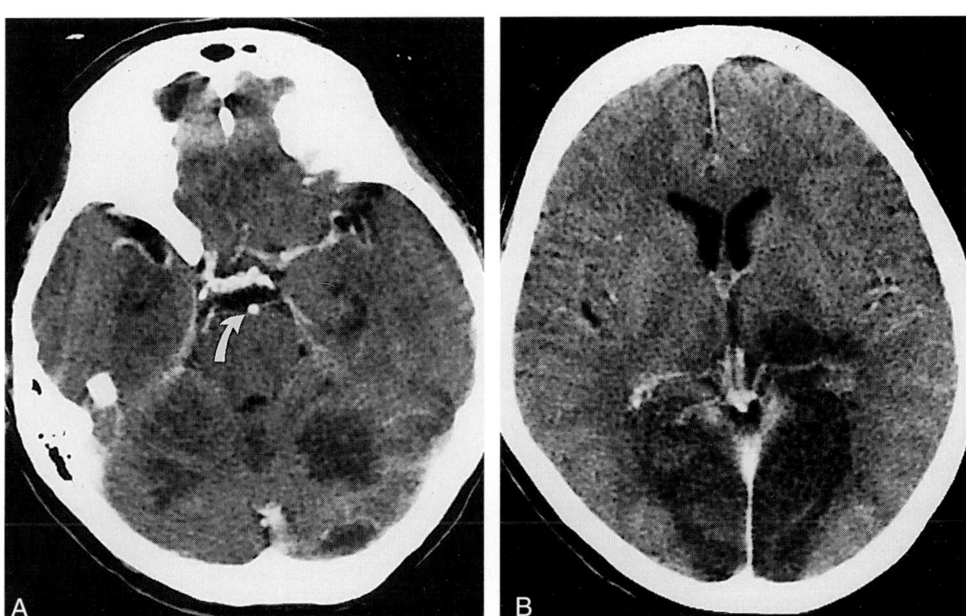

Figure 7–64. Vertebrobasilar/posterior cerebral territory infarct. **(A)** Enhanced CT shows multiple areas of infarction in the territory of both superior cerebellar arteries. The basilar artery (arrow) shows greater enhancement than the carotid branches due to sluggish flow. **(B)** Infarction is present in the left thalamus (supplied by thalamoperforators) and both posterior cerebral artery territories.

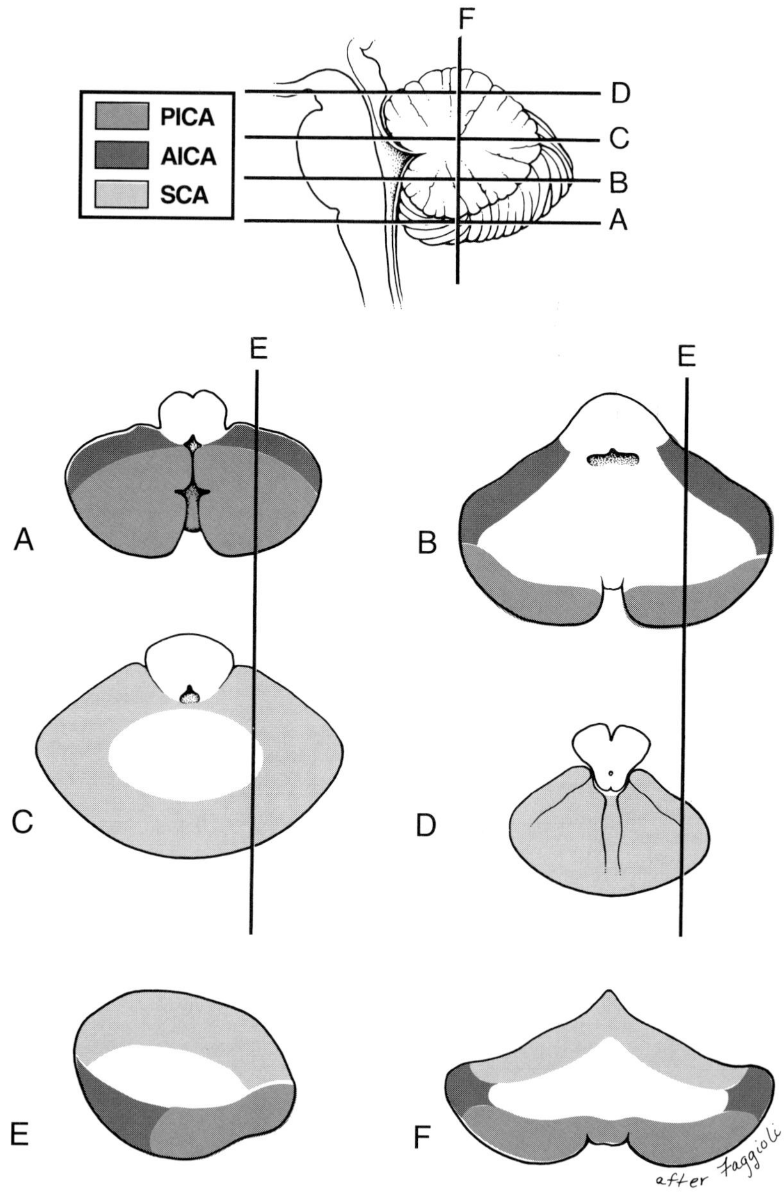

Figure 7–65. Vascular territories of the posterior fossa. Illustrations show **(A–D)** axial, **(E)** sagittal, and **(F)** coronal sections of the cerebellum and brainstem. PICA = posterior inferior cerebellar artery, AICA = anterior inferior cerebellar artery, SCA = superior cerebellar artery. The brainstem is mostly supplied by direct perforating branches of the basilar artery. Unshaded area of the cerebellum is a watershed-type area mostly supplied by the SCA.

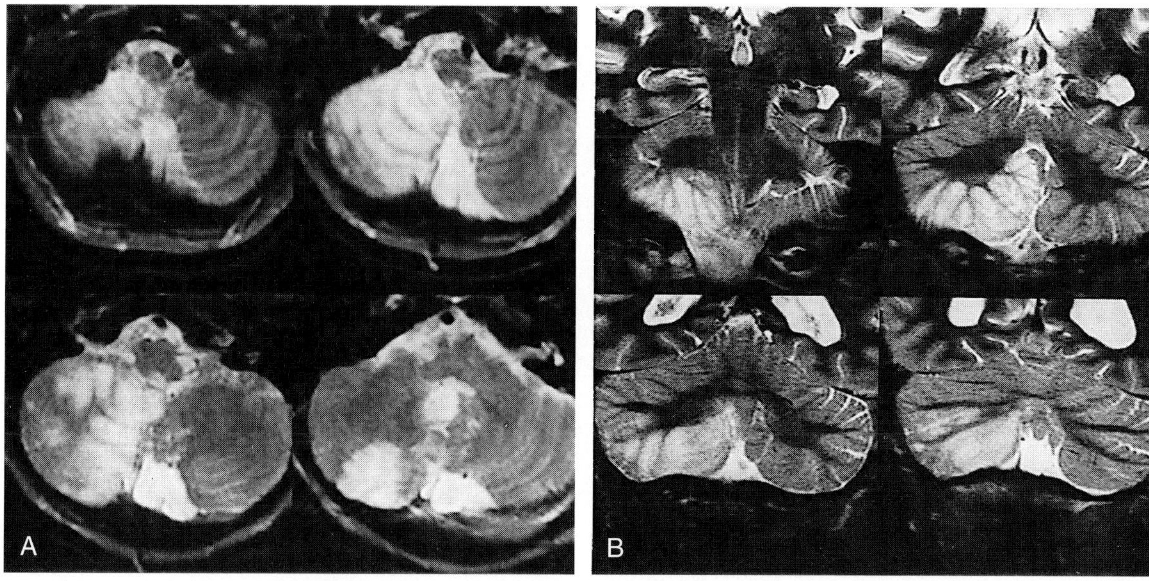

Figure 7–66. Posterior inferior cerebellar artery territory infarct. **(A)** Axial and **(B)** coronal T2-weighted MRI show hyperintense infarction in the territory of the right PICA.

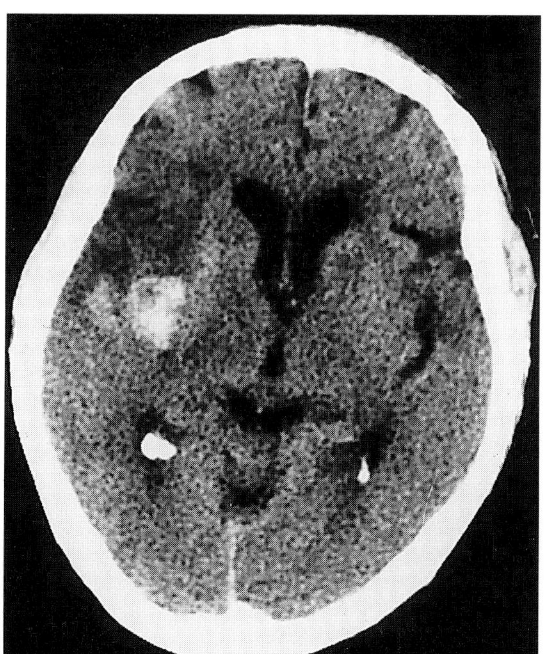

Figure 7–67. Hemorrhagic infarct. Axial unenhanced CT shows a right middle cerebral infarction with hemorrhage in the lentiform nuclei, external capsule, and insular cortex.

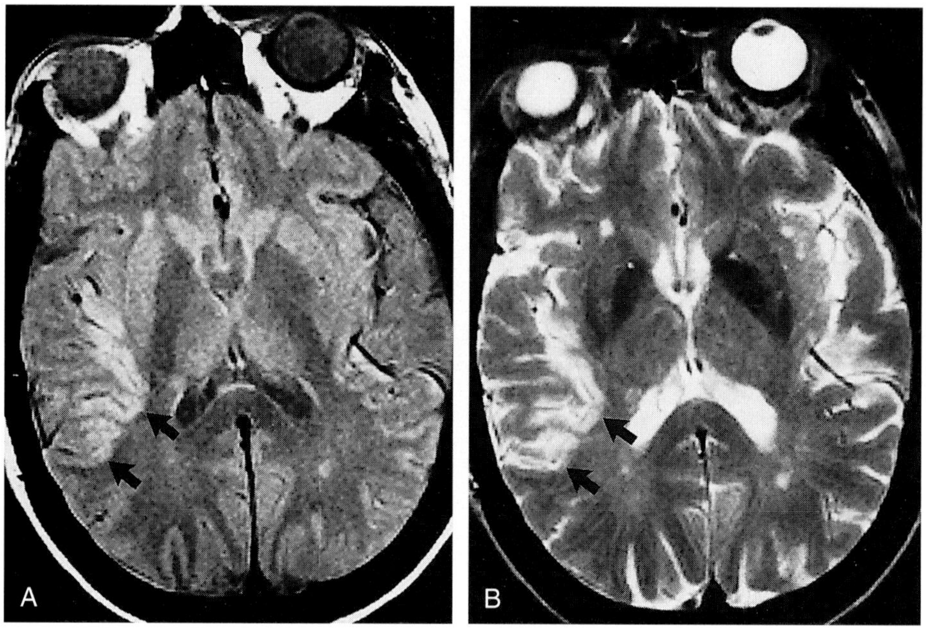

Figure 7–68. Acute infarct. **(A)** Axial PD-weighted and **(B)** T2-weighted MRI show gyral edema (arrows) of the right temporal lobe adjoining the sylvian fissure. Infarct easily could be overlooked in B. The proton-density weighted image A offers better contrast between gyral edema and CSF.

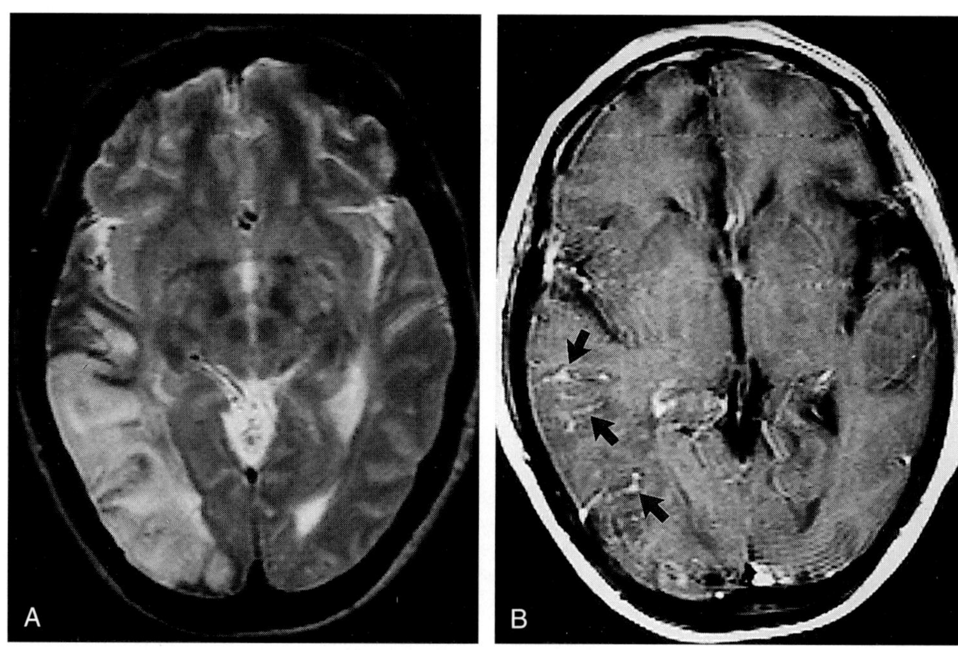

Figure 7–69. Acute infarct (intravascular enhancement sign). **(A)** Axial T2-weighted MRI shows an established infarct in the posterior right middle cerebral territory. **(B)** Axial contrast-enhanced MRI shows extensive enhancement (arrows) within the fissures due to intravascular stasis.

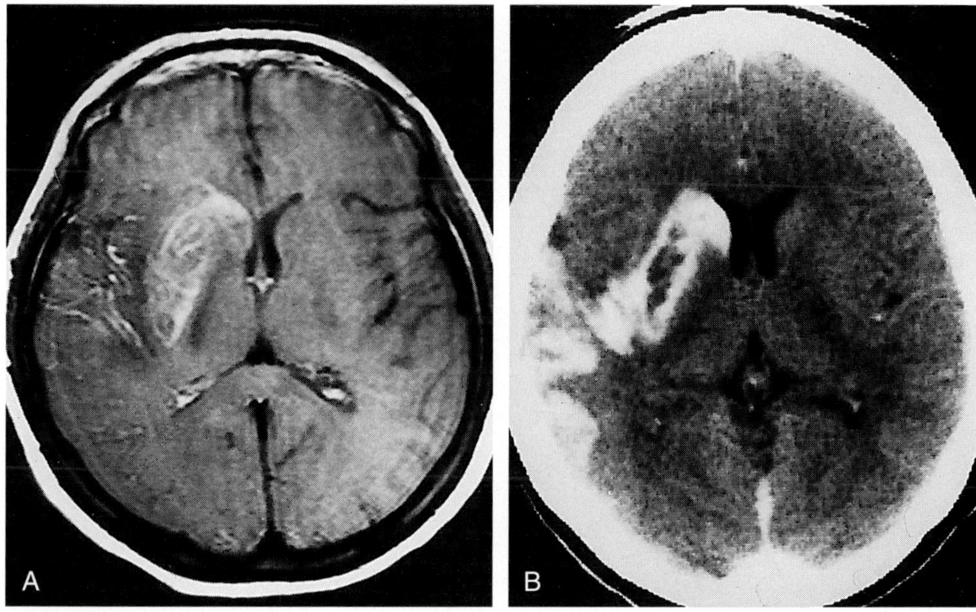

Figure 7–70. Enhancing infarct. **(A)** Axial contrast-enhanced MRI 1 day post-ictus shows intravascular enhancement in the right sylvian fissure and complex enhancement in the right basal ganglia. **(B)** Axial contrast-enhanced CT 10 days later shows solid enhancement in the right caudate head and superficial temporal gyri and ring enhancement in the right globus pallidus.

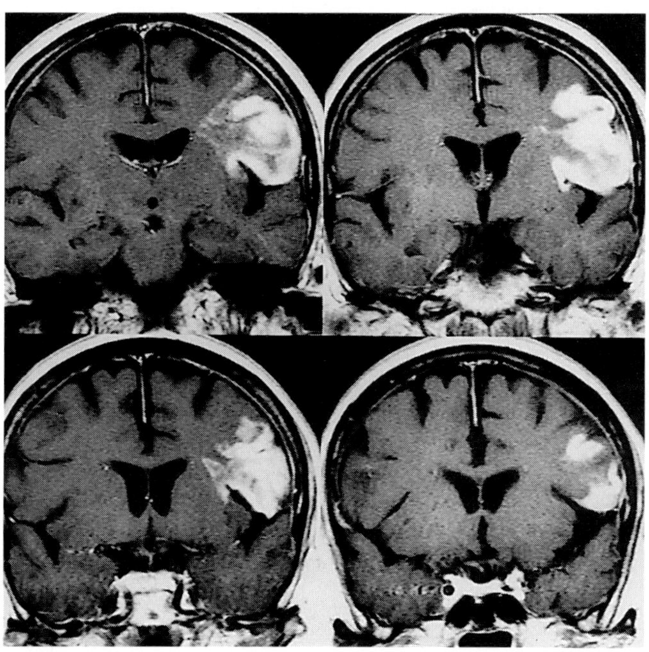

Figure 7–71. Enhancing infarct. Coronal contrast-enhanced MRI shows intense gyral enhancement of the left frontal operculum due to middle cerebral infarction.

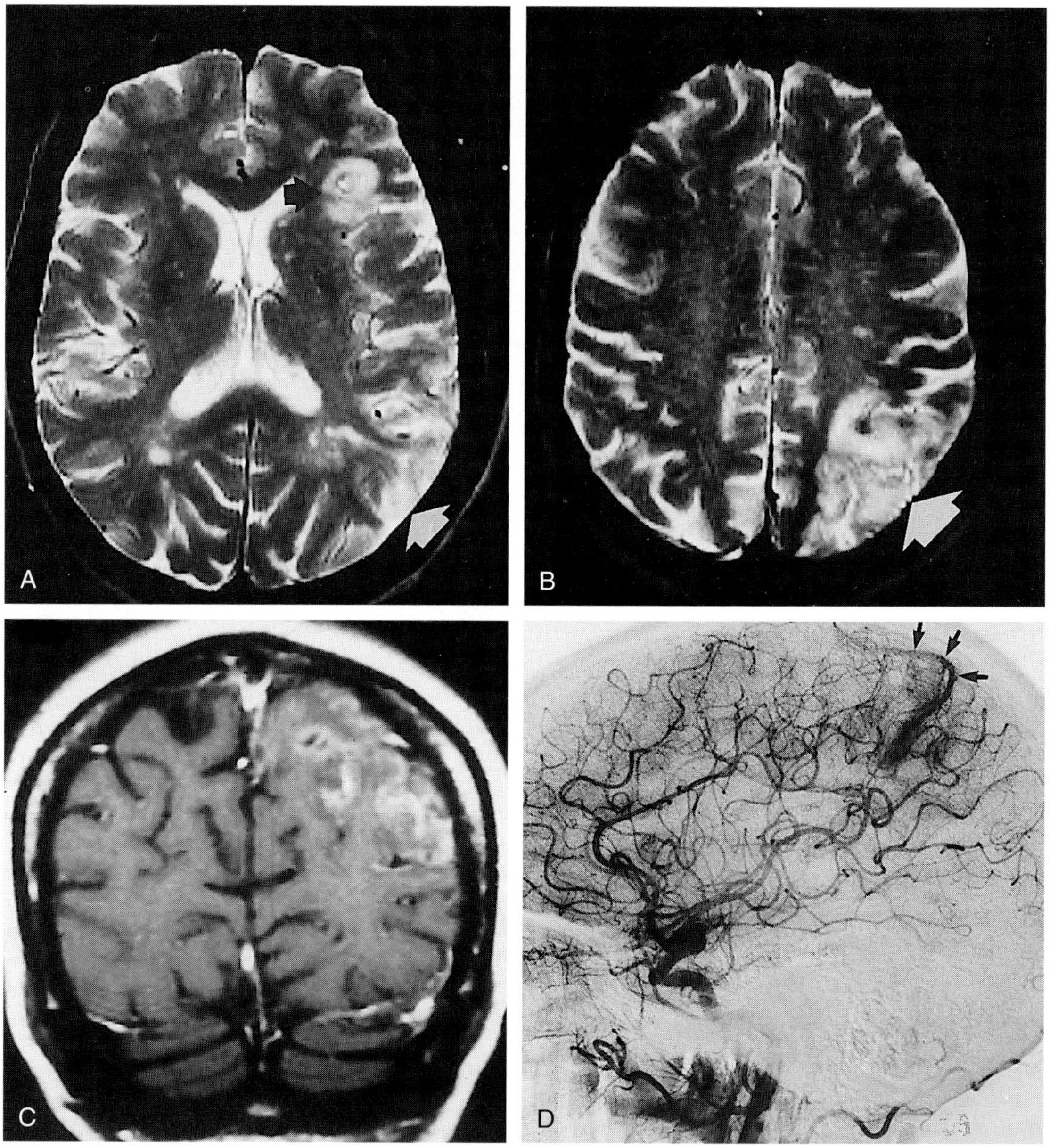

Figure 7–72. Luxury perfusion (multiple infarcts in patient with systemic lupus erythematosus). Axial T2-weighted MRI through **(A)** level of internal cerebral veins and **(B)** centrum semiovale show gyral hyperintensity (arrows) in the left frontal and right parietal lobes. **(C)** Coronal contrast-enhanced MRI shows sulcal effacement and gyral enhancement in the left parietal lobe. **(D)** Left common carotid angiogram (arterial phase) shows parietal staining with an early draining vein (arrows).

Dural Sinus Thrombosis

Occlusion of the cerebral venous sinuses may occur spontaneously without known risk factors or may occur in association with pregnancy and puerperium, use of birth control pills, severe dehydration, hypercoagulable states, or intracranial neoplasms. Cerebral venous hypertension may ensue, leading to venous infarction. The clinical presentation may include headaches, neurologic deficits, altered mental status, or seizures. The symptoms and extent of injury tend to be more severe with occlusion of the superior sagittal or dominant transverse sinus.

CT Findings. Numerous CT findings have been described, including:

- The cord sign—a hyperdense cortical vein on an unenhanced scan.
- The dense vein sign—deep cerebral veins appear enhanced (are dense) on an unenhanced scan.
- The empty delta sign—enhancement of the walls of the sagittal sinus with central hypodensity (filling defect).
- Focal or generalized edema.
- Hemorrhagic infarcts (especially parasagittal).
- Dilated enhanced medullary veins.
- Increased gyral enhancement.
- Increased tentorial enhancement.

The accuracy of CT is quite limited since each of these signs occurs only in a minority and the scan is often completely normal at the time of presentation.

MRI Findings. Routine MRI may show the following:

- Increased signal in venous sinuses due to thrombus. The intraluminal signal intensity varies as a function of age of the clot (see Chapter 1).
- Cortical hyperintensity on T2-weighted images due to edema.
- Dilated medullary veins.
- An intraluminal filling defect or delta sign on contrast-enhanced scans.

The ability of MRI to depict flow (MR angiography) makes it uniquely suited to the noninvasive diagnosis of sinus thrombosis, although not without numerous pitfalls. At present, diagnostic accuracy may be maximized by the use of intravenous contrast with time-of-flight techniques or phase contrast techniques that are especially sensitive to slow flow.

Angiographic Findings. Angiography reveals slow flow with a delayed venous phase and lack of filling of the thrombosed sinus with rerouting of venous drainage to alternate pathways, usually the deep venous system. A filling defect within the sinus is occasionally visible but may be more consistently demonstrated by direct venography.

Differential Diagnosis

See Tables 7–10 and 7–11.

TABLE 7–10 Differential Diagnosis of the Empty Delta Sign

Thrombosis
High splitting of sagittal sinus
Epidural abscess
Arachnoid cyst
Subdural hematoma
Subarachnoid hemorrhage
Delayed scanning following contrast administration (greater than 30 minutes)

TABLE 7–11 Differential Diagnosis of Increased Intravascular Signal on MRI

Thrombosis
Flow-related enhancement (T1 and gradient echo techniques)
Even echo rephasing
Diastolic pseudogating
Use of flow compensation techniques

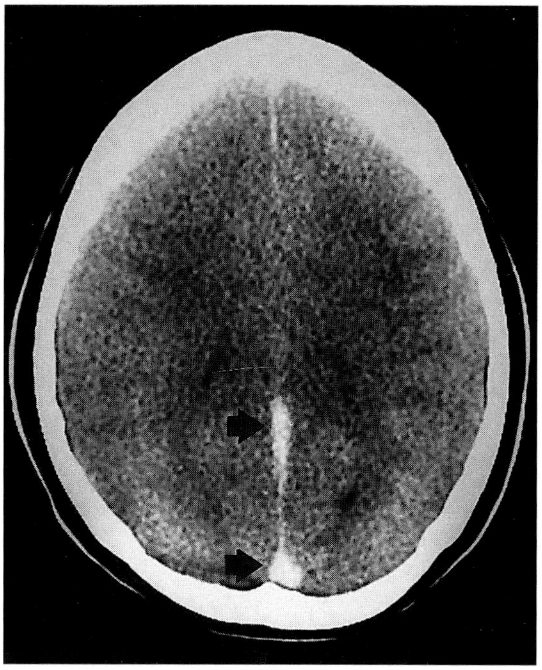

Figure 7–73. Straight sinus thrombosis (dense vein sign). Axial unenhanced CT shows high attenuation (arrows) in the straight and sagittal sinuses.

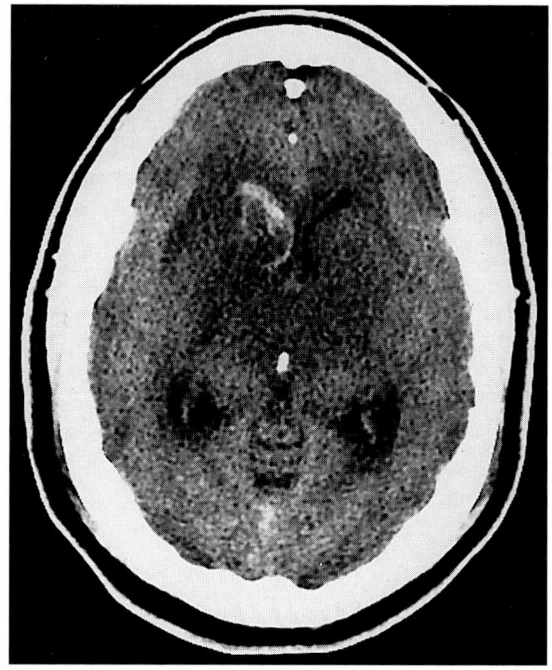

Figure 7–74. Internal cerebral thrombosis (venous infarction). Unenhanced CT shows bilateral thalamic, lentiform, and frontal white matter edema with hemorrhage in the right caudate head.

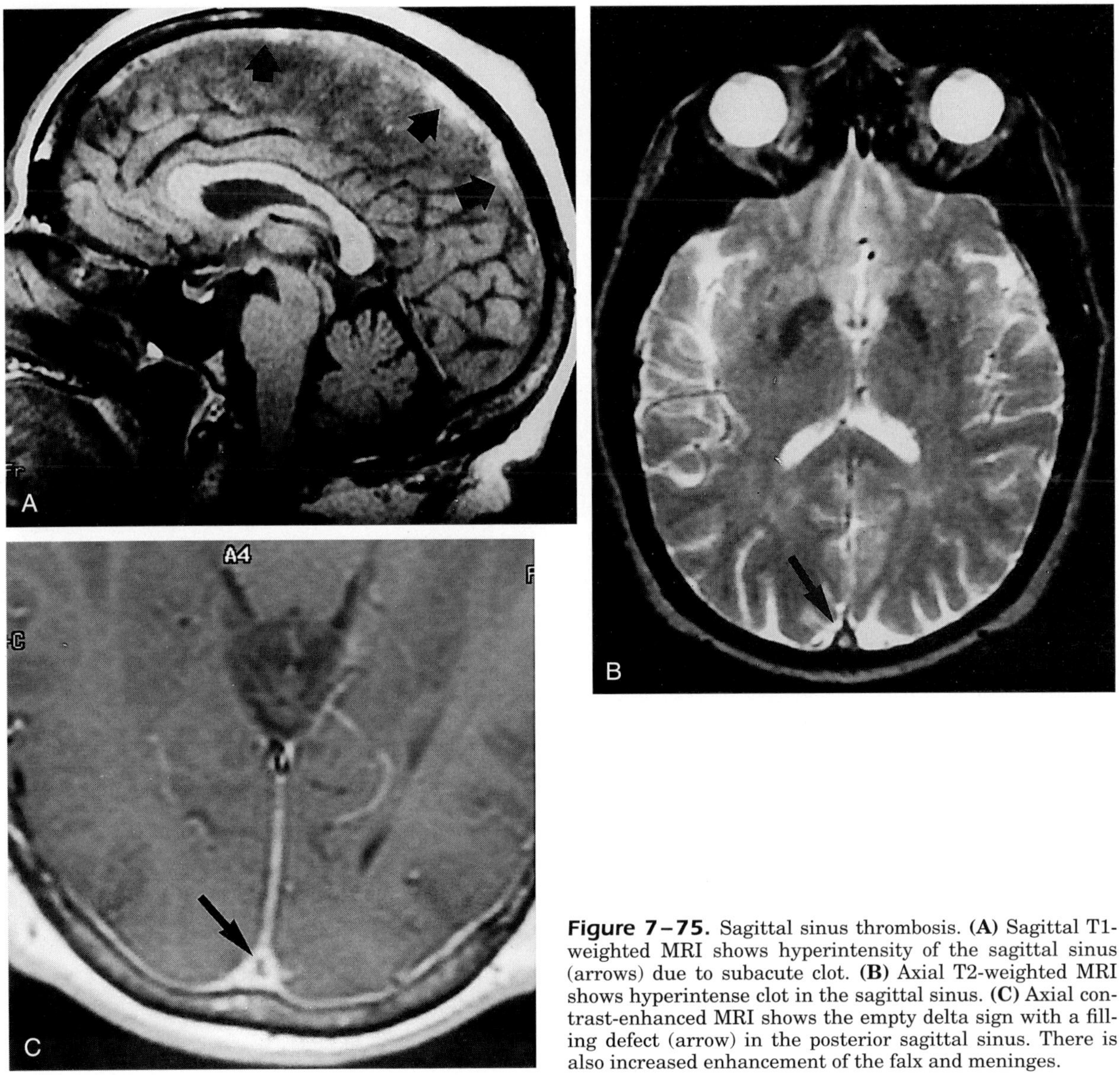

Figure 7–75. Sagittal sinus thrombosis. **(A)** Sagittal T1-weighted MRI shows hyperintensity of the sagittal sinus (arrows) due to subacute clot. **(B)** Axial T2-weighted MRI shows hyperintense clot in the sagittal sinus. **(C)** Axial contrast-enhanced MRI shows the empty delta sign with a filling defect (arrow) in the posterior sagittal sinus. There is also increased enhancement of the falx and meninges.

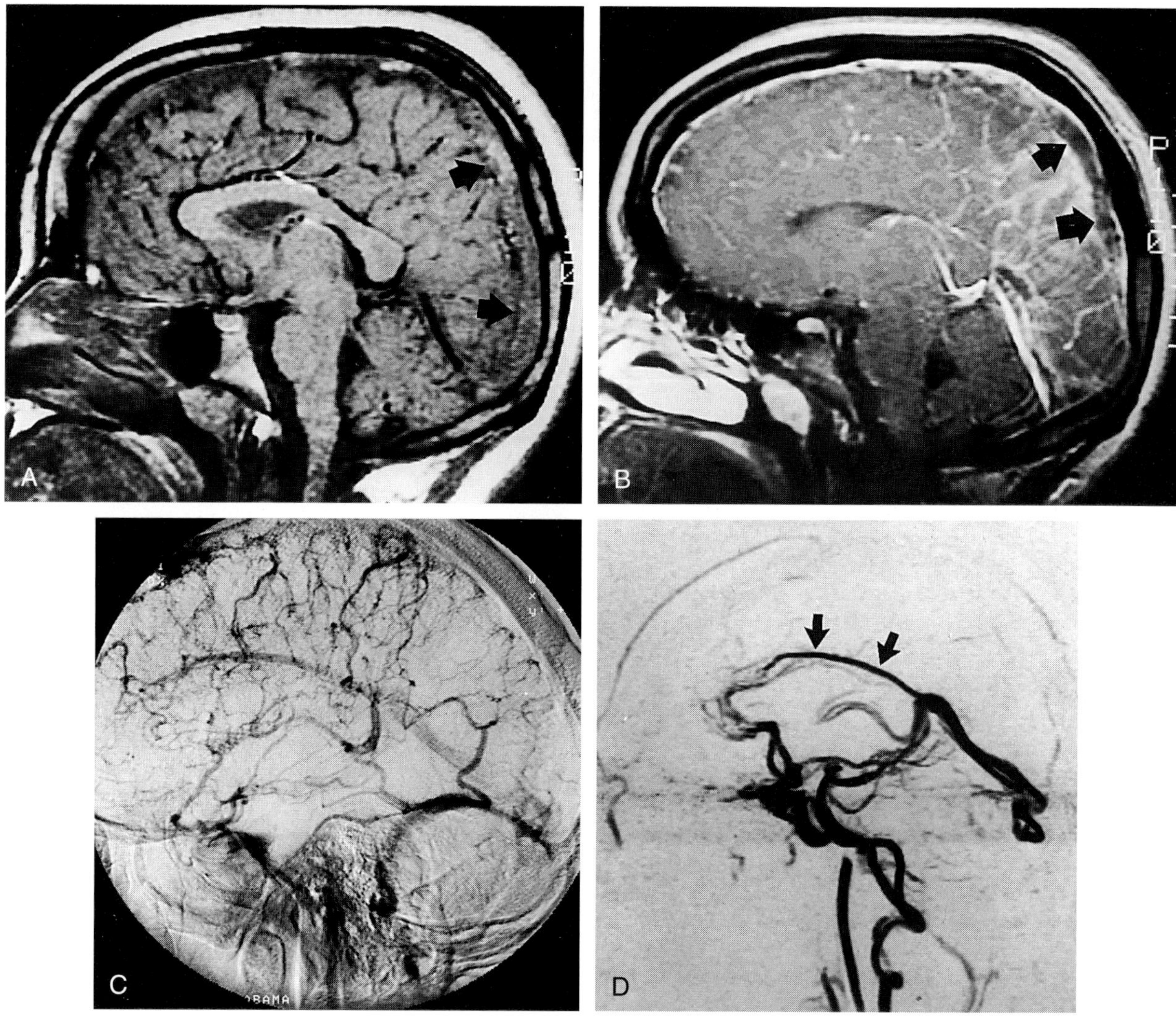

Figure 7–76. Sagittal sinus thrombosis. **(A)** Sagittal T1-weighted MRI shows isointense and mildly hyperintense clot (arrows) in the superior sagittal sinus. **(B)** Contrast-enhanced scan shows a long filling defect (arrows) of the superior sagittal sinus and increased enhancement in the posterior falx. **(C)** Internal carotid angiogram (late venous phase) shows stasis of contrast in frontal and parietal cortical veins with nonfilling of the superior sagittal sinus. **(D)** Phase-contrast MRI angiogram (sagittal projection) shows no signal from the superior sagittal sinus due to absence of flow. Deep venous drainage occurs via the inferior sagittal sinus (arrows) to the straight sinus.

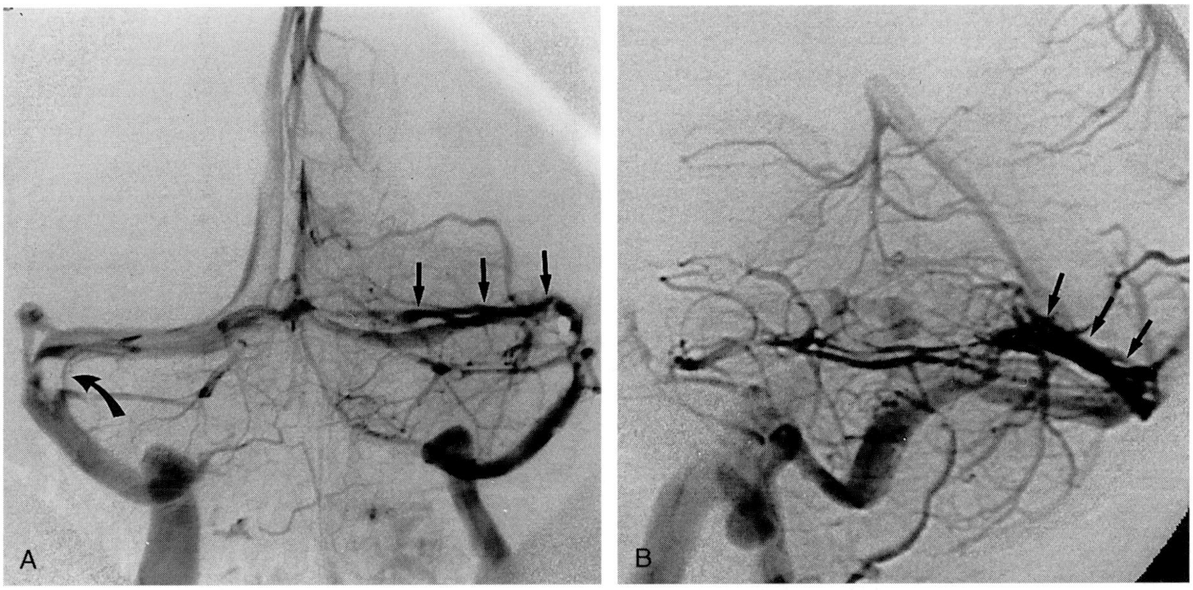

Figure 7–77. Veno-occlusive disease (patient with bilateral temporal lobe hemorrhages). **(A)** Anteroposterior and **(B)** lateral vertebral angiograms (venous phase) show severe stenosis at the juncture of right transverse and sigmoid sinuses (curved arrow). Venous collaterals (straight arrows) above the occluded left transverse sinus are densely opacified due to sluggish drainage into the left sigmoid sinus.

Traumatic

Carotid Cavernous Fistula

The carotid cavernous fistula (CCF) is an infrequent complication of a blunt head injury in which there is a laceration of the intracavernous carotid artery with a direct fistula to the cavernous sinus. Most patients present with pulsatile tinnitus and severe chemosis and proptosis. It may cause palsies of the third, fourth, and sixth cranial nerves. Sequelae of a high-flow CCF include irreversible vision loss due to elevated intraocular pressure, epistaxis, which may be fatal, and cerebral infarction or hemorrhage. The treatment of choice is embolization with detachable balloons.

CT Findings. CT may show an enlarged cavernous sinus that enhances intensely, dilated orbital veins, and proptosis. Related skull base fractures are common and may be a clue to the diagnosis. CT may also show complications such as major vessel infarcts, intracerebral hematoma, or subarachnoid hemorrhage.

MRI Findings. MRI shows an enlarged cavernous sinus with signal void reflecting rapid flow. Proptosis and enlarged orbital veins may be seen. Sections through the sella may show dilated transsellar vascular channels representing venous communications between the two cavernous sinuses.

Angiographic Findings. Angiography shows rapid filling of the cavernous sinus directly from the cavernous internal carotid artery with drainage usually via the superior ophthalmic veins, inferior petrosal veins, and pterygoid plexus. Retrograde drainage to the cortical veins may occur and is an ominous sign. Selective injection of the ipsilateral vertebral artery during compression or temporary occlusion of the affected carotid is particularly helpful in identifying the precise site of the fistula.

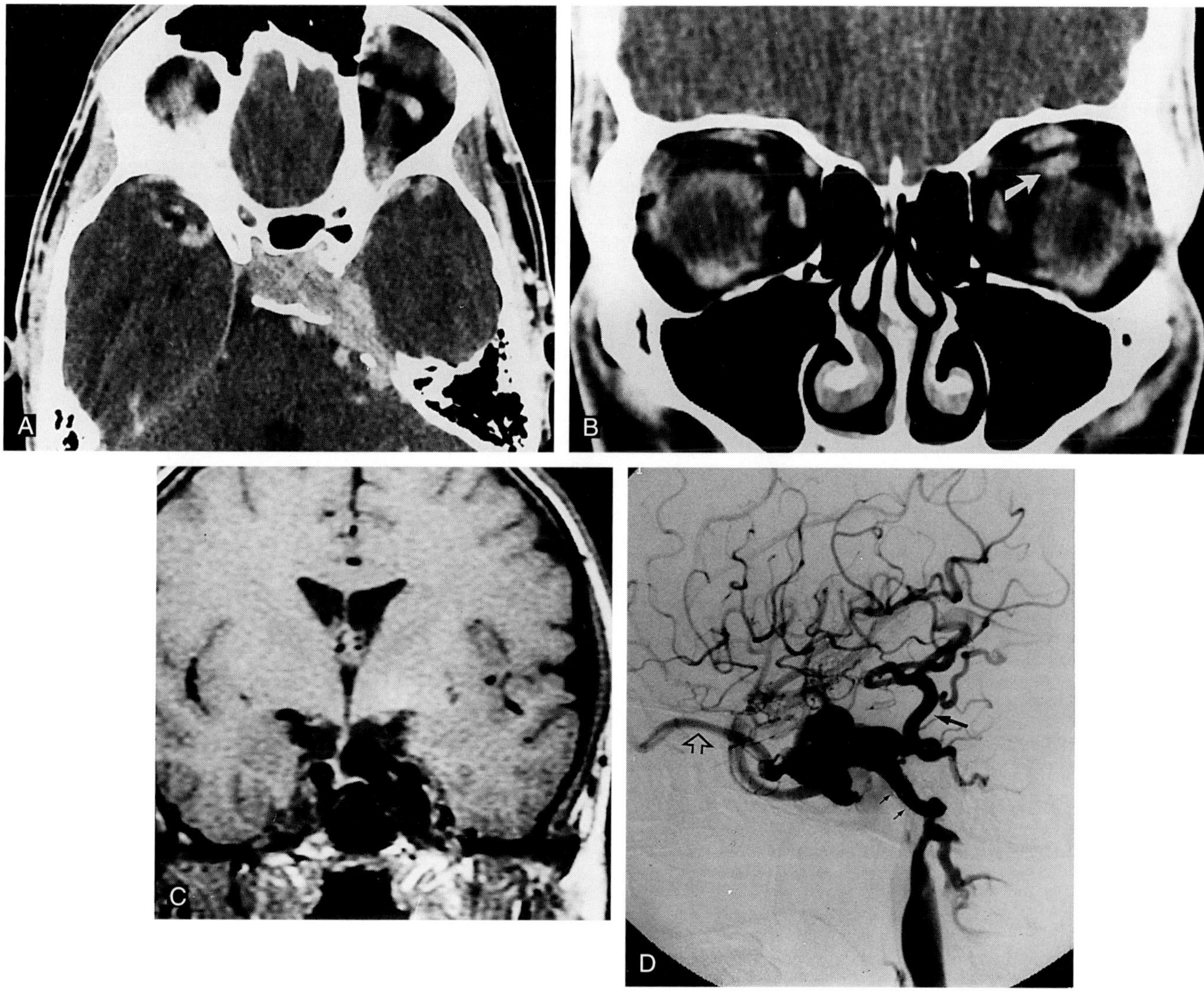

Figure 7–78. Carotid-cavernous fistula. **(A)** Axial contrast-enhanced CT shows an enlarged and enhancing left cavernous sinus with dilated cortical and ophthalmic veins. **(B)** Coronal contrast-enhanced CT shows the dilated left ophthalmic vein (arrow). **(C)** Coronal T1-weighted MRI shows massively enlarged left cavernous sinus bulging into the sella and complete absence of signal due to rapid flow. **(D)** Lateral internal carotid angiogram (early arterial phase) shows shunting of blood to the cavernous sinus. Drainage occurs anteriorly to the ophthalmic vein (open arrow), inferiorly via the inferior petrosal sinus (small arrows), and posteriorly to cortical veins (large arrow).

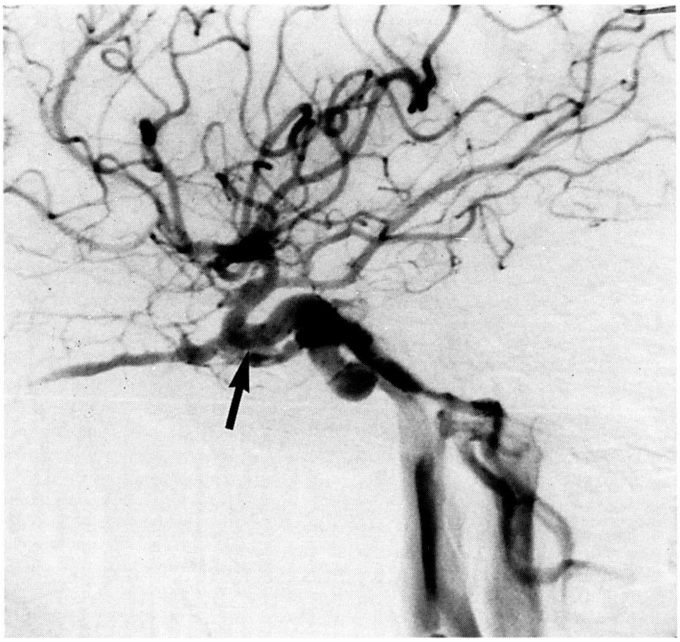

Figure 7–79. Carotid cavernous fistula. Lateral internal carotid angiogram shows precise point of the fistula (arrow). Drainage is anterior to the ophthalmic vein and posterior to the petrosal sinus.

Other Traumatic Vascular Injuries

Both blunt and penetrating trauma to the neck may result in a variety of injuries to the common, internal, and external carotid and the vertebral arteries. Such patients initially present with absent pulse, hematoma, bruit, or neurologic deficit. Any new, delayed, or unexplained neurologic deficit in a trauma victim should prompt consideration of immediate angiography. Any of these injuries may lead to cerebral infarction, although many resolve spontaneously and without incident.

Intimal Tear

Angiographic Findings. An intimal tear is recognized by the presence of a small, often linear intraluminal filling defect projecting from the vessel wall. The formation of thrombus may lead to an even larger convex filling defect. Intimal tears usually resolve spontaneously. The greatest risk is from embolization of associated thrombus.

Dissection

MRI Findings. MRI may show narrowing or occlusion of the vascular lumen, seen as diminution or absence of the normal flow void. Slow flow may produce a train track appearance with bright signal from the periphery of the lumen and central flow void. Abnormal signal due to thrombus may be present in the wall, with the nature of the signal abnormality dependent upon the age of the thrombus.

Angiographic Findings. Angiography reveals tapered narrowing or occlusion of the vessel and typically intimal irregularity in the nearby patent segments. A visible intimal flap or filling of both true and false lumens are specific but rare findings. Associated pseudoaneurysms are frequently present. Dissection may also occur spontaneously in the absence of trauma.

Causes of spontaneous dissection:

- Fibromuscular dysplasia
- Hypertension
- Migraine
- Drug abuse
- Marfan's syndrome

Pseudoaneurysm

CT Findings. Dynamic contrast-enhanced CT shows a mass adjacent to the carotid or vertebral artery that enhances at the same time and to the same degree as the adjacent vessel lumen.

MRI Findings. MRI shows a mass adjacent to the carotid or vertebral artery with signs of flow. The signal is variable depending on the plane of section, pulse sequence, direction of flow, and other factors.

Angiographic Findings. Angiography shows extravasation of contrast beyond the confines of the vessel wall to fill a space that may range from quite small to large, complex, and multilobular. In the larger pseudoaneurysms, contrast may persist for several minutes following injection.

Arteriovenous Fistula

Angiographic Findings. Direct arteriovenous fistulas may arise from the carotid or vertebral arteries and are usually due to penetrating trauma. Angiography shows direct filling of adjacent enlarged veins from the proximal arterial trunk. The carotid usually shunts to the jugular veins, and the vertebral artery shunts to the deep cervical muscular veins and paravertebral venous plexus. Muscular branches of the external carotid and cervical branches of the subclavian artery may also supply these fistulas. Spontaneous arteriovenous fistulas, particularly from the vertebral artery, may occur in patients with neurofibromatosis.

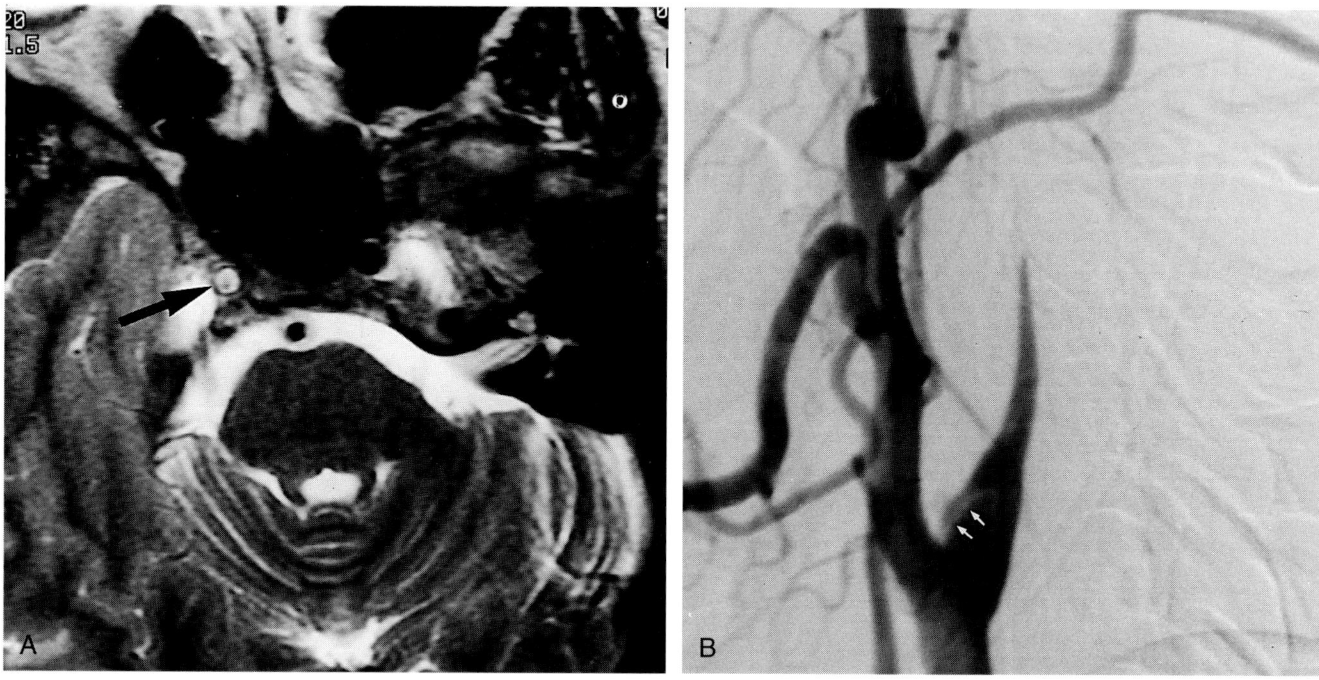

Figure 7–80. Internal carotid dissection. **(A)** Axial T2-weighted MRI shows hyperintense thrombus in the right internal carotid artery (arrow). **(B)** Lateral common carotid angiogram shows a tapered occlusion of the proximal internal carotid artery. An intimal flap is indicated by the arrows.

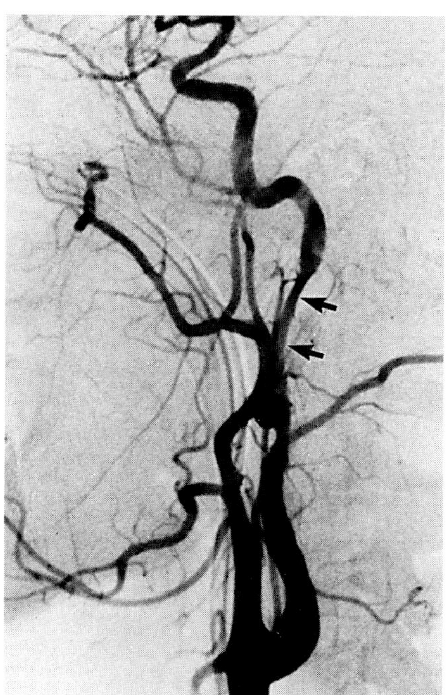

Figure 7–81. Internal carotid dissection. Lateral common carotid angiogram shows a long tapered narrowing (arrows) of the internal carotid artery without occlusion.

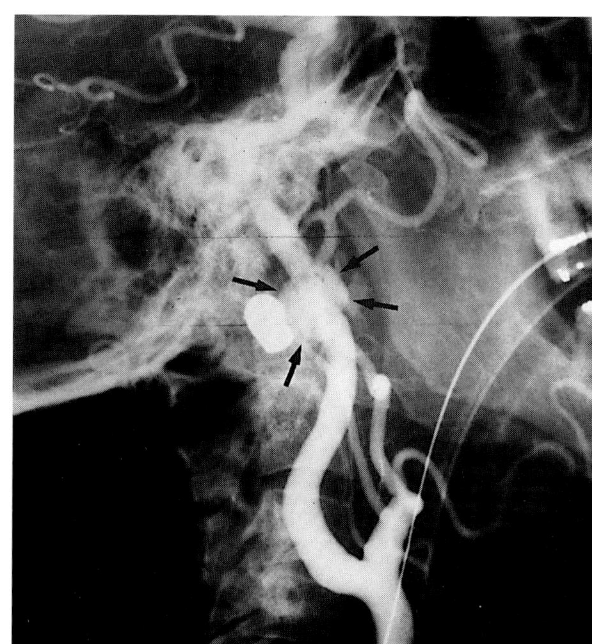

Figure 7–82. Traumatic pseudoaneurysm. Lateral common carotid angiogram. A bullet is superimposed on the odontoid process. Extravasated contrast surrounds the internal carotid artery at this level.

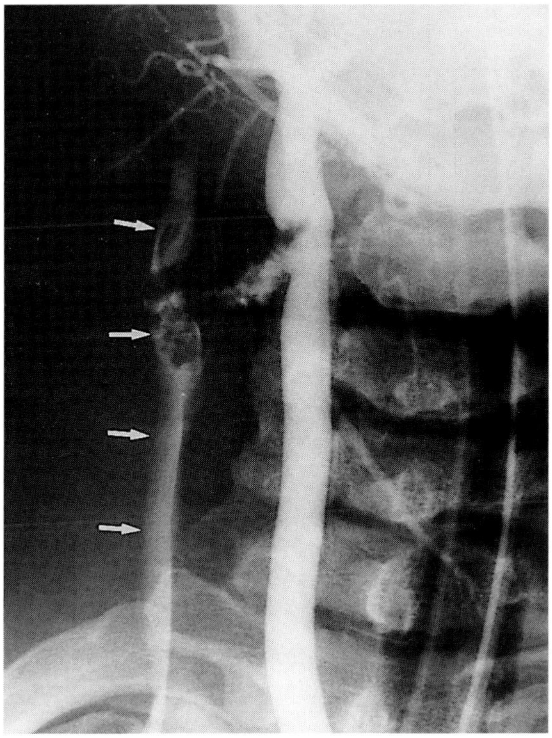

Figure 7–83. Carotid-jugular fistula. There is a laceration of the right common carotid artery with a fistula producing early opacification of the right jugular vein (arrows).

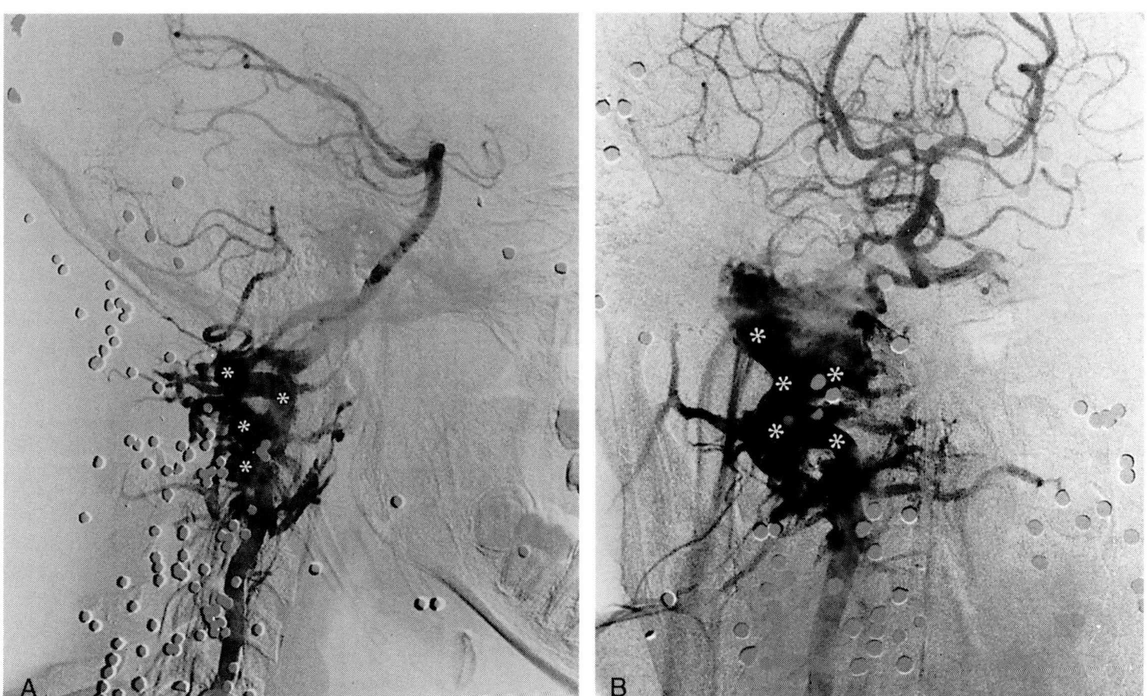

Figure 7–84. Post-traumatic fistula (shotgun injury). **(A)** Lateral and **(B)** AP left vertebral angiograms show extensive shunting from the vertebral artery (asterisks) to deep muscular veins and the paravertebral venous plexus.

Miscellaneous

Vasculitis

CNS vasculitis is a component of many disease processes with varying pathologies and clinical presentations. The common denominator in all is an inflammatory reaction in the vessel walls, especially arterial, with progressive narrowing, occlusion, and secondary infarction. In some conditions, angiography may reveal the primary vascular abnormality, whereas imaging studies in others reveal only the secondary changes of ischemia. Steroid treatment, especially in primary angiitis, may lead to resolution of the vascular abnormalities.

TABLE 7–12 Etiologies of CNS Vasculitis

Condition	Comments
Primary angiitis (granulomatous angiitis)	Affects vessels 200–500 microns in diameter Angiography usually abnormal Cerebral infarcts and hemorrhage No involvement outside CNS
Lupus erythematosus	Angiographically undetectable Affects vessels <100 microns in diameter Atrophy, infarcts, or hemorrhage
Polyarteritis nodosa	Most common systemic vasculitis to affect the CNS CNS affected in 46% of cases
Radiation therapy	A late complication of radiotherapy (years) Affects small and medium-size arteries
Giant cell arteritis (temporal arteritis)	Usually affects temporal artery Intracranial involvement rare
Bacterial meningitis	Tuberculosis and *Haemophilus influenzae* major offending agents Affects arteries at base of brain
Sarcoidosis	Vasculitis rarely encountered Meningeal enhancement on MRI
Drug abuse	Methamphetamine, heroin, and cocaine Angiography may show spasm, narrowing, occlusions, beading, and aneurysms
Behçet's disease	Oral and genital ulcers and multiorgan disease Foci of hyperintensity in brainstem, basal ganglia, thalami, and cerebral hemispheres (T2-weighted MRI) Angiography usually normal

TABLE 7–13 Differential Diagnosis of Segmental Arterial Narrowing

Atherosclerosis
Subarachnoid hemorrhage-induced vasospasm
Vasculitis
Intravenous drug abuse (spasm)
Fibromuscular dysplasia
Neoplasm

CT Findings. CT cannot directly demonstrate the vascular narrowing that is the hallmark of the disease. Typically CT shows the secondary changes of infarction, which may be single or multiple, hemorrhagic or nonhemorrhagic, acute or chronic, and may encompass gray or white matter or both.

MRI Findings. The MRI findings are the same as those for CT but with higher sensitivity for ischemic changes of the deep white matter and posterior fossa. MR angiography currently lacks sufficient spatial resolution to make the diagnosis of vasculitis. Neither CT nor MRI is sufficiently specific to allow a diagnosis of vasculitis, although in a patient with systemic disease, such as lupus, the diagnosis of CNS vasculitis may be inferred with relatively high probability.

Angiographic Findings. With many vasculitides of the CNS, angiography is almost always normal. This is usually because the vessels affected are too small to be seen angiographically. If abnormal, angiography may reveal either cerebral artery narrowing or abnormal focal arterial dilatation. The arterial narrowing may be proximal or distal, focal or diffuse, and smooth or irregular. Alternating areas of narrowing and dilatation are referred to as the "string of beads" sign.

Differential Diagnosis

See Tables 7–12 and 7–13.

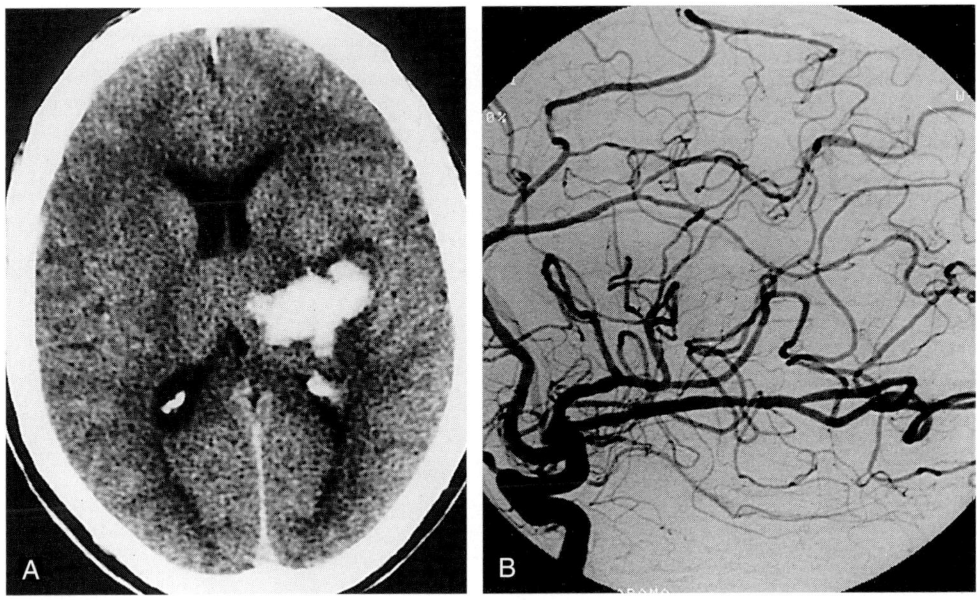

Figure 7–85. Primary angiitis. **(A)** Axial unenhanced CT shows acute hemorrhage in the left thalamus. **(B)** Lateral internal carotid angiogram reveals extensive irregularity of the intracranial vasculature.

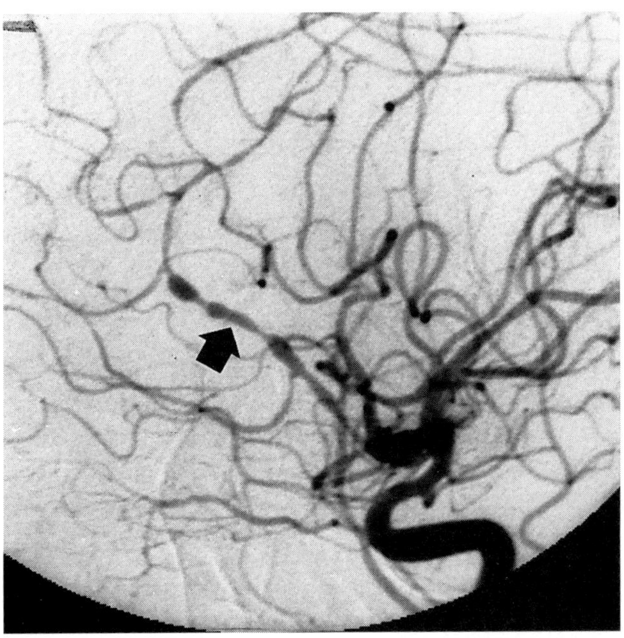

Figure 7–86. Vasculitis. Lateral internal carotid angiogram shows a classic string of beads sign in the anterior cerebral artery (arrow).

Spontaneous Hemorrhage

Primary intracerebral hemorrhage accounts for approximately 10% of all strokes, with an annual incidence in the United States of 15 to 30 cases per 100,000 population. The 30-day mortality rate is approximately 50%. Hypertension is the leading risk factor. Although usually associated with hemorrhage into the basal ganglia or thalamus, hypertension may cause hemorrhage anywhere within the brain. There are many other associated risk factors, such as age, alcohol consumption, and anticoagulants.

Imaging Findings. Either CT or MRI may be employed in the initial detection of primary hemorrhage. The imaging findings of intracerebral hematoma are complex and dependent on time of onset and imaging techniques. This subject is explored in depth in Chapter 1.

For the detection of underlying pathology, contrast-enhanced MRI and angiography tend to be most useful. Angiography is used for macroscopic vascular abnormalities (AVMs, aneurysms, vasculitis), and MRI for conditions such as tumors, cavernomas, infarction, and amyloid angiopathy.

TABLE 7–15 Differential Diagnosis of Nontraumatic Intracerebral Hematoma

Common
- Hypertension
- Embolic infarction
- AVM
- Amyloid angiopathy
- Primary or metastatic tumor

Uncommon
- Bleeding diathesis
- Coagulopathy
- Infection
- Berry or mycotic aneurysm
- Vasculitis
- Cavernous angioma
- Venous sinus thrombosis (venous infarction)

Differential Diagnosis

See Tables 7–14 and 7–15.

TABLE 7–14 Spontaneous Intracerebral Hemorrhage in the Adult

Etiology	Clinical	Distribution	Associated Findings	Angiography
Hypertension	Hypertensive patients	65% basal ganglia and thalamus 20% posterior fossa 15% deep white matter	Intraventricular extension common	Rarely aneurysm of perforating arteries Active extravasation if performed within hours of onset
Embolic infarction	Elderly patients with acute neurologic deficit	Conforms to territory of occluded vessel	Cytotoxic edema in distribution of major cerebral vessel	Abrupt vascular occlusion and intraluminal filling defects
Arteriovenous malformation	Headaches and seizures in young adults	Deep white matter most common	Intraventricular hemorrhage and enlarged vessels near the hematoma	Arteriovenous shunting, nidus, and enlarged feeding and draining vessels
Amyloid angiopathy	Elderly and often demented	Lobar cortex and subcortical white matter	Bleeds may be multiple and of varying ages White matter disease on MRI	No primary vascular abnormalities
Neoplasm	Especially metastases and high grade glial tumors	Lobar subcortical white matter	Many clues on MRI (see Chapter 1)	May reveal tumor vascularity
Mycotic aneurysm	History of endocarditis	Lobar cortex and subcortical white matter	Subarachnoid hemorrhage remote from basal cisterns	Aneurysm, typically in distal cerebral vessels
Berry aneurysm	Sudden onset of severe headaches in young or middle-aged adults	Most often in deep frontal lobe	Subarachnoid hemorrhage nearly always present	Aneurysm, especially middle cerebral

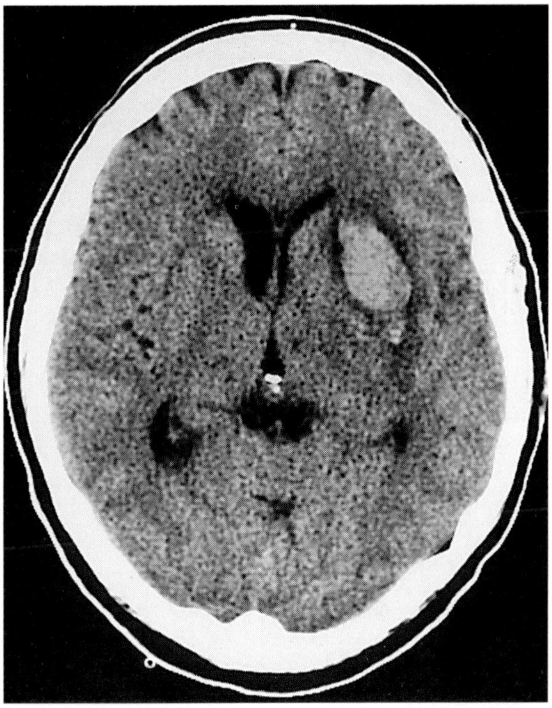

Figure 7–87. Hypertensive hemorrhage. Axial unenhanced CT shows acute hemorrhage in the left putamen and external capsule.

Moyamoya Disease

The term moyamoya applies to both a disease and an angiographic finding. The disease is a condition of unknown etiology most commonly encountered among young girls of Japanese origin. Progressive stenosis leading to occlusion occurs in the supraclinoid internal carotid artery and proximal segments of the anterior and middle cerebral arteries with the development of extensive parenchymal, transdural, and leptomeningeal collaterals to perfuse the ischemic brain. Young children present with seizures, hemiparesis, and movement disorders. Adults typically present with subarachnoid or parenchymal hemorrhage.

An angiographic pattern indistinguishable from primary moyamoya disease may occur idiopathically or as a complication of meningitis, neurofibromatosis, sickle cell disease, Down's syndrome, or radiation treatment.

CT Findings. Intense contrast enhancement in the basal ganglia may be seen related to the tangle of collateral vessels. Larger collaterals may appear as discrete nodular or curvilinear enhancing structures. Secondary findings are common and consist of infarcts and atrophy in children and parenchymal or subarachnoid hemorrhage in adults.

MRI Findings. Both MRI and MR angiography may reveal the primary changes of stenosis or occlusion of the cavernous internal carotid and proximal anterior and middle cerebral arteries, recognized by the absence of normal flow-induced signal changes. The enlarged collaterals in the basal ganglia manifest as multiple small signal voids and are observed in up to 80% of cases. Secondary ischemic changes are usual in children. Adults more typically present with hemorrhage.

Angiographic Findings. Angiography demonstrates narrowing or occlusion of the supraclinoid internal carotid and proximal middle and anterior cerebral arteries. The distal territories are supplied by enlarged intraparenchymal collaterals from the anterior choroidal, posterior communicating, lenticulostriate, and thalamoperforating arteries. A rich network of enlarged collaterals in the basal ganglia results in the dense angiographic staining from which the name moyamoya (puff of smoke) derives. Transdural collaterals may arise from the ophthalmic, tentorial, and middle meningeal arteries. Leptomeningeal collateral vessels may also be seen. The disease is nearly always bilateral, especially in children.

Differential Diagnosis

Angiography is diagnostic.

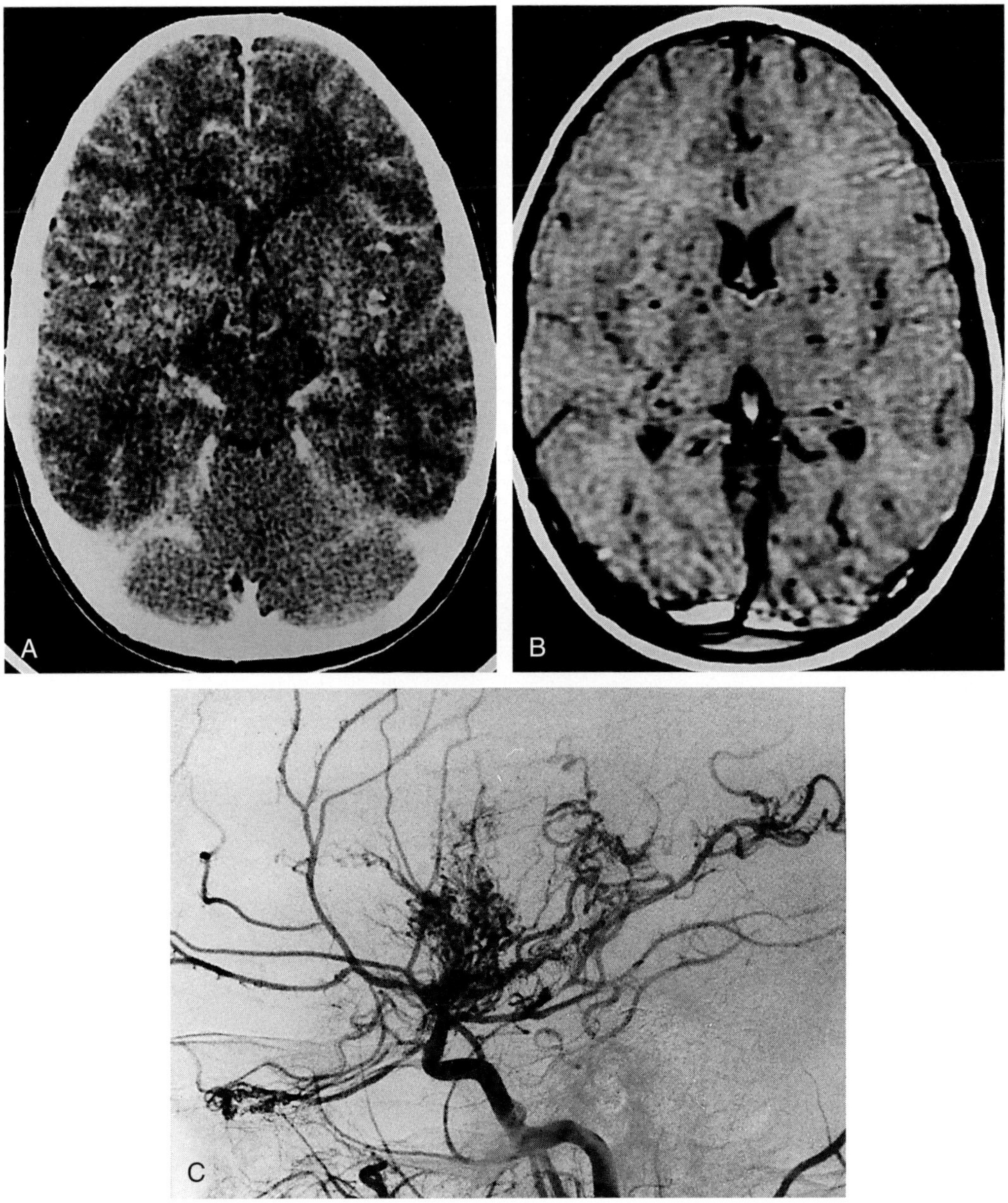

Figure 7–88. Moyamoya disease. **(A)** Axial contrast-enhanced CT shows diffuse punctate enhancement in the basal ganglia bilaterally. **(B)** Axial T1-weighted MRI shows multiple flow voids in the basal ganglia. **(C)** Lateral common carotid angiogram demonstrates occlusion of the internal carotid distal to the posterior communicating artery with opacification of countless lenticulostriate and choroidal collaterals.

Fibromuscular Dysplasia

Fibromuscular dysplasia is a condition affecting large arteries in which fibromuscular proliferation in the intima or media results in alternating areas of stenosis and dilatation. The renal arteries are most often affected, followed by the carotid and vertebral arteries. Females are affected by a 9:1 ratio, with a peak incidence in the fifth decade. Medial, intimal, and subadventitial forms have been described. The medial form accounts for 80–90% of all cases. Patients may present clinically with symptoms of ischemia, or fibromuscular dysplasia may be an incidental finding at angiography. FMD is a risk factor for spontaneous carotid dissection.

MRI Findings. MR angiography may reveal the segmental narrowings and dilatations seen angiographically. There also may be multiple areas of intravascular signal loss due to turbulent flow.

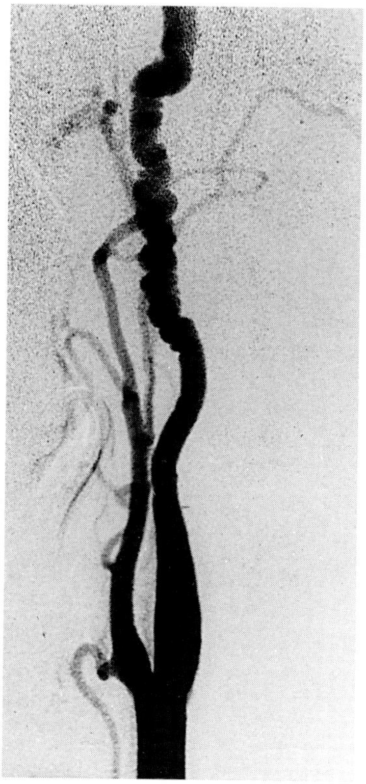

Figure 7–89. Fibromuscular dysplasia. Lateral common carotid angiogram shows the classic string of beads in the high cervical internal carotid artery. (Courtesy of Dr. Pamela Van Tassel, Charleston, SC.)

Angiographic Findings. In 80% of cases, angiography reveals multiple areas of weblike narrowing in the mid and upper cervical internal carotid artery with intervening dilatation, producing the so-called string of beads sign. The changes are most prevalent at the C1-C2 levels. There is bilateral involvement in 65–75% and vertebral artery involvement in 15%. A minority of cases (<10%) demonstrate single or multiple, smooth tubular stenoses of the involved vessel. The least common appearance is that of asymmetric outpouchings, which may lead to aneurysm formation. Coexisting or complicating factors include intracranial berry aneurysms (30%) and spontaneous carotid dissection.

Differential Diagnosis

Angiographically induced vasospasm
Takayasu arteritis

RECOMMENDED READINGS

Common Anomalies

El Gammal,T, Brooks,BS. Conventional MR Neuroangiography. *AJR* 156:1075–1080, 1991.

Schuierer,G, Laub,G, Huk,WJ. MR Angiography of the Primitive Trigeminal Artery: Report on Two Cases. *AJNR* 11: 1131–1132, 1990.

Silbergleit,R, Mehta,BA, Barnes,RD, et al. Persistent Trigeminal Artery Detected with Standard MRI. *J Comput Assist Tomogr* 17:22–25, 1993.

Vein of Galen Malformation

Horowitz,MB, Jungreis,CA, Quisling,RG, Pollack,I. Vein of Galen Aneurysms: A Review and Current Perspective. *AJNR* 15:1486–1496, 1994.

Raybaud,CA, Strother,CM, Hald,JK. Aneurysms of the Vein of Galen: Embryonic Considerations and Anatomical Features Relating to the Pathogenesis of the Malformation. *Neuroradiology* 31:109–128, 1989.

Seidenwurm,D, Berenstein,A, Hyman,A, Kowalski,H. Vein of Galen Malformation: Correlation of Clinical Presentation, Arteriography, and MR Imaging. *AJNR* 12:347–354, 1991.

Neonatal Intracerebral Hemorrhage

Bowerman,RA, Donn,SM, Silver,TM, Jaffe,MH. Natural History of Neonatal Periventricular/Intraventricular Hemorrhage and Its Complications: Sonographic Observations. *AJR* 143: 1041–1052, 1984.

Herman,TE, Siegel,MJ. Intracranial Hemorrhage in the Neonate. *Neuroimaging Clin North Am* 2:107–117, 1992.

Schellinger,D, Grant,EG, Manz,HJ, Patronas,NJ. Intraparenchymal Hemorrhage in Preterm Neonates: A Broadening Spectrum. *AJR* 150:1109–1115, 1988.

Periventricular Leukomalacia

Baker,LL, Stevenson,DK, Enzmann,DR. End-Stage Periventricular Leukomalacia: MR Evaluation. *Radiology* 168: 809–815, 1988.

Barkovich,AJ, Westmark,K, Partridge,C, Sola,A, Ferriero,DM. Perinatal Asphyxia: MR Findings in the First 10 Days. *AJNR* 16:427–438, 1995.

Carson,SC, Hertzberg,BS, Bowie,JD, Burger,PC. Value of Sonography in the Diagnosis of Intracranial Hemorrhage and Periventricular Leukomalacia: A Postmortem Study of 35 Cases. *AJNR* 11:677–683, 1990. *AJR* 155:595–601, 1990.

Schellinger,D, Grant,EG, Richardson,JD. Neonatal Leukoencephalopathy: A Common Form of Cerebral Ischemia. *Radiographics* 5:221–242, 1985.

Volpe,JJ. Current Concepts of Brain Injury in the Premature Infant. *AJR* 153:243–251, 1989.

Arteriovenous Malformation

Chappell,PM, Steinberg,GK, Marks,MP. Clinically Documented Hemorrhage in Cerebral Arteriovenous Malformations: MR Characteristics. *Radiology* 183:719–724, 1992.

Kucharczyk,W, Lemme-Plghos,L, Uske,A, Brant-Zawadski,M, Dooms,G, Norman,D. Intracranial Vascular Malformations: MR and CT Imaging. *Radiology* 156:383–389, 1985.

Mitnick,JS, Pinto,RS, Lin,JP, Rose,H, Lieberman,A. CT of Thrombosed Arteriovenous Malformations in Children. *Radiology* 150:385–389, 1984.

Cavernous Hemangioma

Rapacki,TFX, Brantley,MJ, Furlow,TW, Geyer,CA, Toro,VE, George,ED. Heterogeneity of Cerebral Cavernous Hemangiomas Diagnosed by MR Imaging. *J Comput Assist Tomogr* 14:18–25, 1990.

Sigal,R, Krief,O, Houtteville,JP, Halimi,P, Doyon,D, Pariente,D. Occult Cerebrovascular Malformations: Follow-up with MR Imaging. *Radiology* 176:815–819, 1990.

Venous Angioma

Olson,E, Gilmor,RL, Richmond,B. Cerebral Venous Angiomas. *Radiology* 151:97–104, 1984.

Wilms,G, Bleus,E, Demaeral,P, et al. Simultaneous Occurrence of Developmental Venous Anomalies and Cavernous Angiomas. *AJNR* 16:1247–1254, 1994.

Dural Arteriovenous Fistula

Chen,JC, Tsuruda,JS, Halbach,VV. Suspected Dural Arteriovenous Fistula: Results with Screening MR Angiography in Seven Patients. *Radiology* 183:265–271, 1992.

Cognard,C, Gobin,YP, Pierot,L, et al. Cerebral Dural Arteriovenous Fistulas: Clinical and Angiographic Correlation with a Revised Classification of Venous Drainage. *Radiology* 194:671–680, 1995.

De Marco,JK, Dillon,WP, Halbach,VV, Tsuruda,JS. Dural Arteriovenous Fistulas: Evaluation with MR Imaging. *Radiology* 175:193–199, 1990.

Komiyama,M, Fu,H, Yagura,H, Yasui,T, Hakuba,A, Nishimura,S. MR Imaging of Dural AV Fistulas at the Cavernous Sinus. *J Comput Assist Tomogr* 14:397–401, 1990.

Willinsky,R, Terbrugge,K, Montanera,W, Mikulis,D, Wallace,MC. Venous Congestion and MR Findings in Dural Arteriovenous Malformations with Cortical Venous Drainage. *AJNR* 15:1501–1507, 1994.

Aneurysms

Aoki,S, Sasaki,Y, Machida,T, Ohkubo,T, Minami,M, Sasaki,Y. Cerebral Aneurysms: Detection and Delineation Using 3-D-CT Angiography. *AJNR* 13:1115–1120, 1992.

Heiserman,JE, Bird,CR. Cerebral Aneurysms. *Neuroimaging Clin North Am* 4:799–822, 1994.

Huston,J, Nichols,DA, Luetmer,PH, et al. Blinded Prospective Evaluation of Sensitivity of MR Angiography to Known Intracranial Aneurysms: Importance of Aneurysm Size. *AJNR* 15:1607–1614, 1994.

Korogi,Y, Takahashi,M, Mabuchi,N, et al. Intracranial Aneurysms: Diagnostic Accuracy of Three-dimensional, Fourier Transform, Time-of-Flight Angiography. *Radiology* 193:181–186, 1994.

Olsen,WL, Brant-Zawadski,M, Hodes,J, Norman,D, Newton,TH. Giant Intracranial Aneurysms: MR Imaging. *Radiology* 163:431–435, 1987.

Subarachnoid Hemorrhage

Govaert,P, Van De Velde,E, Vanhaesebrouck,P, De Praeter,C, Leroy,J. CT Diagnosis of Neonatal Subarachnoid Hemorrhage. *Pediatr Radiol* 20:139–142, 1990.

Rinkel,GJE, Wijdicks,EFM, Vermeulen,M, et al. Nonaneurysmal Perimesencephalic Subarachnoid Hemorrhage: CT and MR Patterns That Differ from Aneurysmal Rupture. *AJNR* 12:829–834, 1991. *AJR* 157:1325–1330, 1991.

Watanabe,AT, Mackey,JK, Lufkin,RB. Imaging Diagnosis and Temporal Appearance of Subarachnoid Hemorrhage. *Neuroimaging Clin North Am* 2:53–60, 1992.

Arteriosclerosis

Goldberg,HI. Angiography of Extracranial and Intracranial Occlusive Cerebrovascular Disease. *Neuroimaging Clin North Am* 2:487–507, 1992.

Jacobs,NM, Grant,EG, Schellinger,D, Byrd,MC, Richardson,JD, Cohan,SL. Duplex Carotid Sonography: Criteria for Stenosis, Accuracy, and Pitfalls. *Radiology* 154:385–391, 1985.

Laster,RE, Acker,JD, Halford,HH, Nauert,TC. Assessment of MR Angiography versus Arteriography for Evaluation of Cervical Carotid Bifurcation Disease. *AJNR* 14:681–688, 1993.

Patel,MR, Klufas,RA, Kim,D, Edelman,RR, Kent,KC. MR Angiography of the Carotid Bifurcation: Artifacts and Limitations. *AJR* 162:1431–1437, 1994.

Infarction

Bryan,RN, Levy,LM, Whitlow,WD, Killian,JM, Preziosi,TJ, Rosario,JA. Diagnosis of Acute Cerebral Infarction: Comparison of CT and MR Imaging. *AJNR* 12:611–620, 1991. *AJR* 157:585–594, 1991.

Crain,MR, Yuh,WTC, Greene,GM, et al. Cerebral Ischemia: Evaluation with Contrast-Enhanced MR Imaging. *AJNR* 12:631–639, 1991. *AJR* 157:575–584, 1991.

Elster,AD, Moody,DM. Early Cerebral Infarction: Gadopente-tate Dimeglumine Enhancement. *Radiology* 177:627–632, 1990.

Tomura,N, Uemura,K, Inugami,A, Fujita,H, Higano,S, Shishido,F. Early CT Finding in Cerebral Infarction: Obscuration of the Lentiform Nucleus. *Radiology* 168:463–467, 1988.

Truwit,CL, Barkovich,AJ, Gean-Marton,A, Hibri,N, Norman,D. Loss of the Insular Ribbon: Another Early CT Sign of Acute Middle Cerebral Artery Infarction. *Radiology* 176:801–806, 1990.

Von Kummer,R, Meyding-Lamade,U, Forsting,M, et al. Sensitivity and Prognostic Value of Early CT in Occlusion of the Middle Cerebral Artery Trunk. *AJNR* 15:9–15, 1994.

Wasserman,BA, Haacke,EM, Li,D. Carotid Plaque Formation and Its Evaluation with Angiography, Ultrasound, and MR Angiography. JMRI 4:515–527, 1994.

Yuh,WTC, Crain,MR, Loes,DJ, Greene,GM, Ryals,TJ, Sato,Y. MR Imaging of Cerebral Ischemia: Findings in the First 24 Hours. *AJNR* 12:621–629, 1991. *AJR* 157:565–573, 1991.

Vascular Territories

Berman,SA, Hayman,LA, Hinck,VC. Correlation of CT Cerebral Vascular Territories with Function: 1. Anterior Cerebral Artery. *AJNR* 1:259–263, 1980.

Berman,SA, Hayman,LA, Hinck,VC. Correlation of CT Cerebral Vascular Territories with Function: II. Posterior Cerebral Artery. *AJNR* 2:219–225, 1981.

Berman,SA, Hayman,LA, Hinck,VC. Correlation of CT Cerebral Vascular Territories with Function: III. Middle Cerebral Artery. *AJNR* 5:161–166, 1984.

Cormier,PJ, Long,ER, Russell,EJ. MR Imaging of Posterior Fossa Infarctions: Vascular Territories and Clinical Correlates. *Radiographics* 12:1079–1096, 1992.

Savoiardo,M, Bracchi,M, Passerini,A, Visciani,A. The Vascular Territories in the Cerebellum and Brainstem: CT and MR Study. *AJNR* 8:199–209, 1987.

Takahasi,S, Goto,K, Fukasawa,H, Kawata,Y, Uemura,K, Suzuki,K. Computed Tomography of Cerebral Infarction Along the Distribution of the Basal Perforating Arteries. Part I: Striate Arterial Group. *Radiology* 155:107–118, 1985.

Takahasi,S, Goto,K, Fukasawa,H, Kawata,Y, Uemura,K, Yaguchi,K. Computed Tomography of Cerebral Infarction Along the Distribution of the Basal Perforating Arteries. Part II: Thalamic Arterial Group. *Radiology* 155:119–130, 1985.

Dural Sinus Thrombosis

Rao,KCVG, Knipp,HC, Wagner,EJ. Computed Tomographic Findings in Cerebral Sinus and Venous Thrombosis. *Radiology* 140:391–398, 1981.

Tsai,FY, Higashida,RT, Matovich,V, Alfieri,K. Acute Thrombosis of the Intracranial Dural Sinuses: Direct Thrombolytic Treatment. *AJNR* 13:1137–1141, 1992.

Virapongse,C, Cazenave,C, Quisling,R, et al. The Empty Delta Sign: Frequency and Significance in 76 Cases of Dural Sinus Thrombosis. *Radiology* 162:779–785, 1987.

Vogl,TJ, Bergman,C, Villringer,A, et al. Dural Sinus Thrombosis: Value of Venous MR Angiography for Diagnosis and Follow-up. *AJR* 162:1191–1198, 1994.

Yuh,WTC, Simonson,TM, Wang,AM, et al. Venous Sinus Occlusive Disease: MR Findings. *AJNR* 15:309–316, 1994.

Zimmerman,RD, Ernst,RJ. Neuroimaging of Cerebral Venous Thrombosis. *Neuroimaging Clin North Am* 2:463–485, 1992.

Carotid-Cavernous Fistula and Other Traumatic Vascular Injuries

Bula,WI, Loes,DJ. Trauma to the Cerebrovascular System. *Neuroimaging Clin North Am* 4:753–772, 1994.

Davis,JM, Zimmerman,RA. Injury of the carotid and vertebral arteries. *Neuroradiology* 25:55–69, 1983.

Elster,AD, Chen,MYM, Richardson,DN, Yeatts,PR. Dilated Intercavernous Sinuses: An MR Sign of Carotid-Cavernous and Carotid-Dural Fistulas. *AJNR* 12:641–645, 1991.

Klufas,RA, Hsu,L, Barnes,PD, Patel,MR, Schwartz,RB. Dissection of the Carotid and Vertebral Arteries: Imaging with MR Angiography. *AJR* 164:673–677, 1995.

Levy,C, Laissy,JP, Raveau,V, et al. Carotid and Vertebral Artery Dissections: Three-dimensional Time-of-Flight MR Angiography and MR Imaging versus Conventional Angiography. *Radiology* 190:97–103, 1994.

Vasculitis

Aisen,AM, Gabrielsen,TO, McCune,WJ. MR Imaging of Systemic Lupus Erythematosis Involving the Brain. *AJR* 144: 1027–1031, 1985. *AJNR* 6:197–201, 1985.

Banna,M, El-Ramahi,K. Neurologic Involvement in Behçet Disease: Imaging Findings in 16 Patients. *AJNR* 12:791–796, 1991. *AJR* 157:867–872, 1991.

Greenan,TJ, Grossman,RI, Goldberg,HI. Cerebral Vasculitis: MR Imaging and Angiographic Correlation. *Radiology* 182: 65–72, 1992.

Harris,KG, Tran,DD, Sickels,WJ, Cornell,SH, Yuh,WTC. Diagnosing Intracranial Vasculitis: The Roles of MR and Angiography. *AJNR* 15:317–330, 1994.

Harris,KG, Yuh,WTC. Intracranial Vasculitis. *Neuroimaging Clin North Am* 4:773–798, 1994.

Landi,JL, Spickler,EM. Imaging of Intracranial Hemorrhage Associated with Drug Abuse. *Neuroimaging Clin North Am* 2:187–194, 1992.

Park,JH, Han,MC, Bettmann,MA. Arterial Manifestations of Behçet Disease. *AJR* 143:821–825, 1984.

Spontaneous Hemorrhage

Gokaslan,ZL, Narayan,RK. Intracranial Hemorrhage in the Hypertensive Patient. *Neuroimaging Clin North Am* 2: 171–186, 1992.

Mathews,VP, Bryan,RN. Intracranial Hemorrhage in Occlusive Vascular Diseases. *Neuroimaging Clin North Am* 2: 221–233, 1992.

Vinters,HV, Duckwiler,GR. Intracranial Hemorrhage in the Normotensive Elderly Patient. *Neuroimaging Clin North Am* 2:153–169, 1992.

Moyamoya Disease

Fujisawa,I, Asato,R, Nishimura,D, et al. Moyamoya Disease: MR Imaging. *Radiology* 164:103–105, 1987.

Satoh,S, Shibuya,H, Matsushima,Y, Suzuki,S. Analysis of the Angiographic Findings in Cases of Childhood Moyamoya Disease. *Neuroradiology* 30:111–119, 1988.

Yamada,I, Matsushima,Y, Suzuki,S. Moyamoya Disease: Diagnosis with Three-dimensional Time-of-flight MR Angiography. *Radiology* 184:773–778, 1992.

Fibromuscular Dysplasia

Furie,DM, Tien,RD. Fibromuscular Dysplasia of Arteries of the Head and Neck: Imaging Findings. *AJR* 162:1205–1209, 1994.

Heiserman,JE, Drayer,BP, Fram,EK, Keller,PJ. MR Angiography of Cervical Fibromuscular Dysplasia. *AJNR* 13: 1454–1457, 1992.

Kliewer,MA, Carroll,BA. Ultrasound Case of the Day. *Radiographics* 11:504–505, 1991.

CHAPTER
EIGHT
Paranasal Sinuses, Nose, and Nasopharynx

Diagnostic imaging plays an important role in the management of many diseases of the sinonasal and nasopharyngeal region, particularly in the diagnosis of infections, tumors, and trauma. This chapter will concentrate on the role of CT and MRI in the evaluation of inflammatory diseases and neoplasia. The evaluation of trauma tends to be relatively straightforward, focusing on the identification of maxillofacial fractures.

Plain radiography of the sinuses is being replaced by CT as more physicians begin to recognize the general inaccuracy of sinus radiographs even with the most skilled interpretation. CT has become the standard for imaging sinonasal inflammatory disease.

A comprehensive treatment of all neoplasms occurring in this region is beyond the scope of this publication. This would include all the more important tumors included herein, plus all benign and malignant tumors of mesenchymal, osseous, cartilaginous, vascular, and neurogenic origin (Table 8–1).

TABLE 8–1 | Masses of the Nose and Paranasal Sinuses

Congenital lesions
Meningoencephalocele
Nasal glioma
Dermoid
Epidermoid
Inflammatory lesions
Sinusitis
Retention cyst
Mucocele
Inflammatory polyp
Antrochoanal polyp
Wegener's granulomatosis
Fibro-osseous lesions
Osteoma
Ossifying fibroma
Fibrous dysplasia
Paget's disease
Chondrosarcoma
Osteosarcoma
Dental lesions
Odontogenic cyst
Ameloblastoma
Benign soft tissue neoplasms
Angiofibroma
Papilloma
Giant cell granuloma
Malignant soft tissue neoplasms
Squamous cell carcinoma
Mucoepidermoid carcinoma
Adenoid cystic carcinoma
Lymphoma
Esthesioneuroblastoma
Rhabdomyosarcoma
Plasmacytoma

Developmental Lesions

Choanal Atresia

Choanal atresia is a congenital malformation in which the nasal cavity on one or both sides does not communicate with the nasopharynx. If the atresia is bilateral, nasal breathing is prevented. Most believe that choanal atresia results from failure of the embryologic nasobuccal membrane to lyse, an event that normally occurs around the seventh gestational week.

The incidence has been estimated at 1 in 7,000 with a 2 to 1 male predominance. From 20–50% of those affected have associated anomalies, including cleft palate, Treacher-Collins syndrome, and cardiovascular and abdominal malformations. The atresia is unilateral in two thirds, usually presenting with nasal stuffiness and mucoid discharge. In one third, the atresia is bilateral. The latter present at birth with immediate respiratory distress, resulting in asphyxiation unless an oral airway is placed.

Radiographic Findings. A plain lateral radiograph with oily contrast instilled into the nose with the patient supine will show obstruction of the choana. This procedure, however, has been rendered obsolete by CT.

CT Findings. CT shows a narrowed choana occluded by a bony plate (80–90%) or membranous web (10–20%). There may be bony thickening of the posterolateral nasal wall and posterior vomer, with both curving toward the obstructed choana.

Differential Diagnosis

Mucosal edema with choanal stenosis may imitate membranous atresia.

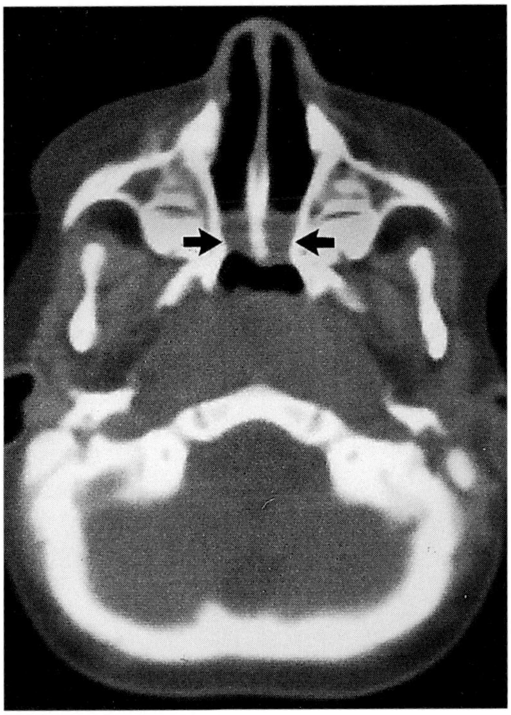

Figure 8–1. Bilateral membranous choanal atresia in a neonate. The choanae are obstructed by soft tissue plugs (arrows).

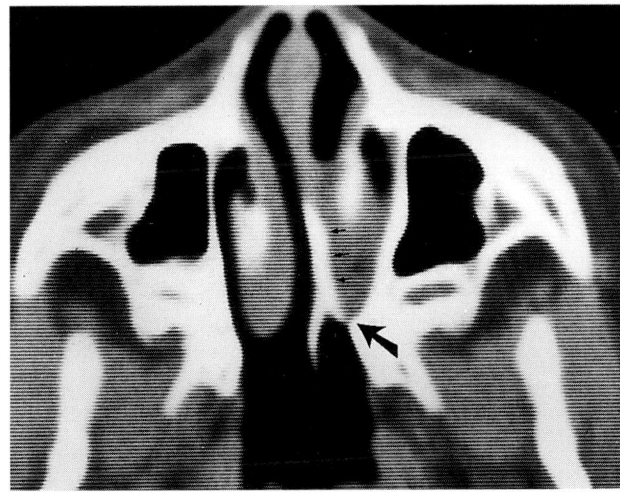

Figure 8–2. Unilateral osseous choanal atresia in an adult. The lateral nasal wall and vomer (small arrows) curve toward the choana with a posterior bony plate (large arrow).

Encephalocele

Nasal encephaloceles are rare congenital malformations. Affected patients typically present in the first year of life with a nasal mass or dimple. The presence of associated sinus tracts may result in intracranial infection, and the vulnerability of exposed dura may lead to chronic CSF rhinorrhea. Associated brain anomalies are common.

CT Findings. About 10% of all encephaloceles involve the skull base and 15% the nose and orbit. With the nasal encephalocele, CT shows a mass in the anterior nasal region composed of herniated brain tissue and meninges. The herniation usually occurs through the foramen cecum (anterior to the crista galli). In such cases, the foramen cecum is always enlarged and the crista galli is hypoplastic or absent. The most common type of basal encephalocele is the sphenopharyngeal encephalocele, which may herniate through a persistent craniopharyngeal canal or ossification defect. Less often encephaloceles may herniate through the ethmoid bone or cribriform plate.

MRI Findings. Sagittal MRI offers better visualization of the herniated brain tissue. MRI also is superior in assessing the commonly associated intracranial anomalies, such as callosal dysgenesis, arachnoid cysts, and lipomas.

Differential Diagnosis

Nasal glioma	No communication with subarachnoid space
Dermoid	Contains fat Dermal sinus usually associated
Epidermoid	Attenuation/signal close to water Dermal sinus usually associated

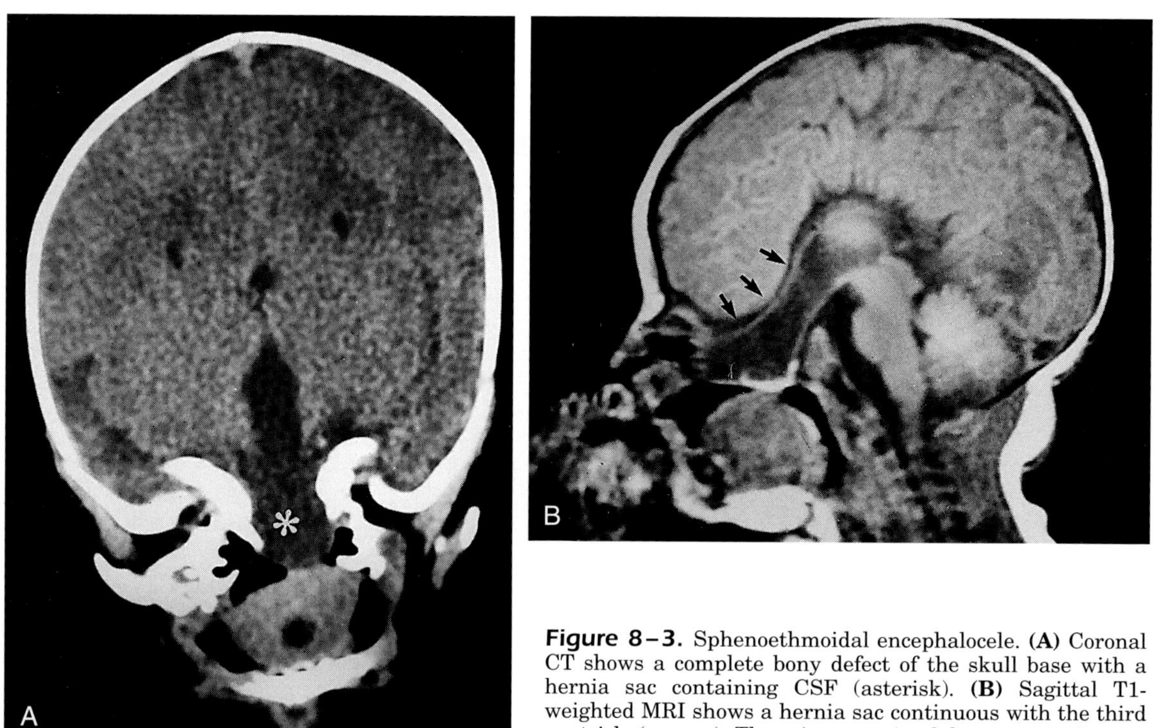

Figure 8–3. Sphenoethmoidal encephalocele. **(A)** Coronal CT shows a complete bony defect of the skull base with a hernia sac containing CSF (asterisk). **(B)** Sagittal T1-weighted MRI shows a hernia sac continuous with the third ventricle (arrows). There is agenesis of the corpus callosum.

Inflammatory Lesions

Abnormalities of the Ostiomeatal Complex

A wide range of anatomic variations commonly occur in the nasal cavity, some of which may predispose to chronic sinusitis. Greatest significance is attached to those conditions that compromise the maxillary ostium, the infundibulum, the hiatus semilunaris, or the middle meatus, collectively referred to as the ostiomeatal complex. The entities described below are most frequently encountered on screening CT of the ostiomeatal complex.

Concha Bullosa

Concha bullosa is the pneumatization of a turbinate, usually the middle. This occurs as an extension of ethmoid sinus pneumatization. Minor pneumatization is extremely common and usually insignificant. When large, it results in narrowing of the middle meatus and infundibulum and distortion of the uncinate process and septum.

Septal Deviation/Septal Spur

Septal deviation refers to any departure of the septum from a straight midline location, but when so defined is present in nearly everyone. It is significant only when there is impingement on adjacent structures. The curvature may be single or double (S shaped) and anterior, posterior, or both. A spur is a triangular bony protuberance of the septum and is usually associated with septal deviation. Both may compromise the middle meatus and are often associated with deformity or asymmetry of adjacent nasal structures.

Enlarged Ethmoid Bulla

This refers to dilatation of the most anterior ethmoid air cells. Enlarged bullae are usually associated with a horizontally displaced uncinate process and may compromise the infundibulum or even prolapse into the middle meatus.

Paradoxic Middle Turbinate

The term refers to a middle turbinate that is convex laterally rather than medially. This may involve the anterior, posterior, or entire turbinate. A paradoxic middle turbinate may become pneumatized or enlarged, leading to compromise of the middle meatus and septal deviation.

Haller Cells

Haller cells are formed by extension of ethmoid pneumatization along the anterior orbital floor and roof of the maxillary sinus. Such cells may compromise or obstruct the infundibulum.

Chronic Mucosal Thickening

Persistent (not reversible with time or medication) mucosal thickening adjacent to the maxillary ostium, infundibulum, or hiatus semilunaris may be a cause of recurrent sinus infection.

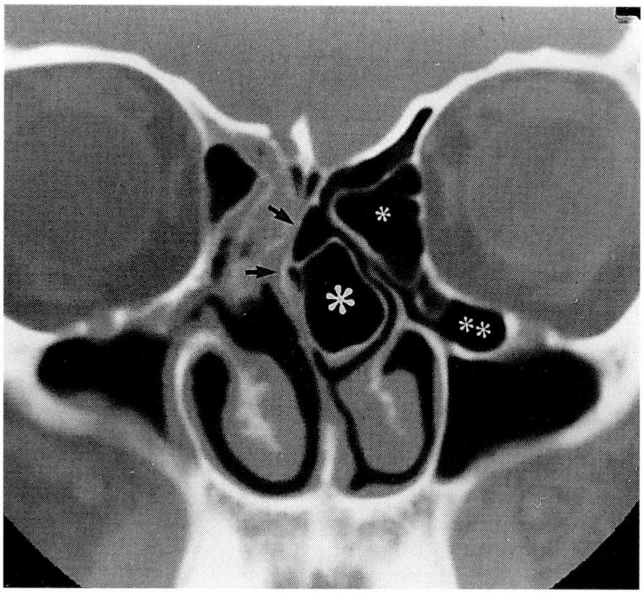

Figure 8–4. Concha bullosa. An expanded and pneumatized middle turbinate (large asterisk) expands the left middle meatus. There is accompanying septal deviation (arrows). Note also enlarged ethnoid bulla (small asterisk) and Haller cell (double asterisk).

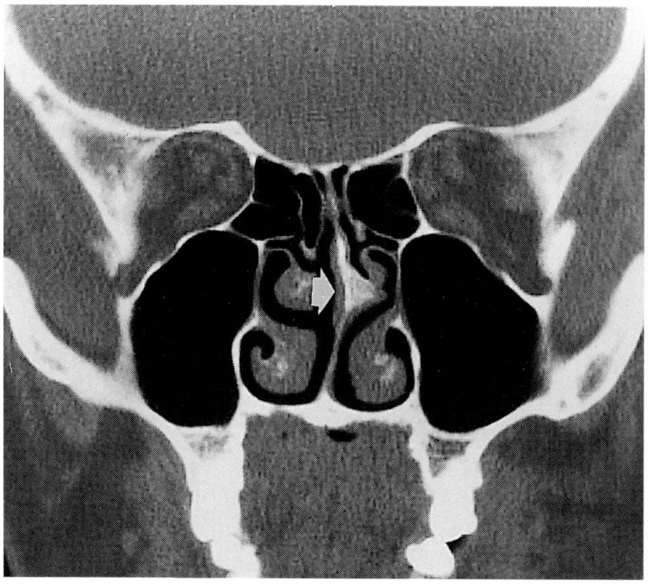

Figure 8–5. Septal spur. A bony spur (arrow) of the septum projects into the left middle meatus. The left middle turbinate is hypoplastic.

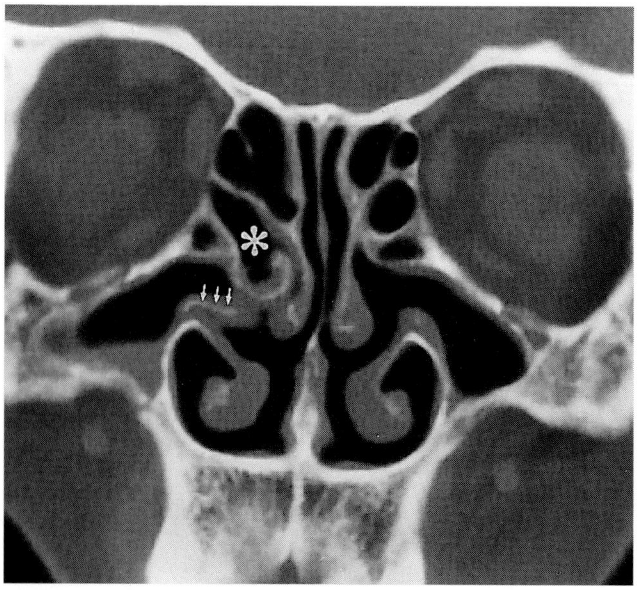

Figure 8–6. Enlarged ethmoid bulla. An enlarged right ethmoid bulla (asterisk) prolapses into the middle meatus. Note the horizontal orientation of the uncinate process (arrows). There is mild mucosal thickening of the infundibulum and hiatus semilunaris.

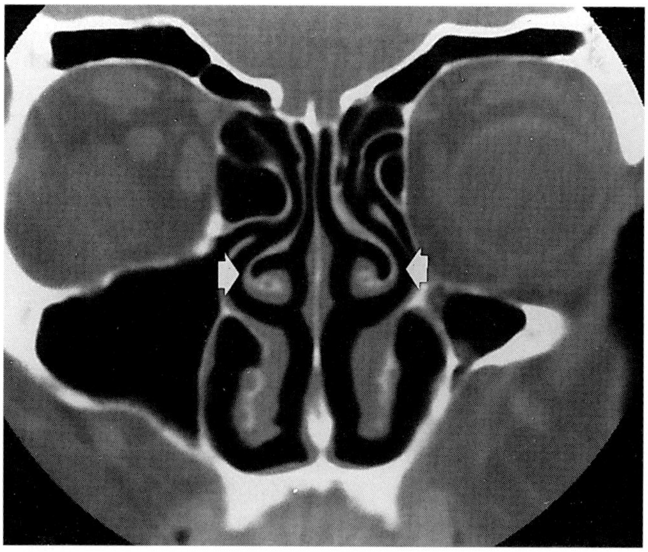

Figure 8–7. Paradoxic middle turbinate (bilateral). The curvatures of the middle turbinates (arrows) are convex laterally rather than medially.

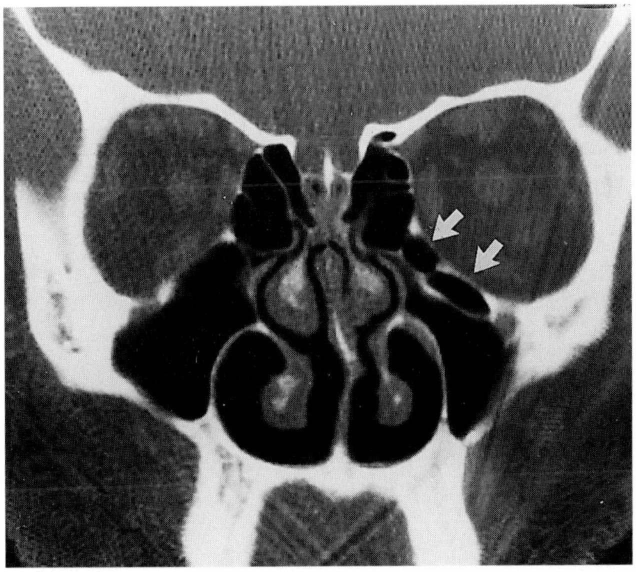

Figure 8–8. Haller cells. There is pneumatization of the floor of the orbit (arrows) in continuity with the ethmoid sinuses. Note also bilateral paradoxic middle turbinates and large ethmoid bullae.

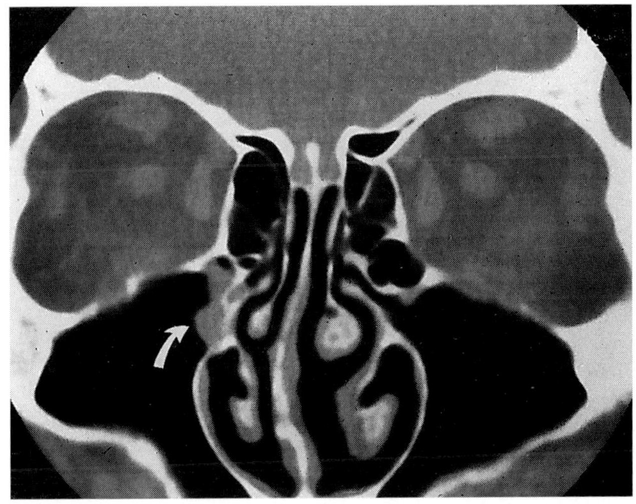

Figure 8–9. Chronic mucosal thickening. Mucosal thickening (curved arrow) obstructs the right maxillary ostium. The normal ostium is seen clearly on the left despite a large ethmoid bulla. Note also the hypoplastic right middle and inferior turbinates, paradoxic left middle turbinate, and septal deviation.

Acute Sinusitis

Acute sinusitis, one of the most common medical afflictions, is an acute bacterial or viral infection of the paranasal sinuses. The bacteria most often involved are *Haemophilus influenzae* and *Streptococcus pneumoniae*. Viral sinusitis usually occurs in the presence of viral rhinitis. Predisposing factors include upper respiratory infections, nasal masses, trauma, nasal anomalies, dental infections, and allergic mucosal edema. Acute sinusitis may in turn lead to osteomyelitis, meningitis, epidural abscess, subdural empyema, and brain abscess. Extracranial spread of infection may lead to a subcutaneous abscess, the so-called Pott's puffy tumor. Acute sinusitis manifests clinically as facial pain, headaches, local tenderness, and purulent nasal drainage.

Radiographic Findings. Sinus radiographs may show air-fluid levels, nodular or smooth mucosal thickening, or complete sinus opacification. Current experience, however, suggests that sinus radiographs are highly unreliable in the diagnosis of sinusitis, with a high rate of both false-positive and false-negative findings.

CT Findings. In contrast with radiography, CT is considered to be highly accurate in the delineation of sinus contents. With sinusitis, CT may show air-fluid levels, nodular or smooth mucosal thickening, or complete opacification by fluid (exudate) or soft tissue (mucosal edema). A concentric ring appearance may occur after intravenous contrast, with thickened enhancing mucosa surrounding unenhancing fluid exudate. The presence of mild mucosal thickening alone, however, is not specific for sinusitis and may be physiologic. Imaging may reveal complications of sinusitis, such as osteomyelitis, subcutaneous abscess, meningitis, epidural abscess, subdural empyema, and brain abscess (see Chapter 3).

TABLE 8–2 Differential Diagnosis of Air-Fluid Level

Acute sinusitis
Hemorrhage
Antral lavage
Barotrauma
CSF leak
Retained uninfected secretions
Large, flaccid retention cyst

TABLE 8–3 Differential Diagnosis of Mucosal Thickening

Acute sinusitis
Chronic sinusitis
Allergic sinusitis
Polyps
Fibrosis
Papilloma
Early carcinoma (without bone invasion)

MRI Findings. With sinusitis, the edematous mucosa and fluid exudate are hyperintense on T2-weighted images and hypointense on T1-weighted images. MRI is extremely sensitive to small degrees of mucosal edema, which may be physiologic. Mucosal thickening of 4 mm or more correlates with symptomatic sinusitis. After intravenous contrast, the inflamed mucosa enhances intensely. Fluid within the sinus lumen and submucosal fluid are usually present and distinct and do not enhance.

With both CT and MRI, one must be alert to possible complications of sinusitis. These include orbital complications such as cellulitis and subperiosteal abscess and intracranial complications such as meningitis, subdural empyema, and brain abscess.

Differential Diagnosis

See Tables 8–2 and 8–3.

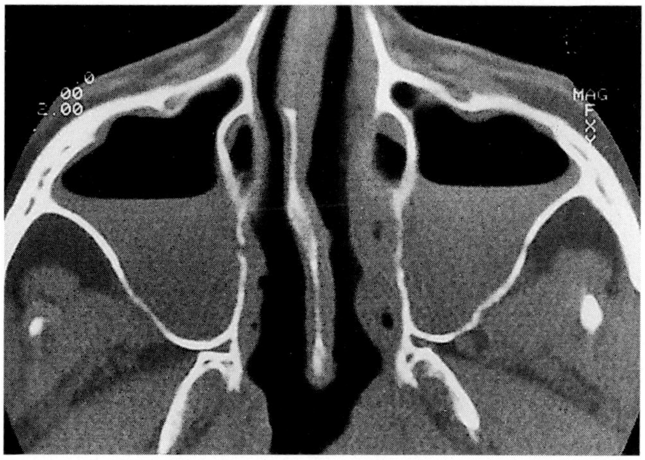

Figure 8–10. Bilateral acute sinusitis. Axial CT shows classic air-fluid levels with mild mucosal edema of the anterior sinus walls.

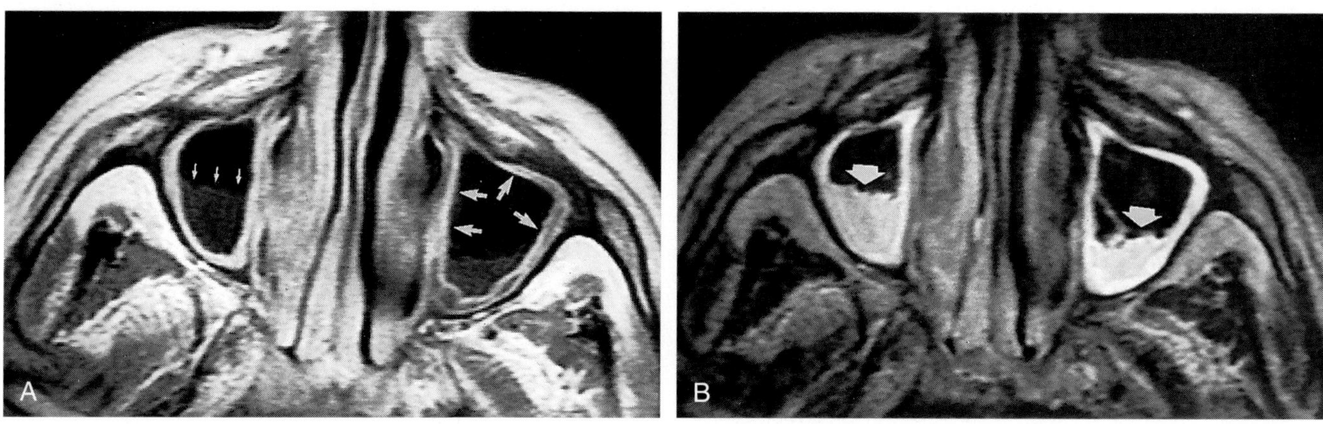

Figure 8–11. Bilateral maxillary sinusitis. **(A)** Axial contrast-enhanced T1-weighted MRI shows bilateral air-fluid levels (small arrows, right sinus) and thickened enhancing mucosa (large arrows, left sinus). **(B)** Axial T2-weighted MRI shows the usual marked hyperintensity of both acute exudate (arrows) and edematous mucosa.

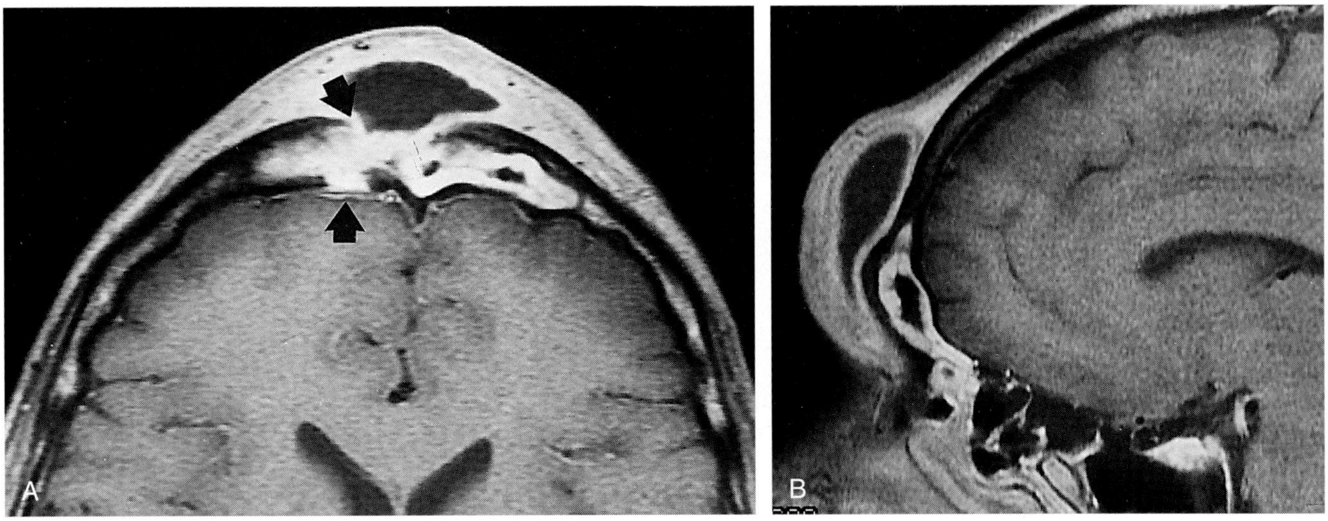

Figure 8–12. Pott's puffy tumor. **(A)** Axial and **(B)** sagittal contrast-enhanced MRI show thickened enhancing mucosa in the frontal sinus, osteomyelitis with erosion of anterior and posterior sinus walls (arrows), and large subcutaneous abscess.

Chronic Sinusitis

Chronic sinusitis is an infection of the paranasal sinuses that persists beyond the acute stage or fails to respond to therapy. As such, it is primarily a clinical diagnosis. Impaired sinus drainage is a predisposing factor.

In contrast to acute sinusitis, anaerobes are more frequently isolated and perhaps the most common etiologic agent. Among children, cystic fibrosis is a common predisposing factor. Chronic sinusitis is characterized by sinus exudates and mucosal edema and inflammation. Over time, reactive sclerosis of the sinus walls and irreversible fibrosis of the sinus lining may develop.

Radiographic Findings. Sinus films may show smooth or irregular mucosal thickening. Sclerosis of the sinus walls and even dystrophic calcification of the mucosa may occur. Similar to acute sinusitis, however, there is a very high rate of both false-positive and false-negative findings relative to CT.

CT Findings. CT demonstrates mucosal thickening, reflecting inflammation or fibrosis. In contrast with acute sinusitis, there is usually sclerosis of the affected sinus walls and possibly dystrophic calcification of the mucosa. With coexistent acute disease, there may be enhancement of the inflamed mucosa.

MRI Findings. Inflamed mucosa even in the chronic stage is usually hyperintense on T2-weighted images. With chronic inflammation, however, the mucosa may become fibrotic, resulting in hypointensity on T2-weighted images.

The fluid secretions within a chronically diseased sinus vary as a function of age. Early on, a high water content produces the expected hypointensity on T1-weighted images and hyperintensity on T2-weighted images. Later on, the contents become hyperintense on T1-weighted images due to increasing protein concentration. In the very late stages, desiccation of the sinus contents may result in marked hypointensity on both T1- and T2-weighted images, even mimicking an aerated sinus. This is one reason why CT is preferable for the routine evaluation of inflammatory disease. Table 8–4 lists the causes of hypointense sinus contents on MRI.

TABLE 8–4 | Causes of Hypointense Sinus Contents on MRI

Desiccated chronic secretions
Mycetoma (*Aspergillus*)
Hemorrhage
Air
Tooth (dentigerous cyst)

Differential Diagnosis

Acute sinusitis	Lack of bone thickening Acute clinical presentation
Polyps	Soft tissue masses in nasal cavity Ethmoid expansion
Fibrosis (inactive disease)	Fibrotic mucosa darker on T2-weighted MRI
Wegener's granulomatosis	Bone sclerosis and erosion both may be present Systemic manifestations

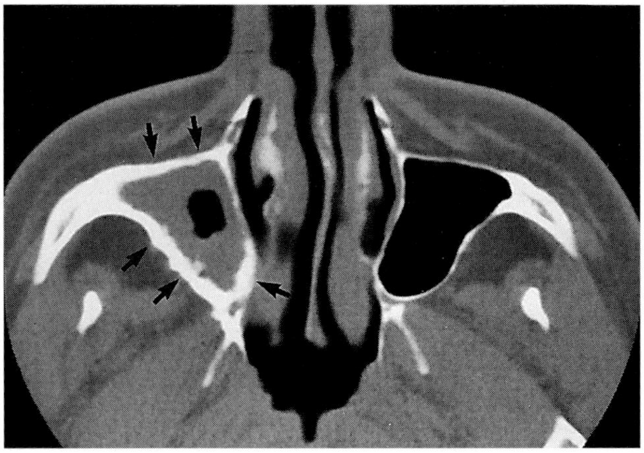

Figure 8–13. Chronic sinusitis. Axial CT shows marked sclerosis of the right maxillary sinus walls (arrows). The mucosal thickening may represent active inflammation or chronic fibrosis.

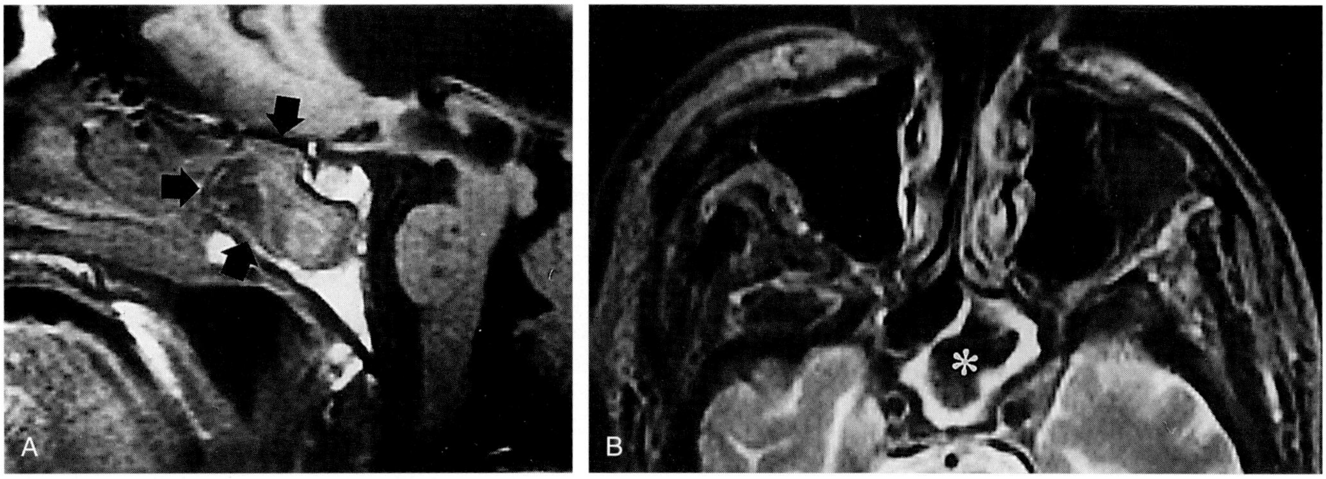

Figure 8–14. Chronic sinusitis. **(A)** Sagittal T1-weighted MRI shows heterogeneous intermediate to high signal intensity in the sphenoid sinus (arrows). **(B)** Axial T2-weighted MRI shows a hyperintense rim of mucosa due to edema with near absence of signal centrally (asterisk). From this sequence it might be erroneously concluded that the sinus contained air rather than inspissated secretions.

Fungal Sinusitis

Various species of *Aspergillus* are the most common fungi to cause sinusitis. Aspergillus sinusitis manifests clinically as a chronic sinusitis that does not improve with antibiotics or irrigation. In 90% of cases, *Aspergillus fumigatus* is the offending organism. Aspergillus sinusitis may be noninvasive, invasive, or fulminant. Although it usually occurs in otherwise healthy patients and causes little morbidity, a fulminant infection may develop in immunocompromised patients.

Patients present with nasal discharge and sinus pain. In immunosuppressed patients, the infection may become highly invasive, resulting in bone destruction. The diagnosis is established by histologic examination with fungal stains of the sinus contents.

Radiographic Findings. Sinus films may show unilateral opacification of the maxillary sinus with calcifications in approximately 50%. Sometimes the sphenoid or ethmoid sinuses are involved.

CT Findings. There are a variety of clinical syndromes related to aspergillosis of the sinuses. Fulminant disease occurs in immunocompromised hosts and they present with rapid soft tissue, orbital, and intracranial invasion. Patients with localized sinusitis present with sinusitis often limited to the maxillary antrum, with formation of a central mycetoma. The mycetoma may become densely calcified. Patients with allergic aspergillus sinusitis present with pansinusitis (usually asymmetrical), sinus expansion and facial deformity, polyps, and hyperdense sinus contents on CT. It may be difficult to distinguish from inflammatory polyposis, which tends to be bilateral.

MRI Findings. T2-weighted images typically show hyperintense mucosal edema with central hypointensity or signal void due to a mycetoma.

Differential Diagnosis

Sinonasal polyposis is the process most likely to be confused with allergic aspergillus sinusitis and the two may be indistinguishable. The central high attenuation on CT and hypointensity on T2-weighted MRI tend to be more consistent and prominent in aspergillus sinusitis. Fulminant aspergillus infection may mimic mucormycosis or malignancy. See Table 8–2.

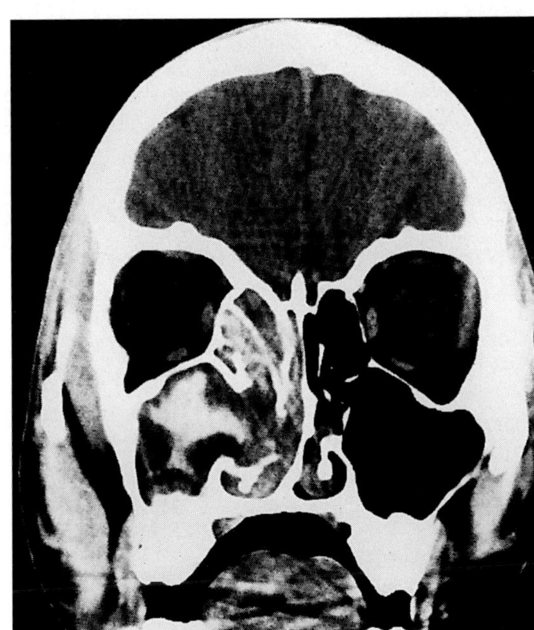

Figure 8–15. Allergic sinus aspergillosis. Coronal CT shows the right ethmoid and maxillary sinuses expanded by a mass with peripheral low attenuation and very high central attenuation.

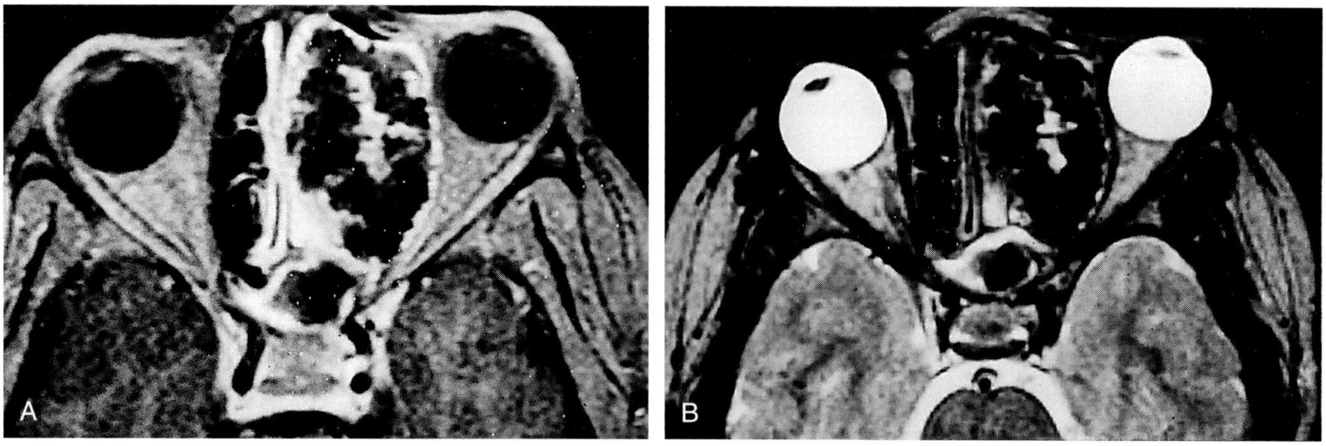

Figure 8–16. Allergic sinus aspergillosis. Axial **(A)** enhanced T1-weighted and **(B)** T2-weighted MRI show left ethmoid sinus expansion with markedly hypointense contents. The signal loss is greater on the T2-weighted sequence. (Courtesy of Dr. Pamela Van Tassel, Charleston, SC.)

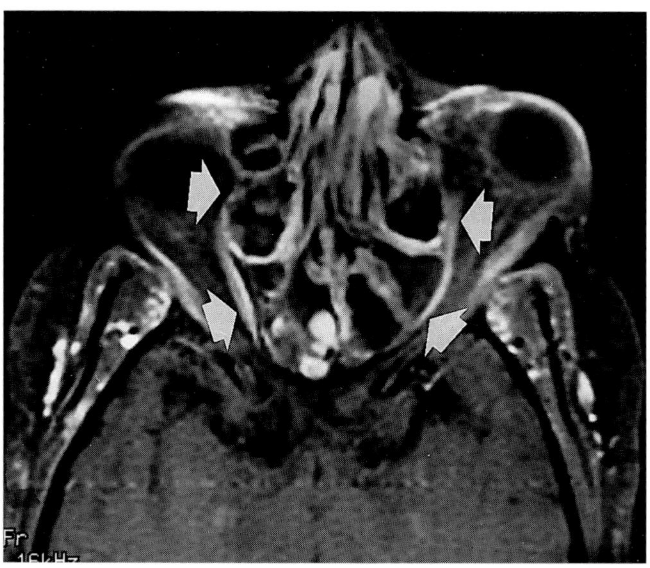

Figure 8–17. Allergic sinus aspergillosis. Axial contrast-enhanced MRI (T1-weighted with fat suppression) shows hypointense ethmoid sinus contents outlined by brightly enhancing mucosa (arrows).

Retention Cyst

The most common mass of the maxillary sinus, retention cysts result from the obstruction of ducts draining mucous glands. Retention cysts are considered a complication of sinusitis, with an incidence of approximately 10%. A common incidental finding on CT scans or sinus radiographs, retention cysts most often are asymptomatic. When very large, they may behave like a mucocele.

Radiographic Findings. Radiographs show a smooth, round soft tissue mass, usually in the floor of the maxillary antrum.

CT Findings. Retention cysts are a common incidental finding on CT, occurring in up to 10% of the normal population. CT scans show a smooth spherical mass of homogeneous water density adherent to the sinus wall. Retention cysts may be single or multiple. Most arise in the floor of the maxillary antrum. The sinus is not airless, as opposed to a mucocele or sinus opacified by exudate. A persistent rim of air and lack of sinus expansion distinguish the retention cyst from a mucocele. Larger cysts become somewhat flaccid and may approximate an air-fluid level in the axial plane with the patient supine. Change of position or higher sections will prove the fluid is not free within the sinus.

MRI Findings. Most retention cysts are homogeneously hyperintense on T2-weighted images. The signal intensity on T1-weighted images is a function of protein concentration. Most are hypointense but may become hyperintense with increasing age or protein concentration.

Differential Diagnosis	
Intrasinus polyp	Usually multiple
Periapical cyst	Floor of maxillary sinus
	Visible continuity with dental root
	Bony defect of maxilla
Mucocele	Sinus remodeling and expansion must be present to diagnose
Sinusitis	More extensive mucosal abnormality
	Symptoms of pain, nasal discharge

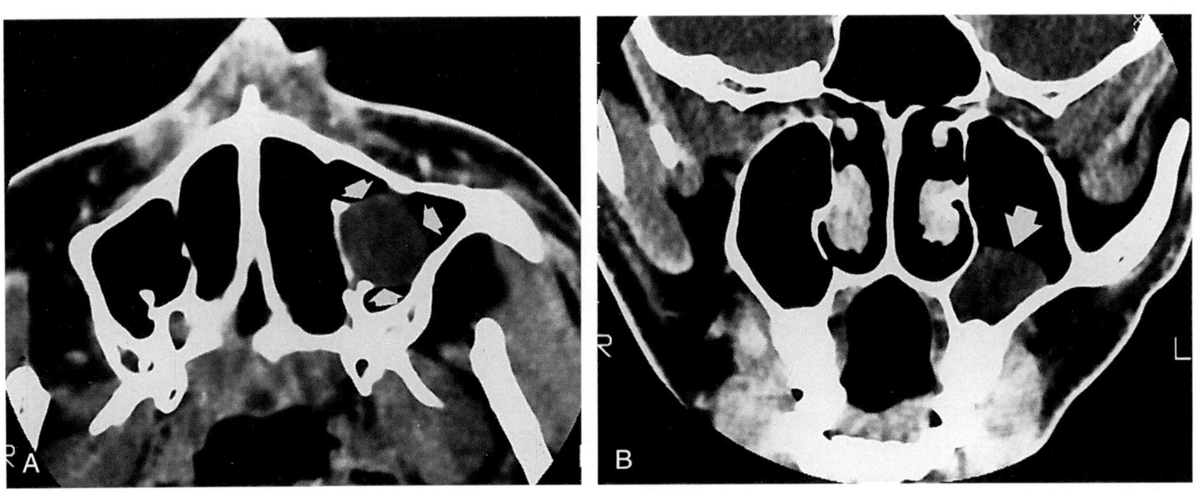

Figure 8–18. Retention cyst. **(A)** Axial and **(B)** coronal contrast-enhanced CT show a sharply defined rounded mass (arrows) in the left maxillary sinus of homogeneous attenuation nearly equal to water. The mass does not enhance.

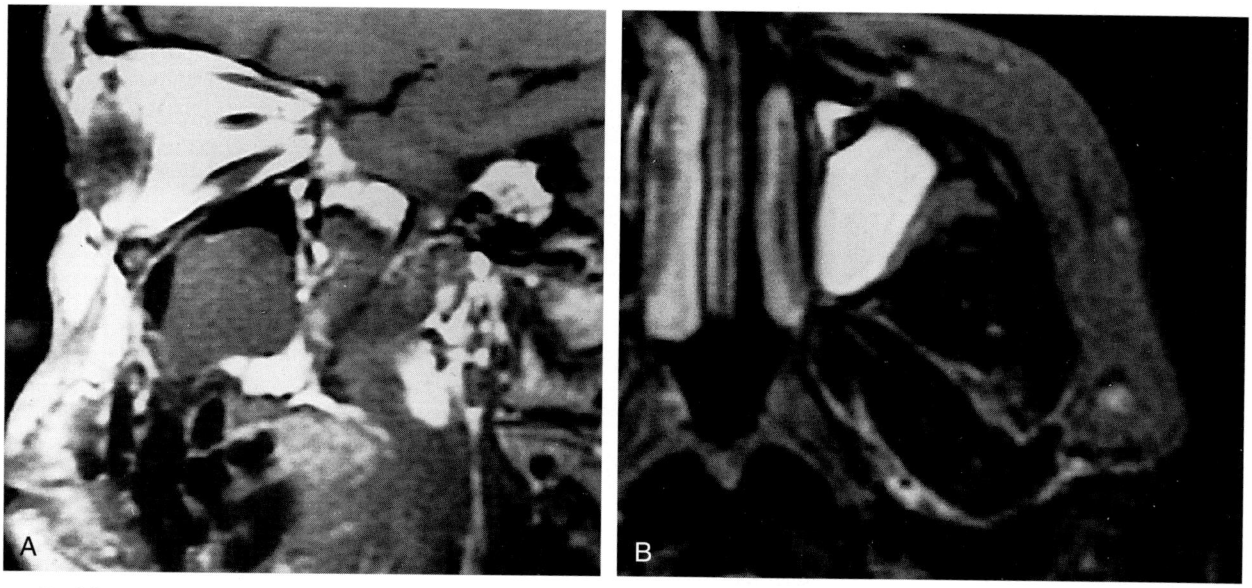

Figure 8–19. Retention cyst. Left maxillary sinus mass (arrows) is homogeneously isointense with water on **(A)** T1-weighted and **(B)** T2-weighted sequences.

Mucocele

A mucocele is an expanded fluid-filled sinus resulting from obstruction of the sinus ostium with continued mucous secretion. It is lined by sinus mucosa. The ostial obstruction may be due to antecedent nasal polyps, inflammatory mucosal thickening, or tumor.

Patients with mucoceles clinically present with headaches, unilateral proptosis, and nasal stuffiness. Local pain is unusual. About two thirds of mucoceles occur in the frontal sinus and one third in the ethmoids. They occur occasionally in the maxillary sinus and rarely in the sphenoid. Table 8–1 lists the masses of the nose and paranasal sinuses.

Radiographic Findings. Sinus films show an opacified expanded sinus. Progressive accumulation of secretions leads at first to bone remodeling and sclerosis of the wall, followed by erosion of the walls as expansion progresses.

CT Findings. CT shows an airless fluid-filled sinus. Sinus expansion is the most specific finding, as progressive mucous secretion causes steady growth of the mucocele. Early on, there may be reactive sclerosis of the sinus walls. Continued expansion leads eventually to pressure erosion of the bony walls and septa. Rim enhancement may occur after intravenous contrast, especially if the mucocele has become infected (a mucopyocele).

Since a mucocele is caused by obstruction of the sinus ostium, the CT scan should be scrutinized for predisposing conditions. Most mucoceles arise secondary to allergic or inflammatory disease, but many sinonasal tumors coexist with mucoceles.

MRI Findings. Mucoceles exhibit variable signal intensity on both T1- and T2-weighted images depending on age of the patient and protein concentration (see MRI Findings, Chronic Sinusitis). Contrast-enhanced MRI may be particularly effective at distinguishing mucocele from neoplasm. An uncomplicated mucocele will show only a thin rim of enhancement. Solid enhancement, although not specific, may indicate the presence of tumor.

Differential Diagnosis

Acute sinusitis	Absence of bone remodeling
Retention cyst	Absence of bone remodeling
Polyp	More diffuse enhancement
Adenocarcinoma	More diffuse enhancement
Mucopyocele	Thick peripheral enhancement

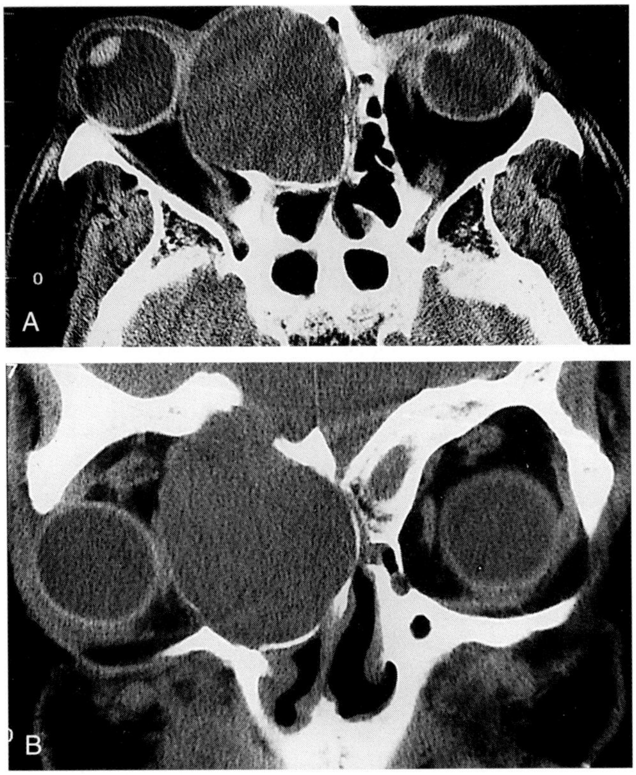

Figure 8–20. Ethmoid mucocele. Axial **(A)** and coronal **(B)** CT show massive expansion of the right ethmoid sinus by a homogeneously hypodense mass. The right optic globe is laterally displaced. The lamina papyracea is eroded and there is an erosion of the floor of the anterior cranial fossa. Portions of the medial and inferior walls show a displaced but smooth and intact bony rim. A small left frontal mucocele is also present.

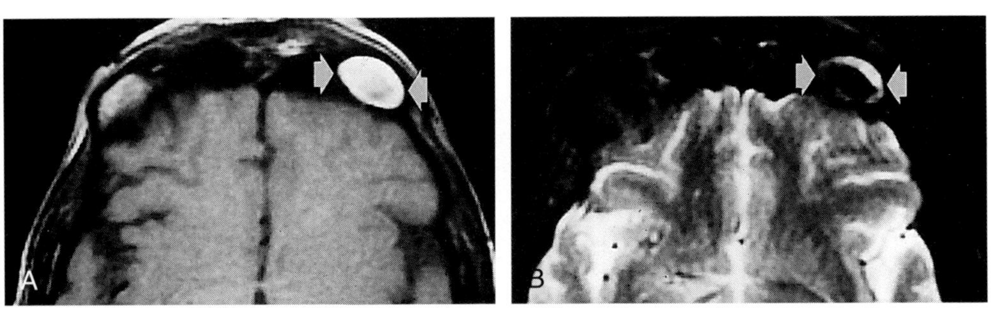

Figure 8–21. Mucocele. **(A)** There is expansion of a lateral frontal sinus air cell on the left. The contents are hyperintense on T1-weighted images (arrows) due to high protein content. **(B)** The contents become hypointense on T2-weighted images (arrows) due to dehydration.

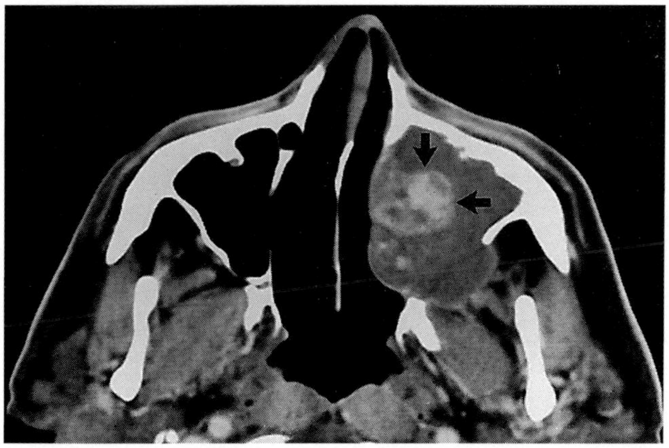

Figure 8–22. Secondary mucocele. Axial contrast-enhanced CT shows an expanded left maxillary antrum with erosion of the posterior wall. A hyperdense mass (arrows) occluding the ostium is an infarcted benign polyp.

Nasal Polyps

The most common mass of the nasal cavity, nasal polyps develop from chronic inflammation of upper respiratory mucosa, resulting in the formation of polyps composed of edematous mucosa. Histologic examination reveals edema, inflammatory cells, and fibrous proliferation.

The frequency of nasal polyps in the general population is approximately 4%. Patients present with nasal stuffiness and sometimes hypertelorism. Sixty percent of patients are male, and children are rarely affected. Predisposing factors include atopy, cystic fibrosis, chronic infection, and asthma. The latter may be present in up to 71% of patients with polyps. When polyps occur in children, consideration should be given to undiagnosed cystic fibrosis.

CT Findings. The CT appearance is somewhat variable. Polypoid soft tissue masses in the nasal cavity are almost always present. CT may also show enlargement of the maxillary infundibulum (89% of cases) or decreased attenuation (deossification) of the ethmoid trabecula (63%) and nasal septum (37%). Cascading, fingerlike soft tissue masses of high attenuation in the sinonasal cavity with a mucoid background are the most specific appearance but virtually indistinguishable from allergic aspergillosis. There may be expansion and opacification of the ethmoids with preservation of the septa (sometimes referred to as a polypoid mucocele). As the ethmoids expand, the lamina papyracea bulges convexly toward the orbits. The antrochoanal polyp is an inflammatory polyp that arises within the maxillary sinus and grows out the infundibulum into the nasal cavity. Expansion of the infundibulum is its distinguishing feature. Most polyps exhibit a slight degree of contrast enhancement.

MRI Findings. Polyps exhibit low to intermediate signal intensity on T1-weighted images and high signal intensity on T2-weighted images. Moderate diffuse enhancement is seen after intravenous contrast. Older chronic polyps may manifest very heterogeneous MRI signal characteristics.

Differential Diagnosis

Allergic sinus aspergillosis
Chronic sinusitis/rhinitis
Papilloma
Esthesioneuroblastoma
Angiofibroma

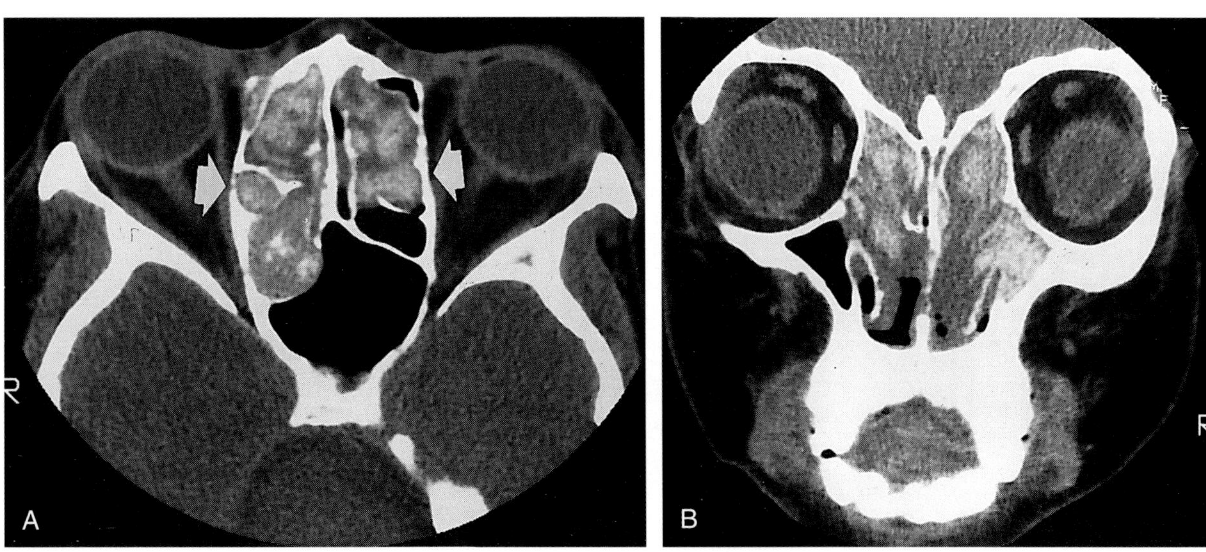

Figure 8–23. Sinonasal polyposis. **(A)** Axial and **(B)** coronal CT show expansion of the ethmoid sinuses, lateral bowing of the lamina papyraceae (arrows), and cascading fingerlike projections in the nasal cavity, an appearance almost specific for polyps.

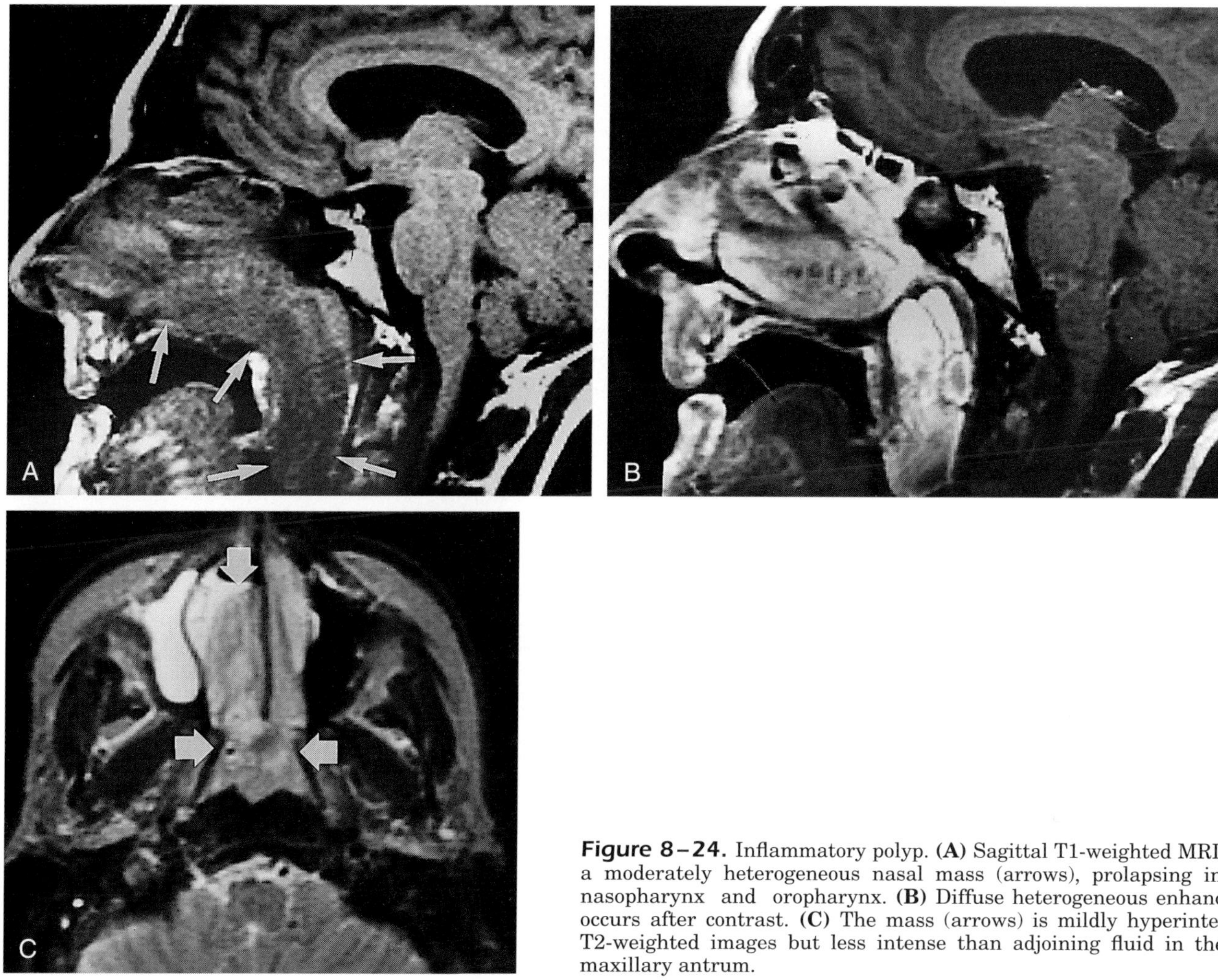

Figure 8–24. Inflammatory polyp. **(A)** Sagittal T1-weighted MRI shows a moderately heterogeneous nasal mass (arrows), prolapsing into the nasopharynx and oropharynx. **(B)** Diffuse heterogeneous enhancement occurs after contrast. **(C)** The mass (arrows) is mildly hyperintense on T2-weighted images but less intense than adjoining fluid in the right maxillary antrum.

Wegener's Granulomatosis

Wegener's granulomatosis is an immunologically mediated disease characterized by granulomatous inflammation and a necrotizing vasculitis. In Wegener's original description, the disease consisted of necrotizing granulomas of the upper and lower respiratory tracts, systemic vasculitis, and focal necrotizing glomerulitis.

Wegener's granulomatosis affects the nose and sinuses, lungs, and kidneys. Patients often present with epistaxis or nasal obstruction. Other common symptoms include vague nasal pain, weakness, chills, and cough. With advanced disease, symptoms may reflect pulmonary or renal involvement. Nasal involvement occurs in 91%, favoring the turbinates. The sinuses are affected in 95%, affecting in decreasing order the maxillary, ethmoid, frontal, and sphenoid sinuses. Secondary staphyloccocal infections are common. At one time, the 2-year survival was less than 10%. With the current use of cytotoxic and immunosuppressive therapy, the prognosis is now excellent.

CT Findings. CT shows mucosal thickening, air-fluid levels, or a soft tissue mass involving the nose and sinuses. The disease is usually bilateral. Additional findings include destruction of the nasal septum, turbinates, and medial antral wall and reactive sclerosis of antral walls, which may be severe. The orbits are often involved, with concomitant orbital masses in 10–15%.

MRI Findings. MRI shows hyperintense mucosal thickening on T2-weighted images. Bone destruction may be seen but is better assessed with CT. Sinus fibrosis may be present and tends to be hypointense on both T1- and T2-weighted images.

TABLE 8–5 Differential Diagnosis of Bone Erosion (Nose and Sinuses)

Vasculitis
Osteomyelitis
Mucormycosis
Sarcoidosis
Wegener's granulomatosis
Cocaine abuse
Carcinoma
Lymphoma
Sarcoma
Metastasis

Differential Diagnosis

See Table 8–5.

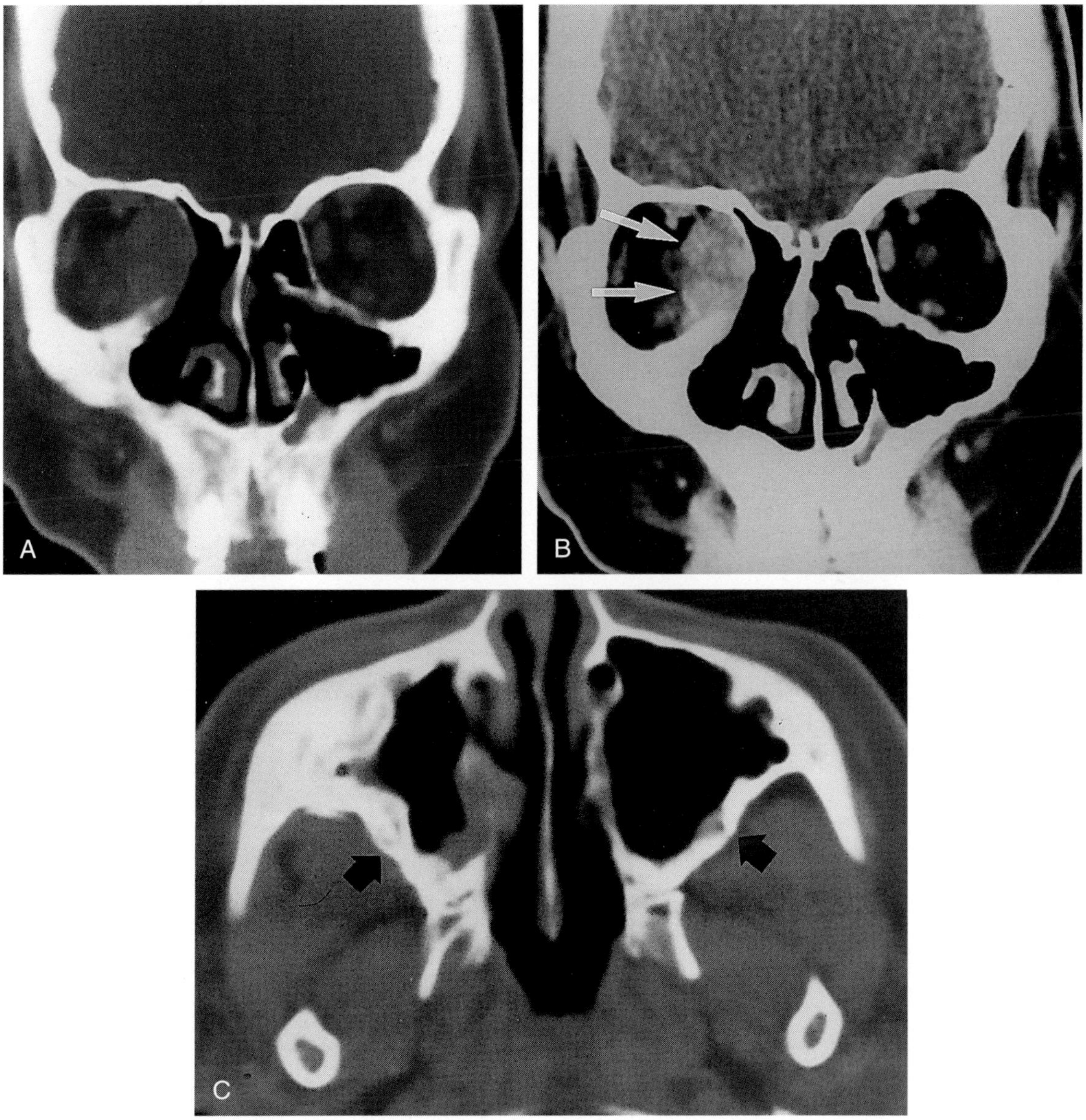

Figure 8–25. Wegener's granulomatosis. **(A)** Coronal CT (bone window) shows erosion of the middle turbinates, lateral nasal wall, medial right orbital wall, and extensive ethmoid sinus erosion. **(B)** Soft tissue window of **A** shows an enhancing mass in the right orbit (arrows). **(C)** Axial CT shows marked sclerosis of both maxillary sinus walls (arrows).

Fibro-osseous Lesions

Osteoma

An osteoma is a slow-growing tumor composed of mature cortical bone. It is the most common osseous tumor of the maxilla and mandible. Most osteomas arising in the sinuses occur in the frontal sinus, followed by the ethmoid and maxillary sinuses. Osteomas have been divided into three groups based on their architecture and degree of mineralization: ivory, mature, and fibrous.

Osteomas are usually asymptomatic throughout life and commonly an incidental finding on radiographs or CT scans. Patients normally present between the ages of 15 and 40 years. Those patients with osteomas in the frontal or ethmoid sinuses may present with headaches. Frontal osteomas may invade the posterior wall of the sinus, leading to CSF rhinorrhea or pneumocephalus. Osteomas also may occlude the sinus ostia, causing sinusitis or mucocele formation.

CT Findings. CT shows an intrasinus mass often attached to the sinus wall by a short pedicle. Osteomas are a common incidental finding on CT and usually small. Eighty percent are located in the frontal sinus. Their CT attenuation is a function of the degree of mineralization. Ivory osteomas are denser than adjacent bone. Fibrous osteomas are lower and more variable in density.

MRI Findings. On MRI, osteomas appear inhomogeneous and are of low to intermediate signal intensity on all sequences. Mild enhancement is seen with intravenous contrast. The MRI appearance is nonspecific. CT is preferred for diagnosis because of the inability of MRI to characterize the typical heavy mineralization.

Differential Diagnosis	
Nonossifying fibroma	Expansile bone lesion Less mineralized than osteoma and much less common
Rhinolith	Foreign body in nasal cavity May be heavily calcified Very rare
Gardner's syndrome	Multiple facial osteomas and intestinal polyposis

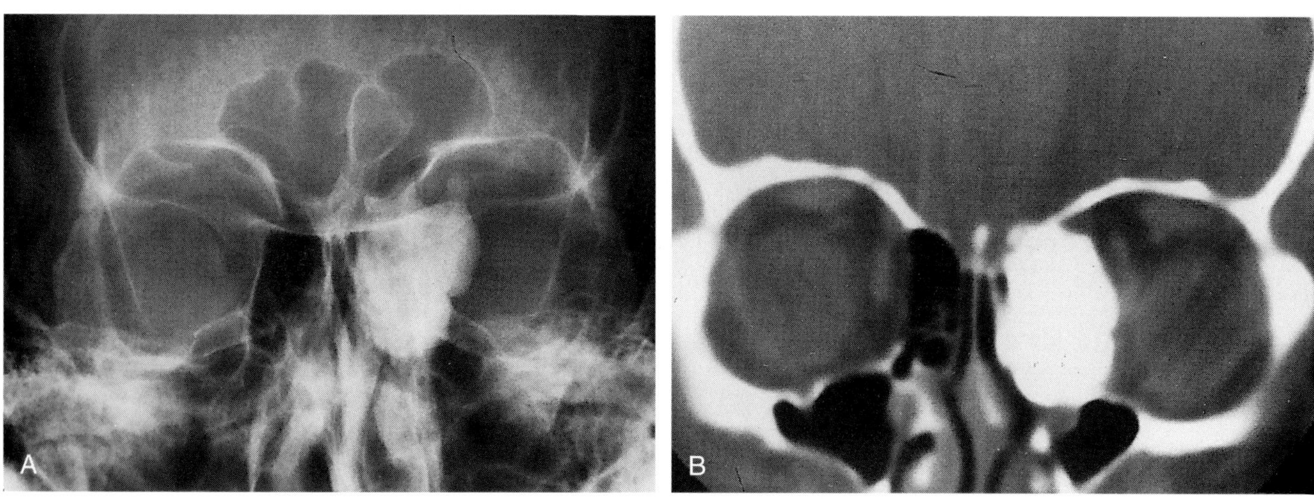

Figure 8–26. Ivory osteoma. **(A)** AP radiograph and **(B)** coronal CT show a very dense expansile mass in the left ethmoids composed of solid cortical bone.

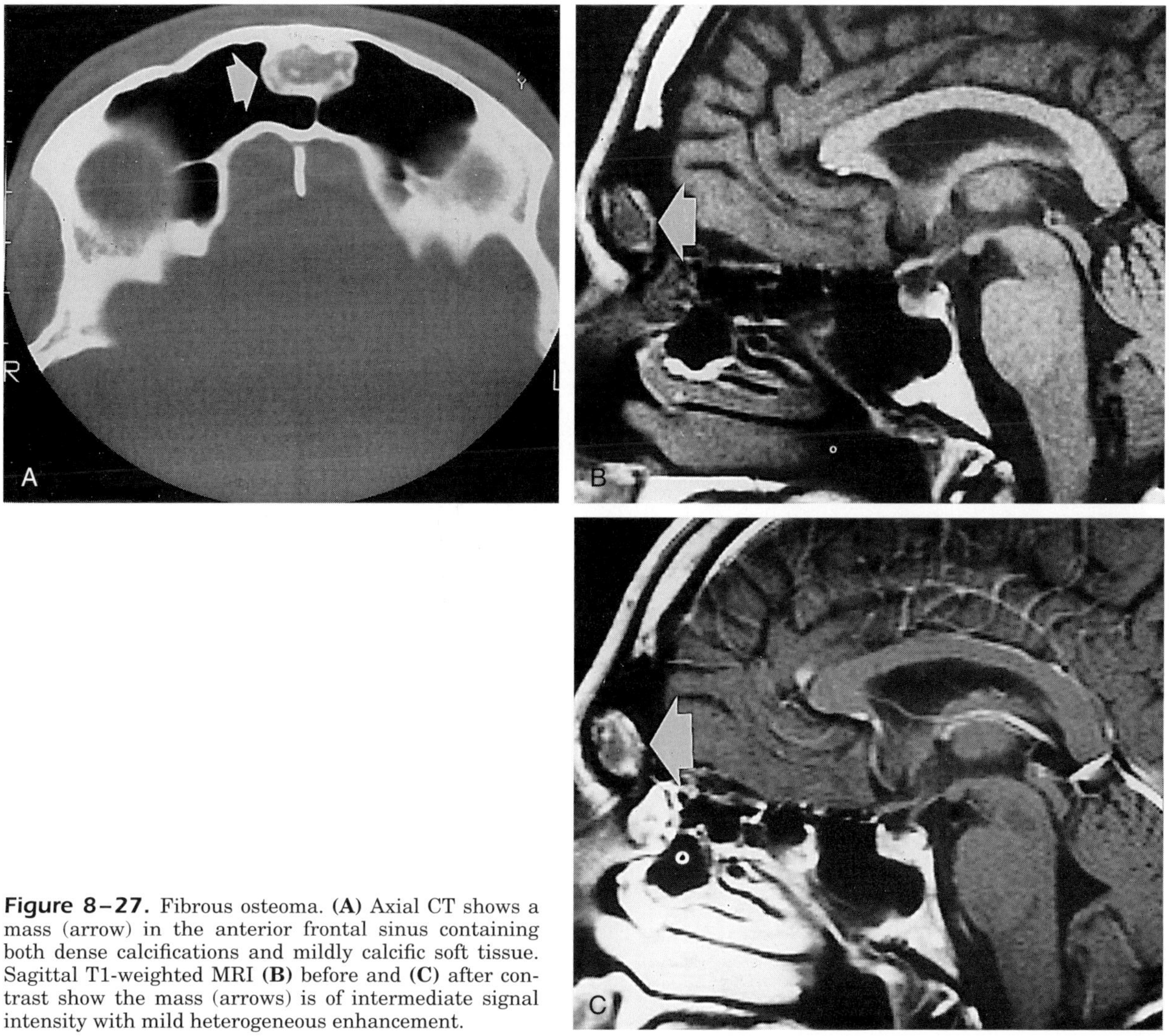

Figure 8–27. Fibrous osteoma. **(A)** Axial CT shows a mass (arrow) in the anterior frontal sinus containing both dense calcifications and mildly calcific soft tissue. Sagittal T1-weighted MRI **(B)** before and **(C)** after contrast show the mass (arrows) is of intermediate signal intensity with mild heterogeneous enhancement.

Fibrous Dysplasia

Fibrous dysplasia is a condition in which normal medullary bone is replaced by a proliferation of fibro-osseous tissue. Affected patients present with progressive enlargement of the affected bone, causing facial deformity. Malignant degeneration to sarcoma occurs in about 0.5%.

Patients with fibrous dysplasia most commonly present with involvement of a single bone (monostatic fibrous dysplasia). The maxilla and mandible are the most commonly affected bones in the head and neck. Polyostotic fibrous dysplasia is less common and almost always unilateral. Facial deformity resulting from diffuse bilateral facial bone involvement is termed leontiasis ossea. Albright's syndrome is the association of polyostotic fibrous dysplasia, skin pigmentation, and precocious puberty.

CT Findings. CT shows a thickened bone with intact cortical rim. The osseous matrix may be fibrous (soft tissue attenuation), irregularly mineralized, or homogeneously mineralized (ground glass appearance). Advanced disease may obliterate the sinus lumen.

MRI Findings. On MRI, fibrous dysplasia has been noted to manifest hypointensity in the marrow on T1-weighted images (similar to skeletal muscle). The appearance on T2-weighted images is more variable, with hyperintensity most commonly identified.

TABLE 8–6 **Differential Diagnosis of Bone Thickening (Nose and Sinuses)**

Fibrous dysplasia
Paget's disease
Metastasis
Chronic sinusitis
Thalassemia
Wegener's granulomatosis
Meningioma
Osteoma
Nonossifying fibroma

Differential Diagnosis

Monostotic fibrous dysplasia must be distinguished from nonossifying fibroma, osteoma, and hyperostosis due to meningioma. Conditions that may cause multiple facial bone thickening are listed in Table 8–6.

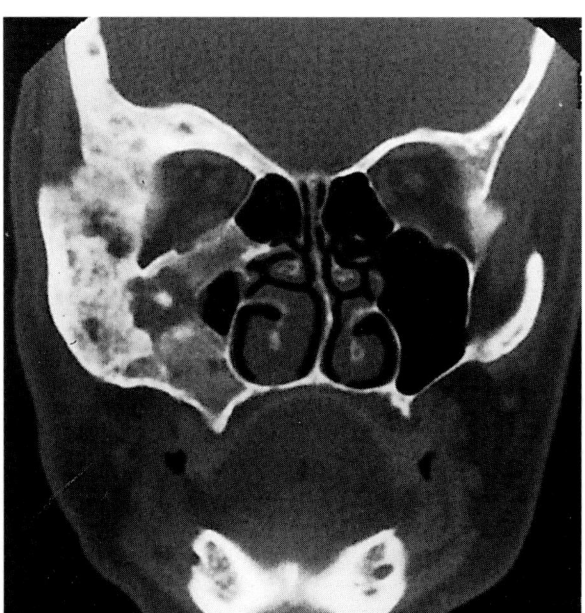

Figure 8–28. Polyostotic fibrous dysplasia. Coronal CT shows extensive thickening of the right zygoma, maxilla, and frontal bone with varying degrees of mineralization.

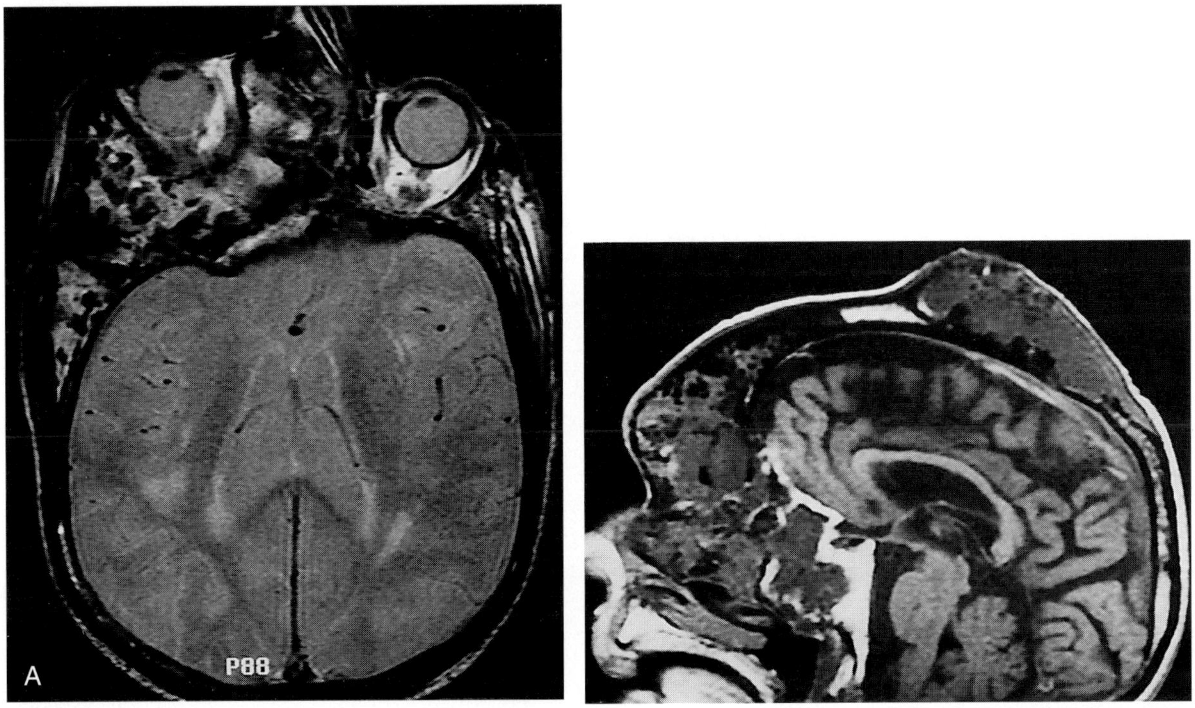

Figure 8–29. Leontiasis ossea. **(A)** Axial PD-weighted MRI shows massive thickening of the right bony orbit, right ethmoids, and right middle cranial wall with mixed areas of high and low signal intensity. **(B)** Sagittal midline T1-weighted scan shows massive thickening of the ethmoids, sphenoids, frontal bone, and skull apex. Marked hypointensity corresponds to sclerotic bone, intermediate signal intensity corresponds to fibrous tissue, and hyperintense areas are probably fatty marrow.

Benign Tumors

Angiofibroma

The most common benign nasopharyngeal neoplasm, the angiofibroma is a vascular tumor composed of ectatic capillaries and fibrous connective tissue. Affected patients present at a median age of 15 years with symptoms of nasal stuffiness and recurrent, severe epistaxis. Angiofibromas occur almost exclusively in young males and normally regress during adulthood. They usually arise from the posterolateral wall of the nasal cavity near the sphenopalatine foramen and may spread into the nasal cavity, retromaxillary space, and maxillary sinus.

CT Findings. CT shows a soft tissue mass of the nasal cavity, nasopharynx, sinuses, or parapharyngeal spaces with intense enhancement following intravenous contrast. Bone erosion and displacement is common. A virtually pathognomonic finding is the antral sign—anterior bowing of the posterior maxillary sinus wall and posterior bowing of the pterygoid plates due to an expansile mass in the pterygopalatine fossa.

Most angiofibromas arise near the sphenopalatine foramen and initially cause enlargement of the foramen and erosion of the adjacent medial pterygoid plate. They spread via adjacent fissures and foramina throughout the nasopharynx and may spread into the orbit or cranium by way of the superior and inferior orbital fissures.

MRI Findings. MRI shows a homogeneous mass of intermediate signal intensity on T1-weighted images and moderate hyperintensity on T2-weighted images. Signal voids are usually observed due to extreme vascularity of these tumors. Intense enhancement occurs with intravenous contrast.

Angiographic Findings. Angiography in all cases shows a highly vascular mass with predominantly external carotid supply by way of the internal maxillary, ascending pharyngeal, and ascending palatine branches. The feeding arteries are often dilated and tortuous, and there is rapid venous filling.

Differential Diagnosis

The finding of a soft tissue mass in the nasal cavity of an adolescent male with epistaxis is nearly pathognomonic. The diagnosis is confirmed by angiography. Other conditions that may occur in this area include capillary hemangioma, inverting papilloma, esthesioneuroblastoma, polyposis, and meningioma.

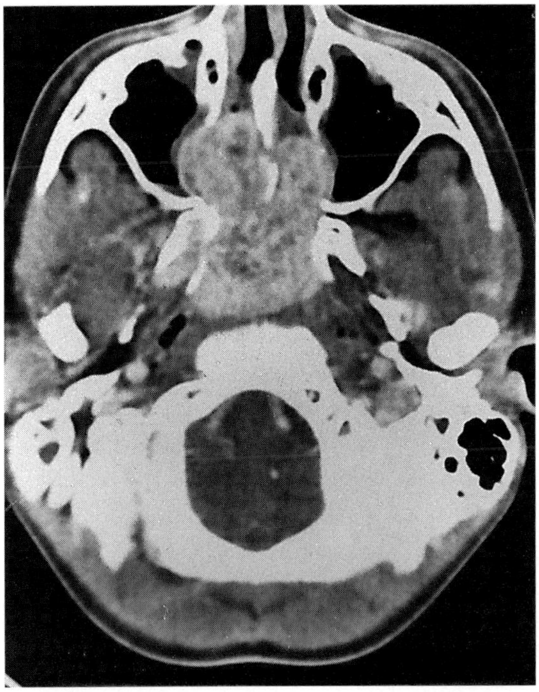

Figure 8–30. Juvenile nasopharyngeal angiofibroma. Axial contrast-enhanced CT shows an enhancing mass expanding the posterior nasal cavity and extending through the choanae into the nasopharynx and right pterygoid fossa.

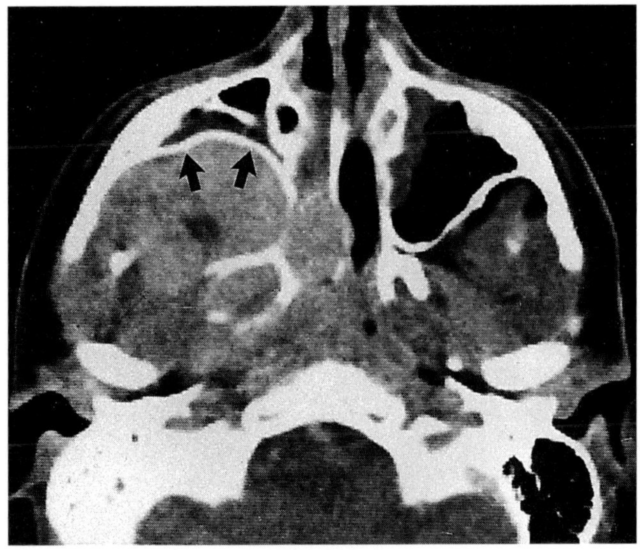

Figure 8–31. Juvenile nasopharyngeal angiofibroma. Axial contrast-enhanced CT shows a large enhancing mass in the right posterior nasal cavity, pterygoid fossa, and retromaxillary space. The marked anterior bowing of the posterior right maxillary sinus wall (arrows) is called the antral sign.

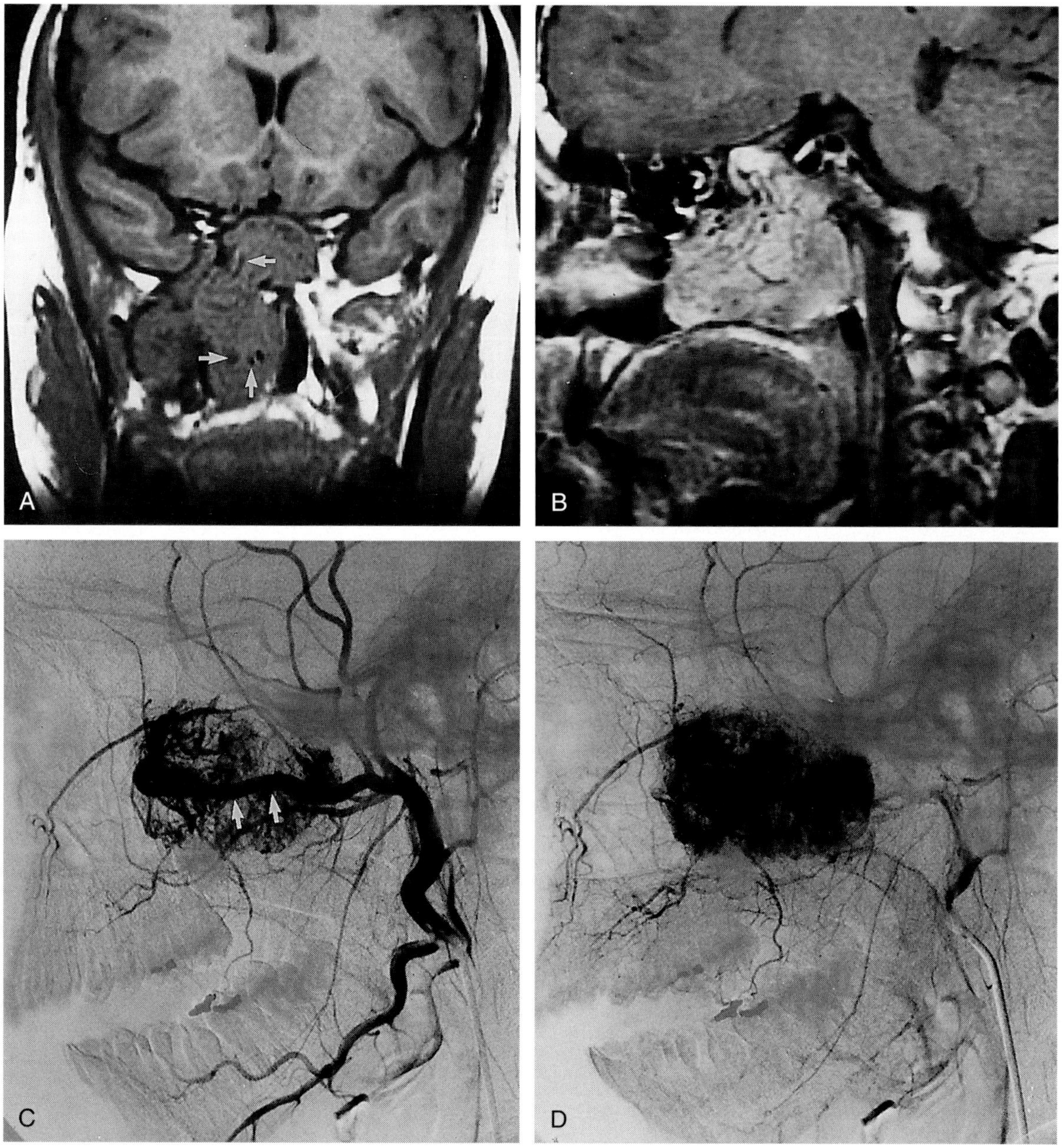

Figure 8–32. Juvenile nasopharyngeal angiofibroma. **(A)** Coronal T1-weighted MRI shows a mass of intermediate signal intensity occupying the posterior nasal cavity, pterygoid fossa, and sphenoid sinus. Multiple punctate and linear signal voids (arrows) point to the vascularity of the tumor. **(B)** Sagittal postcontrast scan shows intense enhancement. Multiple linear signal voids are still visible. **(C)** Arterial and **(D)** capillary phases of external carotid angiogram show early and intense tumor staining. The bulk of the tumor is supplied by the internal maxillary artery (arrows).

Papilloma

The most common nasal papillomas are the inverted papilloma and fungiform papilloma. The inverted papilloma is a neoplasm of the nasal cavity composed of a core of vascular connective tissue covered by well-differentiated stratified squamous epithelium. The term inverted applies to its endophytic growth pattern, tending to grow beneath and elevate the nasal mucosa. Papillomas are much less common than allergic polyps, with a 2.7% relative incidence.

Inverted papillomas occur most commonly in males 40 to 70 years old. They usually arise from the lateral nasal wall near the ethmoids and are typically unilateral. With continued growth, they commonly extend into the maxillary and ethmoid sinuses. Patients may present with nasal stuffiness or obstruction, epistaxis, or anosmia. Secondary bacterial sinusitis may develop and contribute to the patient's symptoms.

The average rate of associated malignancy is about 13%, including both those in whom malignant disease coexists at the time of diagnosis or subsequently develops, particularly squamous cell carcinoma. The rate of postoperative recurrence is approximately 35–40%.

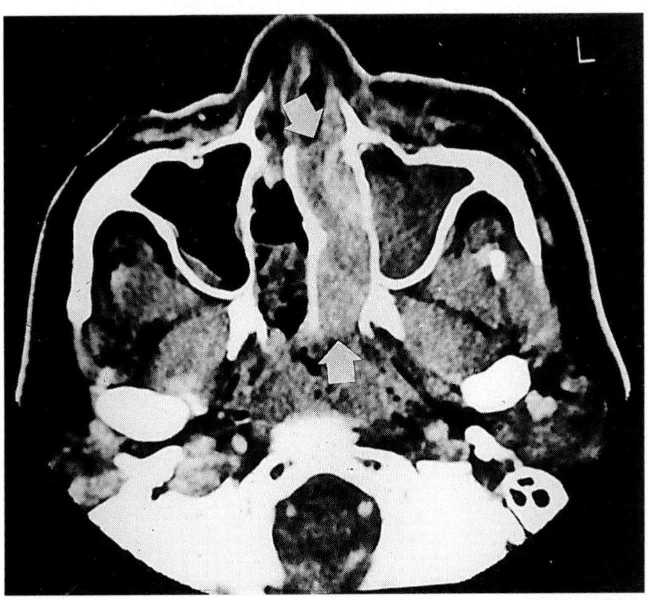

Figure 8–33. Inverted papilloma. Axial CT with contrast shows an enhancing mass (arrows) filling the left nasal cavity. The bony margins and septum are intact and somewhat sclerotic. There are retained secretions in the left maxillary antrum secondary to the obstructing mass.

CT Findings. CT shows a unilateral soft tissue mass, ranging from a small polypoid intranasal mass to a large nasal mass with maxillary or ethmoid sinus involvement and bony remodeling. Most inverted papillomas arise from the lateral nasal wall. Typically the mass deviates but does not cross the nasal septum. Calcifications are occasionally present. Aggressive bone erosion sometimes may be seen in the sphenoid sinus and floor of the anterior cranial fossa, simulating malignancy.

MRI Findings. Inverted papillomas tend to be isointense to hyperintense to muscle on T1-weighted images and isointense to hypointense to fat on T2-weighted images. Moderate, solid, and inhomogeneous enhancement is seen following intravenous contrast.

Differential Diagnosis

Polyposis
Esthesioneuroblastoma
Adenocarcinoma
Squamous cell carcinoma

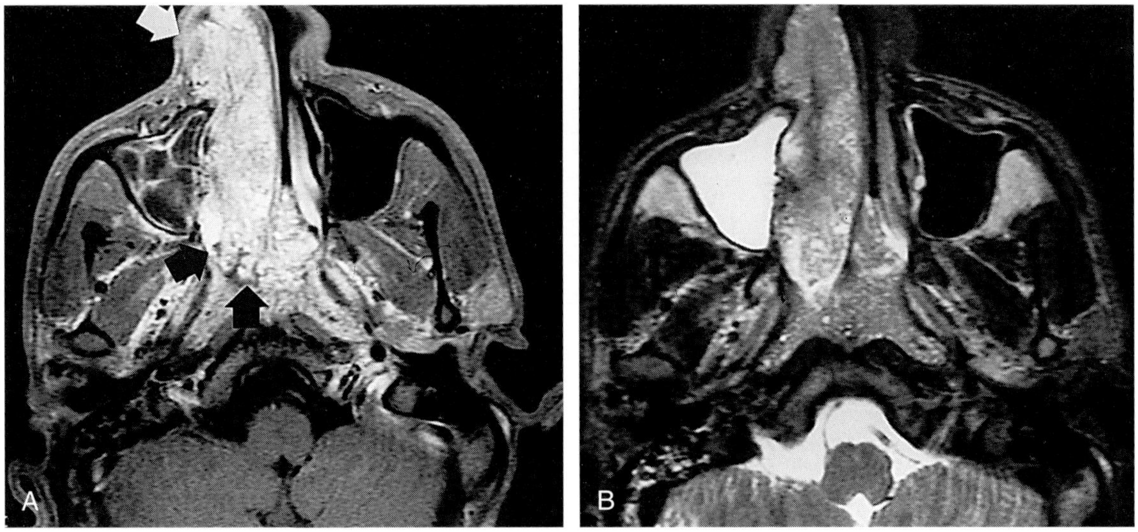

Figure 8–34. Squamous papilloma. **(A)** Axial T1-weighted MRI with contrast shows a mass (arrows) expanding the right nasal cavity with intense diffuse enhancement. The tumor extends into the nasal vestibule and through the choana. Note linear mucosal enhancement in the right maxillary sinus. (The mucosa is displaced by submucosal edema.) **(B)** On axial T2-weighted MRI the mass is of intermediate signal intensity and easily distinguished from hyperintense secretions in the right maxillary sinus.

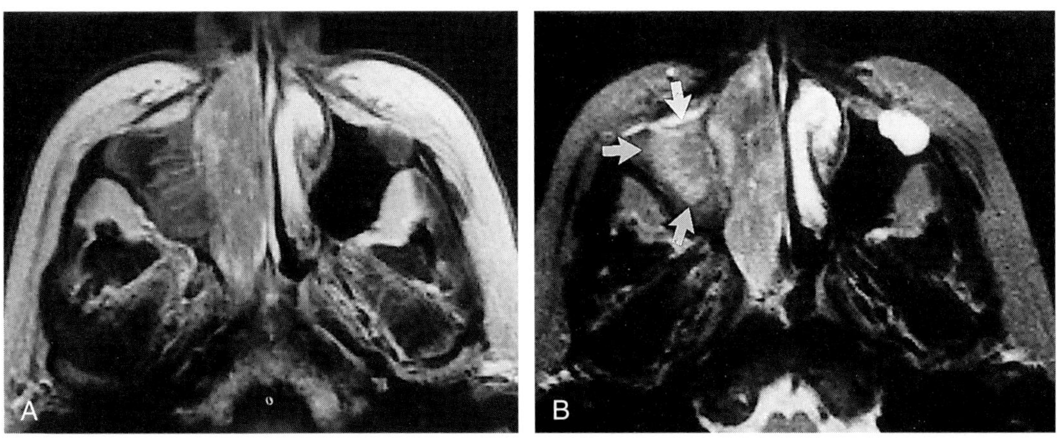

Figure 8–35. Inverted papilloma with maxillary sinus invasion. **(A)** Axial T1-weighted MRI with contrast shows a mass in the right nasal cavity with diffuse enhancement and extending into the right maxillary sinus. **(B)** On axial T2-weighted MRI the mass is of intermediate signal intensity and isointense with tumor in the right maxillary sinus (arrows). There is a hyperintense retention cyst in the left maxillary sinus.

Thornwaldt Cyst

The Thornwaldt cyst is a very common congenital cystic mass of the midline nasopharynx resulting from obstruction of a persistent pharyngeal bursa. (The pharyngeal bursa is an embryonic connection between the nasopharynx and the notochord.) Most Thornwaldt cysts are an incidental finding and do not warrant treatment. They may occasionally become infected and require surgical drainage.

CT Findings. CT shows a midline low attenuation spherical mass up to 3 cm in diameter. These cysts occur only in the high nasopharynx and are usually situated between the longus capitis muscles. Focal calcifications are occasionally seen. They do not enhance with contrast.

MRI Findings. MRI shows a well-circumscribed midline mass in the above-mentioned location. Most are uniformly hyperintense on both T1- and T2-weighted images; however, variations in protein content and possible hemorrhage result in occasional deviations from this appearance. Enhancement is not seen after intravenous contrast.

Differential Diagnosis

Adenoid retention cyst
Second branchial cleft cyst
Rathke's cleft cyst
Encephalocele

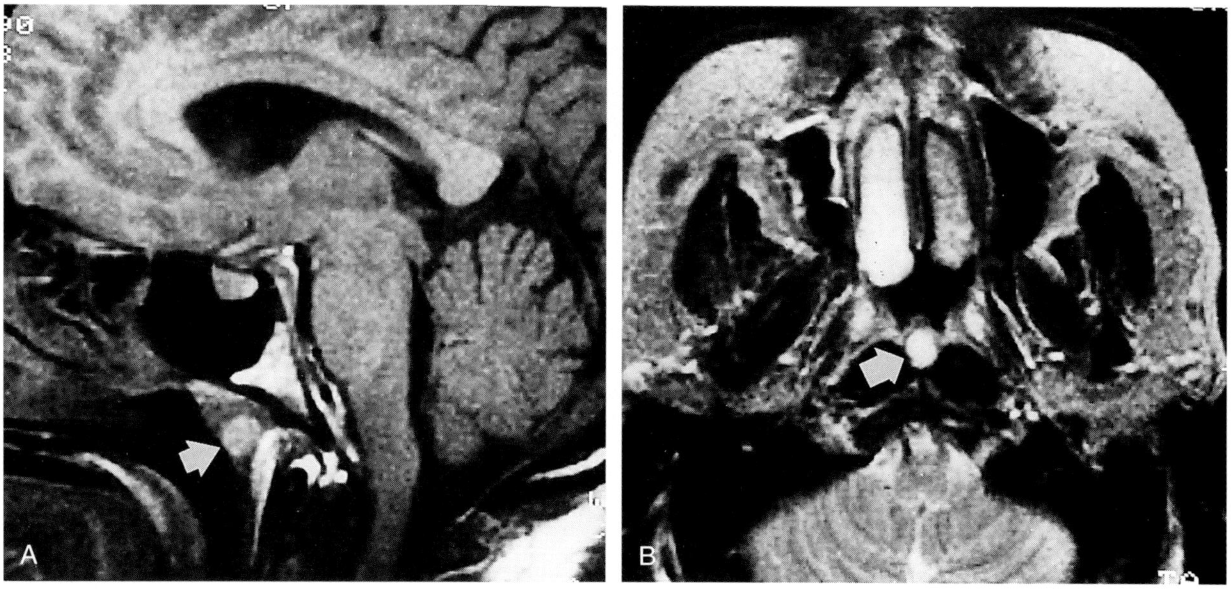

Figure 8–36. Thornwaldt cyst. **(A)** Sagittal T1-weighted MRI shows a round mildly hyperintense submucosal mass (arrow) in the roof of the nasopharynx. **(B)** On axial T2-weighted MRI the mass (arrow) remains hyperintense.

Schwannoma and Neurofibroma

The most common primary nerve sheath tumors are the neurofibroma and schwannoma. Both are common in the head and neck region. Schwannomas (neurilemmomas, neuromas, neurinomas, peripheral fibroblastomas) are slow-growing benign encapsulated tumors arising from Schwann cells. They tend to displace and compress the nerve of origin. Neurofibromas are slow-growing benign unencapsulated tumors that expand and infiltrate the nerve of origin. Patients with both tumors may present with a neck mass or with symptoms of compression or neural compromise.

CT Findings. CT shows a smoothly marginated mass hypodense relative to skeletal muscle and with moderate inhomogeneous enhancement. Neurofibromas may exhibit lower attenuation on precontrast CT compared with schwannomas. Both schwannomas and neurofibromas may arise from any cranial or peripheral nerve, although most cervicofacial schwannomas arise in or involve the carotid sheath. Schwannomas enhance heterogeneously after intravenous contrast due to the frequent presence of cystic or necrotic areas. Cystic changes are rare in neurofibromas.

MRI Findings. On MRI, schwannomas and neurofibromas exhibit intermediate signal intensity on T1-weighted images and hyperintensity on T2-weighted images. Neurofibromas often contain central hypointensity on T2-weighted images caused by a dense fibrous core. Enhancement tends to be homogeneous in neurofibromas and heterogeneous in schwannomas.

Angiographic Findings. On selective angiography, schwannomas are moderately hypervascular. They are characterized by tortuous and irregular tumor vessels, by the absence of arteriovenous shunting, and in particular by "puddles" of contrast 1 to 4 mm in size appearing in the late arterial phases and persisting into the late venous phases.

Differential Diagnosis

See Table 8–7.

TABLE 8–7 **Differential Diagnosis of Parapharyngeal Space Masses**

	Carotid Displacement	Precontrast and Postcontrast Attenuation (CT)	Fat Plane Deep to Parotid	MRI	Angiography
Parotid tumor	Posterior	Nonspecific Smaller tumors homogeneous Larger tumors heterogeneous	Absent	Heterogeneous Well-differentiated tumors may be bright on T2-weighted images	Hypovascular
Carotid paraganglioma	Posterior	Marked enhancement	Intact	Flow voids	Hypervascular
Vagal paraganglioma	Anterior	Marked enhancement	Intact	Flow voids	Hypervascular
Schwannoma	Anterior	Moderate enhancement	Intact	Nonspecific	Moderately vascular Venous puddles
Neurofibroma	Anterior	Hypodense precontrast	Intact	Nonspecific	Hypovascular
Metastasis	Normal	Nonspecific Occasionally ring enhancement	Variable	Nonspecific	Variable (usually hypovascular)

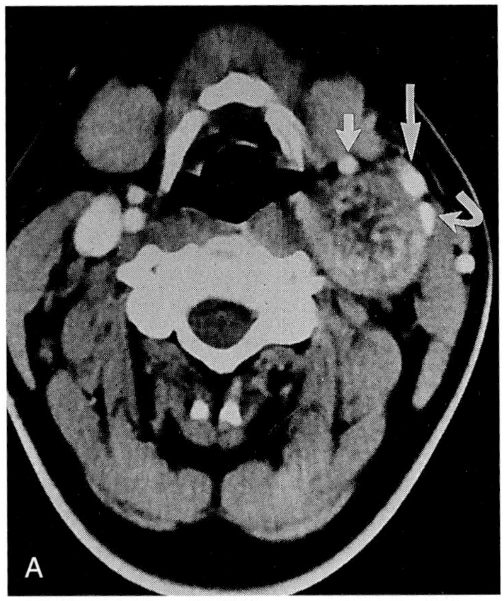

Figure 8–37. Schwannoma. **(A)** Axial contrast-enhanced CT shows a well-defined mass in the left carotid sheath with inhomogeneous enhancement. Short arrow indicates external carotid artery, long arrow indicates internal carotid artery, and curved arrow indicates internal jugular vein. **(B)** Sagittal T1-weighted MRI shows a mass of intermediate intensity (asterisk) displacing the internal carotid (arrows) anteriorly. **(C)** Coronal contrast-enhanced MRI shows inhomogeneous enhancement of the mass (arrows) and smooth margins. **(D)** Early arterial and **(E)** late venous lateral common carotid angiograms show the tumor is supplied by small muscular branches (open arrow) of the ascending pharyngeal artery and a posterior branch (solid arrow) of the superior thyroid artery. Late phase shows staining of the tumor (large arrows) and venous puddling (small arrows).

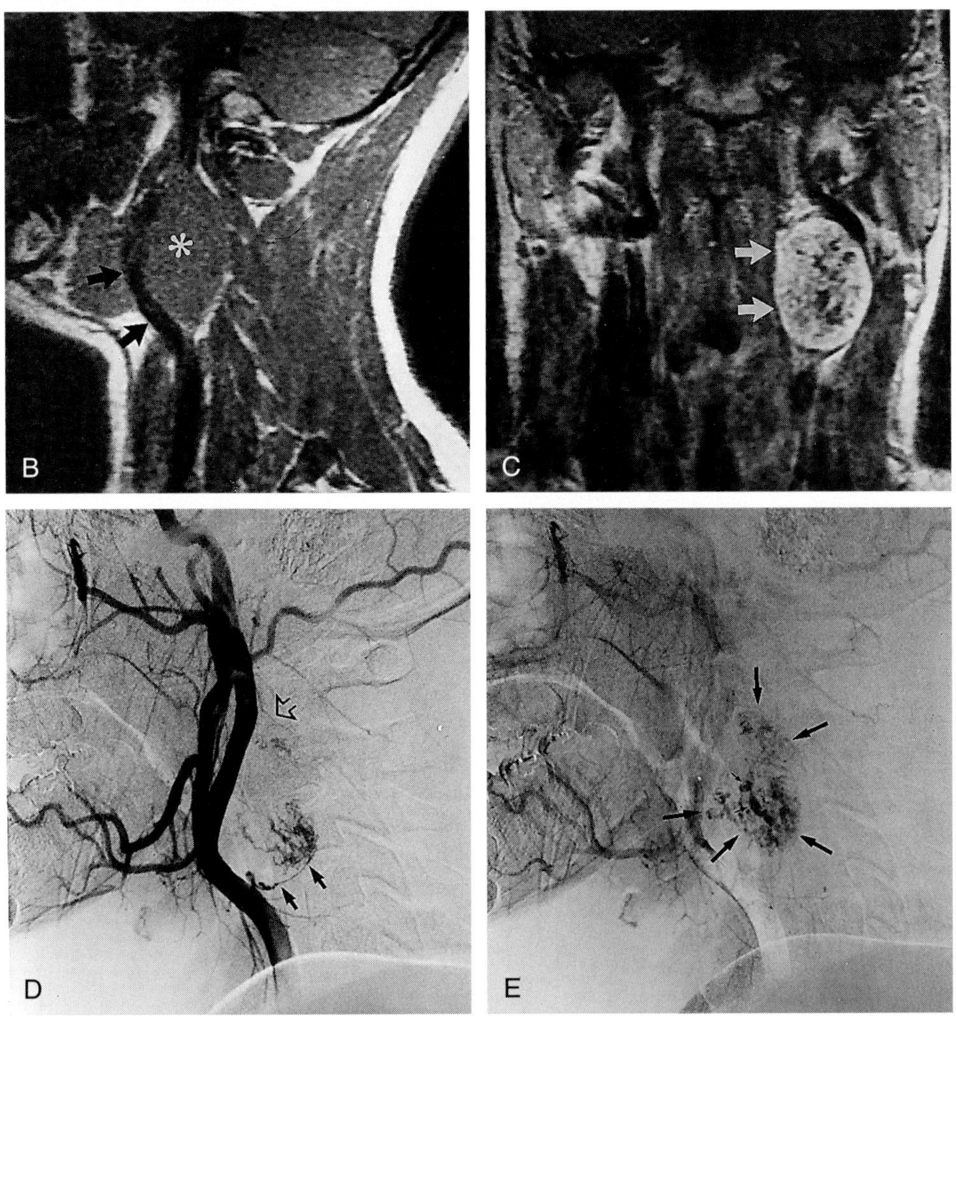

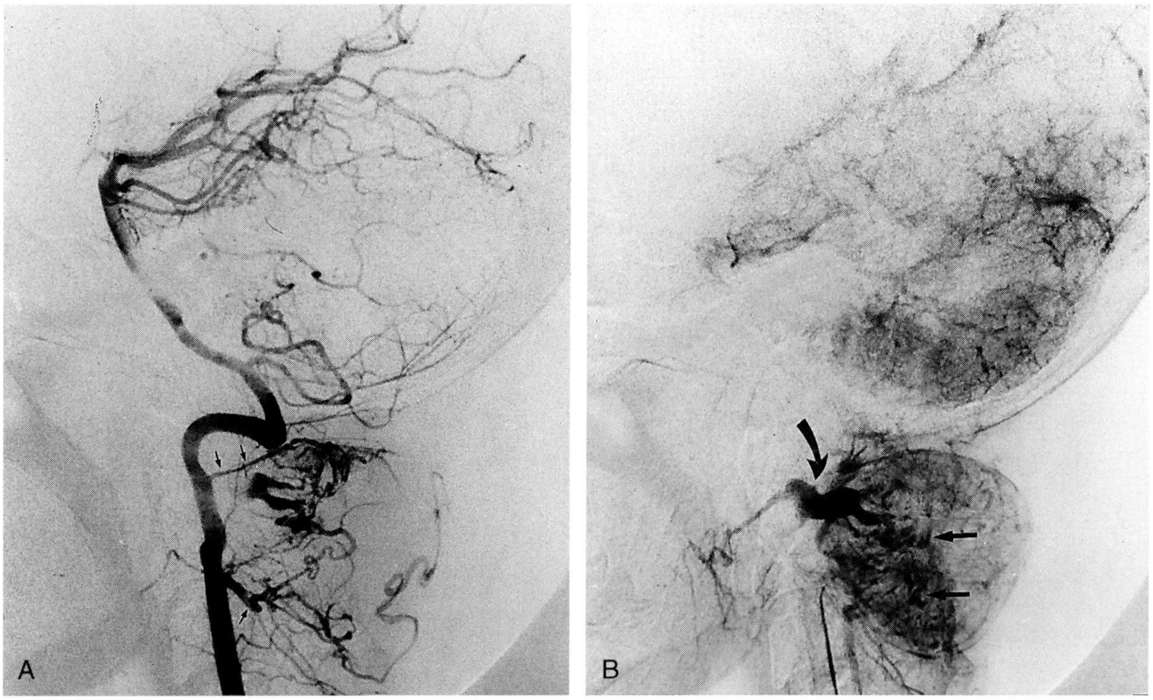

Figure 8–38. Schwannoma. **(A)** Early and **(B)** late lateral vertebral angiograms show the tumor is supplied by enlarged muscular branches of the vertebral artery (small arrows). A large venous varix (curved arrow) along with smaller areas of venous puddling (large straight arrows) appear in the early venous phase.

Paraganglioma

Synonyms: Glomus tumor (glomus vagale, glomus jugulare), carotid body tumor, chemodectoma.

The paraganglioma is a tumor, usually benign, of the autonomic paraganglia and is pathogenetically related to the adrenal pheochromocytoma. As with pheochromocytoma, about 10% are multiple, and 10% become malignant. In the neck, paragangliomas of vagal origin are most common, followed by those of the carotid body. The mean age at presentation is about 45 years. Tumors of carotid origin show no sex predilection, whereas vagal and jugular tumors are more common in females. The treatment of choice is preoperative embolization followed by surgical resection.

CT Findings. CT shows a smooth well-defined mass isodense to muscle in the parapharyngeal space. It exhibits intense contrast enhancement on dynamic scans and rapid washout if enhancement is plotted against time. The internal carotid is displaced anteriorly with paragangliomas of vagal origin (more common) and posteriorly with those of carotid body origin. Splaying of the carotid bifurcation is the hallmark of a carotid body tumor.

MRI Findings. Paragangliomas exhibit intermediate signal intensity on T1-weighted images and intermediate to moderately high signal intensity on T2-weighted images, with multiple small foci of more marked hyperintensity. Scattered serpentine flow voids reveal the vascular nature of the mass and are the most helpful diagnostic feature. Intense homogeneous enhancement occurs with intravenous contrast.

Angiographic Findings. Angiography consistently reveals a hypervascular mass with enlarged feeding vessels and dense homogeneous staining. Most paragangliomas are supplied by the external carotid artery via the ascending pharyngeal artery, the superior thyroid artery, the occipital artery, and a small direct branch, the artery to the carotid body.

Differential Diagnosis

See Table 8–7.

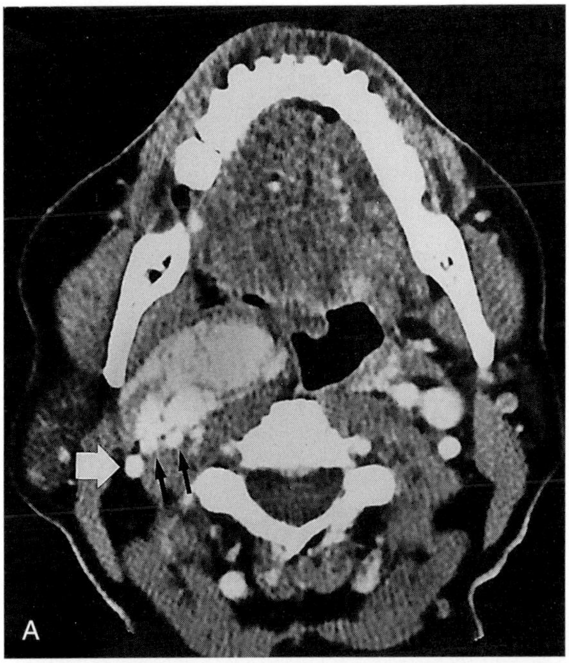

Figure 8–39. Vagal paraganglioma. **(A)** Axial contrast-enhanced CT shows a well-defined and intensely enhancing mass in the right carotid space on dynamic CT. Thick white arrow indicates jugular vein and thin black arrows indicate enlarged branches of external carotid. **(B)** Early arterial phase of lateral carotid angiogram shows the faintly opacified internal carotid (arrows) is displaced anteriorly, a feature of vagal paragangliomas. Open arrow points to an enlarged occipital artery, which was the major feeding vessel. **(C)** Late arterial phase shows intense tumor staining throughout the mass.

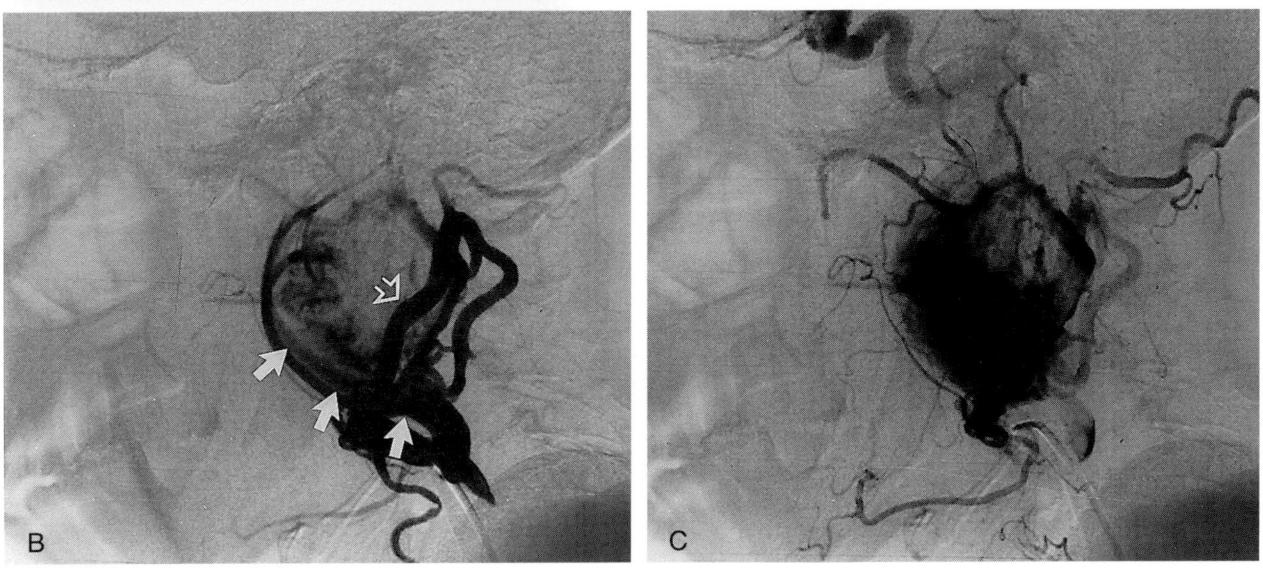

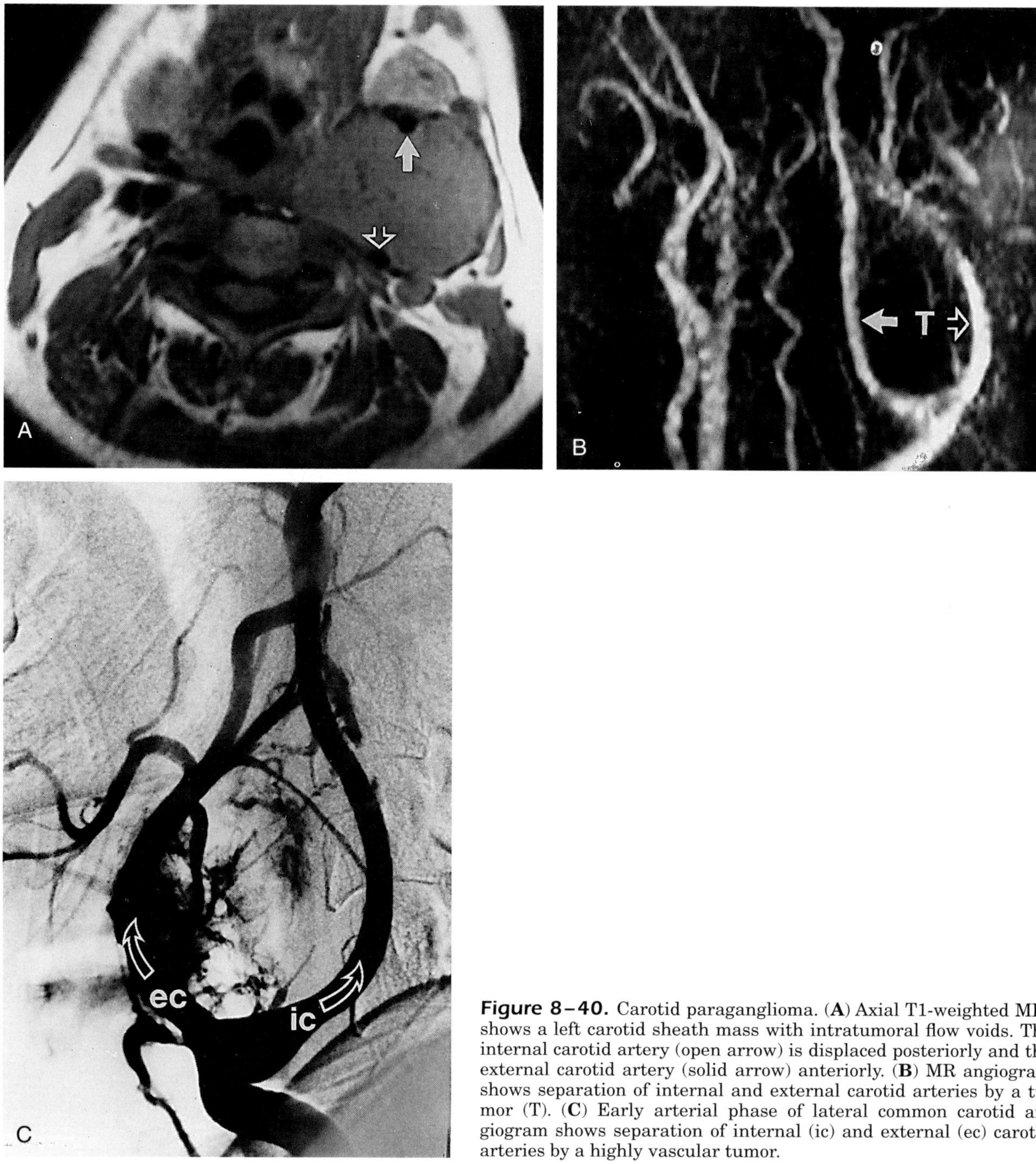

Figure 8–40. Carotid paraganglioma. (**A**) Axial T1-weighted MRI shows a left carotid sheath mass with intratumoral flow voids. The internal carotid artery (open arrow) is displaced posteriorly and the external carotid artery (solid arrow) anteriorly. (**B**) MR angiogram shows separation of internal and external carotid arteries by a tumor (T). (**C**) Early arterial phase of lateral common carotid angiogram shows separation of internal (ic) and external (ec) carotid arteries by a highly vascular tumor.

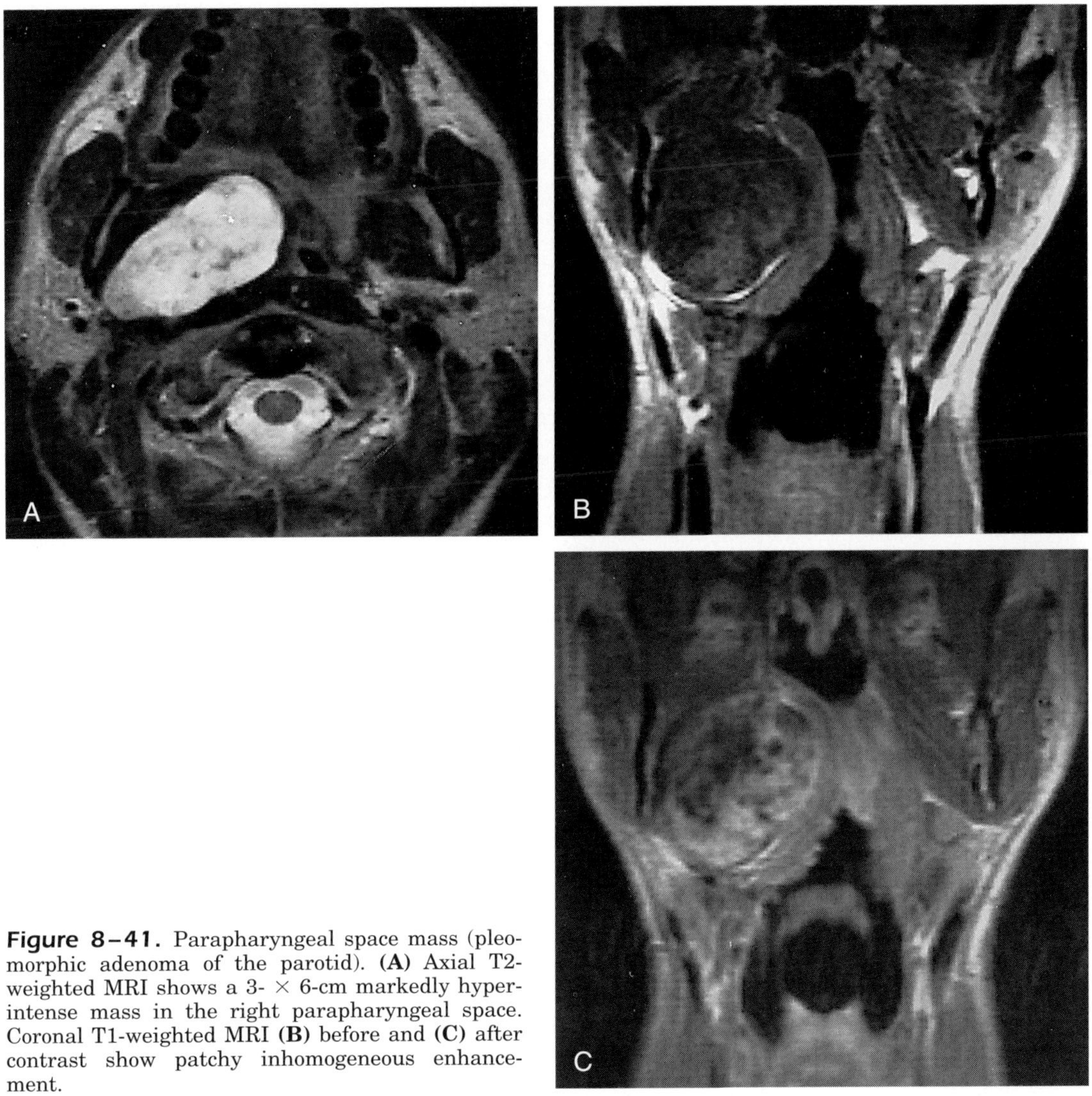

Figure 8–41. Parapharyngeal space mass (pleomorphic adenoma of the parotid). **(A)** Axial T2-weighted MRI shows a 3- × 6-cm markedly hyperintense mass in the right parapharyngeal space. Coronal T1-weighted MRI **(B)** before and **(C)** after contrast show patchy inhomogeneous enhancement.

Malignant Tumors

Squamous Cell Carcinoma

Squamous cell carcinoma is the most common malignant neoplasm of the nose and sinuses, comprising 50–60% of all malignant sinus lesions. Males are more commonly affected by a ratio of 2:1, with an average age of 60 years. About 60–80% originate in the maxillary antra, followed by the nasal cavity and ethmoid sinuses. The maxillary antrum is involved either primarily or secondarily in 80%.

Common presenting symptoms of all malignant sinus lesions include facial or dental pain, nasal obstruction, and epistaxis. Other symptoms include diplopia, epiphora, facial swelling, malocclusion, trismus, neck mass, hearing loss, and facial numbness. Risk factors for developing squamous cell carcinoma of the sinus include certain occupations (particularly those involving exposure to nickel), chronic sinusitis, and inverted papilloma. The disease is usually advanced by the time the patient presents with bone destruction, which is seen at diagnosis in 80%. The cumulative survival rate with combined radiation and surgery is approximately 25–30%.

CT Findings. Most paranasal sinus carcinomas arise in the maxillary antrum, followed by the ethmoid sinus. CT shows an irregular soft tissue mass with minimal to moderate contrast enhancement. Bone destruction is seen early and often. As the tumor grows, it destroys bone in its path, leaving small fragments behind. Bone remodeling or expansion is not seen. Local invasion is the rule, with extension to the nasal cavity, the orbits, other sinuses, the masticator space, the oral cavity, the pterygopalatine fossa, and the skull base, in decreasing order of frequency. Nodal metastases are first seen in the lateral retropharyngeal and jugulodigastric nodes. Associated sinusitis or retained secretions are common due to ostial obstruction.

MRI Findings. MRI shows a soft tissue mass of intermediate signal intensity on T1-weighted images and low to intermediate intensity on T2-weighted images. T2-weighted images help to differentiate hypointense tumors from hyperintense inflammation and secretions. The signal intensity remains moderately homogeneous throughout. The mass enhances moderately with intravenous contrast, and fat suppression techniques aid in differentiating enhanced tumors from fat in the adjacent soft tissues. Perineural invasion, seen as an enlarged enhancing cranial nerve, is best diagnosed with MRI.

Differential Diagnosis

The most important role of imaging is to distinguish inflammatory disease and benign tumors from malignant disease (Table 8–8). It is not usually possible on the basis of imaging alone to differentiate the various primary malignancies in this region.

TABLE 8–8 Inflammatory Versus Malignant Sinus Disease

	Inflammatory Disease	Malignant Disease
Relative incidence	Extremely common	Rare
Sinus size	Normal or small	Expanded
Bone wall	Thinned or sclerotic	Destruction
Infratemporal extension	Never	May be present
Nasal extension	Sometimes	Common
Contrast enhancement	Smooth and linear or none	Irregular and solid or nodular
T2-weighted MRI	Markedly hyperintense (>95%) Exceptions: inspissated secretions, fibrosis, and fungal infections may be hypointense	Hypointense to mildly hyperintense (95%) Exceptions: well-differentiated adenocarcinomas (mucoepidermoid, adenoid cystic) may be quite hyperintense

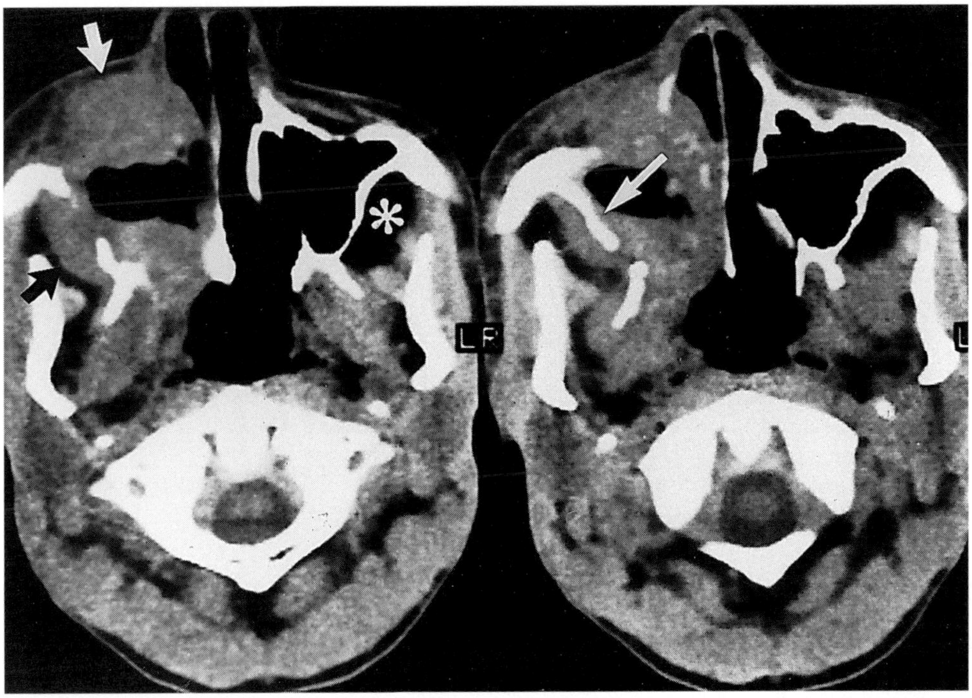

Figure 8–42. Squamous cell carcinoma. Axial contrast-enhanced CT shows an irregular soft tissue mass of the right maxillary sinus with destruction of anterior, medial, and posterior walls. Note infiltration of the malar soft tissue (white arrow), nasal cavity, and masticator space (black arrow). Asterisk indicates normal retroantral fat pad. Typical malignant pattern is indicated by bone erosion without displacement, as seen in the posterior maxillary sinus wall (long white arrow).

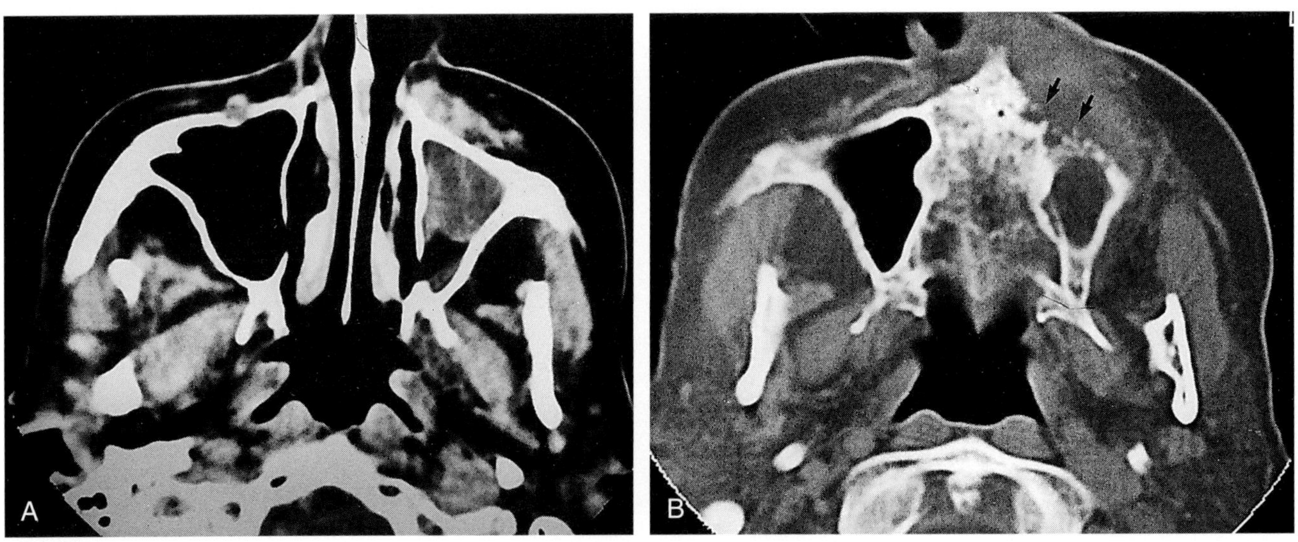

Figure 8–43. Squamous cell carcinoma. **(A)** Axial contrast-enhanced CT shows a mass in the anterior left maxillary sinus and infiltrating the malar soft tissue. **(B)** Bone windows show erosion (arrows) of the anterior floor of the maxillary sinus and hard palate.

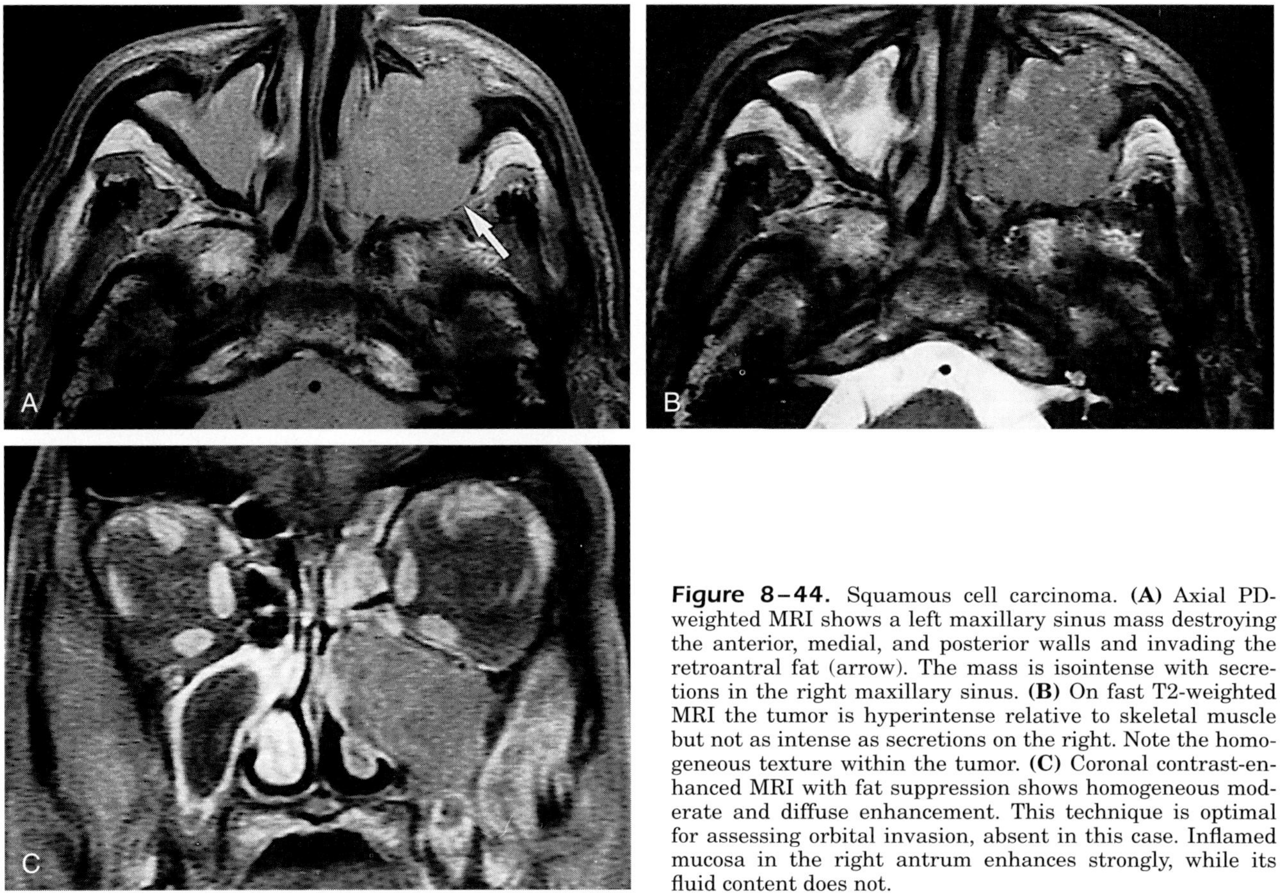

Figure 8–44. Squamous cell carcinoma. **(A)** Axial PD-weighted MRI shows a left maxillary sinus mass destroying the anterior, medial, and posterior walls and invading the retroantral fat (arrow). The mass is isointense with secretions in the right maxillary sinus. **(B)** On fast T2-weighted MRI the tumor is hyperintense relative to skeletal muscle but not as intense as secretions on the right. Note the homogeneous texture within the tumor. **(C)** Coronal contrast-enhanced MRI with fat suppression shows homogeneous moderate and diffuse enhancement. This technique is optimal for assessing orbital invasion, absent in this case. Inflamed mucosa in the right antrum enhances strongly, while its fluid content does not.

Adenoid Cystic Carcinoma

Adenoid cystic carcinoma (ACC) is the most common malignant tumor of the minor salivary glands. The others are mucoepidermoid carcinoma, adenocarcinoma, and malignant pleomorphic adenoma. ACC may arise in the infratemporal fossa, parapharyngeal space, palate, parotid gland, sinuses, nasal cavity, or retropharyngeal space.

About 10% of malignant sinonasal tumors are glandular in origin. The most common adenocarcinoma of the upper respiratory tract, ACC arises from small submucosal salivary glands. It is slow growing but locally invasive, spreading along nerve sheaths. Up to 20% metastasize, especially to the lungs.

ACC most often starts in the ethmoids and nasal vault. It is more common in men ages 30 to 60 years, who most often present with nasal obstruction and epistaxis. Patients may develop cranial nerve deficits or dull pain due to perineural invasion. The short-term prognosis is good, with a 5-year survival of 75%. Late recurrence is common, however, and the 15-year survival drops to 25%.

CT Findings. ACC initially expands the sinus walls as it grows, remodeling bone without breakthrough, thus potentially resembling a mucocele. Attenuation within the tumor is usually inhomogeneous due to cystic degeneration, necrosis, or serous and mucous collections. A mottled appearance often has been noted. More cellular tumors tend to be homogeneous in attenuation.

MRI Findings. ACC appears as a poorly defined mass with infiltrative margins. It is homogeneous and isointense to skeletal muscle on T1-weighted images and enhances diffusely with intravenous contrast. The signal intensity on T2-weighted images is more variable. Hyperintensity on T2-weighted images correlates with low cellularity and a better prognosis. Hypointensity correlates with more cellular tumors and a worse prognosis.

TABLE 8–9 **Malignant Sinonasal Neoplasms**

Tumor	Relative Percentage
Carcinomas	
Squamous cell carcinoma	33.5
Undifferentiated carcinoma	17
Lymphoepithelioma	2
Adenoid cystic carcinoma	11.5
Adenocarcinoma	8
Others	
Lymphoma	6
Malignant melanoma	4.5
Esthesioneuroblastoma	4.5
Plasmacytoma	2
Rhabdomyosarcoma	1.5
Other	9.5
	100.0%

*From: Weber, AL, Stanton, AC. Malignant Tumors of the Paranasal Sinuses: Radiologic, Clinical, and Histopathologic Evaluation of 200 Cases. *Head Neck Surg* 6:761–776, 1984. © 1984. Reprinted by permission of John Wiley & Sons, Inc.

Differential Diagnosis

Early or less aggressive adenocarcinoma may resemble mucocele, with expansion of an airless sinus. However, a mucocele will show only thin rim enhancement and usually a more homogeneous texture. Adenocarcinoma is less easily distinguished from other primary malignancies in this region. See Tables 8–5, 8–8, and 8–9.

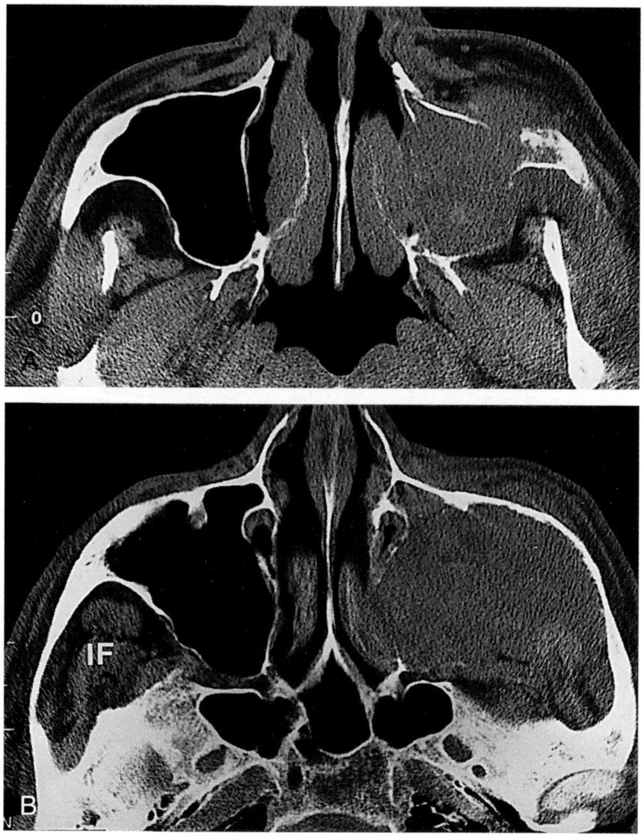

Figure 8–45. Adenocarcinoma (undifferentiated). **(A,B)** Axial CT shows a large soft tissue mass filling and expanding the left maxillary antrum with irregular bone destruction. The tumor invades the malar soft tissues and the infratemporal fossa (IF = normal right infratemporal fossa).

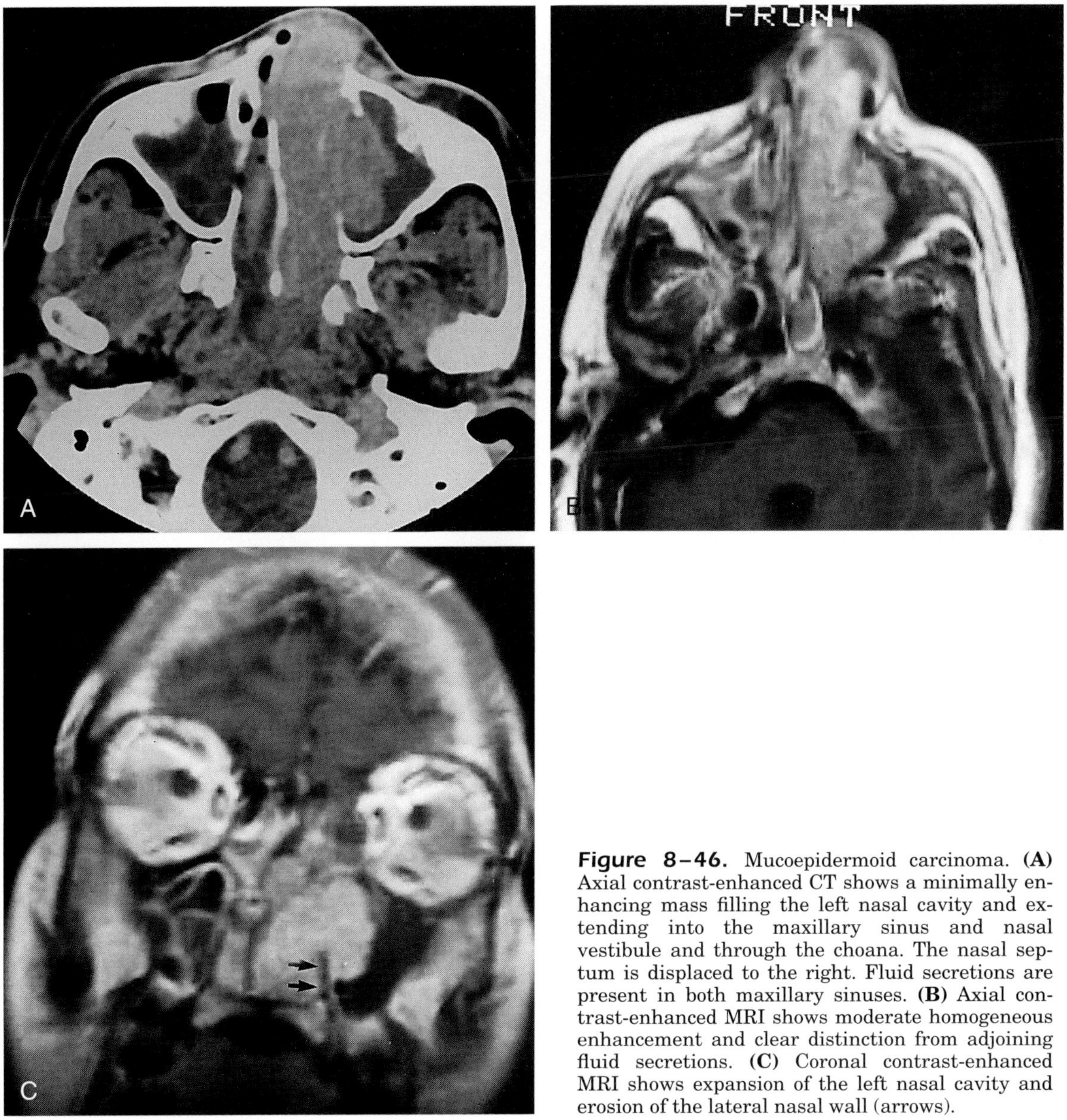

Figure 8–46. Mucoepidermoid carcinoma. **(A)** Axial contrast-enhanced CT shows a minimally enhancing mass filling the left nasal cavity and extending into the maxillary sinus and nasal vestibule and through the choana. The nasal septum is displaced to the right. Fluid secretions are present in both maxillary sinuses. **(B)** Axial contrast-enhanced MRI shows moderate homogeneous enhancement and clear distinction from adjoining fluid secretions. **(C)** Coronal contrast-enhanced MRI shows expansion of the left nasal cavity and erosion of the lateral nasal wall (arrows).

Lymphoma

Lymphoma is the second most common tumor of the head and neck after squamous cell carcinoma. Primary head and neck lymphomas may be either Hodgkin's or non-Hodgkin's and nodal or extranodal. Extranodal Hodgkin's lymphoma is rare. Both non-Hodgkin's lymphoma and an extranodal site of origin are more common in this area. The major extranodal sites are Waldeyer's ring, the paranasal sinuses, the orbits, and the nasal cavity, although lymphoma may arise virtually anywhere.

CT Findings. CT shows a homogeneous mass with mild enhancement. Hodgkin's lymphoma occurs almost exclusively in lymph nodes (most cases) or Waldeyer's ring. The more common non-Hodgkin's lymphoma occurs in Waldeyer's ring or the paranasal sinuses. Both bone expansion and erosion are encountered. Bone destruction is less common and less severe than that typically seen with the more common squamous cell carcinoma. Lymph node enlargement is usually moderate (1 to 2 cm) but may be massive (up to 10 cm) in non-Hodgkin's lymphoma. Central necrosis is seldom seen in involved lymph nodes, which also may help to distinguish it from carcinoma.

MRI Findings. On MRI, lymphomas exhibit homogeneous intermediate signal intensity on both T1- and T2-weighted images and moderate uniform enhancement with intravenous contrast. The margins are usually sharp, and bone invasion is less common than with carcinomas.

Differential Diagnosis

See Tables 8–5, 8–8, and 8–9.

Features favoring lymphoma versus carcinoma:

- Multiple large bilateral lymph nodes without central necrosis
- More than one extranodal, extralymphatic site involved
- Enlarged nodes not in usual pathway of spread for carcinoma (submental, submandibular, retropharyngeal, posterior triangle)

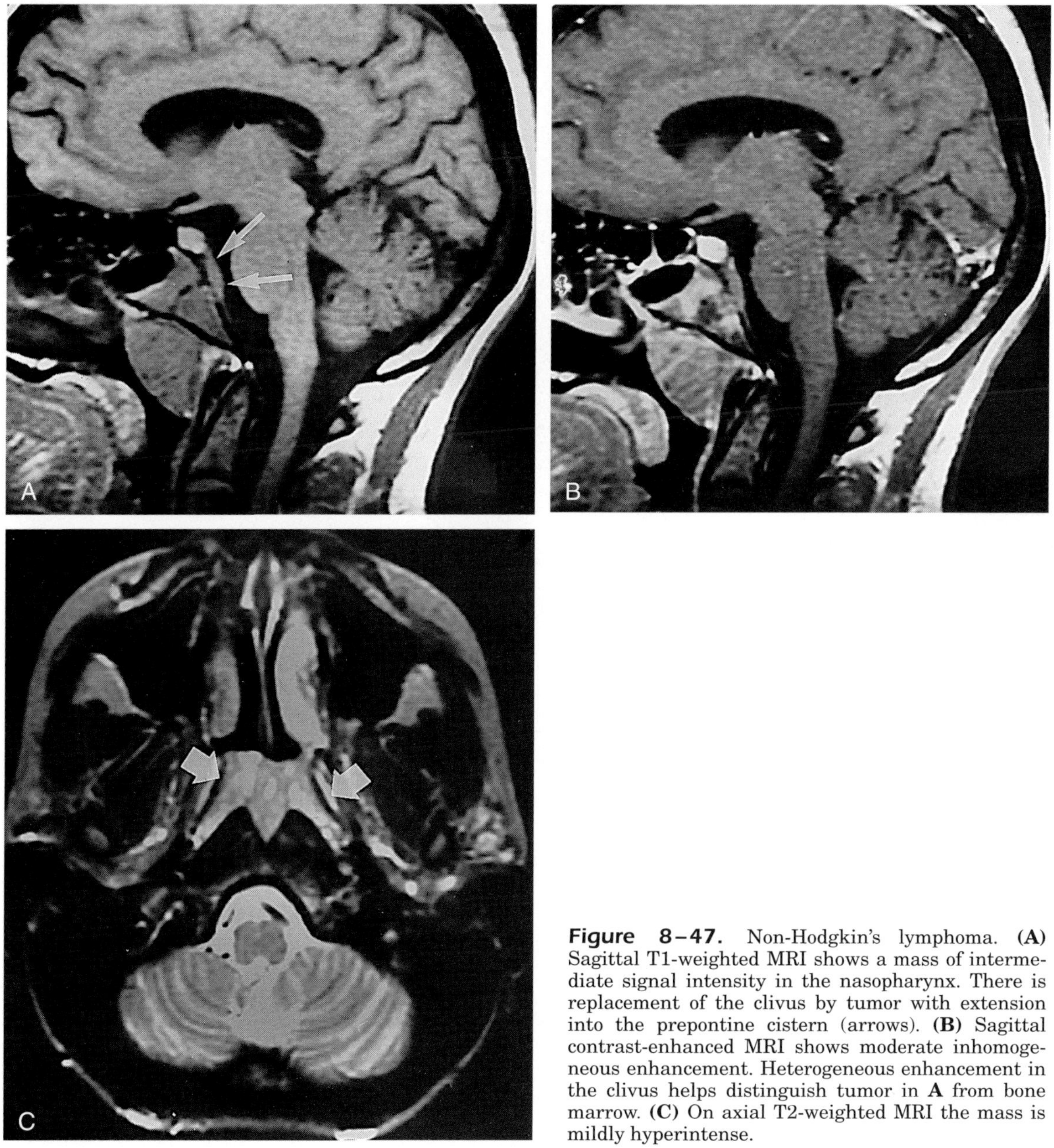

Figure 8–47. Non-Hodgkin's lymphoma. **(A)** Sagittal T1-weighted MRI shows a mass of intermediate signal intensity in the nasopharynx. There is replacement of the clivus by tumor with extension into the prepontine cistern (arrows). **(B)** Sagittal contrast-enhanced MRI shows moderate inhomogeneous enhancement. Heterogeneous enhancement in the clivus helps distinguish tumor in **A** from bone marrow. **(C)** On axial T2-weighted MRI the mass is mildly hyperintense.

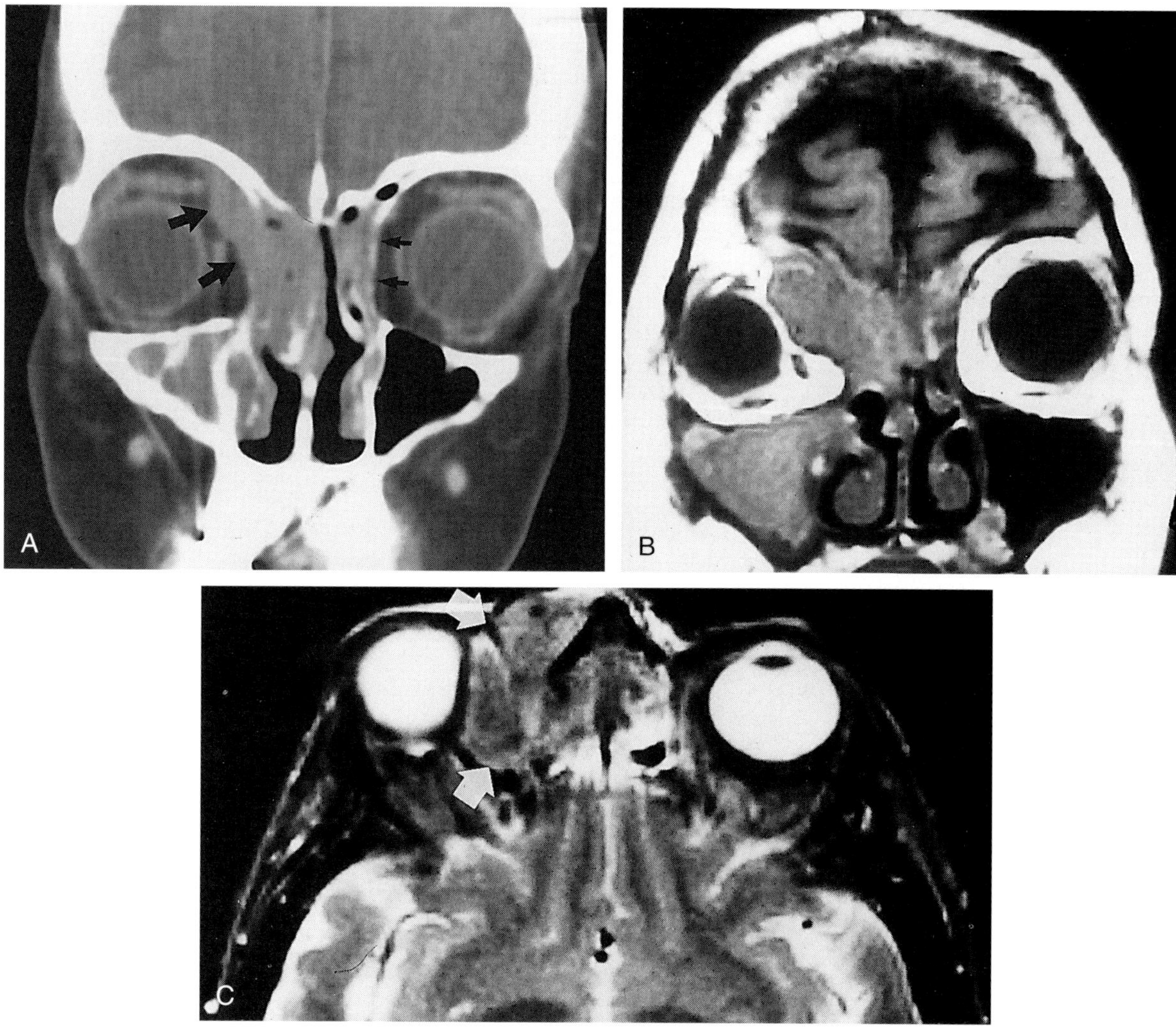

Figure 8–48. Non-Hodgkin's lymphoma. **(A)** Coronal contrast-enhanced CT shows a homogeneously enhancing mass of the right ethmoids with destruction of the lamina papyracea and invasion of the right orbit (large arrows). Small arrows indicate normal left lamina papyracea. **(B)** Coronal T1-weighted MRI shows a soft tissue mass of intermediate intensity involving the right orbit, right ethmoids, and right maxillary sinus. **(C)** On axial T2-weighted MRI, tumor mass (arrows) in the right ethmoids is of intermediate signal intensity.

Rhabdomyosarcoma

The most common malignant neoplasm of the upper respiratory tract among children, rhabdomyosarcoma occurs only occasionally in adults. About 78% of affected individuals are less than 12 years old. An aggressive neoplasm, it is characterized by extremely rapid growth and frequently advanced at the time of diagnosis. In the head and neck area, the orbit is the most common site of origin, followed by the sinonasal region. Affected patients may present with nasal bleeding, rhinorrhea, nasal obstruction, otalgia, or ear obstruction. The 3-year survival is approximately 70% with combined therapy. Metastases occur by hematogenous, lymphatic, direct, and meningeal spread.

CT Findings. CT shows a poorly defined inhomogeneous mass that distorts soft tissue planes and destroys bone. Little or moderate enhancement occurs after contrast. Intracranial involvement and cervical adenopathy are common.

MRI Findings. Most rhabdomyosarcomas are isointense with muscle on T1-weighted images and hyperintense on T2-weighted images. Marked enhancement occurs with intravenous contrast. They may be homogeneous to markedly heterogeneous and occasionally contain areas of hemorrhage. Common associated findings include intracranial invasion, bone destruction, and metastatic adenopathy.

Differential Diagnosis

Esthesioneuroblastoma	Arises in upper nasal cavity, usually midline Much less common in the first decade of life
Metastatic neuroblastoma	Common tumor in the first decade and frequently metastasizes to bone Usually first manifests somewhere other than the facial region
Nasal polyposis	May cause extensive bone resorption and remodeling Much slower progression Ethmoid expansion and hypertelorism common
Angiofibroma	Almost exclusively in adolescent males May cause extensive bone erosion Hypervascular on MRI and angiography

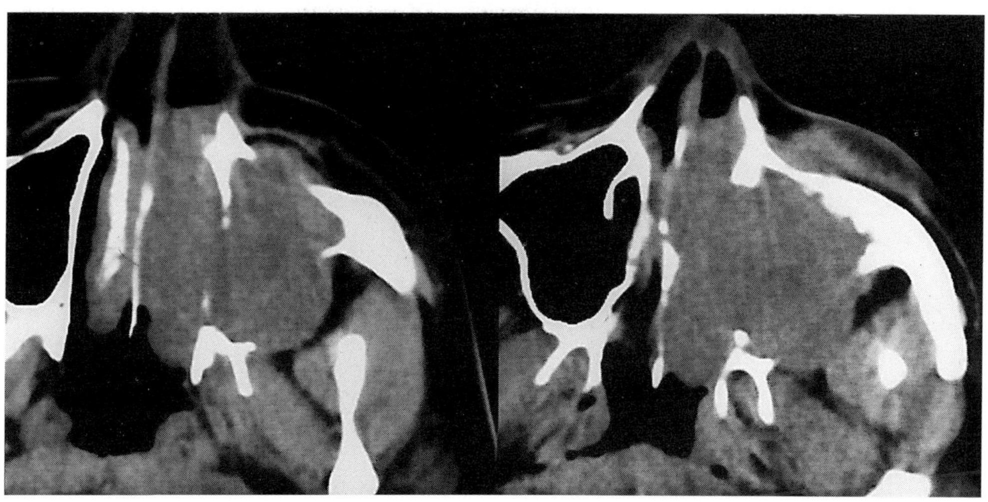

Figure 8–49. Rhabdomyosarcoma. Unenhanced CT shows a soft tissue mass of the left maxilla. There is destruction of the anterior, medial, and posterior maxillary sinus walls with invasion of the retroantral fat pad and nasal cavity.

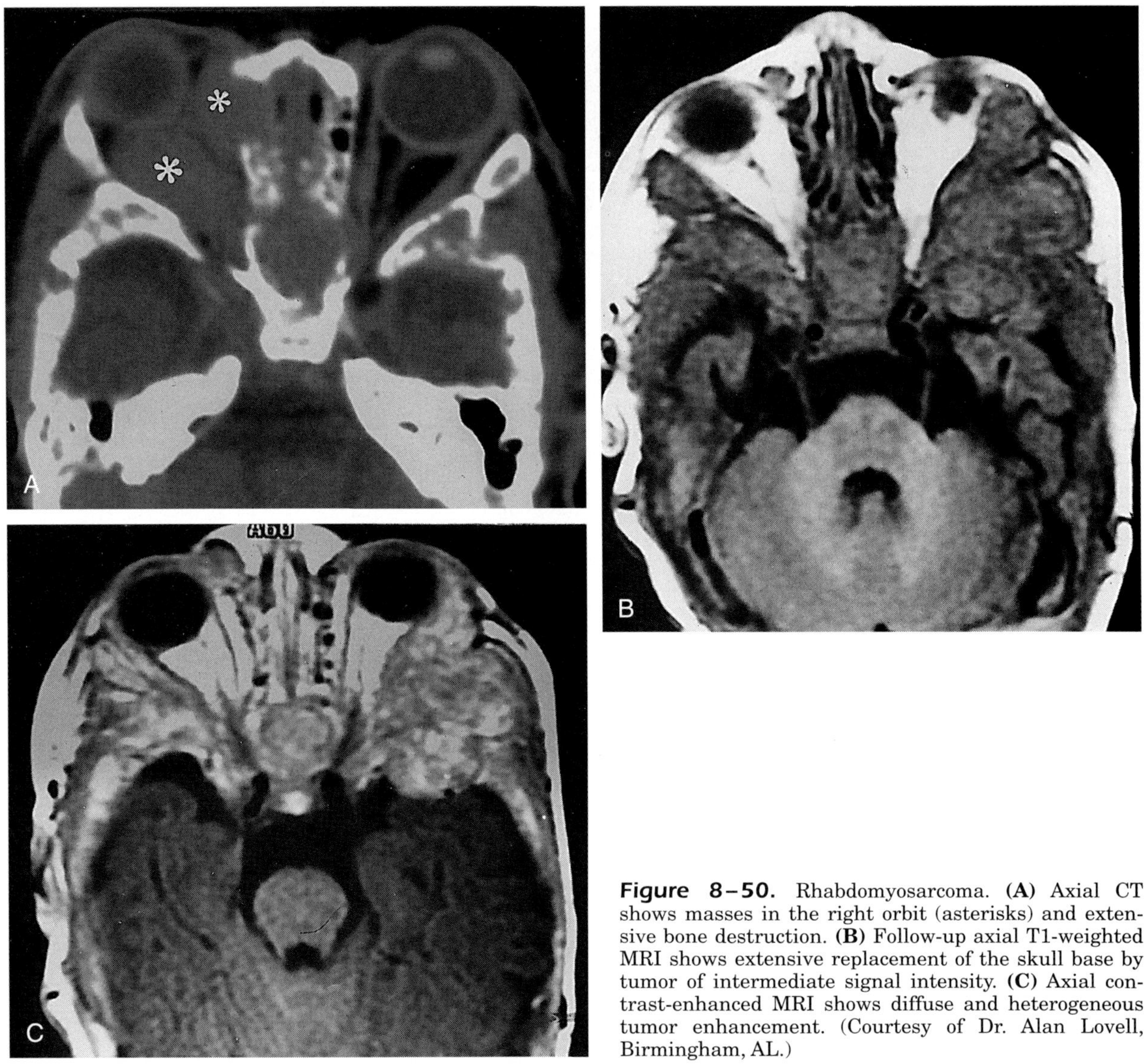

Figure 8–50. Rhabdomyosarcoma. **(A)** Axial CT shows masses in the right orbit (asterisks) and extensive bone destruction. **(B)** Follow-up axial T1-weighted MRI shows extensive replacement of the skull base by tumor of intermediate signal intensity. **(C)** Axial contrast-enhanced MRI shows diffuse and heterogeneous tumor enhancement. (Courtesy of Dr. Alan Lovell, Birmingham, AL.)

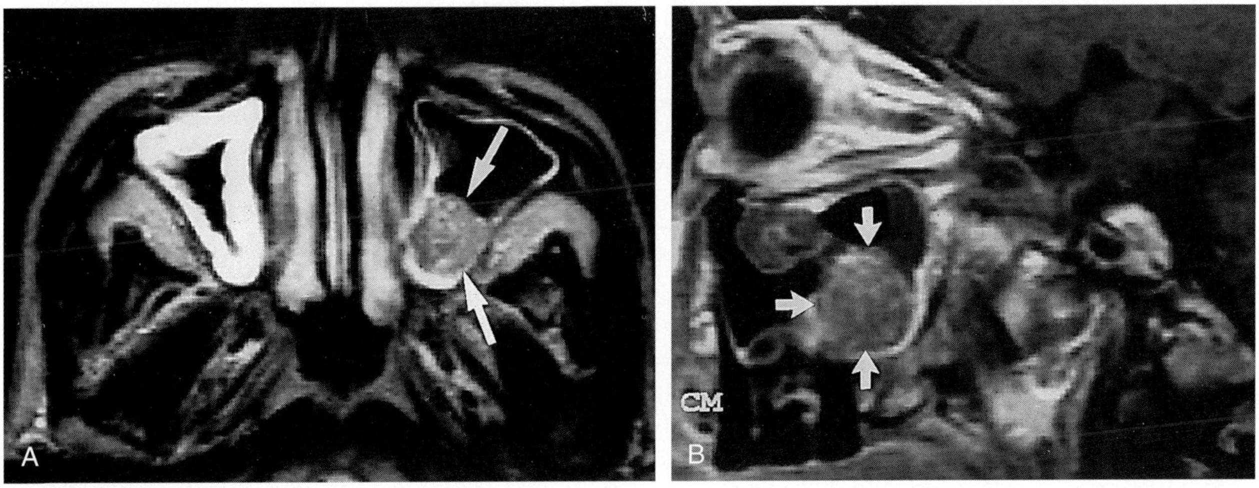

Figure 8–51. Rhabdomyosarcoma. **(A)** Axial T2-weighted MRI shows a mildly hyperintense mass (arrows) of the left maxillary sinus, which is easily distinguished from the markedly hyperintense inflamed mucosa. **(B)** Sagittal contrast-enhanced MRI shows very mild enhancement of the tumor (arrows).

Esthesioneuroblastoma

Synonyms: Olfactory neuroblastoma, esthesioneurocytoma, neuroendocrine carcinoma.

Esthesioneuroblastoma is a rare malignant tumor of the olfactory epithelium, which derives from the neural crest. It is now widely regarded as part of the spectrum of primitive neuroectodermal tumors. It occurs over a wide age range, with a mean age in the fourth or fifth decade and a slight male predominance. Nasal obstruction and epistaxis are the usual presenting complaints, with metastases to cervical nodes or more distant sites in 20%.

CT Findings. The most common appearance is a homogeneous mass in the upper nasal cavity that both remodels and destroys bone and exhibits moderate uniform enhancement. Calcification may be present. Infrequently an exuberant hyperostosis may be encountered. Intracranial and intraorbital extension is very common.

MRI Findings. Esthesioneuroblastomas tend to be isointense with muscle on T1-weighted images and moderately hyperintense on T2-weighted images. There may be hyperintense foci on T2-weighted images due to necrosis. Moderate diffuse enhancement is seen following intravenous contrast.

Differential Diagnosis

See Tables 8–5, 8–8, and 8–9. A site of origin high in the nasal cavity and intracranial extension are the two most distinctive features of esthesioneuroblastoma but are not specific.

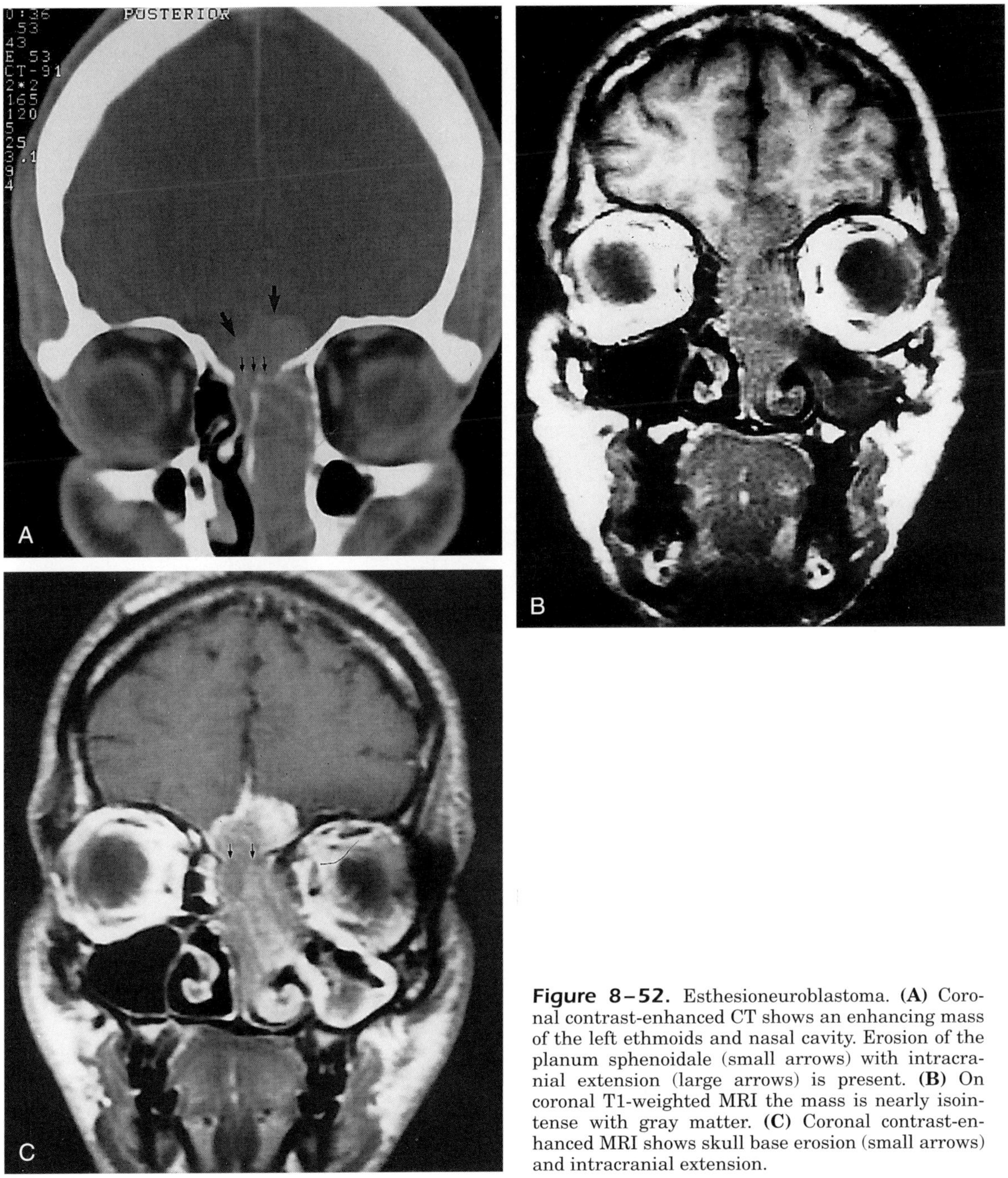

Figure 8–52. Esthesioneuroblastoma. **(A)** Coronal contrast-enhanced CT shows an enhancing mass of the left ethmoids and nasal cavity. Erosion of the planum sphenoidale (small arrows) with intracranial extension (large arrows) is present. **(B)** On coronal T1-weighted MRI the mass is nearly isointense with gray matter. **(C)** Coronal contrast-enhanced MRI shows skull base erosion (small arrows) and intracranial extension.

Squamous Cell Carcinoma of the Nasopharynx

Squamous cell carcinoma accounts for 80% of epithelial malignant tumors of the nasopharynx. Although generally rare, its incidence is markedly increased in persons of southern Chinese ancestry. Patients often present with cervical adenopathy. Other symptoms include serous otitis from obstruction of the eustachian tubes and nerve deficits. Progressive infiltration of surrounding structures, including the skull base, is a hallmark of the disease.

Radiotherapy is the treatment of choice and yields a 3-year survival of 50–70%.

CT Findings. The earliest CT finding is thickening or asymmetry of the nasopharyngeal mucosa at the fossa of Rosenmüller (pharyngeal recess). Nasopharyngeal carcinoma grows submucosally, not into the nasopharyngeal cavity. As the mass enlarges, there is direct spread to the contralateral side, the parapharyngeal spaces with early invasion of the levator palati muscle (>80%), the sphenoid sinus, the nasal fossa, the ethmoid sinus, and the base of the skull (30–50%). Middle cranial fossa invasion (up to 50%) usually occurs by way of the foramen lacerum or foramen ovale. Associated findings include serous otitis media and mucosal thickening of the maxillary antra. The tumor enhances moderately after intravenous contrast.

MRI Findings. MRI shows a mass of the nasopharynx and parapharyngeal space. Carcinoma exhibits intermediate signal intensity on both T1- and T2-weighted images, with irregular margins, inhomogeneous texture, and areas of central necrosis. Moderate enhancement is seen after intravenous contrast.

Differential Diagnosis

Lymphoid hyperplasia (enlarged adenoids) is the most frequently encountered benign mass of the nasopharyx. It is distinguished by the preservation of mucosal contours, preservation of parapharyngeal fat space, midline symmetry, and lack of bone erosion. Other common malignant tumors in the nasopharynx include adenoid cystic carcinoma, metastatic carcinoma (especially from the maxillary sinus), and lymphoma.

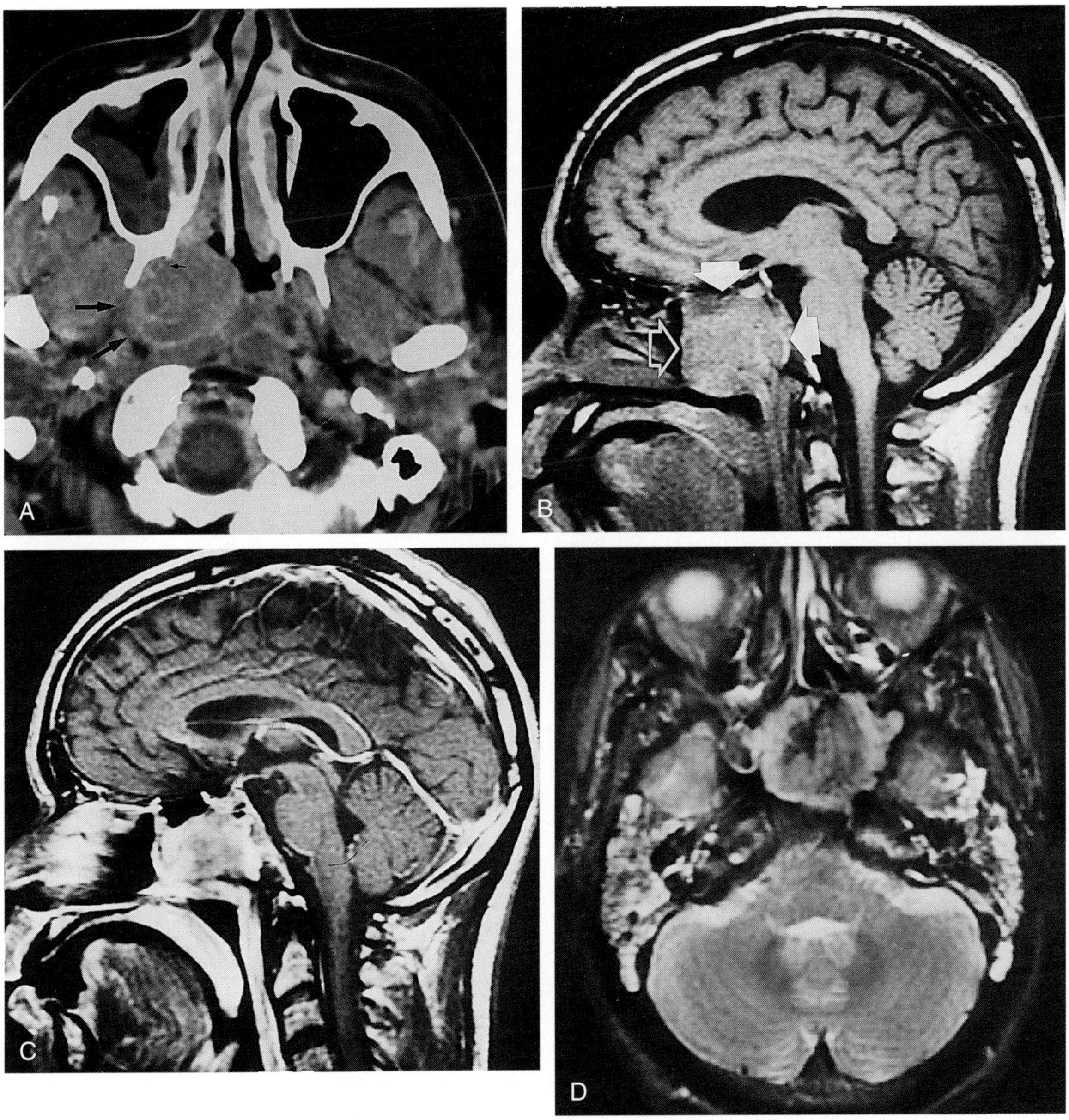

Figure 8–53. Nasopharyngeal carcinoma (squamous cell). **(A)** Axial contrast-enhanced CT shows a mildly enhancing mass of the right nasopharynx with extension to the parapharyngeal space and contralateral spread. The medial pterygoid plate is eroded (small arrow). Note the mucosal thickening of the right maxillary sinus, a common associated finding. **(B)** Sagittal T1-weighted MRI shows a bulky nasopharyngeal mass with extension into the nasal cavity (open arrow) and invasion of the sphenoid and clivus (solid arrows). **(C)** Sagittal contrast-enhanced MRI shows moderate diffuse enhancement. **(D)** On axial T2-weighted MRI the mass exhibits heterogeneous signal characteristics. Note the bilateral serous otitis and mastoiditis.

RECOMMENDED READINGS

Choanal Atresia

Castillo,M. Congenital Abnormalities of the Nose: CT and MR Findings. *AJR* 162:1211–1217, 1994.

Harner,SG, McDonald,TJ, Reese,DF. The Anatomy of Congenital Choanal Atresia. *Otolaryngol Head Neck Surg* 89:7–9, 1981.

Tadmor,R, Ravid,M, Millet,D, Leventon,G. Computed Tomographic Demonstration of Choanal Atresia. *AJNR* 5: 743–745, 1984.

Encephalocele

Barkovich,AJ, Vandermarck,P, Edwards,MSB, Cogen,PH. Congenital Nasal Masses: CT and MR Imaging Features in 16 Cases. *AJNR* 12:105–116, 1991. *AJR* 156:587–598, 1991.

Naidich,TP, Osborn,RE, Bauer,BS, McLone,DG, Kernahan,DA, Zaparackas,ZG. Embryology and Congenital Lesions of the Midface. In Som,PM, Bergeron,RT: *Head and Neck Imaging*. St. Louis: Mosby–Year Book, 1990, pp 1–50.

Abnormalities of the Ostiomeatal Complex

Babbel,RW, Harnsberger,HR, Sonkens,J, Hunt,S, Recurring Patterns of Inflammatory Sinonasal Disease Demonstrated on Screening Sinus CT. *AJNR* 13:903–912, 1992.

Earwaker,J. Anatomic Variants in Sinonasal CT. *Radiographics* 13:381–415, 1993.

Zinreich,SJ, Kennedy,DW, Rosenbaum,AE, Gayler,BW, Kumar,AJ, Stammberger,H. Paranasal Sinuses: CT Imaging Requirements for Endoscopic Surgery. *Radiology* 163:769–775, 1987.

Acute Sinusitis

Carter,BL, Bankoff,MS, Fisk,JD. Computed Tomographic Detection of Sinusitis Responsible for Intracranial and Extracranial Infections. *Radiology* 147:739–742, 1983.

Glasier,CM, Ascher,DP, Williams,KD. Incidental Paranasal Sinus Abnormalities on CT of Children: Clinical Correlation. *AJNR* 7:861–864, 1986.

Rak,KM, Newell,JD, Yakes,WF, Damiano,MA, Luethke,JM. Paranasal Sinuses on MR Images of the Brain: Significance of Mucosal Thickening. *AJNR* 11:1211–1214, 1990. *AJR* 156:381–384, 1991.

Som,PM, Lawson,W, Biller,HF, Lanzieri,CF. Ethmoid Sinus Disease: CT Evaluation in 400 Cases. Part I. Nonsurgical Patients. *Radiology* 159:591–597, 1986.

Chronic Sinusitis

Dillon,WP, Som,PM, Fullerton,GD. Hypointense MR Signal in Chronically Inspissated Sinonasal Secretions. *Radiology* 174:73–78, 1990.

McAlister,WH, Lusk,R, Muntz,HR. Comparison of Plain Radiographs and Coronal CT Scans in Infants and Children with Recurrent Sinusitis. *AJR* 153:1259–1264, 1989.

Som,PM, Dillon,WP, Curtin,HD, Fullerton,GD, Lidov,M. Hypointense Paranasal Sinus Foci: Differential Diagnosis with MR Imaging and Relation to CT Findings. *Radiology* 176: 777–781, 1990.

Weber,AL. Inflammatory Diseases of the Paranasal Sinuses and Mucoceles. *Otolaryngol Clin North Am* 21:421–437, 1988.

Fungal Sinusitis

Kopp,W, Fotter,R, Steiner,H, Beaufort,F, Stammberger,H. Aspergillosis of the Paranasal Sinuses. *Radiology* 156:715–716, 1985.

Manning,SC, Vuitch,F, Weinberg,AG, Brown,OE. Allergic Aspergillosis: A Newly Recognized Form of Sinusitis in the Pediatric Population. *Laryngoscope* 99:681–685, 1989.

Zinreich,SJ, Kennedy,DW, Malat,J, et al. Fungal Sinusitis: Diagnosis with CT and MR Imaging. *Radiology* 169:439, 1988.

Retention Cyst

Gardner,DG. Pseudocysts and retention cysts of the maxillary sinus. *Oral Surg Oral Med Oral Pathol* 58:561–567, 1984.

Ruprecht,A, Batniji,S, El-Neweihi,E. Mucous retention cyst of the maxillary sinus. *Oral Surg Oral Med Oral Pathol* 62:728–731, 1986.

Mucocele

Han,MH, Chang,KH, Lee,CH, et al. Cystic Expansile Masses of the Maxilla: Differential Diagnosis with CT and MR. *AJNR* 16:333–338, 1995.

Hasso, AN. CT of Tumors and Tumor-like Conditions of the Paranasal Sinuses. *Radiol Clin North Am* 22:119–130, 1984.

Lanzieri,CF, Shah,M, Krauss,D, Lavertu,P. Use of Gadolinium-enhanced MR Imaging for Differentiating Mucoceles from Neoplasms in the Paranasal Sinuses. *Radiology* 178:425–428, 1991.

Van Tassel,P, Lee,Y, Jing,B, De Pena,CA. Mucoceles of the Paranasal Sinuses: MR Imaging with CT Correlation. *AJNR* 10:607–612, 1989.

Nasal Polyps

Drutman,J, Babbel,RW, Harnsberger,HR, Sonkens,JW, Braby,D. Sinonasal Polyposis. *Semin CT US MR* 12:561–574, 1991.

Som,PM, Sacher,M, Lawson,W, et al. Computed Tomography Appearance Distinguishing Benign Nasal Polyps from Malignancies. *J Comput Assist Tomogr* 11:129–133, 1987.

Weissman,JL, Tabor,EK, Curtin,HD. Sphenochoanal Polyps: Evaluation with CT and MR Imaging. *Radiology* 178: 145–148, 1991.

Wegener's Granulomatosis

Lloyd,GAS, Lund,VJ, Phelps,PD, Howard,DJ. Magnetic Resonance Imaging in the Evaluation of Nose and Paranasal Sinus Disease. *Br J Radiol* 60:957–968, 1987.

Simmons,JT, Leavitt,R, Kornblut,AD, Fauci,AS. CT of the Paranasal Sinuses and Orbits in Patients with Wegener's Granulomatosis. *Ear Nose Throat J* 66:134–140, 1987.

Osteoma

Som,PM. Sinonasal Cavity. In Som,PM, Bergeron,RT: *Head and Neck Imaging*. St. Louis: Mosby–Year Book, 1991, pp 51–276.

Weber,AL. Tumors of the Paranasal Sinuses. *Otolaryngol Clin North Am* 21(3):439–454, 1988.

Fibrous Dysplasia

Swartz,JD, Vanderslice,RB, Korsvik,H, et al. High Resolution Computed Tomography: Part 6, Craniofacial Paget's Disease and Fibrous Dysplasia. *Head Neck Surg* 8:40–47, 1985.

Utz,JA, Kransdorf,JJ, Jelinek,JS, Moser,RP, Berrey,BH. MR Appearance of Fibrous Dysplasia. *J Comput Assist Tomogr* 13:845–851, 1989.

Angiofibroma

Lloyd,GAS, Phelps,PD. Juvenile Angiofibroma: Imaging by Magnetic Resonance, CT, and Conventional Techniques. *Clin Otolaryngol* 11:247–259, 1986.

Papilloma

Som,PM, Lawson,W, Lidov,MW. Simulated Aggressive Skull Base Erosion in Response to Benign Sinonasal Disease. *Radiology* 180:755–759, 1991.

Woodruff,WW, Vrabec,DP. Inverted Papilloma of the Nasal Vault and Paranasal Sinuses: Spectrum of CT Findings. *AJR* 162:419–423, 1994.

Yousem,DM, Fellows,DW, Kennedy,DW, Bolger,WE, Kashima,H,

Zinreich,SJ. Inverted Papilloma: Evaluation with MR Imaging. *Radiology* 185:501–505, 1992.

Thornwaldt Cyst

Ford,WJ, Brooks,BS, El Gammal,T. Thornwaldt Cyst: An Incidental MR Diagnosis (letter). *AJNR* 8:922–923, 1987.

Weissman,JL. Thornwaldt Cysts. *Am J Otolaryngol* 13:381–385, 1992.

Schwannoma and Neurofibroma

Abramowitz,J, Dion,JE, Jensen,ME, et al. Angiographic Diagnosis and Management of Head and Neck Schwannomas. *AJNR* 12:977–984, 1991. *AJR* 157:1309–1316, 1991.

Silver,AJ, Mawad,ME, Hilal,SK, Ascherl,GF, Chynn,KY, Baredes,S. Computed Tomography of the Carotid Space and Related Cervical Spaces. Part II: Neurogenic Tumors. *Radiology* 150:729–739, 1984.

Som,PM, Braun,IF, Shapiro,JD, Reede,DL, Curtin,HD, Zimmerman,RA. Tumors of the Parapharyngeal Space and Upper Neck: MR Imaging Characteristics. *Radiology* 164:823–829, 1987.

Paraganglioma

Brismar,J. Angiography of Chemodectomas of the Neck. *Acta Radiol* 21:689–696, 1980.

Som,PM, Braun,IF, Shapiro,MD, Reede,DL, Curtin,HD, Zimmerman,RA. Tumors of the Parapharygeal Space and Upper Neck: MR Imaging Characteristics. *Radiology* 164:823–829, 1987.

Som,PM, Sacher,M, Stollman,AL, Biller,HF, Lawson,W. Common Tumors of the Parapharyngeal Space: Refined Imaging Diagnosis. *Radiology* 169:81–85, 1988.

Squamous Cell Carcinoma

Silver,AJ, Baredes,S, Bello,JA, Blitzer,A, Hilal,SK. The Opacified Maxillary Sinus: CT Findings in Chronic Sinusitis and Malignant Tumors. *Radiology* 163:205–210, 1987.

Som,PM, Shapiro,MD, Biller,HF, Sasaki,C, Lawson,W. Sinonasal Tumors and Inflammatory Tissues: Differentiation with MR Imaging. *Radiology* 167:803–808, 1988.

Weber,AL, Stanton,AC. Malignant Tumors of the Paranasal Sinuses: Radiologic, Clinical, and Histopathologic Evaluation of 200 Cases. *Head Neck Surg* 6:761–776, 1984.

Adenoid Cystic Carcinoma

Sigal,R, Monnet,O, de Baere,T, et al. Adenoid Cystic Carcinoma of the Head and Neck: Evaluation with MR Imaging and Clinical-Pathologic Correlation in 27 Patients. *Radiology* 184:95–101, 1992.

Som,PM, Shapiro,MD, Biller,HF, Sasaki,C, Lawson,W. Sinonasal Tumors and Inflammatory Tissues: Differentiation with MR Imaging. *Radiology* 167:803–808, 1988.

Lymphoma

Harnsberger,HR, Bragg,DG, Osborn,AG, et al. Non-Hodgkin's Lymphoma of the Head and Neck: CT Evaluation of Nodal and Extranodal Sites. *AJNR* 8:673–679, 1987.

Lee,YY, Van Tassel,P, Nauert,C, North,LB, Jing,BS. Lymphomas of the Head and Neck: CT Findings at Initial Presentation. *AJNR* 8:665–671, 1987.

Vogl,T, Dresel,S, Bilaniuk,LT, Grevers,G, Kang,K, Lissner,J. Tumors of the Nasopharynx and Adjacent Areas: MR Imaging with Gd-DTPA. *AJNR* 11:187–194, 1990. *AJR* 154:585–592, 1990.

Rhabdomyosarcoma

Latack,JT, Hutchinson,RJ, Heyn,RM. Imaging of Rhabdomyosarcomas of the Head and Neck. *AJNR* 8:353–359, 1987.

Yousem,DM, Lexa,FJ, Bilaniuk,LT, Zimmerman,RI. Rhabdomyosarcomas in the Head and Neck: MR Imaging Evaluation. *Radiology* 177:683–686, 1990.

Esthesioneuroblastoma

Hurst,RW, Erickson,S, Cail,WS, et al. Computed Tomographic Features of Esthesioneuroblastoma. *Neuroradiology* 31: 253–257, 1989.

Schuster,JJ, Phillips,CD, Levine,PA. MR of Esthesioneuroblastoma (Olfactory Neuroblastoma) and Appearance after Craniofacial Resection. *AJNR* 15:1169–1177, 1994.

Som,PM, Dillon,WP, Sze,G, Lidov,M, Biller,HF, Lawson,W. Benign and Malignant Sinonasal Lesions with Intracranial Extension: Differentiation with MR Imaging. *Radiology* 172: 763–766, 1989.

Squamous Cell Carcinoma of the Nasopharynx

Sham,JST, Cheung,YK, Choy,D, Chan,FL, Leong,L. Nasopharyngeal Carcinoma: CT Evaluation of Patterns of Tumor Spread. *AJNR* 12:265–270, 1991.

Silver,AJ, Mawad,ME, Hilal,SK, Sane,P, Ganti,SR. Computed Tomography of the Nasopharynx and Related Spaces. Part II: Pathology. *Radiology* 147:733–738, 1983.

Vogl,T, Dresel,S, Bilaniuk,LT, Grevers,G, Kang,K, Lissner,J. Tumors of the Nasopharynx and Adjacent Areas: MR Imaging with Gd-DTPA. *AJNR* 11:187–194, 1990. *AJR* 154:585–592, 1990.

CHAPTER
NINE

Temporal Bone

The most complex bone of the human body, the temporal bone is home to auditory and vestibular functions and accommodates the transit of the facial nerve and internal carotid artery. Common signs of temporal bone disorders therefore include hearing loss, tinnitus, vertigo, and facial nerve deficits. Nonspecific symptoms may include pain, discharge, or an enlarging mass. For most cases, CT is the preferred modality in the initial assessment of temporal bone disease due to its high resolution of fine bone anatomy. Only in the evaluation of an adult with acquired sensorineural hearing loss, in whom acoustic neuroma is a consideration, is MRI clearly the initial examination of choice. However, there are many other situations in which MRI is a valuable adjunct. The widespread use of MRI frequently leads to the incidental detection of temporal bone disease, especially inflammatory.

Congenital Abnormalities

Aberrant Carotid Artery

This condition results from atresia of the cervical internal carotid artery. A collateral pathway is formed by hypertrophy of the inferior tympanic artery (ITA), a branch of the ascending pharyngeal. The ITA anastomoses with the caroticotympanic artery in the middle ear, in turn reconstituting the internal carotid artery in the horizontal carotid canal. Affected patients present with pulsatile tinnitus and a mass on otoscopy. Preoperative diagnosis of an aberrant carotid artery is critical because biopsy may be disastrous.

TABLE 9–1 Differential Diagnosis of Pulsatile Tinnitus

Aberrant carotid artery
Dehiscent jugular bulb
Paraganglioma
Carotid-cavernous fistula
Dural arteriovenous fistula
Cerebral AVM
Carotid stenosis

CT Findings. CT is the preferred modality for the initial evaluation of pulsatile tinnitus or a vascular mass. The key CT findings include (1) absence of the vertical carotid canal (anteromedial to the jugular foramen), (2) enlargement of the inferior tympanic canaliculus (anterolateral to the jugular foramen), (3) aberrant course of the artery through the hypotympanum, and (4) dehiscence of the carotid plate, the bony plate separating the normal carotid canal from the hypotympanum.

Angiographic Findings. On an anteroposterior projection, the internal carotid courses more laterally (swings lateral to the cochlea) and is smaller than normal. On a lateral projection, it courses more posteriorly in the temporal bone than normal.

Differential Diagnosis

See Table 9–1.

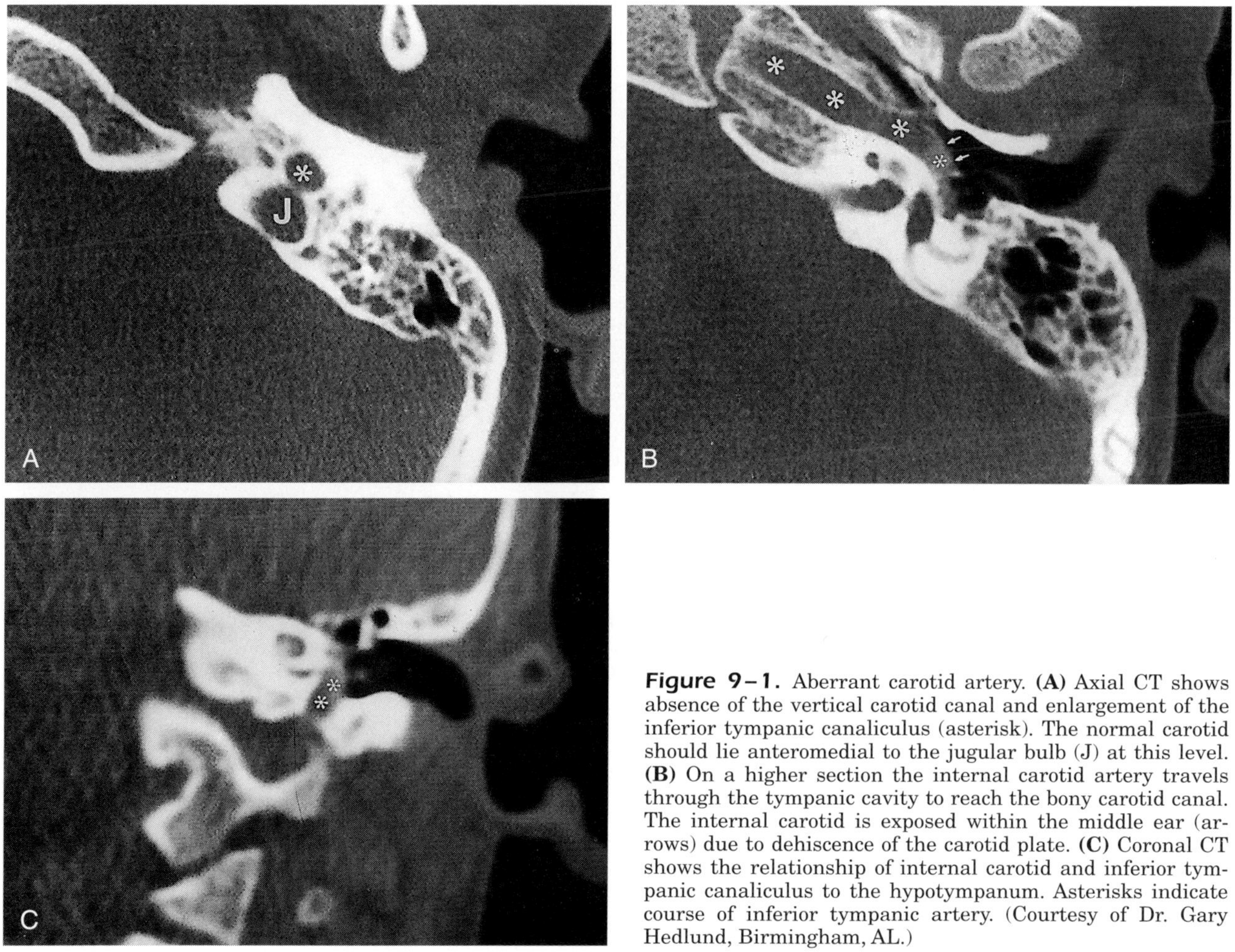

Figure 9–1. Aberrant carotid artery. **(A)** Axial CT shows absence of the vertical carotid canal and enlargement of the inferior tympanic canaliculus (asterisk). The normal carotid should lie anteromedial to the jugular bulb (J) at this level. **(B)** On a higher section the internal carotid artery travels through the tympanic cavity to reach the bony carotid canal. The internal carotid is exposed within the middle ear (arrows) due to dehiscence of the carotid plate. **(C)** Coronal CT shows the relationship of internal carotid and inferior tympanic canaliculus to the hypotympanum. Asterisks indicate course of inferior tympanic artery. (Courtesy of Dr. Gary Hedlund, Birmingham, AL.)

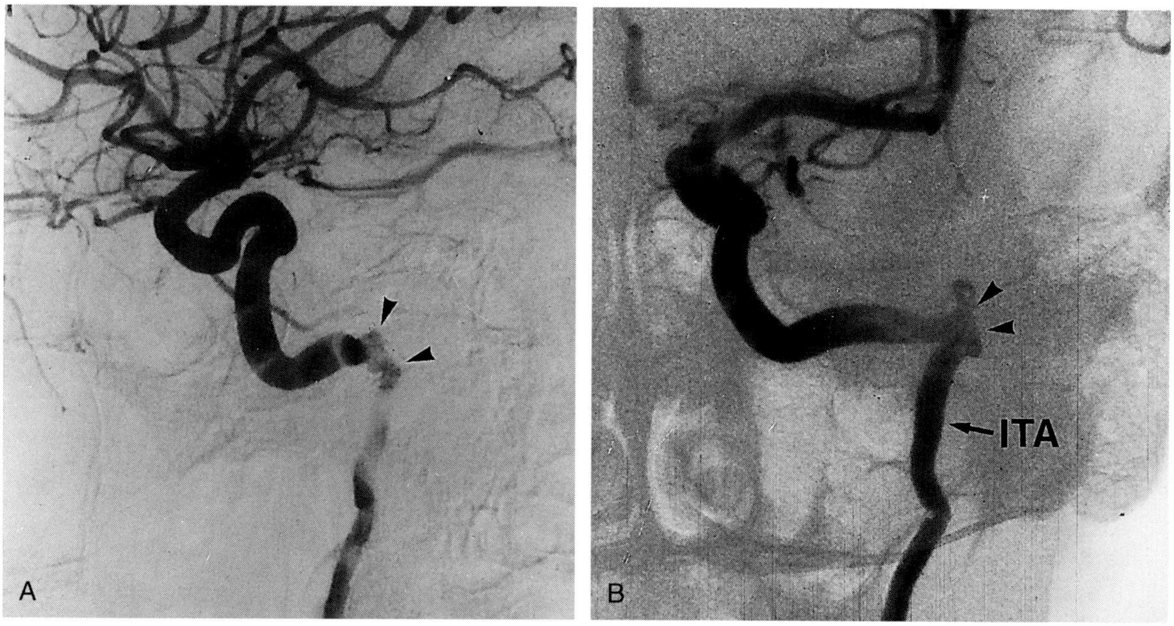

Figure 9–2. Aberrant carotid artery. **(A)** Lateral projection and **(B)** anteroposterior internal carotid angiogram show the internal carotid follows a more lateral and posterior course in its petrous portion (arrowheads) and is small and irregular where it joins the inferior tympanic artery (ITA). (Courtesy of Dr. John Perl, Cleveland, OH.)

Jugular Bulb Variants

Jugular bulb variants are common among the general population. A small minority present clinically with pulsatile tinnitus and a vascular retrotympanic mass. Symptoms are most often due to a dehiscent jugular bulb but may be experienced with a high nondehiscent bulb.

CT Findings. The normal jugular bulb remains below the floor of the hypotympanum. A high jugular bulb extends above this plane and is present in up to 6% of the general population. It is more common on the right, although the right bulb is usually larger anyway. A dehiscent jugular bulb is a high jugular bulb with dehiscence of the jugular plate and protrusion into the hypotympanum. A jugular bulb diverticulum is an enlargement or outpouching of the bulb that extends posteriorly and medially to lie behind the internal auditory canal. The posterior wall of the internal auditory canal may be thinned or eroded.

Angiographic Findings. CT is generally sufficient for the diagnosis. Angiography or venography may be performed to confirm the diagnosis and will show an enlarged and elevated jugular bulb.

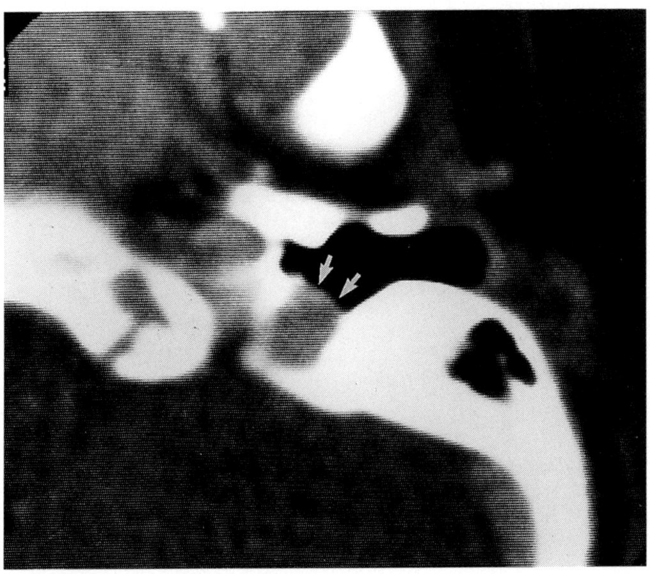

Figure 9–3. Dehiscent jugular bulb. Axial CT shows absence of the jugular plate with the jugular bulb (arrows) freely exposed within the tympanic cavity.

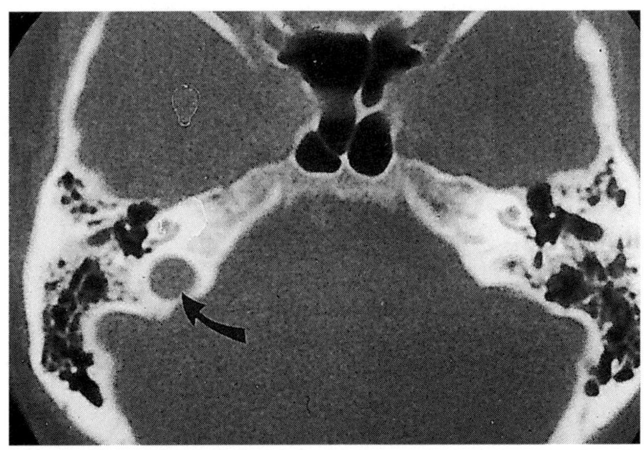

Figure 9–4. High jugular bulb. The right jugular bulb (arrow) ascends to the level of the mesotympanum.

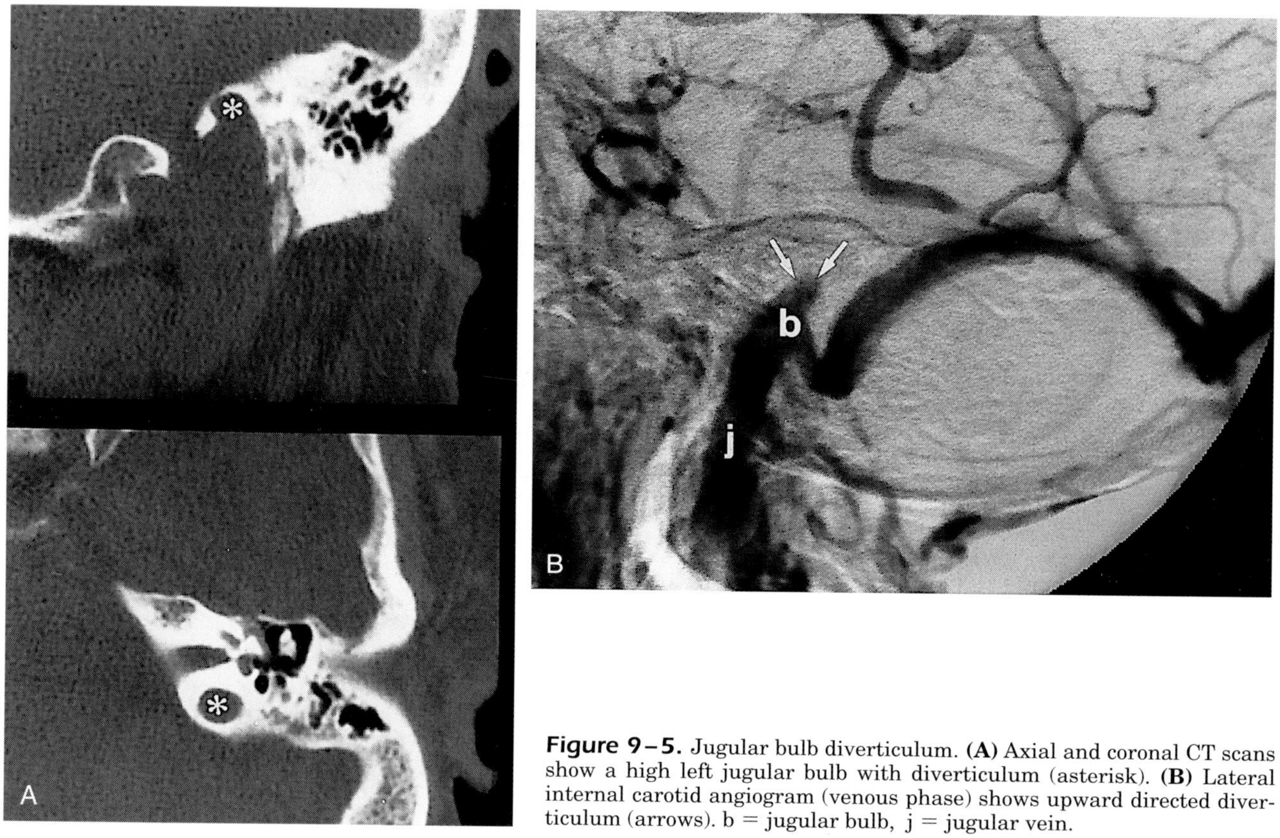

Figure 9–5. Jugular bulb diverticulum. **(A)** Axial and coronal CT scans show a high left jugular bulb with diverticulum (asterisk). **(B)** Lateral internal carotid angiogram (venous phase) shows upward directed diverticulum (arrows). b = jugular bulb, j = jugular vein.

Malformations of Labyrinth

Patients with congenital malformations of the ear present with hearing deficit, deformity of the external ear, CSF leaks, or recurrent meningitis. The inner ear has a separate embryogenesis from the middle and external ears, so malformations tend to involve one or the other but not both. The most common inner ear malformation involves only the soft tissues of the labyrinth (Scheibe malformation) and is not radiographically detectable.

CT Findings. CT remains the primary imaging tool for the investigation of congenital hearing deficit. Interpretation requires the recognition of any deviation from the normal anatomic configuration of the bony labyrinth.

Malformations of the Labyrinth

- Incomplete partition (classic Mondini malformation) (55% of cochlear malformations). The cochlea is small with turns averaging 1.5 (normal is 2.5). The basal turn may be present, but the middle and apical turns form a single cavity with absence of the interscalar septum. The vestibule may be enlarged, and the semicircular canals are deformed in 20%.
- Common cavity (26%). The cochlea and vestibule form a confluent cavity averaging 7 to 10 mm in diameter. The semicircular canals are deformed in 90%.
- Cochlear hypoplasia (15%). The cochlea consists of a small 1- to 3-mm bud. The vestibule may be enlarged, and semicircular canals may be normal or deformed.
- Cochlear aplasia (3%). There is complete absence of the cochlea. The vestibule is present and often enlarged, and the semicircular canals may be normal or deformed.
- Complete labyrinthine aplasia (Michel malformation) (1%). There is complete absence of the cochlea, vestibule, and semicircular canals.

Other Malformations Associated with Congenital Sensorineural Hearing Loss

- Enlarged vestibular aqueduct. This is the most common radiographically detectable inner ear malformation. Associated anomalies are common, especially of the vestibule and semicircular canals. The normal vestibular aqueduct is less than 1.0 mm in diameter; if greater than 1.5 mm, the aqueduct is enlarged.
- Hypoplasia of internal auditory canal (IAC). An IAC less than 3 mm in diameter is hypoplastic and is associated with atresia of the eighth nerve.
- Malformation of lateral semicircular canal. This is also common and may occur in isolation. There is variable enlargement of the lateral semicircular canal or an open pouch.

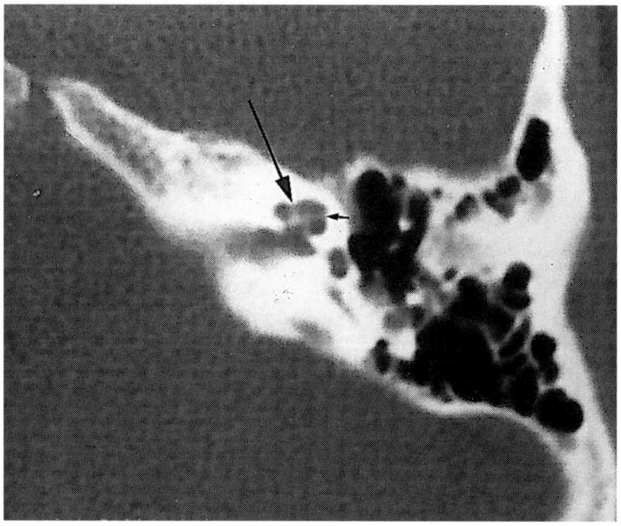

Figure 9-6. Normal cochlea. Axial CT through the cochlea shows the thin bony plates of the interscalar septum (long arrow) separating the second and apical (short arrow) turns of the cochlea. This anatomic feature is absent in the Mondini malformation.

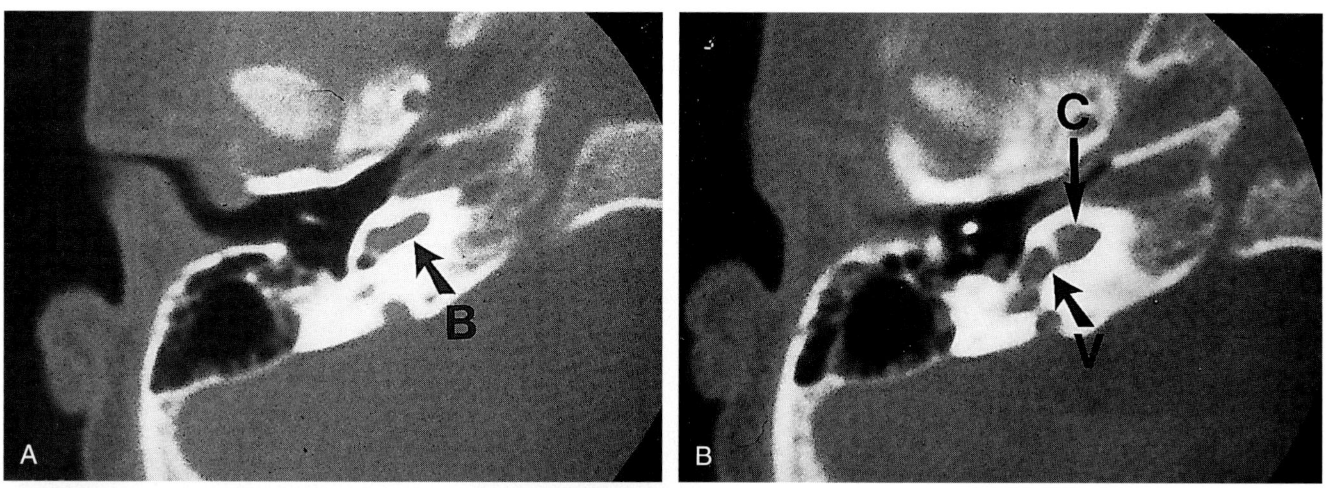

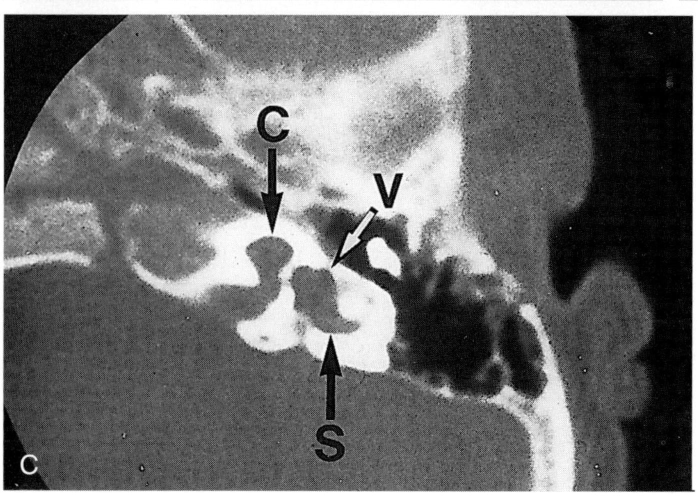

Figure 9-7. Bilateral classic Mondini malformation. **(A,B)** Axial CT of right temporal bone shows an enlarged vestibule. The interscalar septum is absent and the second and apical turns of the cochlea form a single chamber. **(C)** Axial CT of the left temporal bone shows a single apical cavity, enlarged vestibule, and enlarged lateral semicircular canal. B = basal turn of cochlea, C = apex of cochlea, S = lateral semicircular canal, V = vestibule.

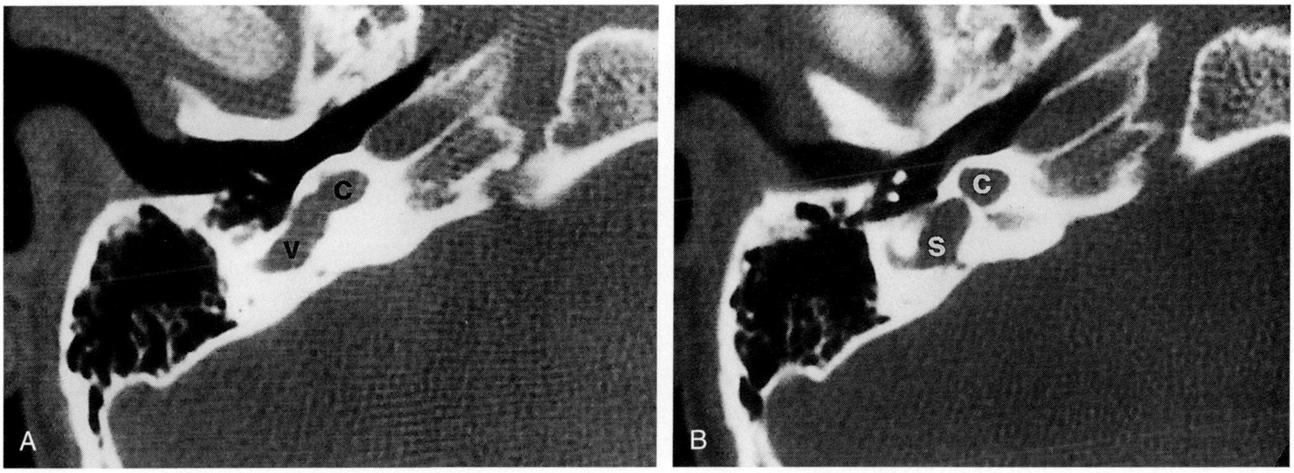

Figure 9–8. Common cavity. **(A,B)** Contiguous axial CT slices show an enlarged vestibule is in wide communication with the cochlear cavity. Cochlear turns are absent and there is deformity of the lateral semicircular canal. c = cochlea, s = lateral semicircular canal, v = vestibule.

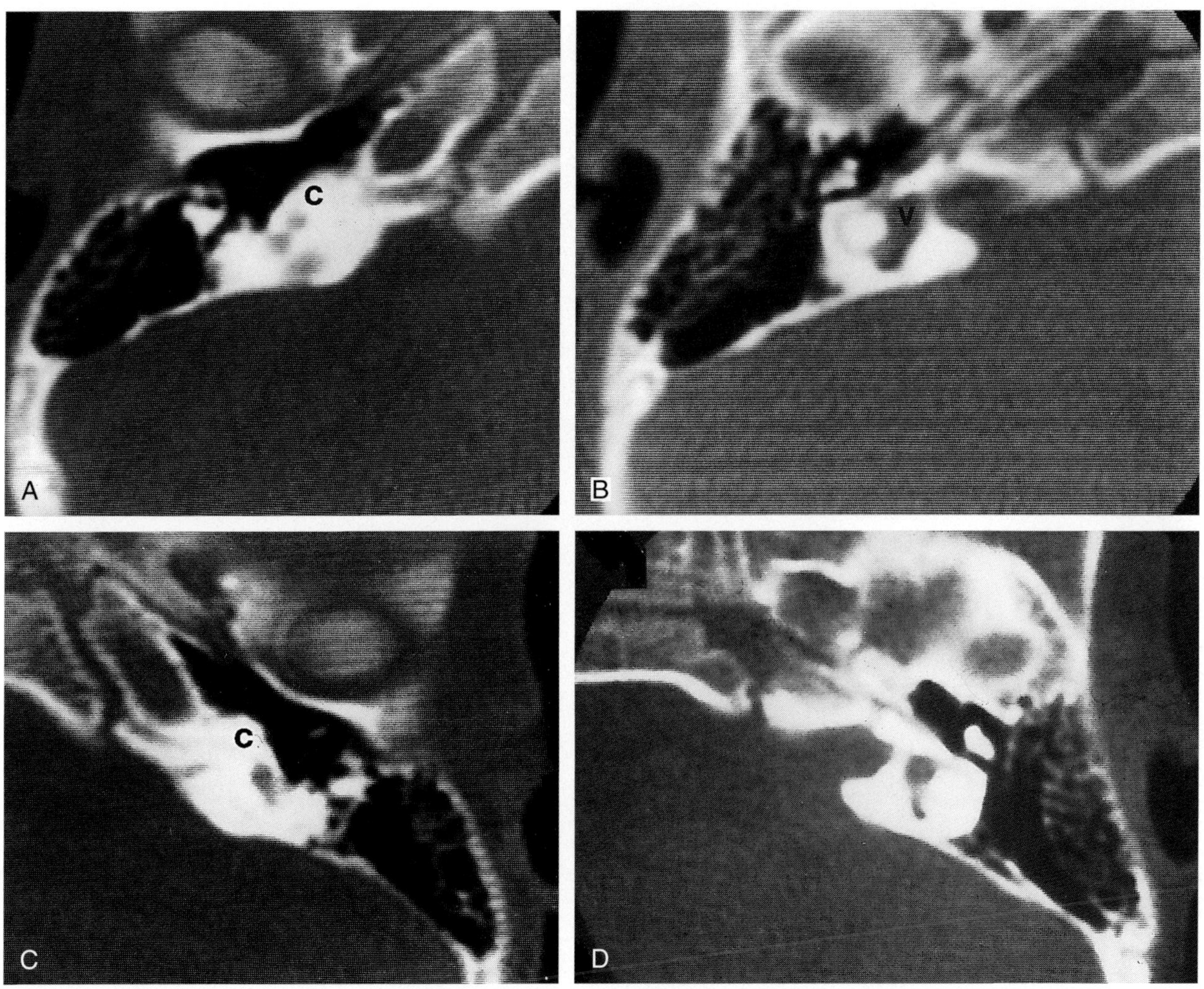

Figure 9–9. Bilateral cochlear aplasia. Axial CT of **(A,B)** right and **(C,D)** left temporal bone show dense bone occupies the expected position of the cochlea (c). The right vestibule (v) is slightly enlarged. (**A** and **C** are through mesotympanum, and **B** and **D** are through epitympanum).

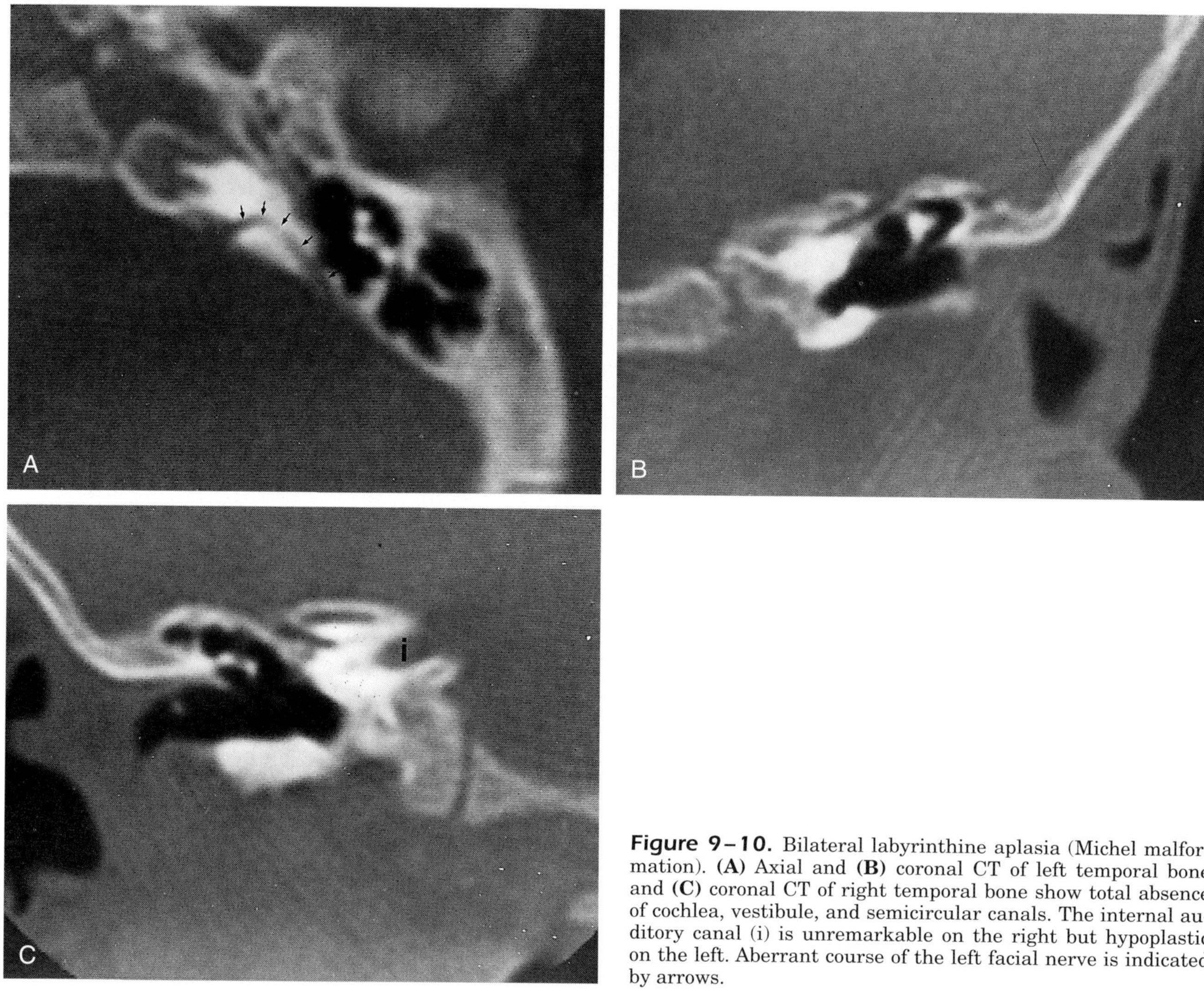

Figure 9–10. Bilateral labyrinthine aplasia (Michel malformation). **(A)** Axial and **(B)** coronal CT of left temporal bone and **(C)** coronal CT of right temporal bone show total absence of cochlea, vestibule, and semicircular canals. The internal auditory canal (i) is unremarkable on the right but hypoplastic on the left. Aberrant course of the left facial nerve is indicated by arrows.

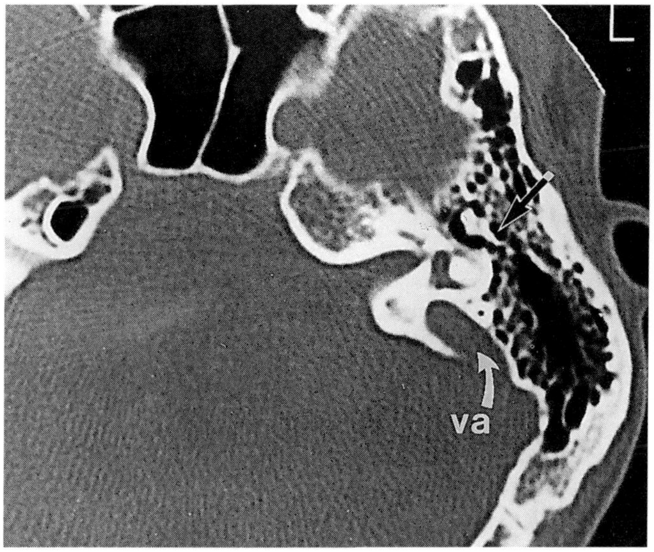

Figure 9–11. Dilated vestibular aqueduct and ossicular fixation. The left vestibular aqueduct (va) is markedly dilated with a diameter of 6 mm. The left incus is affixed to the wall of the epitympanum by a bony strut (straight arrow).

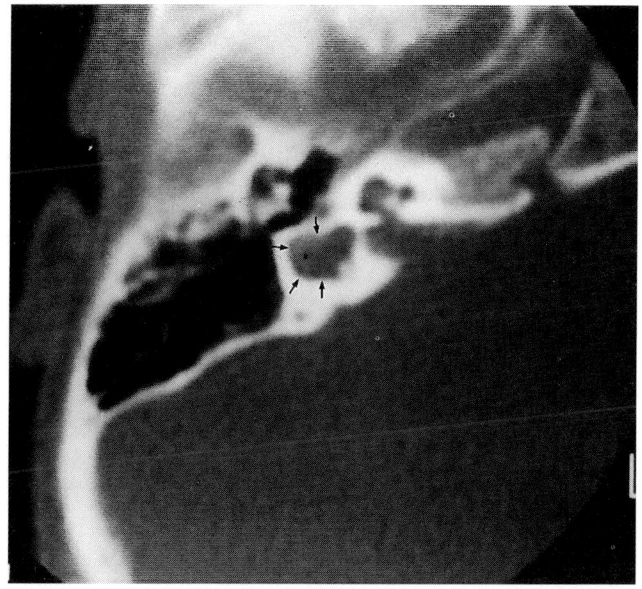

Figure 9–12. Deformity of lateral semicircular canal. An open pouch (arrows) occupies the position of the right lateral semicircular canal.

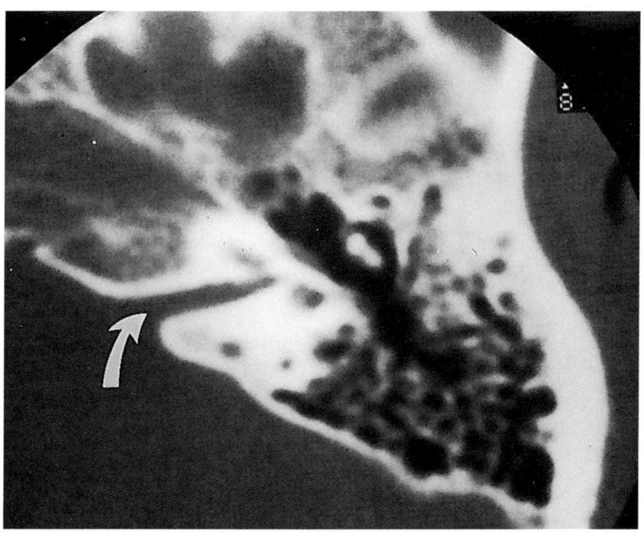

Figure 9–13. Hypoplasia of internal auditory canal. The left internal auditory canal (arrow) is markedly stenotic.

Malformations of Middle and External Ear

Malformations of the middle and external ears are more common than inner ear anomalies. Affected patients usually present with a small deformed pinna (microtia) or conductive hearing deficit. The external auditory canal (EAC) may be stenotic or completely atretic. Complete atresia results in absence of the external auditory meatus. It is usually unilateral by a 6:1 ratio.

CT Findings. CT is the modality best suited for evaluation of these malformations. Prior to surgical correction, the surgeon must know the status of the middle ear and ossicular chain, the status of the inner ear, and whether an atresia is membranous or bony.

- EAC stenosis. In cases of stenosis, CT shows unilateral or bilateral narrowing of the EAC.
- EAC atresia. In atresia, CT may show a bony external auditory canal plugged with soft tissue (membranous atresia) or complete absence of the bony canal. The ossicles are often fused to each other or to the atresia plate. Other abnormalities may include hypoplasia of the middle ear cleft, anterior displacement of the facial nerve, and absence of the round window.
- Ossicular anomalies. Congenital malformations of the ossicles may also occur in isolation. The more common ones are absence or fixation of the stapes, fusion of the malleus to the incus, and deformity of the long process of the incus.

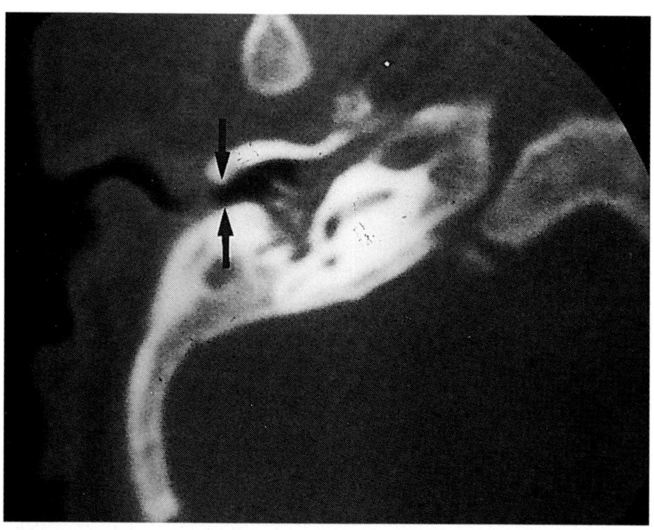

Figure 9–14. EAC stenosis. Axial CT of right temporal bone shows marked stenosis (arrows) of the bony portion of the right external auditory canal.

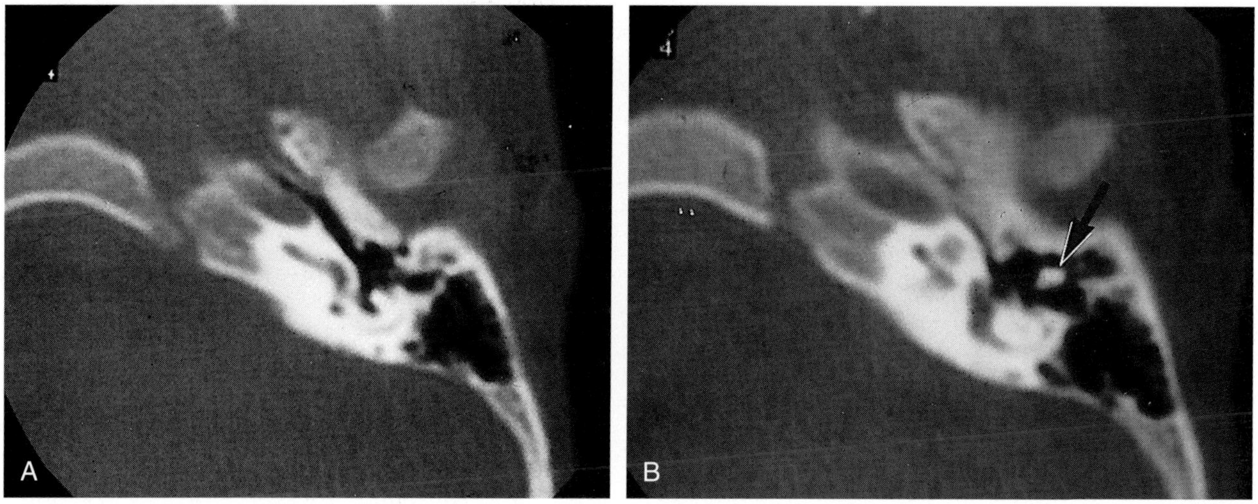

Figure 9–15. Atresia of external auditory canal. Axial CT through left **(A)** mesotympanum and **(B)** epitympanum show complete absence of the left bony external auditory canal. The external auditory canal normally lies in the same axial plane as the mesotympanum. The middle ear cleft is normal in size but the ossicles (arrow) appear fused in **B**.

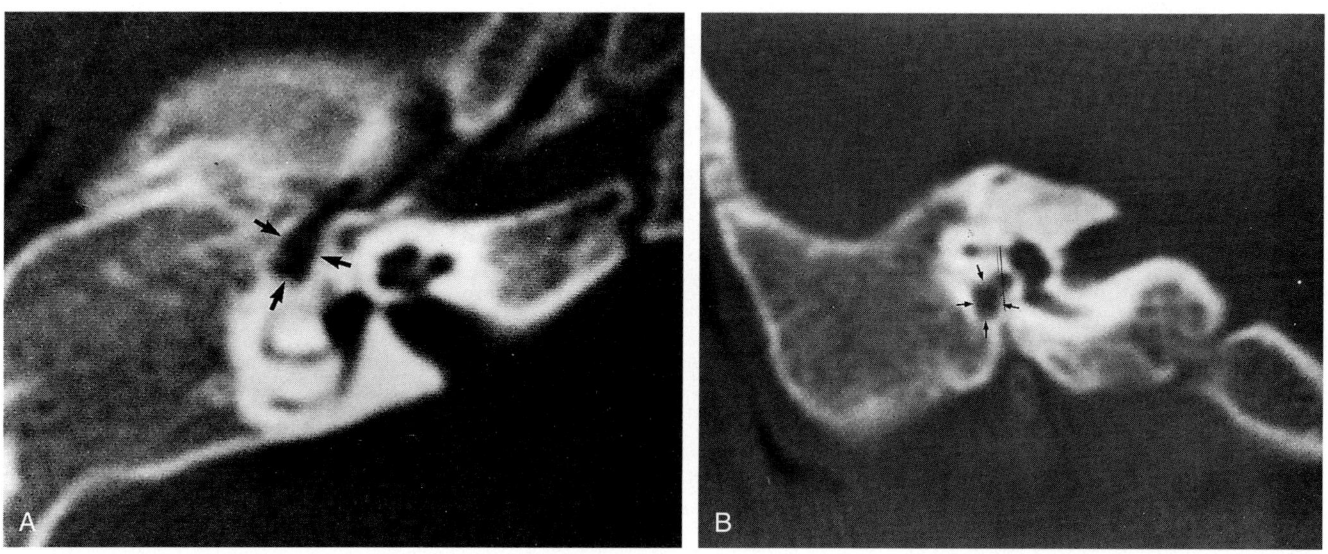

Figure 9–16. Atresia of external auditory canal. **(A)** Axial and **(B)** coronal CT of right temporal bone show complete absence of the bony external auditory canal. The middle ear cleft (arrows) is severely hypoplastic, and the ossicles are absent.

Inflammatory Diseases

Otomastoiditis

Bacterial infection of the middle ear and mastoid (acute otomastoiditis) is a common condition that normally does not necessitate diagnostic imaging. It is a common incidental finding, however, on studies performed for other reasons. Diagnostic imaging plays a key role in diagnosing its complications, which may include subperiosteal abscess, labyrinthitis, meningitis, brain abscess, and dural sinus thrombosis.

CT Findings. In acute otitis or mastoiditis, some or all of the air spaces are opacified by fluid or mucosal edema. The presence of air-fluid levels is pathognomonic for effusion. Coalescent mastoiditis is characterized by erosion of bony walls and septae. With repeated bouts of infection, the mastoid becomes sclerotic and the air cells may be obliterated. Manifestations of chronic otomastoiditis include cholesteatoma, granulation tissue, cholesterol granuloma, ossification of the labyrinth, and ossicular erosion or fixation.

MRI Findings. Acute disease is markedly hyperintense on T2-weighted images and of intermediate intensity on T1-weighted images. Chronically retained secretions may manifest more variable signal intensity. Contrast-enhanced scans may show enhancement of inflamed mucosa, although this finding is less prominent than that typically seen in the sinuses.

TABLE 9–2 Differential Diagnosis of Opacified Middle Ear

Otitis media/serous otitis
Granulation tissue
Cholesteatoma
Cholesterol cyst
Paraganglioma
Hemorrhage
Brain herniation

Differential Diagnosis

See Table 9–2.

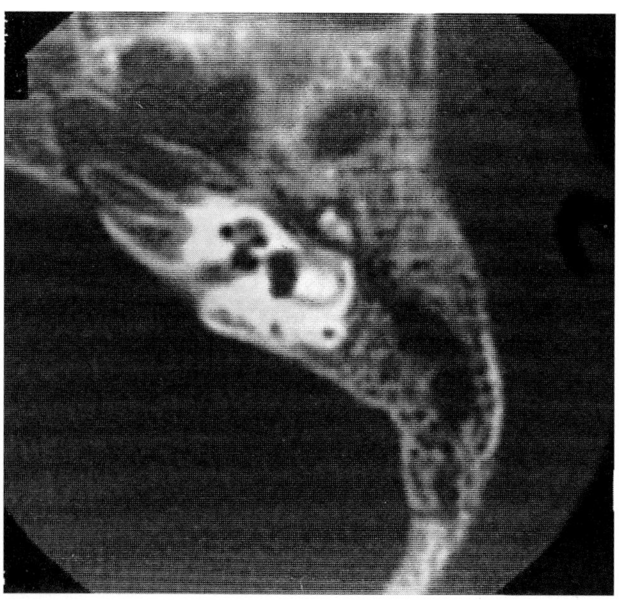

Figure 9–17. Coalescent mastoiditis. Axial CT of left temporal bone shows opacification of mastoid air cells, rarefaction and erosion of mastoid septa, and marked periauricular soft tissue swelling (Pott's puffy tumor).

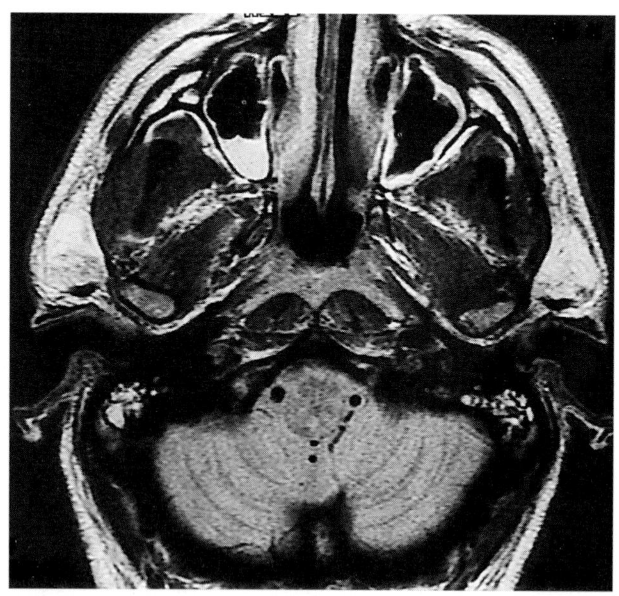

Figure 9–18. Simple mastoiditis. Axial PD-weighted MRI shows right maxillary sinusitis. High signal coming from both mastoids indicates fluid accumulation within mastoid air cells.

Cholesteatoma

A cholesteatoma is an expanding mass of keratinous debris lined by stratified squamous epithelium that is histologically identical to the epidermoid. Congenital cholesteatomas are rare; most (>95%) are acquired as a complication of chronic otomastoiditis. Acquired cholesteatomas are believed to originate from retraction pockets of the tympanic membrane and usually begin in Prussak's space, the portion of epitympanum between the scutum and head of the malleus or body of incus.

CT Findings. The classic CT appearance is a nondependent soft tissue mass arising from the tympanic membrane with ossicular displacement and erosion. Cholesteatomas do not enhance with contrast. Secondary findings relate to progressive bone erosion and may include destruction of the ossicles, facial nerve canal, labyrinth (particularly the lateral semicircular canal), mastoid, or floor of the middle cranial fossa. Intracranial infections and CSF leaks are rare complications.

MRI Findings. The majority of cholesteatomas are of intermediate intensity on T1-weighted images and hyperintense on T2-weighted images. MRI is ineffective for the assessment of subtle bony erosion.

Differential Diagnosis

See Table 9–2. Bone erosion is the hallmark of cholesteatoma that serves to distinguish it from uncomplicated otomastoiditis. Contrast-enhanced MRI can aid in distinguishing cholesteatoma, which does not enhance, from granulation tissue and tumor, which do.

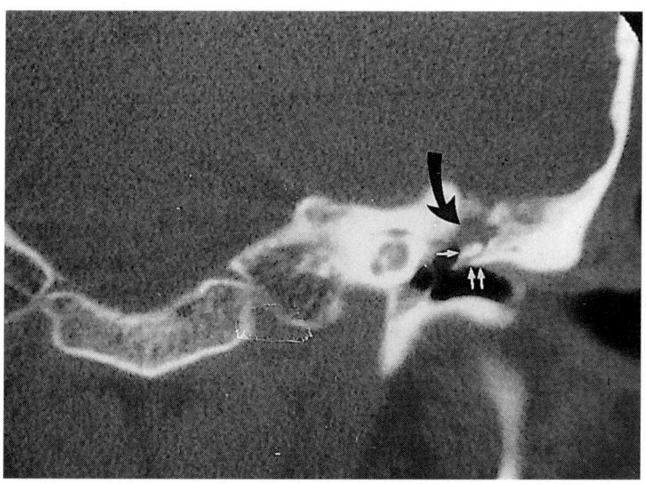

Figure 9–19. Attic cholesteatoma (early). A soft tissue mass (arrow) fills the attic (epitympanum). The malleus (small arrow) is pressed laterally against the scutum (double arrow).

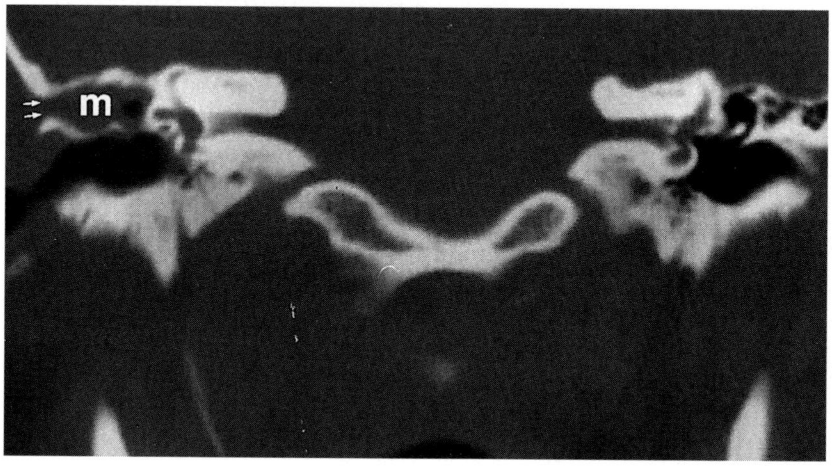

Figure 9–20. Attic cholesteatoma (advanced). Soft tissue mass (m) fills the right attic and adjoining mastoid. The ossicles are destroyed, mastoid septa are eroded, and there is dehiscence of the lateral wall of the mastoid (arrows). The left side is normal.

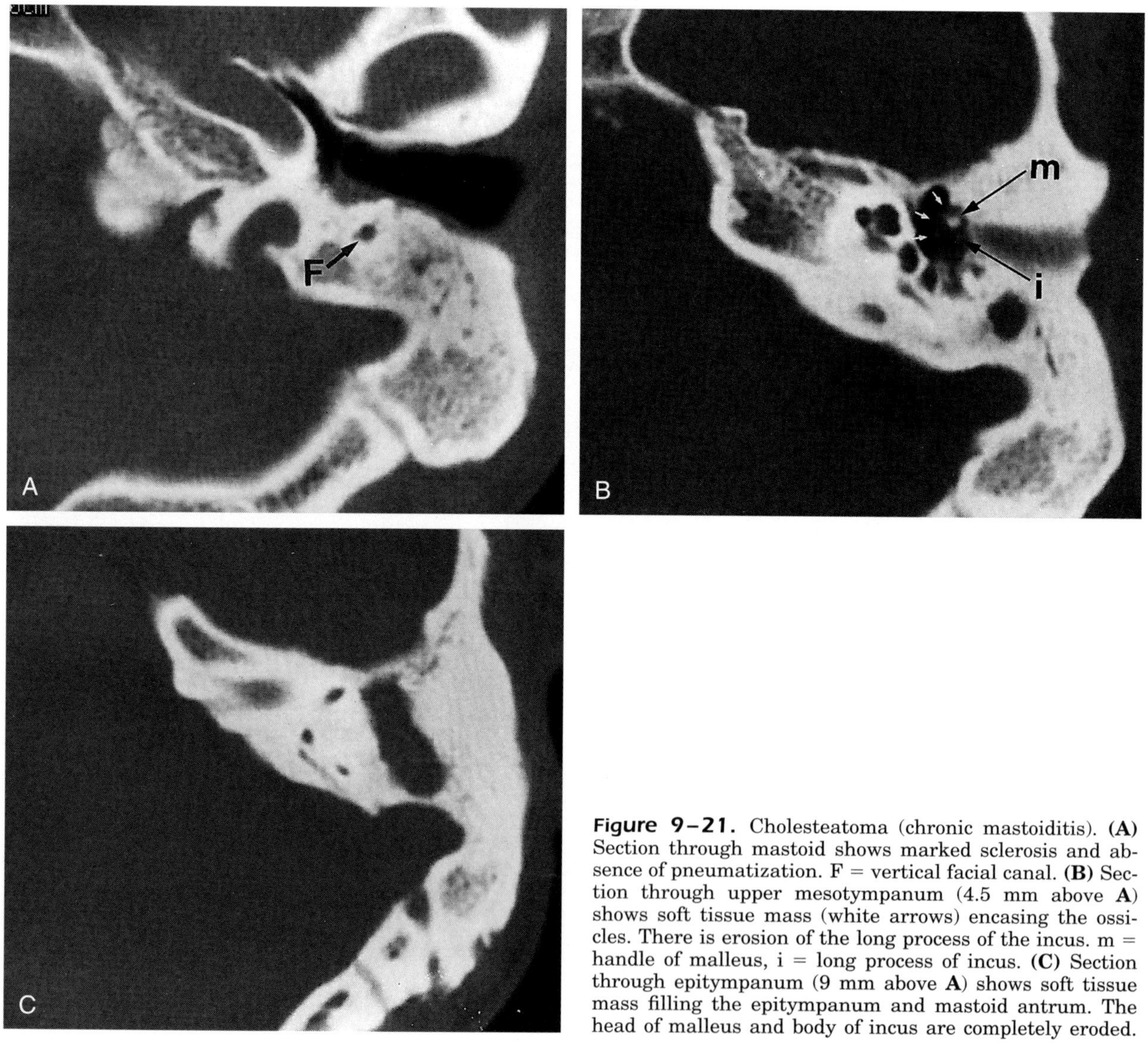

Figure 9–21. Cholesteatoma (chronic mastoiditis). **(A)** Section through mastoid shows marked sclerosis and absence of pneumatization. F = vertical facial canal. **(B)** Section through upper mesotympanum (4.5 mm above **A**) shows soft tissue mass (white arrows) encasing the ossicles. There is erosion of the long process of the incus. m = handle of malleus, i = long process of incus. **(C)** Section through epitympanum (9 mm above **A**) shows soft tissue mass filling the epitympanum and mastoid antrum. The head of malleus and body of incus are completely eroded.

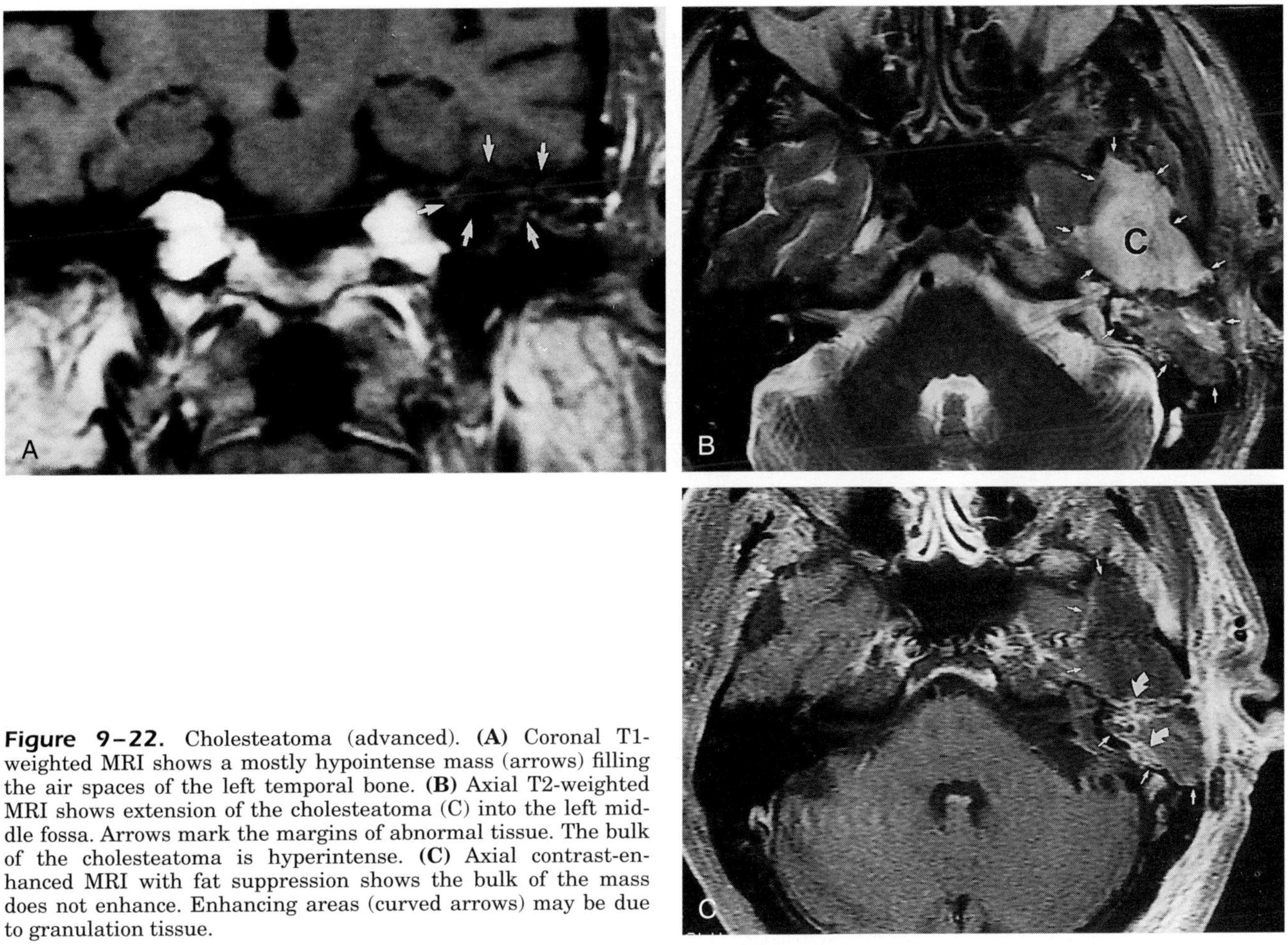

Figure 9–22. Cholesteatoma (advanced). **(A)** Coronal T1-weighted MRI shows a mostly hypointense mass (arrows) filling the air spaces of the left temporal bone. **(B)** Axial T2-weighted MRI shows extension of the cholesteatoma (C) into the left middle fossa. Arrows mark the margins of abnormal tissue. The bulk of the cholesteatoma is hyperintense. **(C)** Axial contrast-enhanced MRI with fat suppression shows the bulk of the mass does not enhance. Enhancing areas (curved arrows) may be due to granulation tissue.

Cholesterol Granuloma

Cholesterol granuloma is a complication of chronic otomastoiditis that only rarely causes sufficient mass effect to require therapeutic intervention. It is composed of cholesterol crystals and blood breakdown products lined by giant cells, macrophages, and blood vessels. A gradually progressive conductive hearing loss is the usual symptom of those that come to clinical attention.

CT Findings. CT shows a nonenhancing soft tissue mass, sometimes with bone erosion. These lesions arise in pneumatized portions of the temporal bone, usually the squamous or mastoid segments. Cholesterol cysts may produce large punched out bone defects with contents that appear hypodense relative to brain.

MRI Findings. MRI shows a temporal bone mass with hyperintensity on both T1- and T2-weighted sequences. The bright signal on T1 sequences has been attributed to byproducts of hemoglobin breakdown and is the most specific feature of cholesterol cysts.

TABLE 9–3 **Differential Diagnosis of Expansile Masses in the Temporal Bone**

Differential Diagnosis of Expansile Masses in the Temporal Bone
Cystic
Epidermoid
Cholesterol cyst
Dermoid
Solid
Cholesteatoma
Paraganglioma
Schwannoma
Histiocytosis X
Fibrous dysplasia

Differential Diagnosis

See Table 9–3.

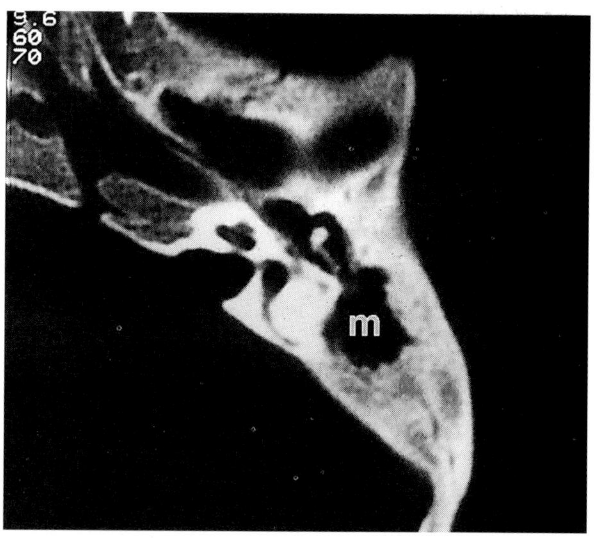

Figure 9–23. Cholesterol granuloma. Axial CT of left temporal bone shows a soft tissue mass (m) filling the left mastoid antrum. This is indistinguishable from cholesteatoma on CT but might be differentiated by T1-weighted MRI.

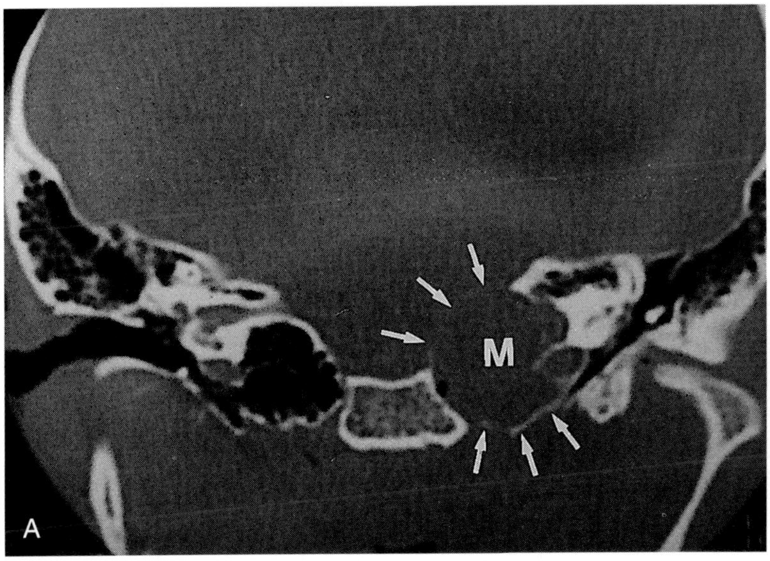

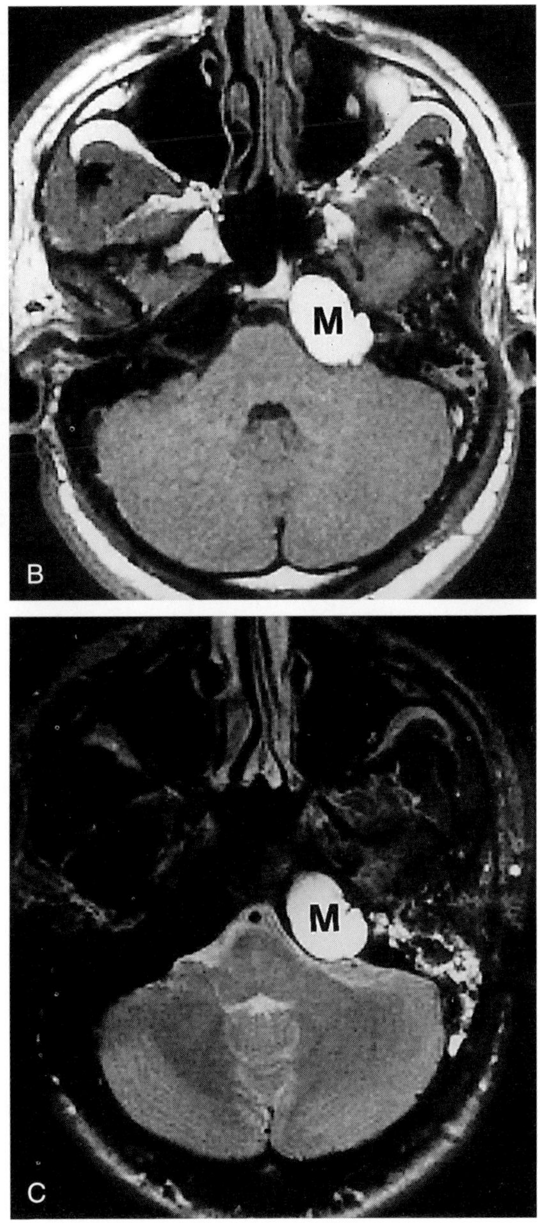

Figure 9–24. Cholesterol granuloma of petrous apex. **(A)** Coronal CT shows an expansile mass (M) of the left petrous apex with a very thin bony shell (arrows). **(B)** On axial T1-weighted MRI the mass is extremely hyperintense. **(C)** The mass remains extremely hyperintense on T2-weighted images. Otomastoiditis is also present on the left.

Osseous and Dysplastic Diseases

Paget's Disease

Synonym: Osteitis deformans.

Paget's disease is a primary bone disorder of unknown etiology characterized by abnormal bone remodeling leading to osseous deformity. Its prevalence increases with age, affecting 10% of those over 85 years old. Its early phase (also referred to as active, destructive, resorptive, or osteolytic phases) demonstrates hypervascularity and active osteoclastic activity. This proceeds to a mixed phase, with active new bone formation. The late phase (sclerotic, quiescent) is defined by thick and sclerotic but relatively inactive bone. A mixed conductive and sensorineural hearing loss is a common manifestation of Paget's disease of the skull.

CT Findings. CT shows generalized demineralization of the temporal bone, which is usually bilateral but can be asymmetric. The process most often begins at the petrous apex and proceeds laterally. Changes elsewhere in the calvarium are nearly always present and are related to the stage of disease. In the resorptive phase, diminished attenuation of the bone and calvarial thickening occur. In the sclerotic phase, the thickened calvarium becomes very dense. Basilar invagination may develop. In contrast with fibrous dysplasia, Paget's disease is usually bilateral and spares the facial bones.

TABLE 9–4 Differential Diagnosis of Sclerotic Temporal Bone

Paget's disease
Fibrous dysplasia
Osteoma
Osteopetrosis
Chronic otomastoiditis

MRI Findings. As on CT, there is thickening of the affected bone with expansion of the diploic space. On MRI, Paget's disease manifests as variable signal intensity on T1- and T2-weighted images, which may correlate with the stage of disease. The resorptive phase tends to be hypointense on T1-weighted images and hyperintense on T2-weighted images, whereas the sclerotic phase demonstrates hypointensity on both T1- and T2-weighted images. Increased marrow enhancement has been noted in the active phase. The clinical utility of MRI for this condition is limited to the assessment of complications, such as basilar invagination or cranial nerve compression.

Differential Diagnosis

See Table 9–4.

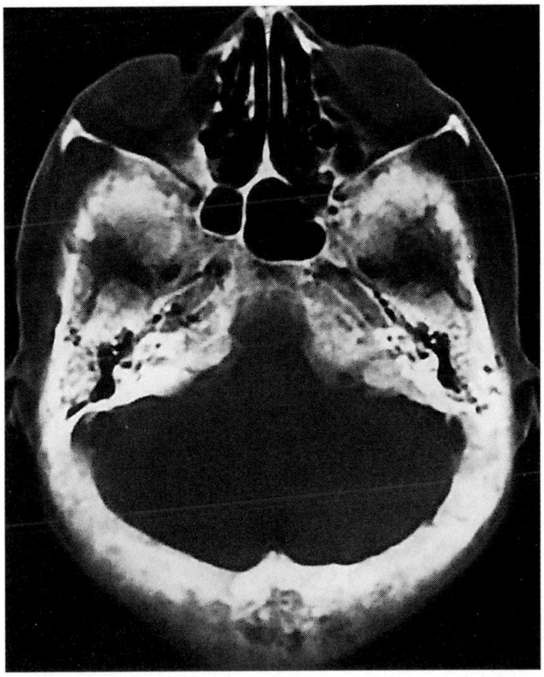

Figure 9–25. Paget's disease (sclerotic phase). Axial CT shows diffuse thickening and sclerosis of the bones of the calvarium and skull base.

Fibrous Dysplasia

Fibrous dysplasia of the facial bones was discussed in Chapter 8. In contrast with Paget's disease, fibrous dysplasia affects facial bones much more than the skull, is found in younger patients, and is usually unilateral.

CT Findings. CT shows smooth expansion of a normally mineralized temporal bone, usually around the external auditory canal and perhaps the mastoid but usually sparing the inner ear. It may lead to obliteration of air spaces and stenosis of the external auditory canal. Localized proliferation of fibrous tissue may occasionally produce punched out defects in the bone. Facial bone involvement is most common, particularly the sphenoid, ethmoid, maxillary, and frontal bones. The occipital and temporal bones are less frequently involved.

MRI Findings. On MRI, fibrous dysplasia has been reported to manifest hypointensity in the marrow on T1-weighted images (similar to skeletal muscle). The appearance on T2-weighted images is variable, with hyperintensity seen most commonly.

Differential Diagnosis

See Tables 9–3 and 9–4.

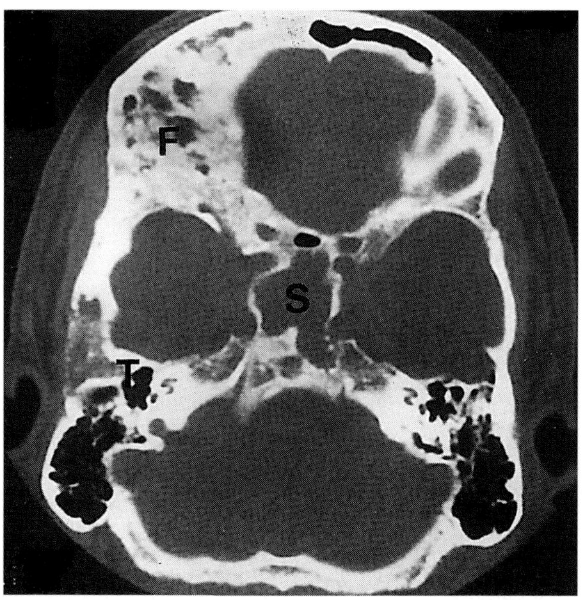

Figure 9–26. Fibrous dysplasia. There is mixed sclerosis and lucency (the latter representing fibrous tissue) involving frontal (F), temporal (T), and sphenoid (S) bones.

Otosclerosis

Synonym: Otospongiosus.

Otosclerosis is a disorder of endochondral bone that initially causes endochondral bone resorption, later followed by lamellar new bone formation and remodeling. This condition has been observed only in the human temporal bone. Sclerosis and fixation of the stapes footplate and oval window often result in conductive hearing loss. The less common cochlear form may cause a sensorineural hearing loss. Otosclerosis is a common disorder and one of the leading causes of acquired conductive hearing loss. It is bilateral in 80–90% and usually presents between the ages of 20 and 40 years. It is more common in females and Caucasians.

CT Findings. CT is the primary imaging modality for the assessment of conductive hearing loss. There are two types of otosclerosis, fenestral and cochlear. Fenestral otosclerosis is more common and on CT shows thickening or ossification of the stapes footplate and margins of the oval window. Cochlear otosclerosis is almost always associated with the fenestral type but is less common. CT shows demineralization of the otic capsule, especially around the cochlea. Generalized bony overgrowth does not occur in this condition.

Differential Diagnosis

Differential diagnosis of demineralization of the otic capsule:

- Cochlear otosclerosis
- Paget's disease
- Osteogenesis imperfecta

Differential diagnosis of sclerosis of the oval window:

- Fenestral otosclerosis
- Osteogenesis imperfecta
- Postinflammatory ossicular fixation (tympanosclerosis)

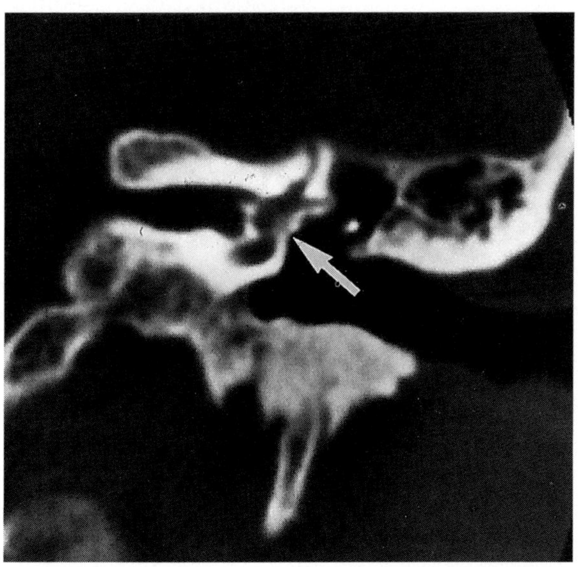

Figure 9–27. Fenestral otosclerosis. Coronal CT shows dense sclerosis of the stapes footplate obliterating the oval window (arrow). (Courtesy of Dr. H. Ric Harnsberger, Salt Lake City, UT.)

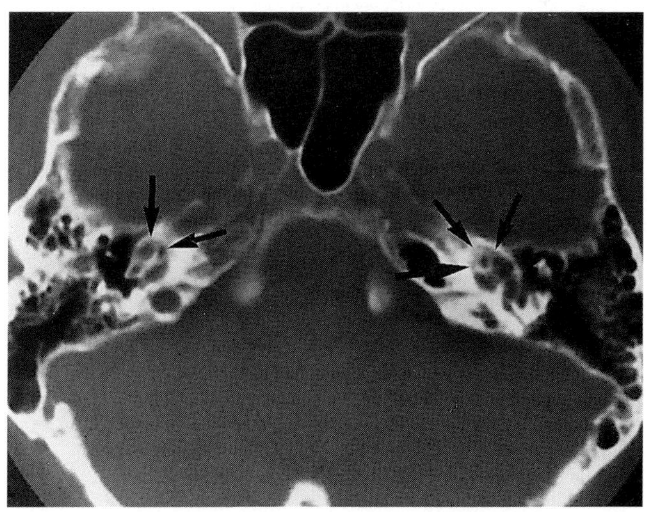

Figure 9–28. Cochlear otosclerosis. Axial CT shows bilateral demineralization of the otic capsule (arrows) surrounding the cochleae. (Courtesy of Dr. H. Ric Harnsberger, Salt Lake City, UT.)

Trauma

Fractures and Ossicular Dislocations

Injuries to the temporal bone and its contents are common accompaniments of severe head injury. They may go unsuspected or patients will present with hemotympanum, otorrhagia, CSF leaks, hearing loss, or facial nerve deficits. CT is the primary modality for the diagnosis of temporal bone injuries. The main radiologically detectable lesions include fractures and disruption of the ossicular chain. The major complications of temporal bone trauma are listed in the box.

Conductive hearing loss
Sensorineural hearing loss
Labyrinthine dysfunction
Perilymphatic fistula
Facial nerve paralysis
CSF leaks
Meningocele
Encephalocele

Transverse fractures occur perpendicular to the long axis of the temporal bone. There is a high probability of sensorineural hearing loss and facial nerve deficit secondary to injury of the seventh and eighth cranial nerves. Transverse fractures account for only about 10% of temporal bone fractures.

Longitudinal/oblique fractures are more or less parallel to the long axis of the temporal bone. They are seven to eight times more common than transverse fractures, and patients are more likely to present with CSF otorrhea and a conductive hearing loss.

Ossicular disruption (dislocation) is a break in the ossicular chain and also presents with conductive hearing loss. Most disruptions involve the incus, with separation of the incus from the stapes (incudostapedial disruption) more common than separation of the incus from the malleus (incudomalleal disruption).

CT Findings. Routine head CT may show opacification of the middle ear or mastoid, air in the temporomandibular joint fossa, or pneumocephalus but is rarely adequate to diagnose temporal bone fractures. The preceding findings should prompt a directed temporal bone examination, which will demonstrate most osseous and ossicular injuries. Thin section (2 mm or less) high-resolution CT scans are essential for adequate evaluation of temporal bone trauma. With appropriate scanning technique, fracture lines are clearly evident. Incudostapedial disruption is present when there is more than 1 mm separation between the incus and stapes. Incudomalleal separation is present when there is any significant separation of the head of the malleus from the body of the incus.

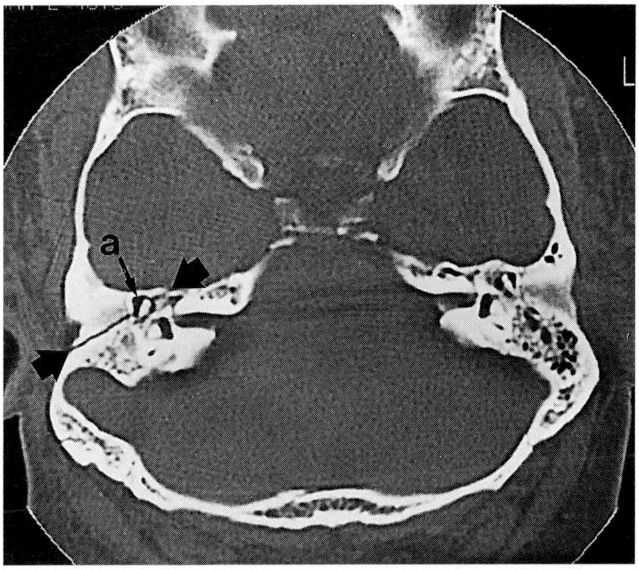

Figure 9–29. Longitudinal fracture. A fracture line (between arrows) extends parallel to the long axis of the right temporal bone passing through the attic (a).

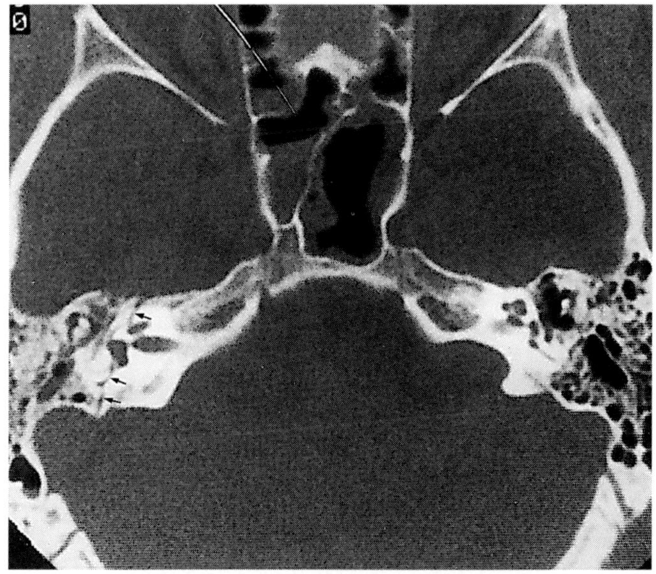

Figure 9–30. Transverse fracture. A fracture line (arrows) passes perpendicular to the long axis of the temporal bone through the otic capsule and labyrinth.

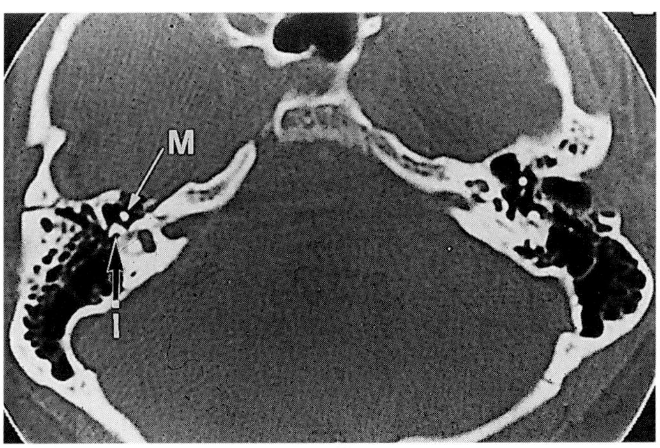

Figure 9–31. Incudomalleal disruption. There is a small longitudinal fracture anterior to the mastoid air cells. The incus (I) is rotated and posteriorly displaced relative to the malleus (M).

Neoplasms

Langerhans Cell Histiocytosis

Synonym: Histiocytosis X.

Langerhans cell histiocytosis is a condition of abnormal proliferation of histiocytes, resulting in destructive bone lesions and functional impairment of involved organs. The etiology is not established but is believed to be a dysfunction of immune regulation. The presentation is variable, with the following three syndromes reflecting the increasing severity of disease and with a considerable overlap between them:

Eosinophilic granuloma

- Age 5–15 years
- Usually unifocal bone defect
- Skull most commonly affected
- Excellent prognosis

Hand-Schüller-Christian syndrome

- Age 1 to 5 years
- Multifocal bone lesions
- Involvement of lymph nodes, skin, and viscera
- Diabetes insipidus due to hypothalamic involvement

Letterer-Siwe syndrome

- Infancy up to 2 years of age
- Disseminated histiocytosis of skeleton, skin, and viscera
- Rapid clinical course and frequently fatal
- May respond to multidrug chemotherapy

CT Findings. CT shows bone destruction with an associated soft tissue mass. The margins of bone erosion are usually sharp but not sclerotic. Moderate contrast enhancement is seen, often with focal unenhancing areas within the mass. Skull lesions are typically round or ovoid and sharply defined. Bilateral temporal bone involvement or multiple calvarial lesions in a child are strongly suggestive of histiocytosis.

MRI Findings. MRI may show soft tissue masses that are hypointense on T1-weighted images and hyperintense on T2-weighted images, associated with bone destruction, and manifesting homogeneous or heterogeneous contrast enhancement. Intracranial involvement is manifested by intensely enhancing meningeal or parameningeal nodules, especially involving the hypothalamus.

TABLE 9–5 Destructive Lesions of the Temporal Bone in Children

Congenital cholesteatoma
Acquired cholesteatoma
Histiocytosis X
Rhabdomyosarcoma
Adenocarcinoma
Squamous cell carcinoma

Differential Diagnosis

The differential diagnosis of destructive lesions of the temporal bone is given in Tables 9–5 and 9–6. Bilateral temporal bone involvement or multiple calvarial defects in a child are strongly suggestive of histiocytosis.

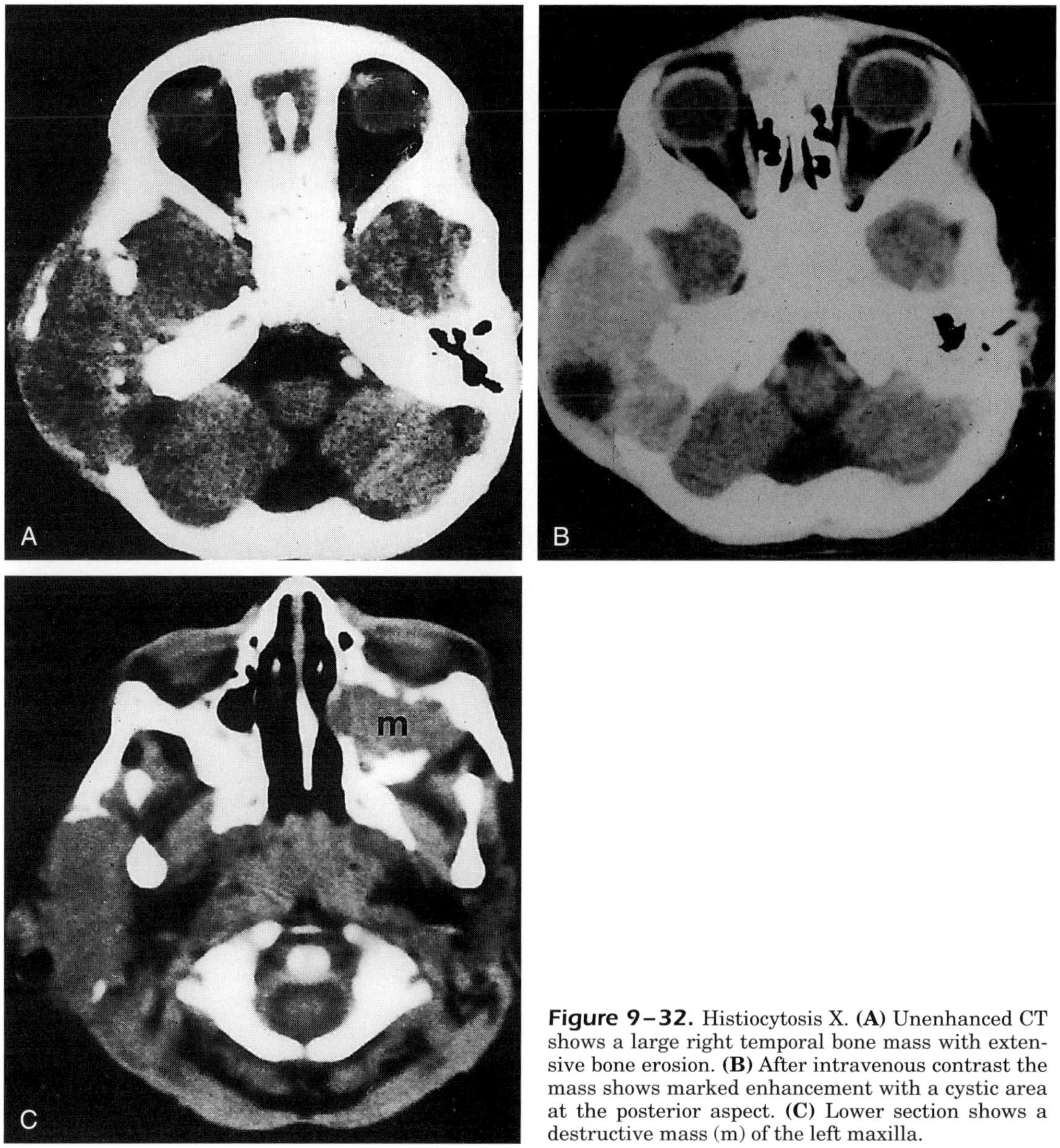

Figure 9–32. Histiocytosis X. **(A)** Unenhanced CT shows a large right temporal bone mass with extensive bone erosion. **(B)** After intravenous contrast the mass shows marked enhancement with a cystic area at the posterior aspect. **(C)** Lower section shows a destructive mass (m) of the left maxilla.

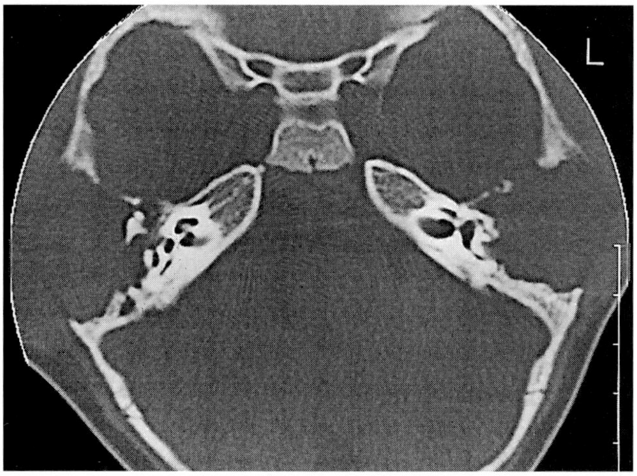

Figure 9–33. Histiocytosis X. Axial CT shows the characteristic appearance of bilateral soft tissue masses with sharply marginated bone erosion.

Paragangl ioma

Synonym: Glomus tumor.

Paragangliomas are the most common neoplasms of the middle ear. Among all temporal bone neoplasms, they are second only to schwannomas in frequency. They arise from neuroectodermal derivatives, the branchial paraganglia, and are closely related to pheochromocytomas. Clinically, temporal bone paragangliomas occur with pulsatile tinnitus or hearing loss and are about twice as common in females, peaking in the fifth decade. Deficits of the 9th, 10th, and 11th cranial nerves occur with tumors in the jugular fossa. There is a lower incidence of multicentricity (about 2%) than is seen with carotid and vagal tumors.

Paragangliomas of the temporal bone have traditionally been divided into tympanic and jugular types, depending on the site of origin. However, many tumors involve both the jugular fossa and middle ear, and the distinction is often irrelevant.

CT Findings. With tympanic paragangliomas, CT shows an enhancing soft tissue mass, usually small, arising over the cochlear promontory. Bone erosion is uncommon. The tumor tends to spread along natural air spaces and canals.

Jugular paragangliomas are much more common than purely tympanic lesions and tend to be larger upon presentation. The earliest and most common CT finding is erosion of the jugular plate, the bony wall between the jugular bulb and middle ear. Isolated dehiscence of the jugular plate, however, may be a normal variant. From its site of origin, the jugular paraganglioma may grow into the middle ear, jugular vein, or posterior fossa or produce progressive erosion of contiguous osseous structures.

MRI Findings. Paragangliomas are of intermediate signal intensity on T1-weighted images and moderately hyperintense on T2-weighted images. They enhance intensely following contrast administration. A distinctive MRI feature of larger paragangliomas is the presence of signal voids from enlarged vessels within these hypervascular tumors.

Angiographic Findings. Carotid angiography reveals a hypervascular mass that appears in the middle to late arterial phase and disappears in the venous phase. Blood supply is usually via the inferior tympanic branch or posterior division of the ascending pharyngeal artery and the auricular or occipital arteries, with less frequent supply by deep cervical arteries and the internal carotid and vertebral systems. Larger jugular lesions may show occlusion of the ipsilateral sigmoid sinus or jugular vein.

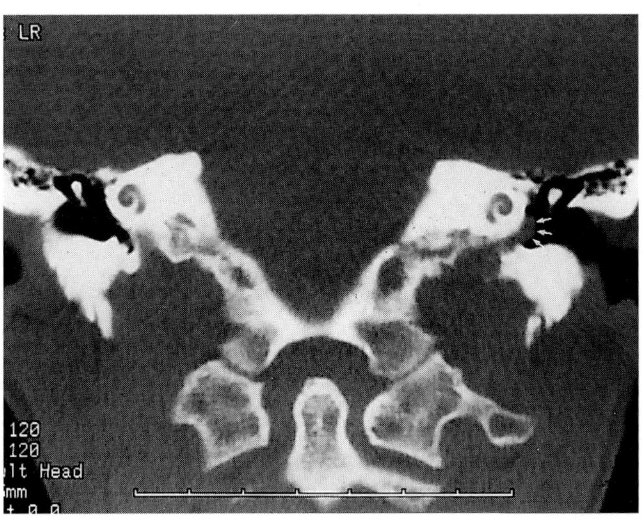

Figure 9–34. Tympanic paraganglioma. Coronal CT shows a soft tissue mass (arrows) in the left middle ear overlying the promontory. The right side is normal.

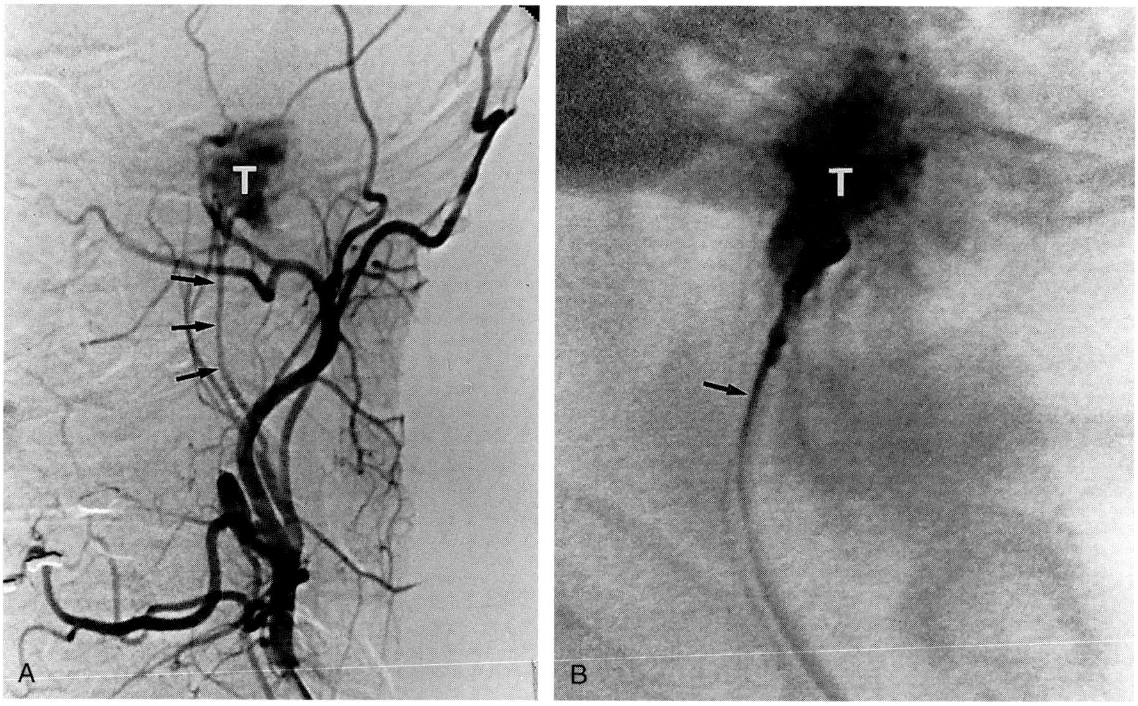

Figure 9–35. Jugular paraganglioma. **(A)** Left external carotid (LAO projection) and **(B)** selective ascending pharyngeal (lateral) angiograms show dense tumor stain (T) supplied by the ascending pharyngeal artery (arrows).

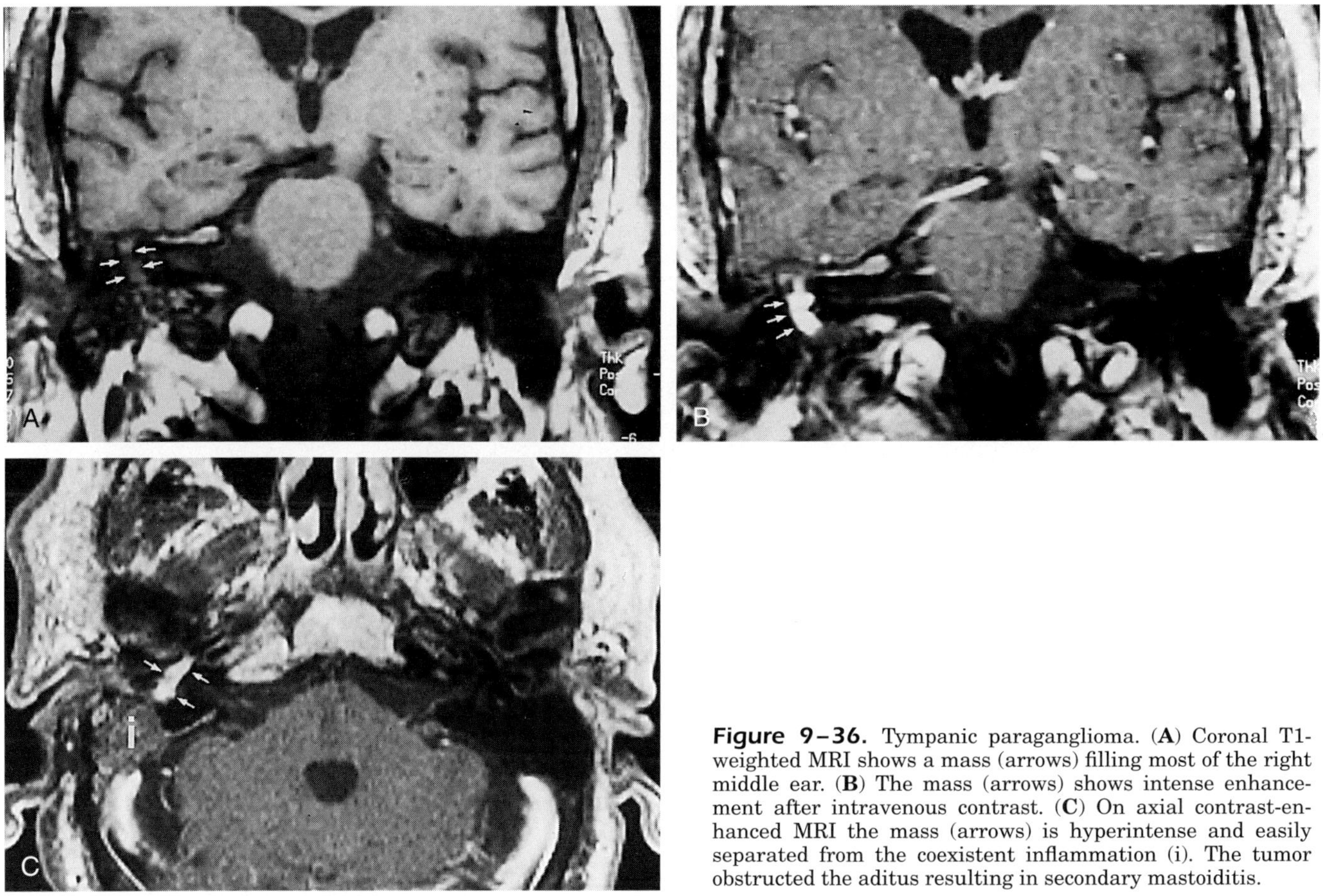

Figure 9–36. Tympanic paraganglioma. (**A**) Coronal T1-weighted MRI shows a mass (arrows) filling most of the right middle ear. (**B**) The mass (arrows) shows intense enhancement after intravenous contrast. (**C**) On axial contrast-enhanced MRI the mass (arrows) is hyperintense and easily separated from the coexistent inflammation (i). The tumor obstructed the aditus resulting in secondary mastoiditis.

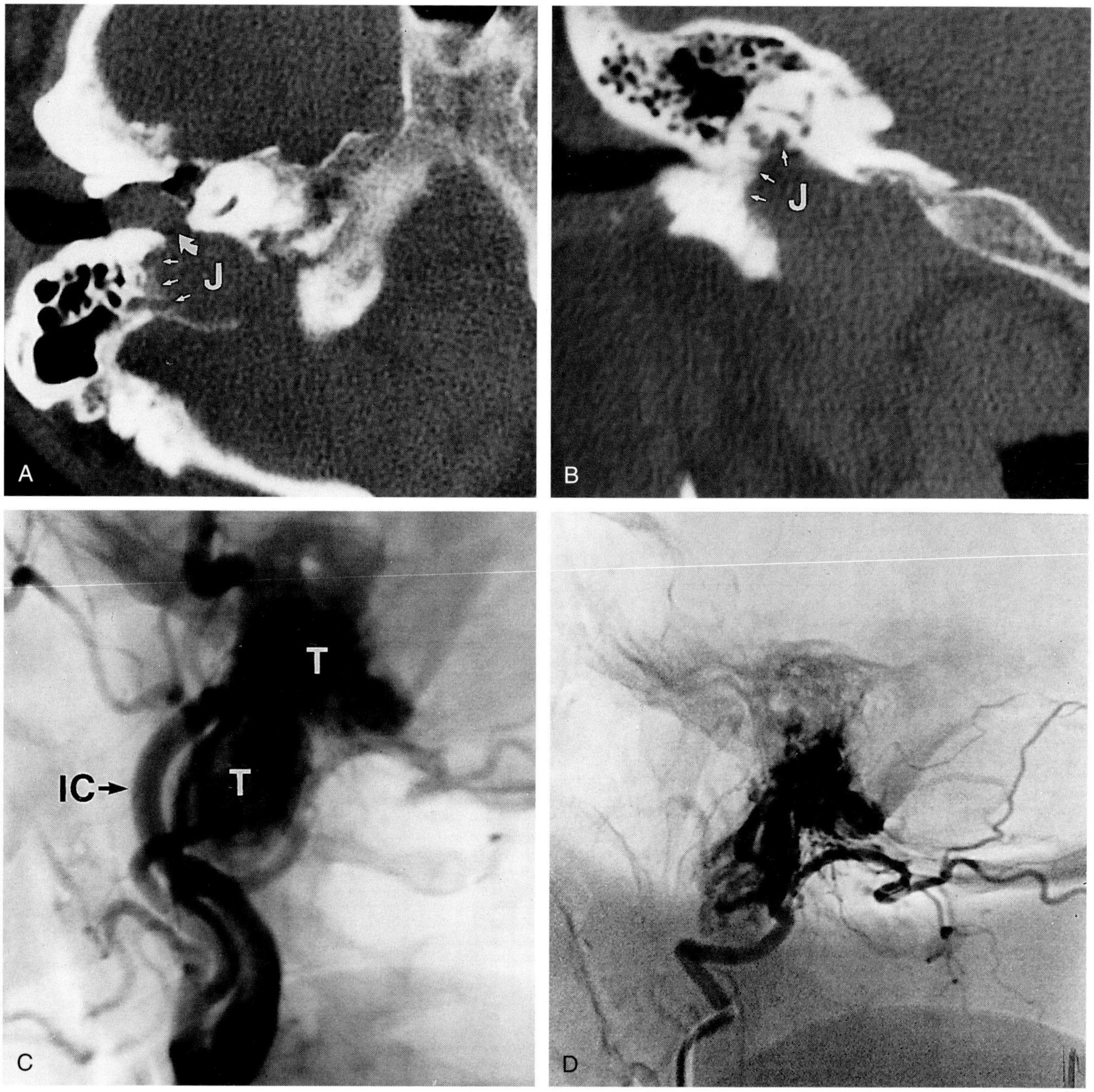

Figure 9–37. Jugular paraganglioma. **(A)** Axial CT shows enlargement of the jugular bulb (J) with irregular marginal bony erosion (small arrows). The tumor has penetrated the jugular plate (curved arrow) and extended into the tympanic cavity and external auditory canal. **(B)** Coronal scan shows erosion (small arrows) of the bony margins of the jugular bulb. **(C)** Common carotid angiogram shows staining of a large tumor (T) and anterior displacement of the internal carotid artery (IC). **(D)** Selective occipital artery angiogram (the dominant feeding vessel) shows dense staining of tumor in the the temporal bone and upper jugular vein.

Rhabdomyosarcoma

Rhabdomyosarcomas are the most common primary malignancy of the head and neck in children, excluding brain tumors. Although most arise in the orbits or nasopharynx, rhabdomyosarcomas are also the most common primary malignancy of the temporal bone in children. There are three histologic subtypes: embryonal, alveolar, and pleomorphic. The embryonal subtype is most common in the head and neck. Patients with rhabdomyosarcomas of the temporal bone commonly present with symptoms of chronic otitis, with rapid development of facial nerve and other cranial nerve deficits.

CT Findings. CT shows a homogeneous soft tissue mass with variable but homogeneous enhancement. Bone destruction is present in two thirds and may be extensive. Cervical lymph node metastases are present in 12–50%.

MRI Findings. Rhabdomyosarcomas are slightly hyperintense relative to muscle on T1-weighted images and markedly hyperintense on T2-weighted images. Intense homogeneous contrast enhancement is seen with intravenous contrast. MRI is superior to CT for the evaluation of parameningeal and intracranial involvement, whereas CT is superior for the evaluation of bone destruction.

Differential Diagnosis

See Table 9–5.

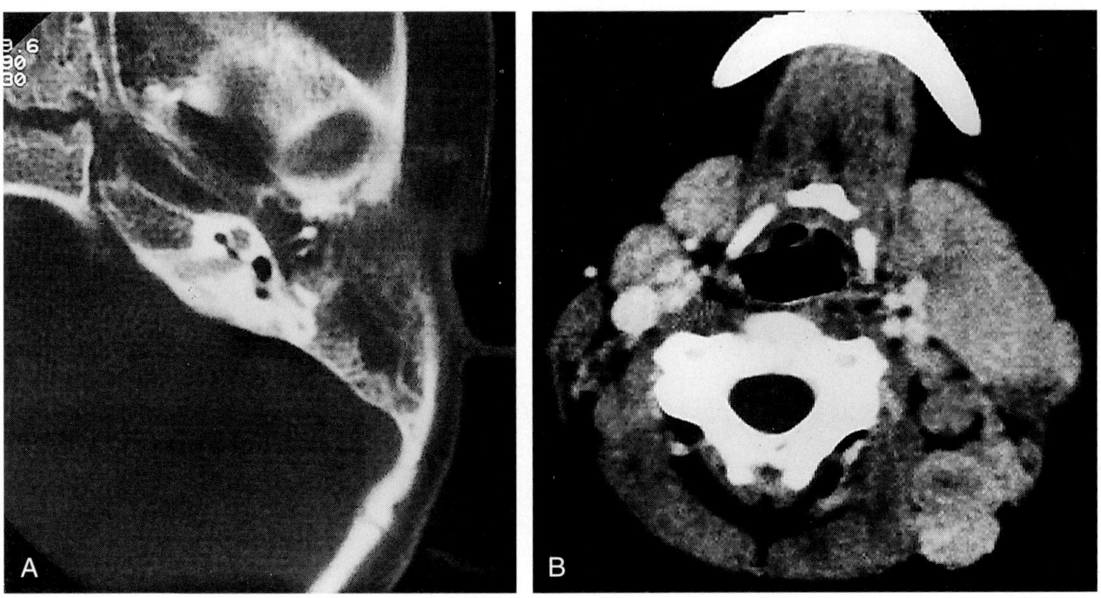

Figure 9–38. Rhabdomyosarcoma. **(A)** Axial CT of the left temporal bone shows irregular bone destruction involving the anterior mastoid and external auditory canal. **(B)** Contrast-enhanced CT at level of hyoid shows extensive bilateral adenopathy.

Squamous Cell Carcinoma

Squamous cell carcinoma is the most common malignant tumor of the temporal bone but is still an uncommon condition. It usually arises in the external auditory canal, and patients present with otalgia and persistent ear drainage that is often bloody. The peak incidence is in the fifth to seventh decades. Carcinoma spreads via direct extension into the parotid gland, posterior auricular sulcus, pinna, and middle ear. Adenopathy is uncommon, and distant metastases are rare.

CT Findings. CT shows a soft tissue mass with or without bone destruction. It enhances with contrast, but this is difficult to appreciate owing to the high attenuation of adjacent bone. Carcinoma initially spreads superficially into the parotid gland, temporomandibular joint, or mastoid and later involves the middle ear structures. Destruction of the tegmen tympani or sinodural plate leads to intracranial involvement.

MRI Findings. MRI shows a mass in the external auditory canal of intermediate signal intensity on T1-weighted images and mildly hyperintense on T2-weighted images. It enhances uniformly with intravenous contrast. MRI is less effective at demonstrating the bone erosion, but enhanced MRI is superior to CT in showing intracranial, nasopharyngeal, and perineural invasion.

TABLE 9–6 Differential Diagnosis of Destructive Temporal Bone Mass

Squamous cell carcinoma
Malignant external otitis
Cholesteatoma
Histiocytosis
Neuroma
Sarcoma
Paraganglioma
Metastasis
Rhabdomyosarcoma

Differential Diagnosis

See Tables 9–6 and 9–7.

TABLE 9–7 **Inflammatory and Neoplastic Processes of the Temporal Bone**

Condition	Location	Texture	Bone Destruction	Enhancement	Comments
Otitis/mastoiditis	Tympanic cavity and mastoid air cells	CT: Opacification of air cells and possible air-fluid levels MRI: Hyperintense on T2-weighted images	May develop if untreated beginning with septa	Usually none on CT or MRI	Very common Often an incidental finding on cranial MRI or CT
Cholesteatoma	Tympanic cavity in continuity with tympanic membrane About 80% begin in Prussak's space	CT: Soft tissue mass MRI: Isointense to brain on T1-weighted images and hyperintense on T2-weighted images	Common (50–75%) Usually begins with ossicles and scutum	None	Bone erosion and ossicular displacement help to distinguish from otitis
Granulation tissue	Tympanic cavity	CT: Soft tissue mass MRI: Isointense to hyperintense on T1 weighted images- and hyperintense on T2-weighted images	Possible	Consistently enhances on MRI but not CT	May coexist with cholesteatoma and cholesterol granuloma or occur in isolation
Cholesterol granuloma	Petrous apex or tympanic cavity	CT: Ovoid soft tissue mass MRI: Hyperintense on T1-weighted images (the most distinguishing feature) and T2-weighted images	Middle ear: rare Petrous apex: bone expansion with smooth, sharp margins	Granulation tissue at margins may enhance on MRI	Far more common than epidermoid in petrous apex
Paraganglioma	Tympanic cavity (cochlear promontory) or jugular bulb	CT: Soft tissue mass MRI: Intermediate signal intensity on T1-weighted images, intermediate to high intensity on T2-weighted images, and signal voids	Nearly always present with jugular lesions, with expansion and irregularity of the jugular bulb margins	Enhances intensely on CT or MRI	Hypervascular mass on angiography Second most common temporal bone tumor
Histiocytosis	Not localized Typically large Frequently other cranial lesions are present	CT: Soft tissue mass MRI: Hypointense on T1-weighted images and hyperintense on T2-weighted images	A hallmark of this lesion Margins may be sharp, giving punched out appearance	Moderate enhancement, sometimes with nonenhancing foci	Typically appears in children 1–5 years old
Carcinoma	External auditory canal	CT: Soft tissue mass MRI: Intermediate on T1-weighted images and mildly hyperintense on T2-weighted images	Erosion of external auditory canal	Enhances with contrast	Most common malignant neoplasm of the temporal bone
Rhabdomyosarcoma	Anywhere within temporal bone Typically large	CT: Soft tissue mass with intracranial or extracranial spread MRI: Intermediate on T1-weighted images and markedly hyperintense on T2-weighted images	Usually present and extensive	Enhances with contrast	Most common temporal bone neoplasm in children
Schwannoma	Eighth (usually) or seventh cranial nerve Most commonly in IAC	CT: Soft tissue mass MRI: Hypointense or isointense to brain on T1-weighted images and hyperintense on T2-weighted images	Smooth expansion of bone along course of nerve	Enhances intensely on CT and MRI	Most common temporal bone neoplasm

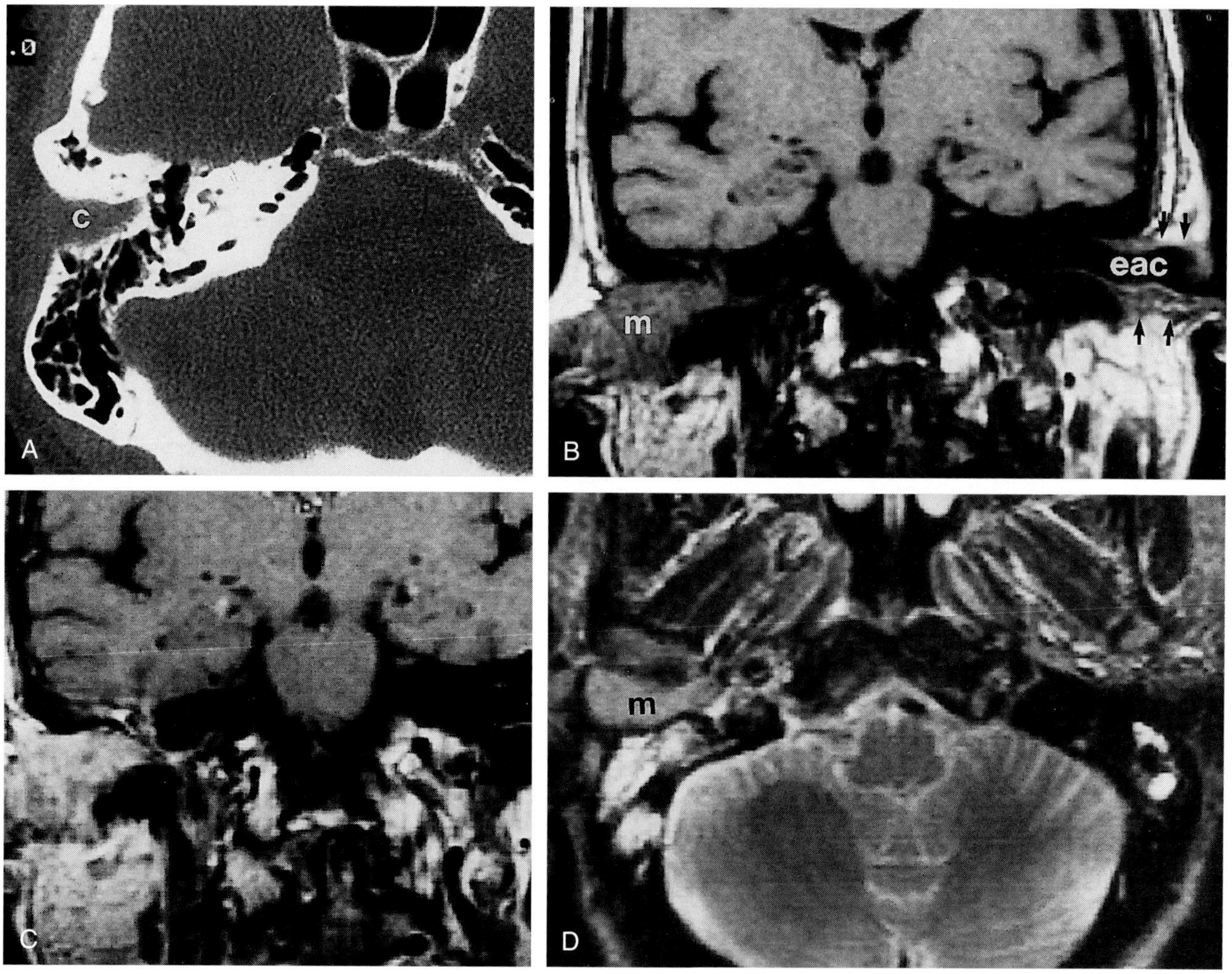

Figure 9–39. Carcinoma of external auditory canal. **(A)** Axial CT shows a soft tissue mass filling the right external auditory canal (c). The posterior wall appears slightly irregular. **(B)** Coronal T1-weighted MRI shows a large mass (m) of intermediate signal intensity occupying the right external auditory canal. The bulk of the mass occupies the cartilaginous canal with cartilaginous invasion and infiltration of adjoining soft tissue. Note normal left external auditory canal (eac) with thin cartilaginous walls (arrows). **(C)** On coronal contrast-enhanced MRI the mass shows homogeneous enhancement. **(D)** On axial T2-weighted MRI the mass is mildly hyperintense. Otomastoiditis developed subsequent to the CT.

RECOMMENDED READINGS

General

Mark,AS, Seltzer,S, Harnsberger,HR. Sensorineural Hearing Loss: More than Meets the Eye? *AJNR* 14:37–45, 1993.

Swartz,JD. Current Imaging Approach to the Temporal Bone. *Radiology* 171:309–317, 1989.

Aberrant Carotid Artery

Lo,WWM, Solti-Bohman,LG, McElveen,JT. Aberrant Carotid Artery: Radiologic Diagnosis with Emphasis on High-resolution Computed Tomography. *Radiographics* 6:985–993, 1985.

Remley,KB, Harnsberger,HR, Jacobs,JM, Smoker,WRK. The Radiologic Evaluation of Pulsatile Tinnitus and the Vascular Tympanic Membrane. *Semin Ultrasound CT MR* 10:236–250, 1989.

Jugular Bulb Variants

Lo,WWM, Solti-Bohman,LG. High Resolution CT of the Jugular Foramen: Anatomy and Vascular Variants and Anomalies. *Radiology* 150:743–747, 1984.

Overton,SB, Ritter,FN. A High Placed Jugular Bulb in the Middle Ear: A Clinical and Temporal Bone Study. *Laryngoscope* 83:1986–1991, 1973.

Malformations of Labyrinth

Jackler,RK, Luxford,WM, House,WF. Congenital Malformations of the Inner Ear: A Classification Based on Embryogenesis. *Laryngoscope* 97(3 Pt 2 Suppl 40):2–14, 1987.

Mafee,MF, Charletta,D, Kumar,A, Belmont,H. Large Vestibular Aqueduct and Congenital Sensorineural Hearing Loss. *AJNR* 13:805–819, 1992.

Urman,SM, Talbot,JM. Otic Capsule Dysplasia: Clinical and CT Findings. *Radiographics* 10:823–838, 1990.

Malformations of Middle and External Ear

Eelkema,EA, Curtin,JD. Congenital Anomalies of the Temporal Bone. *Semin Ultrasound CT MR* 10:195–212, 1989.

Jahrsdoerfer,RA. Clinical Aspects of Temporal Bone Anomalies. *AJNR* 13:821–825, 1993.

Otomastoiditis

Holliday,RA. Inflammatory Diseases of the Temporal Bone: Evaluation with CT and MR. *Semin Ultrasound CT MR* 10: 213–235, 1989.

Holliday,RA, Reede,DL. MRI of Mastoid and Middle Ear Disease. *Radiol Clin North Am* 27:283–299, 1989.

Mafee,MF, Singleton,EL, Valvassori,GE, Espinosa,GA, Kumar,A, Aimi,K. Acute Otomastoiditis and Its Complications: Role of CT. *Radiology* 155:391–397, 1985.

Cholesteatoma

Holliday,RA. Inflammatory Diseases of the Temporal Bone: Evaluation with CT and MR. *Semin Ultrasound CT MR* 10: 213–235, 1989.

Ishii,K, Takahashi,S, Kobayashi,T, Matsumoto,K, Ishibashi,T. MR Imaging of Middle Ear Cholesteatomas. *J Comput Assist Tomogr* 15:934–937, 1991.

Martin,N, Sterkers,O, Nahum,H. Chronic Inflammatory Disease of the Middle Ear Cavities: Gd-DTPA-enhanced MR Imaging. *Radiology* 176:399–405, 1990.

Swartz,JD. Cholesteatomas of the Middle Ear: Diagnosis, Etiology, and Complications. *Radiol Clin North Am* 22:15–35, 1984.

Cholesterol Granuloma

Lo,WWM, Solti-Bohman,LG, Brackmann,DE, Gruskin,P. Cholesterol Granuloma of the Petrous Apex: CT Diagnosis. *Radiology* 153:705–711, 1984.

Martin,N, Sterkers,O, Mompoint,D, Nicolas,J, Nahum,H. Cholesterol Granulomas of the Middle Ear Cavities: MR Imaging. *Radiology* 172:512–525, 1989.

Paget's Disease and Fibrous Dysplasia

Brown,EW, Megerian,CA, McKenna,MJ, Weber,A. Fibrous Dysplasia of the Temporal Bone: Imaging FIndings. *AJR* 164: 679–682, 1995.

Ginsberg,LE, Elster,AD, Moody,DM. MRI of Paget Disease with Temporal Bone Involvement Presenting with Sensorineural Hearing Loss. *J Comput Assist Tomogr* 16:314–316, 1992.

Swartz,JD, Vanderslice,RB, Korsvik,H, et al. High Resolution Computed Tomography: Part 6, Craniofacial Paget's Disease and Fibrous Dysplasia. *Head Neck Surg* 8:40–47, 1985.

Utz,JA, Kransdorf,MJ, Jelinek,JS, Moser,RP, Berrey,BH. MR Appearance of Fibrous Dysplasia. *J Comput Assist Tomogr* 13:845–851, 1989.

Otosclerosis

Mafee,MF, Henrikson,GC, Deitch,RL, et al. Use of CT in Stapedial Otosclerosis. *Radiology* 156:709–714, 1985.

Swartz,JD. Otosclerosis, Diagnosis, and Differential Diagnosis. *Semin Ultrasound CT MR* 10:251–261, 1989.

Swartz,JD, Mandell,DW, Berman,SE, Wolfson,RJ, Marlowe,FI, Popky,GL. Cochlear Otosclerosis (Otospongiosis): CT Analysis with Audiometric Correlation. *Radiology* 155:147–150, 1985.

Fractures and Ossicular Dislocations

Betz,BW, Wiener,MD. Air in the Temporomandibular Joint Fossa: CT Sign of Temporal Bone Fracture. *Radiology* 180: 463–466, 1991.

Dolan,KD. Temporal Bone Fractures. *Semin Ultrasound CT MR* 10:262–279, 1989.

Gentry,LR. Temporal Bone Trauma: Current Perspectives for Diagnostic Evaluation. *Neuroimaging Clin North Am* 1:319–340, 1991.

Swartz,JD, Zwillenberg,S, Berger,AS. Acquired Disruptions of the Incudostapedial Articulation: Diagnosis with CT. *Radiology* 171:779–781, 1989.

Langerhans Cell Histiocytosis

Cunningham,MJ, Curtin,HD, Butkiewicz,BL. Histiocytosis of the Temporal Bone: CT Findings. *J Comput Assist Tomogr* 12:70–74, 1988.

Ragland,RL, Moss,DS, Duffis,AW, Wolf,D, Knorr,JR. CT and MR Findings in Diffuse Cerebral Histiocytosis: Case Report. *AJNR* 12:525–526, 1991.

Stull,MA, Kransdorf,MJ, Devaney,KO. Langerhans Cell Histiocytosis of Bone. *Radiographics* 12:801–823, 1992.

Paraganglioma

Chakeres,DW, LaMasters,DL. Paragangliomas of the Temporal Bone: High-Resolution CT Studies. *Radiology* 150:749–753, 1984.

Larson,TC, Reese,DF, Baker,HL, McDonald,TJ. Glomus Tympanicum Chemodectomas: Radiographic and Clinical Characteristics. *Radiology* 163:801–806, 1987.

Lo,WWM, Solti-Bohman,LG, Lambert,PR. High Resolution CT in the Evaluation of Glomus Tumors of the Temporal Bone. *Radiology* 150:737–742, 1984.

Vogl,T, Bruning,R, Schedel,H, et al. Paragangliomas of the

Jugular Bulb and Carotid Body: MR Imaging with Short Sequences and Gd-DTPA Enhancement. *AJNR* 10:823–827, 1989. *AJR* 153:583–587, 1989.
Vogl,TJ, Juergens,M, Balzer,J, et al. Glomus Tumors of the Skull Base: Combined Use of MR Angiography and Spin-Echo Imaging. *Radiology* 192:103–110, 1994.

Rhabdomyosarcoma

Castillo,M, Pillsbury,HC. Rhabdomyosarcoma of the Middle Ear: Imaging Features in Two Children. *AJNR* 14:730–733, 1993.
Scotti,G, Harwood-Nash,D. Computed Tomography of Rhabdomyosarcomas of the Skull Base in Children. *J Comput Assist Tomogr* 6:33–39, 1982.

Squamous Cell Carcinoma

Arriaga,M, Curtin,H, Takahashi,H, Hirsch,BE, Kamerer,DB. Staging Proposal for External Auditory Meatus Carcinoma Based on Preoperative Clinical Examination and Computed Tomography Findings. *Ann Otol Rhinol Laryngol* 99: 714–721, 1990.
Bird,CR, Hasso,AN, Stewart,CE, Hinshaw,DB, Thompson,JR. Malignant Primary Neoplasms of the Ear and Temporal Bone Studied by High-Resolution Computed Tomography. *Radiology* 149:171–174, 1983.
Friedman,DP, Rao,VM. MR and CT of Squamous Cell Carcinoma of the Middle Ear and Mastoid Complex. *AJNR* 12:872–874, 1991.

CHAPTER TEN

Orbits

The usual indication for imaging of the orbits is the work-up of a mass lesion. The presence of abundant retro-orbital fat allows effective delineation of orbital masses by CT. MRI is more susceptible to motion, as well as more time consuming and expensive. Nonetheless, MRI is occasionally helpful, particularly because of its ability to image in any plane. With intraocular lesions, MRI has shown greater efficacy in distinguishing tumor from subretinal effusions through the use of T2-weighted sequences.

Localization of a lesion within the orbit is the first step toward a differential diagnosis. This is readily accomplished through the use of both axial and coronal imaging. The major disorders related to each anatomic compartment are presented in the following sections.

Disorders of the Optic Globe

See Table 10–1 and Diagram 10–1.

Coloboma

A coloboma is a congenital defect of the sclera associated with a characteristic outpouching of the inferonasal globe. The defect may extend from the optic nerve to the pupil. It results from failure of the embryonic ocular fissure to close, an event that normally occurs in the sixth week of gestation. Colobomas most often arise as a spontaneous defect but can be associated with a variety of malformations, including trisomy 13, agenesis of the corpus callosum, and cleft lip or palate.

CT Findings. CT shows a cone-shaped deformity of the posterior globe, usually in the inferonasal direction. The uveoscleral rim is thinned with decreased enhancement after intravenous contrast. Colobomas are bilateral in 60%. The globe may be either larger or smaller than normal. Retinal cysts may form, invariably accompanied by microphthalmos. Retinal detachment may also occur.

MRI Findings. MRI shows the same morphologic features in the globe as does CT. MRI is superior to CT in the demonstration of associated malformations such as callosal agenesis and encephaloceles.

TABLE 10–1 | Intraocular Masses

Cause	Distinguishing Features
Melanoma	Mildly to markedly hyperintense on T1-weighted images Hypointense on T2-weighted images
Metastasis	Hypointense to vitreous on T2-weighted images Slightly hyperintense on T1-weighted images
Retinoblastoma	Isointense to slightly hyperintense on T1-weighted images Calcifications on CT
Hemangioma	Intense contrast enhancement Isointense to vitreous on T2-weighted images
Retinal detachment	Usually hyperdense on CT Hyperintense or isointense to vitreous on T1-and T2-weighted images V-shaped with apex at optic disc No contrast enhancement
Choroidal detachment	Hyperintense on T2-weighted images Does not extend to optic disc

TABLE 10–2 | Differential Diagnosis of Enlarged Optic Globe

Cause	Features
Buphthalmos	(Congenital glaucoma) Increased AP diameter
Macrophthalmos	Associated with neurofibromatosis All diameters increased
Myopia	Increased AP diameter
Staphyloma	Nonenhancing posterior bulge
Coloboma	Inferonasal deformity with optic nerve head widening

TABLE 10–3 | Differential Diagnosis of Small Optic Globe

Cause	Features
Microphthalmos	CNS, palatal, and digital anomalies
Persistent hyperplastic primary vitreous	Hyperdense vitreous and cone-shaped density behind lens
Phthisis bulbi	Dense calcification of sclera
Coloboma	Inferonasal deformity with optic nerve head widening

Differential Diagnosis

See Tables 10–2 and 10–3. A staphyloma is a congenital or acquired outpouching of the sclera, which may involve any portion of the globe. In this condition, the uvea is thinned with diminished enhancement.

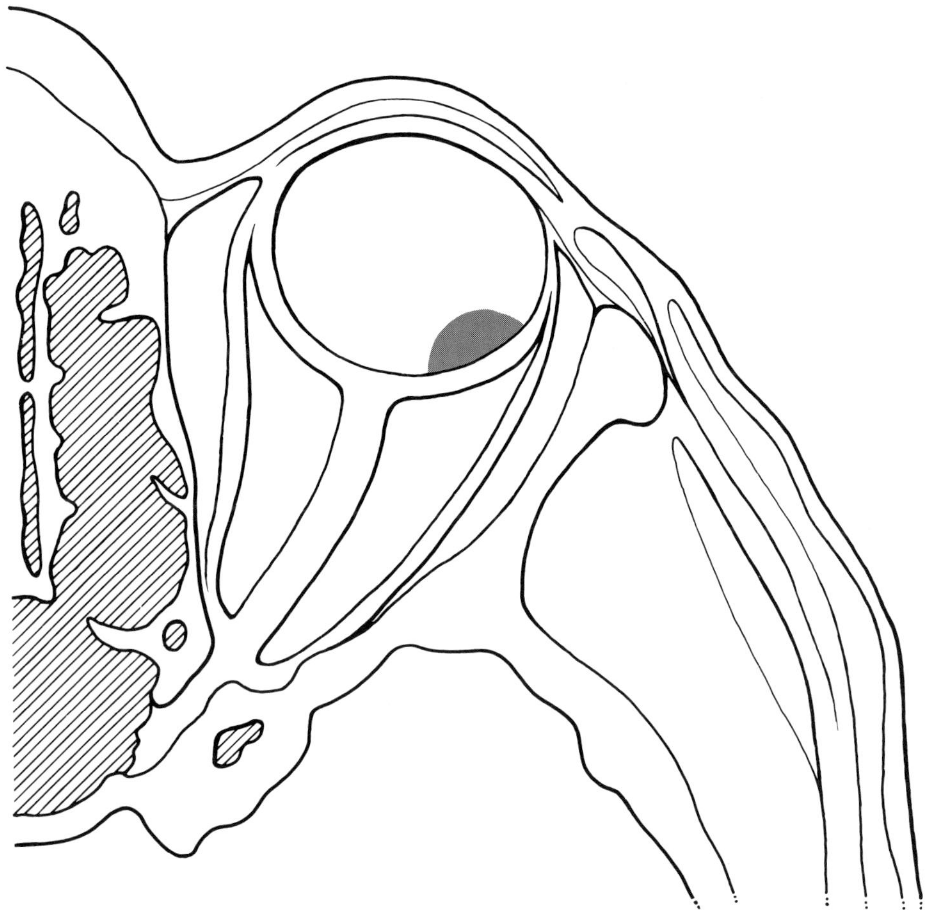

Diagram 10–1. Intraocular mass. The usual intraocular mass arises from or involves the retina or uvea.

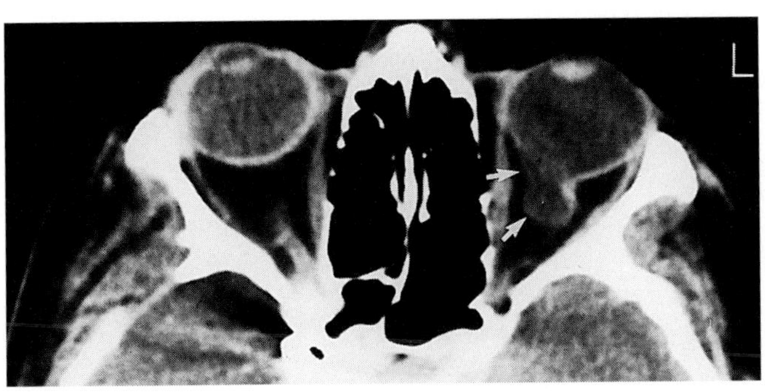

Figure 10–1. Coloboma. CT shows an inferonasal outpouching (arrows) of the left globe.

Drusen

Synonym: Hyaline bodies.

Optic disc drusen consist of an accumulation of acellular hyalinelike material on or near the optic disc. They commonly become calcified. Drusen may occur secondary to many intraocular conditions or as a primary process, particularly in the elderly. The usual complaint is a visual field defect due to optic nerve damage. However, drusen may be an incidental finding on CT.

Imaging Findings. CT shows a focal discrete and superficial calcification of the optic disc usually less than 1 mm thick and often bilateral (up to 73%). Optic disc hemorrhage may occasionally be seen. MRI findings have not been described. However, MRI is quite insensitive to small amounts of calcification.

TABLE 10–4 Differential Diagnosis of Ocular Calcifications

Drusen
Phthisis bulbi
Osteoma
Senile scleral plaque
Retinoblastoma

Differential Diagnosis

See Table 10–4. Calcification limited to the optic disc is nearly specific for drusen.

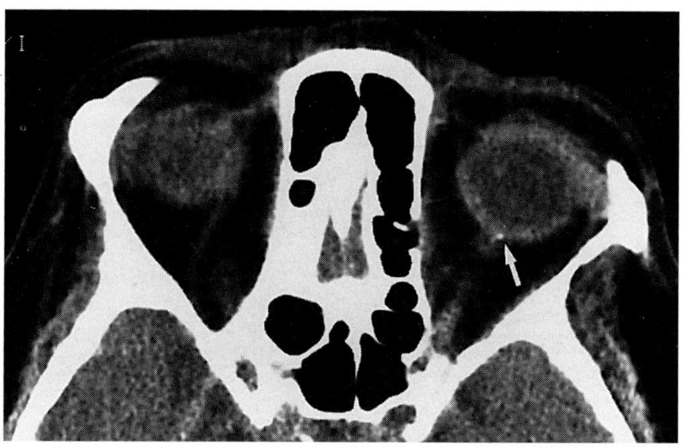

Figure 10–2. Drusen. There is a discrete calcification (arrow) on the lateral margin of the left optic disc.

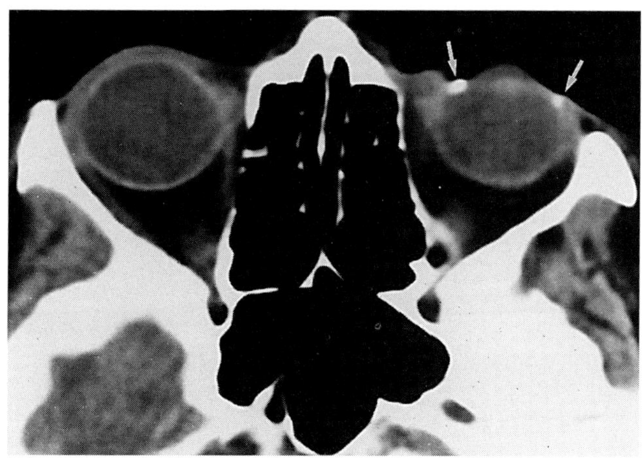

Figure 10–3. Senile plaques. Calcified scleral plaques as seen in the left globe (arrows) are an occasional incidental finding in the elderly.

Phthisis Bulbi

Phthisis bulbi denotes a chronically degenerated globe with shrinkage and tissue disorganization. It most commonly occurs as a result of trauma or severe intraocular inflammation. Pathology reveals a small globe (less than 20 mm in diameter) with scleral thickening and irregularity, disorganization of intraocular contents, and osseous metaplasia in the subretinal space.

CT Findings. CT shows a small and deformed globe, characteristically with heavy subretinal calcification or ossification. The vitreous may be of increased attenuation.

MRI Findings. The globe is small, with an irregular band of hypointensity in a retinal or subretinal configuration representing calcification. Alterations in the vitreous result in increased signal on T1- and proton-density–weighted images.

TABLE 10–5 Differential Diagnosis of Altered Vitreous (Altered Signal on MRI, Hyperdense on CT)

Phthisis bulbi
Persistent hyperplastic primary vitreous
Retinal detachment
Choroidal detachment
Hemorrhage
Silicone oil injection
Coats' disease
Toxocara canis endophthalmitis

Differential Diagnosis

See Tables 10–4 and 10–5. Calcification of a shrunken globe is nearly specific.

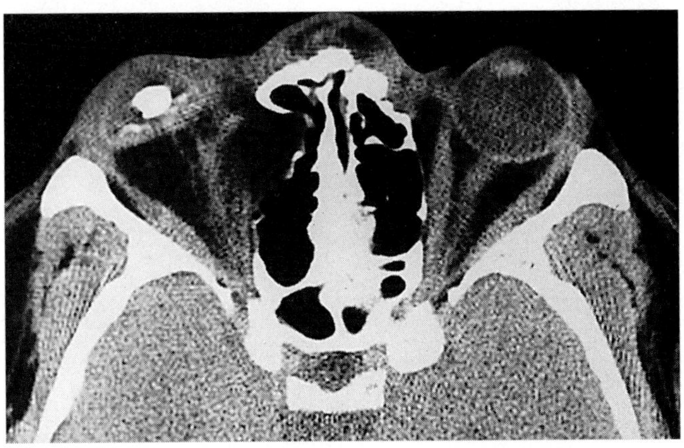

Figure 10–4. Phthisis bulbi (post-traumatic). The right globe is shrunken with dense ossification. Note the old blowout fracture of the right medial orbital wall. (Courtesy of Dr. Pamela Van Tassel, Charleston, SC.)

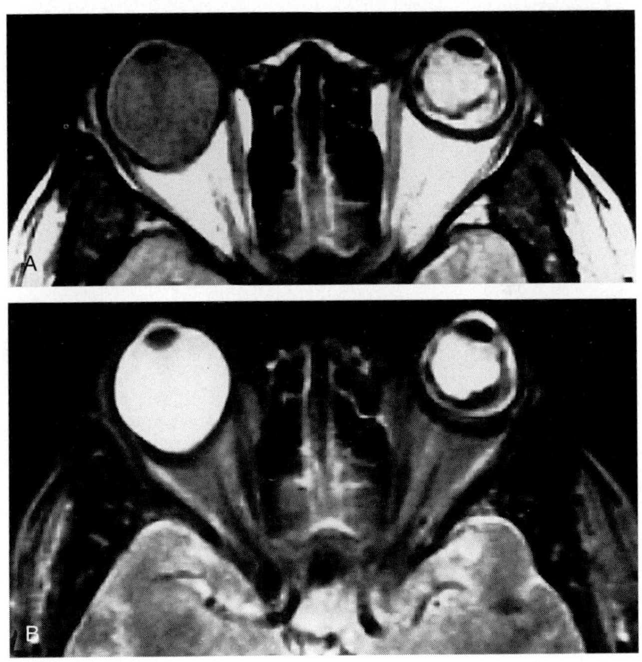

Figure 10–5. Phthisis bulbi. **(A)** Axial PD-weighted and **(B)** T2-weighted MRI show a small left globe with hyperintense vitreous due to T1 shortening and a hypointense rind of ossification.

Retinal Detachment

Retinal detachment is the separation of the sensory retina from the retinal pigment epithelium with a subsequent accumulation of fluid in the subretinal space. The principal role of imaging is to clarify the etiology, particularly if underlying neoplasm is suspected.

Imaging Findings. The retina itself is usually too thin to resolve. Subretinal fluid tends to be hyperdense on CT and hyperintense on MRI relative to the vitreous. Smaller detachments form a V-shape, with the apex directed toward the optic disc. Larger detachments may replace the entire vitreous cavity.

TABLE 10–6 | Causes of Retinal Detachment

Causes of Retinal Detachment
Intraocular tumor
Retrolental fibroplasia
Diabetic retinopathy
Toxocara endophthalmitis
Chorioretinitis (CMV, toxoplasmosis)
Coats' disease
Trauma

Differential Diagnosis

See Tables 10–1, 10–5, and 10–6.

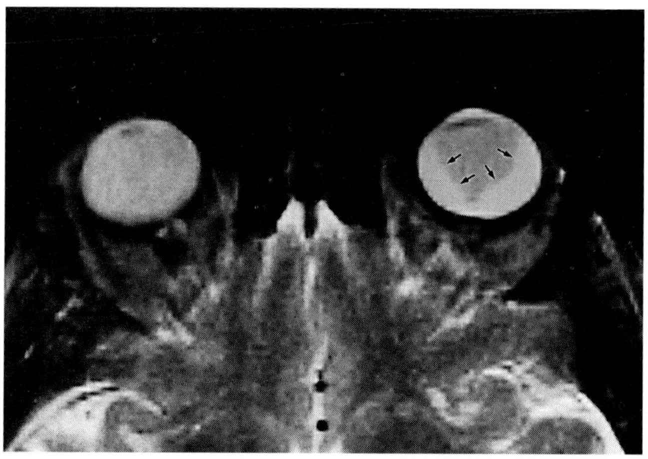

Figure 10–6. Retinal detachment. MRI shows hyperintense subretinal effusion (arrows) forming cone with apex directed toward the optic disc.

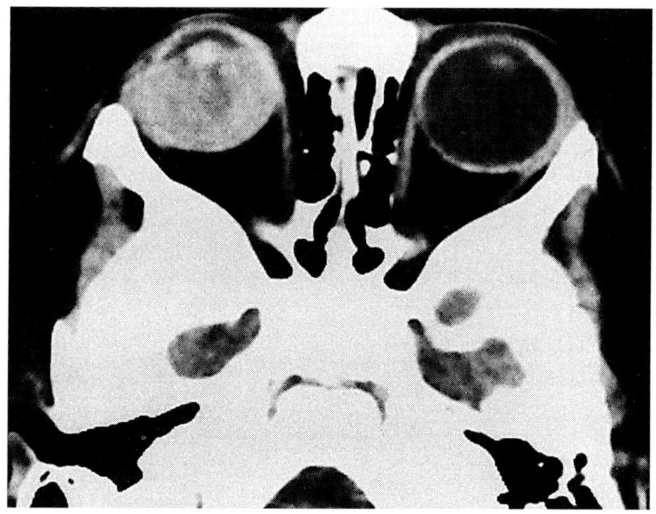

Figure 10–7. Coats' disease. CT shows a hyperdense right vitreous due to hemorrhagic or proteinaceous subretinal exudate filling the posterior chamber.

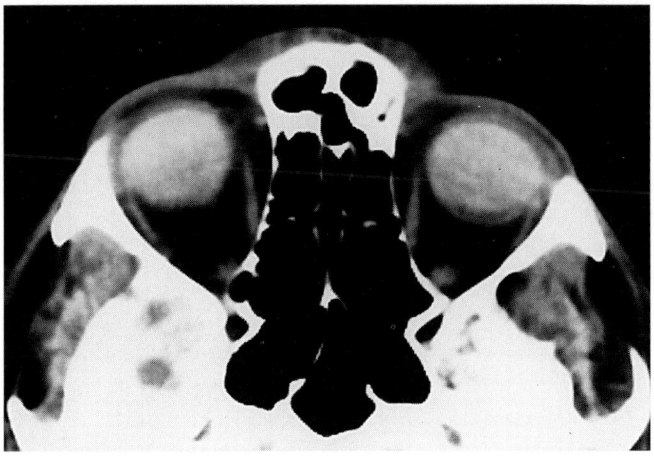

Figure 10–8. Intraocular silicone oil (retinal detachment due to (CMV) retinitis). CT shows bilateral hyperdense posterior chambers. The intraocular silicone oil is placed to stabilize the detached retina.

Retinoblastoma

Retinoblastoma is one of the more common childhood malignancies and the most common intraocular tumor in children. It arises from neuroectodermal precursor cells destined to become retinal photoreceptors. The hereditary form is autosomal dominant with incomplete (60–90%) penetrance and often bilateral. Overall, retinoblastoma is bilateral in 25–30% of cases. Unilateral retinoblastoma is usually not familial. Both sporadic and familial forms are attributed to a mutation on the long arm of chromosome 13. Most patients present with leukokoria (white pupil) before the age of 3. Long-term survival of 80% or better may be anticipated following enucleation. The syndrome of trilateral retinoblastoma consists of bilateral retinoblastomas and intracranial pineoblastoma.

CT Findings. CT shows a slightly hyperdense intraocular mass with moderate contrast enhancement. Calcifications are present in 90%. Associated retinal detachments and effusions are common. Intravenous contrast aids in distinguishing the tumor from subretinal effusions.

MRI Findings. MRI is less sensitive than CT due to its inability to visualize calcifications. Retinoblastoma is isointense to slightly hyperintense relative to vitreous on T1-weighted images and hypointense on T2-weighted images. Subretinal hemorrhage or effusion is somewhat easier to distinguish from tumor on MRI by virtue of its more homogeneous signal characteristics relative to the tumor itself.

Differential Diagnosis

The differential diagnosis includes conditions of children that present with leukocoria and intraocular mass: persistent hyperplastic primary vitreous, retrolental fibroplasia, *Toxocara canis* granuloma, and Coats' disease.

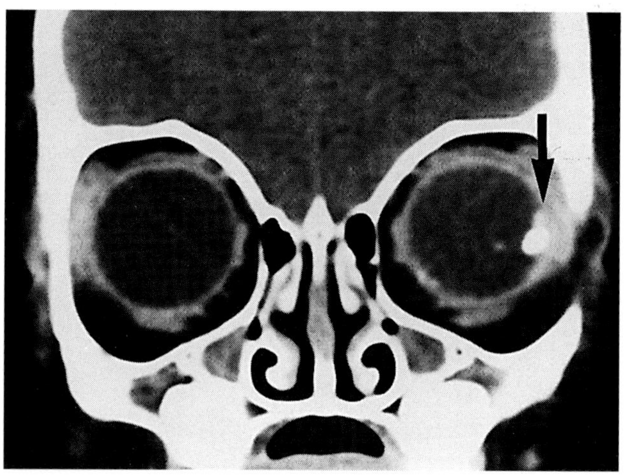

Figure 10–9. Retinoblastoma. Coronal CT shows a small mostly calcified mass (arrows) on the lateral wall of the left globe.

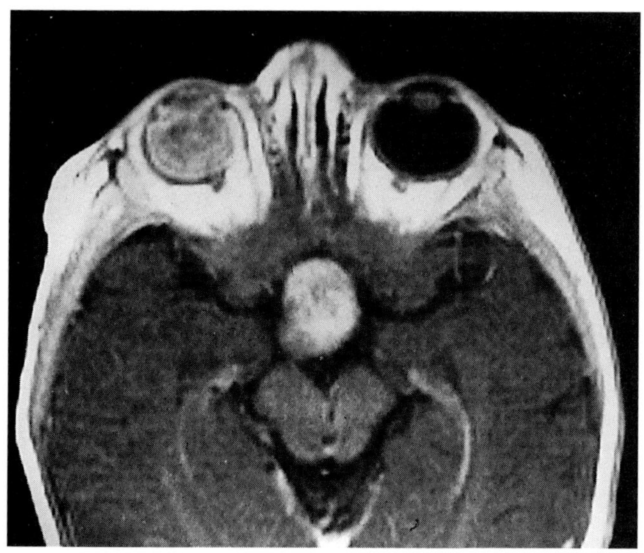

Figure 10–10. Retinoblastoma. Contrast-enhanced MRI shows an enhancing mass filling the right globe with metastasis to the suprasellar region. (Courtesy of Dr. Loretta Shearer, Louisville, KY.)

Melanoma

Malignant melanoma is the most common primary intraocular neoplasm. Only metastases are more common. It usually presents between the ages of 30 and 70 and is rare in blacks. Most cases arise in the choroid (85%), followed by the ciliary body and iris. Patients may present with visual field defects due to retinal detachment. The prognosis depends on tumor size, with mortality ranging from 13% for tumors less than 10 mm to 70% for tumors more than 12 mm in diameter. In advanced disease, metastases may be found in the liver (92%), lungs (31%), and bone (23%).

CT Findings. CT shows a round, oval, or crescentic hyperdense mass projecting into the vitreous and exhibiting mild to moderate contrast enhancement. Associated retinal detachments are difficult to distinguish from, and may conceal, the actual tumor. Advanced tumors may show invasion of the sclera with retro-ocular extension.

MRI Findings. MRI reveals a choroid mass bulging into the vitreous. Melanotic melanoma is characteristically hyperintense to markedly hyperintense on T1-weighted images and hypointense relative to the vitreous on T2-weighted images. Moderate enhancement is seen following intravenous contrast. There is a high frequency of associated retinal detachment. Subretinal fluid if present also tends to be hyperintense on T1-weighted images but may be separated from the tumor by its higher signal intensity on T2-weighted images.

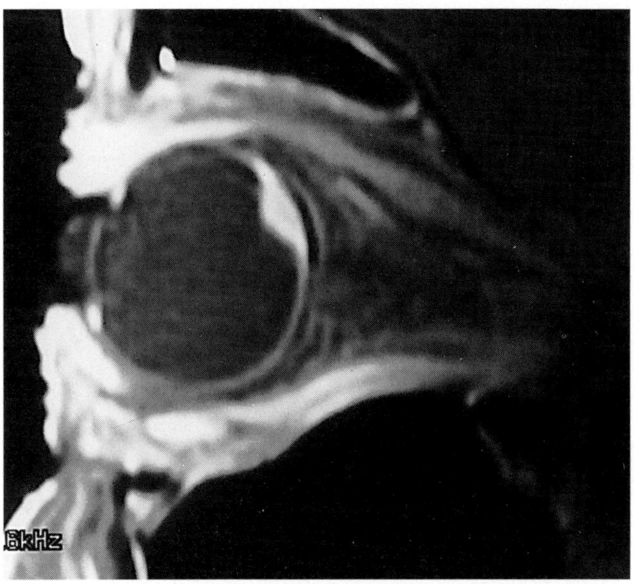

Figure 10–11. Melanoma. Contrast-enhanced MRI shows a hyperintense, smoothly convex mass on the posterior choroid. The mass was nearly as hyperintense prior to contrast administration.

Differential Diagnosis

See Table 10–1.

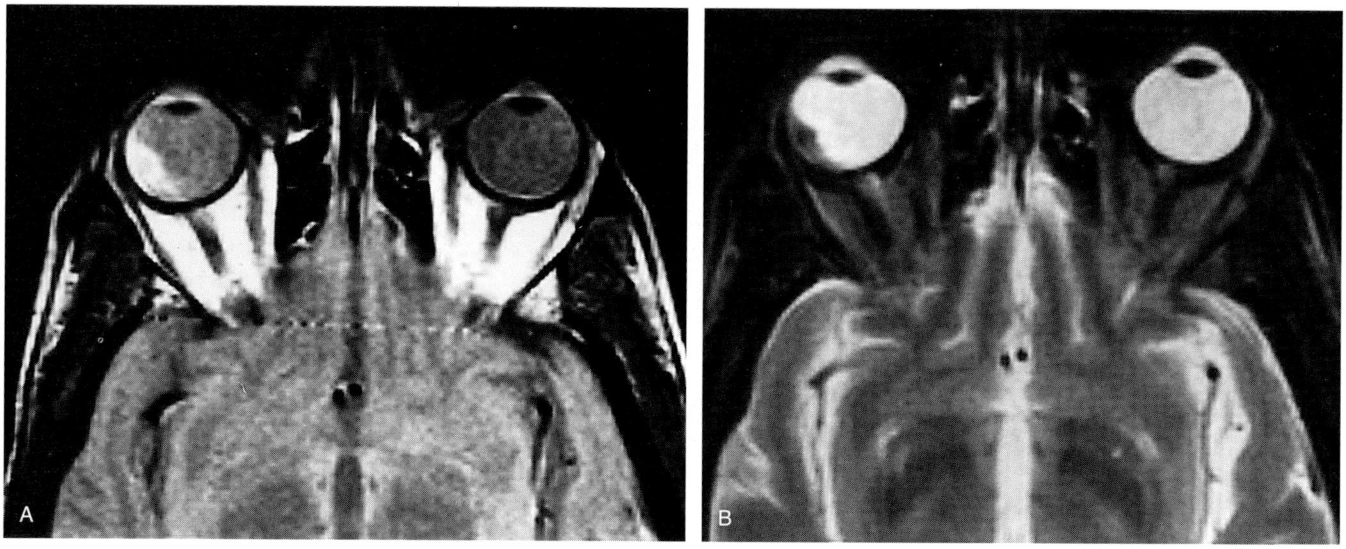

Figure 10–12. Melanoma. **(A)** PD-weighted MRI shows a hyperintense mass of the right choroid. **(B)** Hypointensity of the mass on T2-weighted images enables differentiation from subretinal effusion, which would be hyperintense.

Metastasis

Metastases from systemic malignancies may deposit anywhere within the orbit. The choroid is the most common site probably due to its rich vascularity. The most common sources are breast carcinoma in women, lung carcinoma in men, and neuroblastoma in children. Choroidal metastases often precipitate a secondary retinal detachment with resulting visual impairment.

CT Findings. CT shows an enhancing mass with irregular margins. The globe (choroid or retina) is the most common site, but choroidal metastases are usually small and frequently indetectable by imaging. Associated retinal detachments may be present. Metastases may also occur in the extraocular muscles, intraconal or extraconal space, or orbital bony wall and on CT appear as an irregular soft tissue mass with invasion of adjacent structures.

MRI Findings. The same general principles apply as with CT. Metastases are typically isointense to muscle on T1-weighted images and variable on T2-weighted images. A solitary mass of an extraocular muscle that is hyperintense on T2-weighted images is more likely to be a metastasis than thyroid disease or a pseudotumor.

Differential Diagnosis

The differential diagnosis depends on the mass's location within the orbit. See Tables 10–1, 10–9, 10–10, and 10–11. Most patients with orbital metastases have a known primary malignancy with systemic metastases.

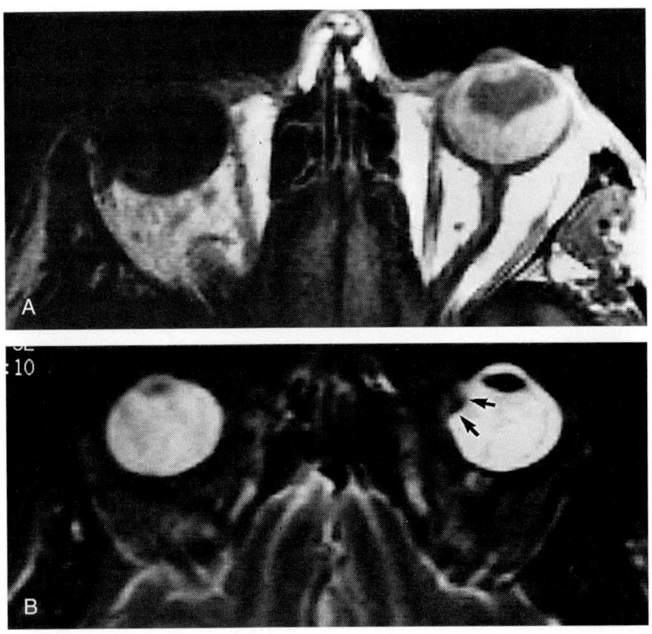

Figure 10–13. Choroidal metastasis (adenocarcinoma). **(A)** Axial T1-weighted image shows left retinal detachment with hyperintense subretinal effusions. **(B)** T2-weighted image shows a hypointense mass on the medial aspect (arrows) and enables separation of tumor from subretinal effusion.

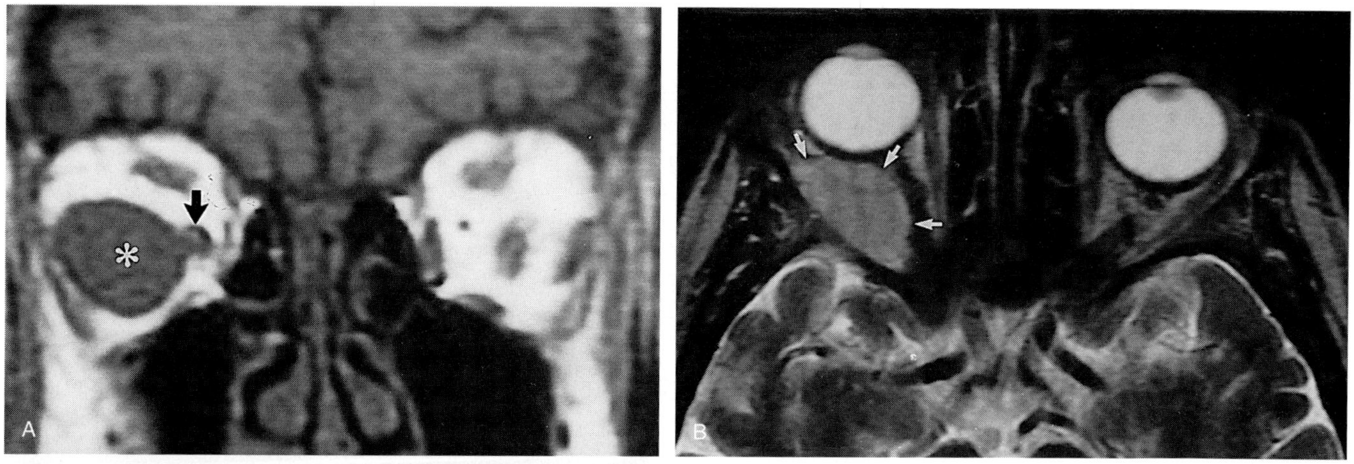

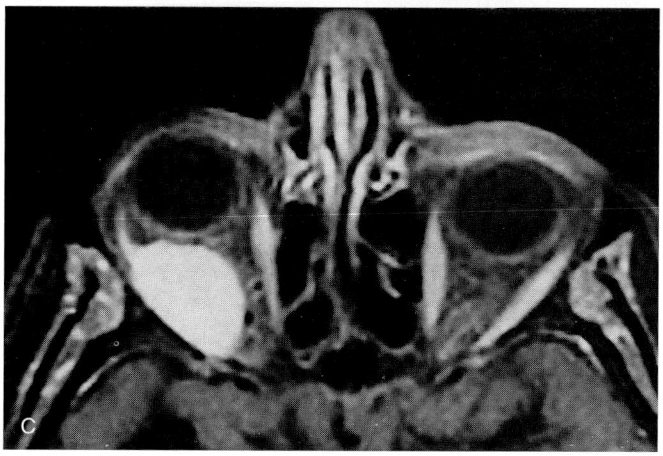

Figure 10–14. Intraorbital metastasis (leiomyosarcoma). **(A)** Coronal T1-weighted image shows a well-defined isointense (with muscle) mass (asterisk) arising from the right lateral rectus muscle. Arrow points to optic nerve. **(B)** On axial T2-weighted sequence the mass (arrows) is mildly hyperintense. **(C)** Contrast-enhanced scan with fat suppression shows marked enhancement of the mass. The prominent enhancement of the extraocular muscles is normal.

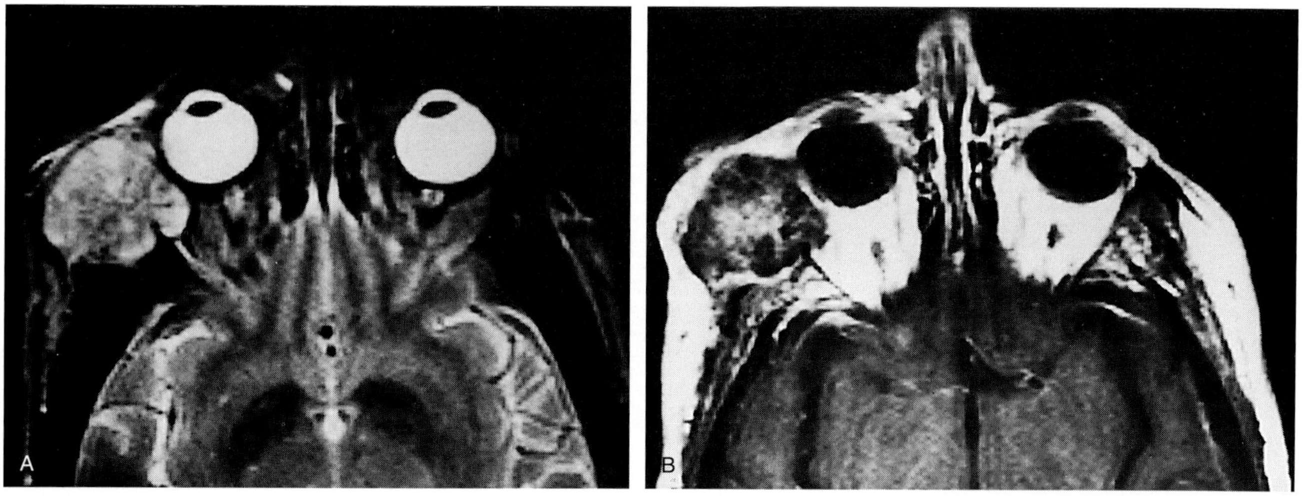

Figure 10–15. Orbital wall metastasis (breast carcinoma). Axial **(A)** T2-weighted and **(B)** contrast-enhanced MRI show a hyperintense enhancing mass arising from and destroying the right lateral orbital wall.

Disorders of the Optic Nerve

Optic Neuritis

Inflammatory demyelination of the optic nerve may occur in association with multiple sclerosis or systemic viral diseases such as varicella or herpes. Less common causes include lupus, ischemia, syphilis, and sarcoid. Patients present with pain and diminished visual acuity. Optic neuritis is the initial manifestation of multiple sclerosis in 15% of cases. The probability that a patient newly diagnosed with isolated optic neuritis will ultimately develop multiple sclerosis is approximately 30% for males and 75% for females. Radiation-induced optic neuritis presents as rapid, painless visual loss 1 to 3 years following radiotherapy near the optic nerves or chiasm.

TABLE 10–7 | Optic Nerve and Sheath Masses

Cause	Features
Optic glioma	Usually children Diffuse swelling of optic nerve and sheath with tortuosity and buckling of the nerve
Meningioma	Usually adults Tram track and donut signs Occasionally calcified
Optic neuritis	Diffuse swelling of optic nerve and sheath Enhancement on MRI Intracranial MS in up to 50%
Pseudotumor	Multifocal disease Painful orbit
Papilledema	Distended nerve sheath (CSF) on MRI with normal optic nerve

TABLE 10–8 | Differential Diagnosis of Distended Optic Nerve Sheath

Idiopathic
Elevated intracranial pressure
Arachnoid cyst
Optic atrophy
Orbital apex obstruction

CT Findings. CT is usually normal but may show an enlarged enhancing optic nerve with irregular borders.

MRI Findings. MRI shows enlargement and hyperintensity of the optic nerve on T2-weighted images, with enhancement of the nerve following intravenous contrast. Up to 50% may have intracranial findings of multiple sclerosis at the time of diagnosis. Later stages may show optic nerve atrophy with a small nerve surrounded by a sleeve of CSF.

Differential Diagnosis

See Tables 10–7 and 10–8 and Diagram 10–2.

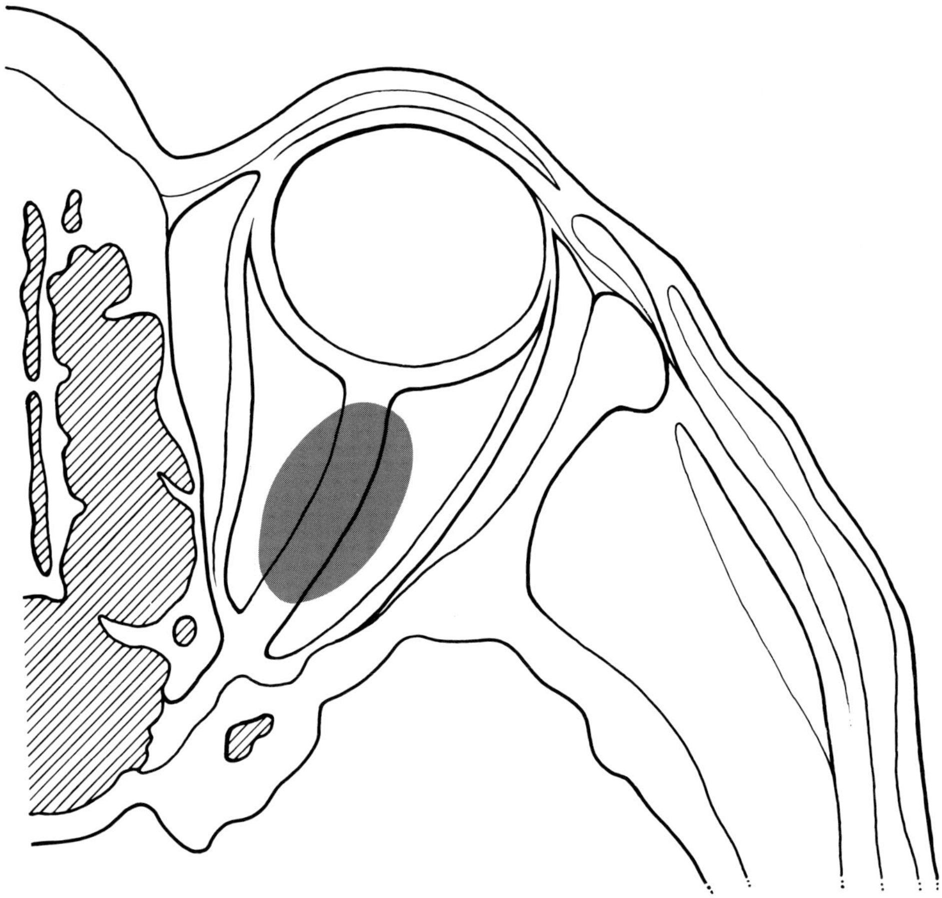

Diagram 10–2. Optic nerve or sheath mass. Primary masses of the optic nerve or sheath enlarge the entire nerve or result in a focal mass.

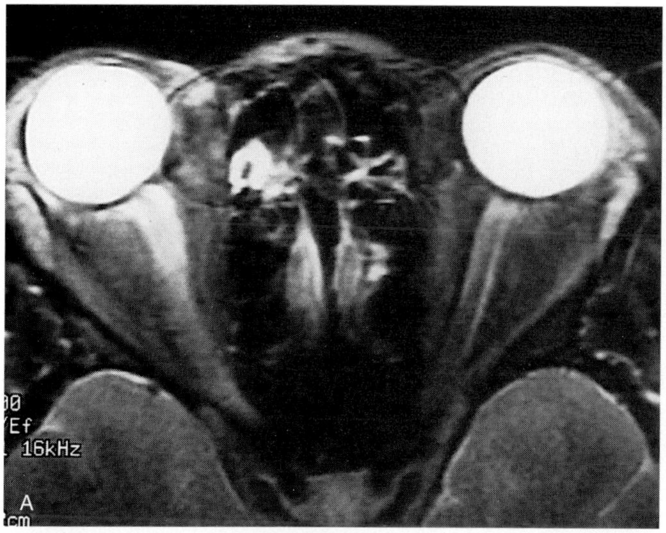

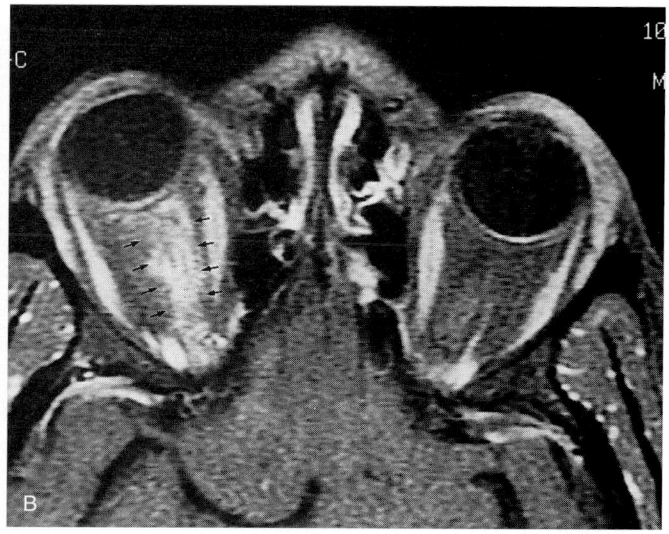

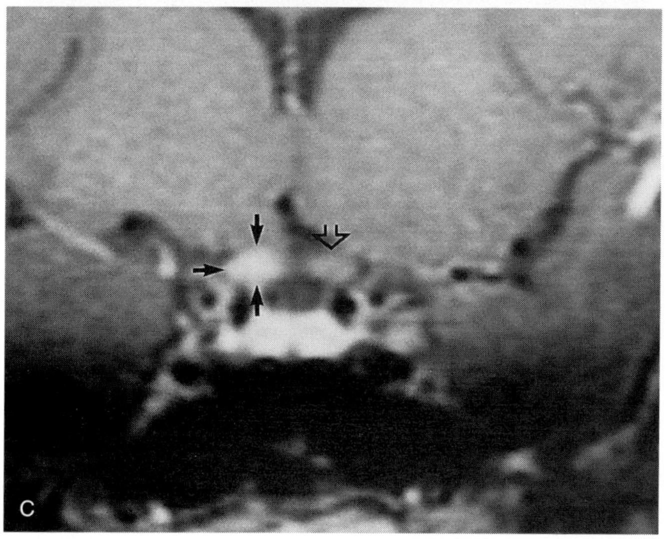

Figure 10–16. Optic neuritis. **(A)** Axial T2-weighted MRI shows marked hyperintensity in and around the right optic nerve. (Compare to normal left optic nerve and sheath.) **(B)** Contrast-enhanced MRI with fat suppression shows marked enhancement of the right optic nerve and sheath (arrows). **(C)** Coronal contrast-enhanced MRI through the sella shows enhancement of the prechiasmatic right optic nerve (arrows). Open arrow points to normal left optic nerve.

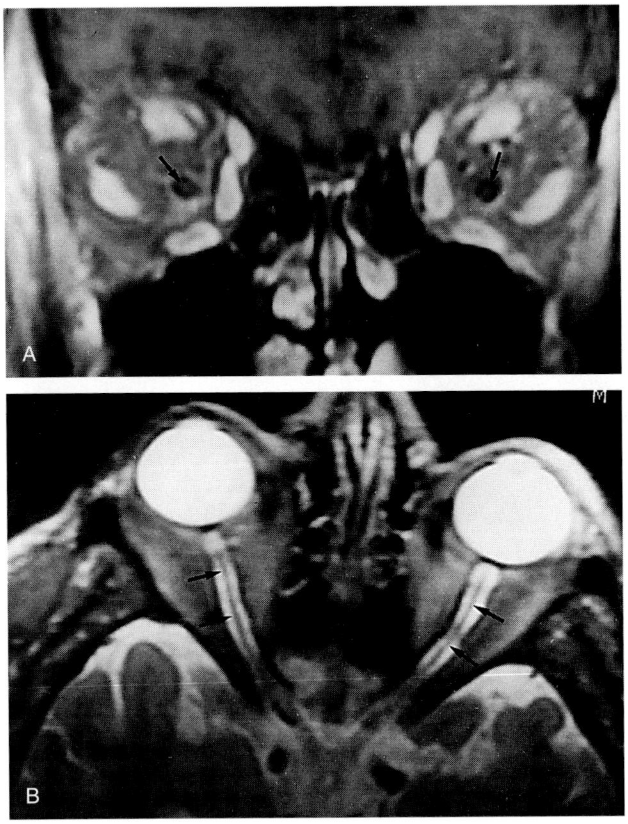

Figure 10–17. Optic atrophy due to radiation-induced optic neuritis. Both **(A)** coronal T1-weighted and **(B)** axial T2-weighted MRI show bilaterally atrophic optic nerves (arrows) surrounded by prominent CSF-filled nerve sheath. The CSF is hypointense relative to the nerve in **A** and markedly hyperintense in **B**.

Optic Nerve Glioma

Optic nerve gliomas are rare low-grade astrocytomas of the optic nerves, chiasm, or optic tracts. Such astrocytomas are usually of the juvenile pilocytic type. About 75% are diagnosed before age 10, and 25–50% are associated with type 1 neurofibromatosis. Affected patients present with proptosis or visual loss.

CT Findings. Three typical morphologic patterns are encountered: (1) diffuse thickening of the optic nerve, (2) fusiform thickening of the optic nerve, or (3) a focal mass of the optic nerve. The optic nerve commonly appears kinked. Small hypodensities may be present before or after contrast enhancement. The tumor is multicentric only in patients with neurofibromatosis. In about 25% of cases, the tumor extends posteriorly to involve the chiasm, optic tracts, lateral geniculate bodies, or even optic radiations. Contrast enhancement is usually intense.

MRI Findings. Glioma of the optic nerve is mildly hypointense or isointense to cerebral white matter on T1-weighted images and isointense to mildly hyperintense on T2-weighted images. In contrast, glioma of the chiasm and retrochiasmatic structures is quite hyperintense on T2-weighted images. The pilocytic tumors show marked enhancement after intravenous contrast, best seen in conjunction with fat-suppression techniques.

Differential Diagnosis

See Table 10–7 and Diagram 10–2.

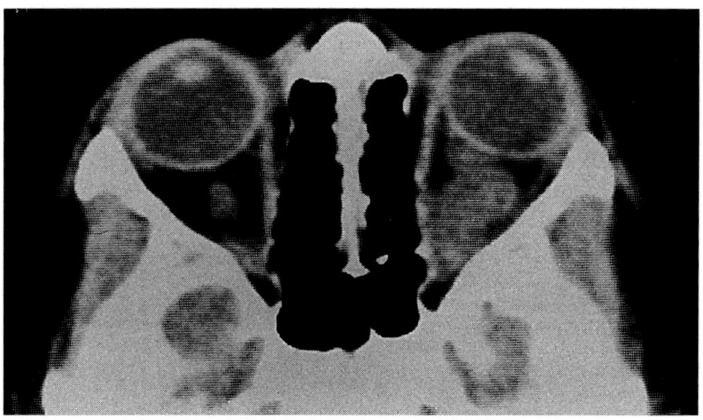

Figure 10–18. Optic glioma. CT shows an enlarged left optic nerve with characteristic buckling.

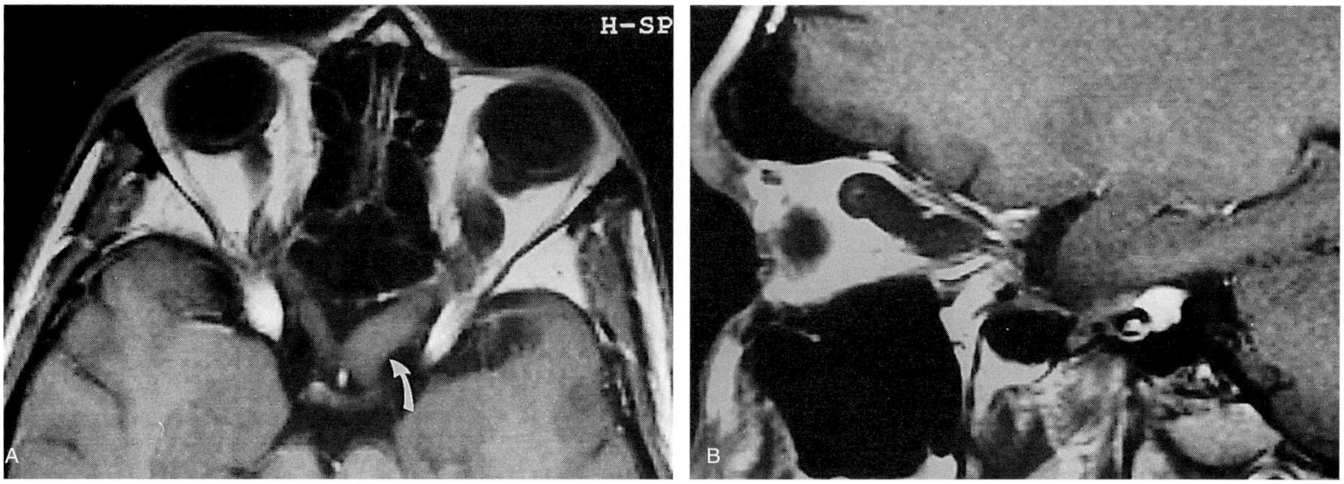

Figure 10–19. Optic glioma. **(A)** Axial and **(B)** sagittal enhanced MRI show enlargement of the left optic nerve extending to the optic chiasm (arrow).

Optic Nerve Meningioma

Meningiomas of the orbit may arise from the optic nerve sheath, the periosteum of the orbital wall, or the spread of intracranial meningiomas via the orbital fissures. Optic nerve sheath meningiomas are more common among women (5 to 1). Some 15% of patients have type 1 neurofibromatosis.

CT Findings. CT shows diffuse, typically uniform thickening of the optic nerve sheath with enhancement. The lower attenuation of the optic nerve within the tumor gives rise to the tram track sign (donut sign on coronal images) present in most cases. Calcifications are seen in a minority. Optic canal widening and intracranial extension may develop. Hyperostosis may occur at the orbital apex.

MRI Findings. MRI shows a thickened optic nerve. The mass is usually isointense with muscle on T1-weighted images and isointense with fat on T2-weighted images. Intracranial extension is seen to better advantage with MRI than with CT. Hyperostosis may develop in the vicinity of the optic canal. Contrast enhancement is constant and best identified with the use of fat suppression techniques.

Differential Diagnosis

See Table 10–7 and Diagram 10–2.

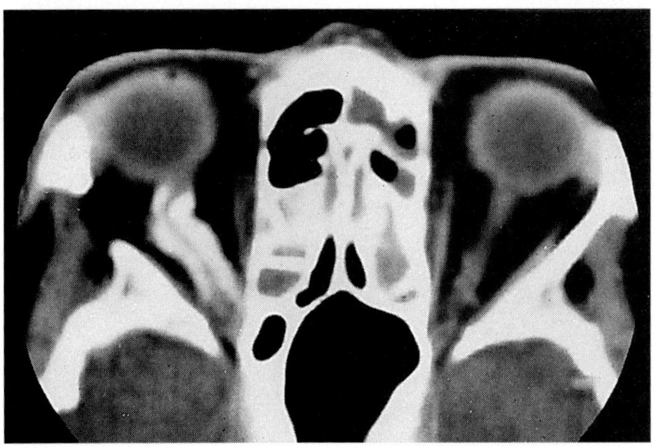

Figure 10–20. Optic nerve meningioma. CT without contrast shows dense calcification of the right optic nerve sheath with sparing of the centrally located optic nerve, a form of tram track sign.

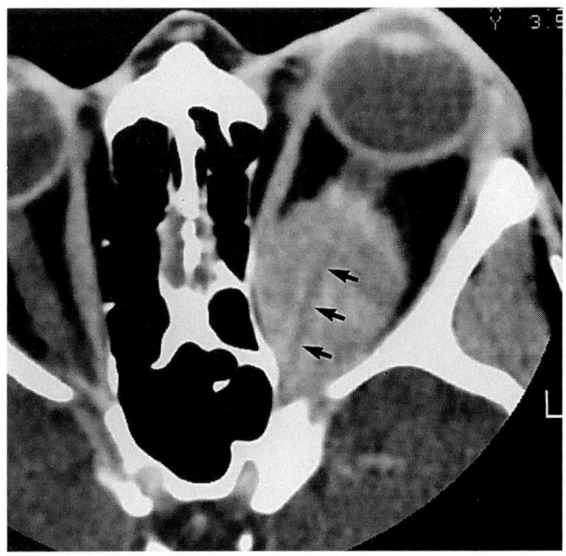

Figure 10–21. Optic nerve meningioma. CT with contrast shows a fusiform, enhancing mass of the left optic nerve. There is sparing of the centrally located optic nerve (arrows), the tram track sign.

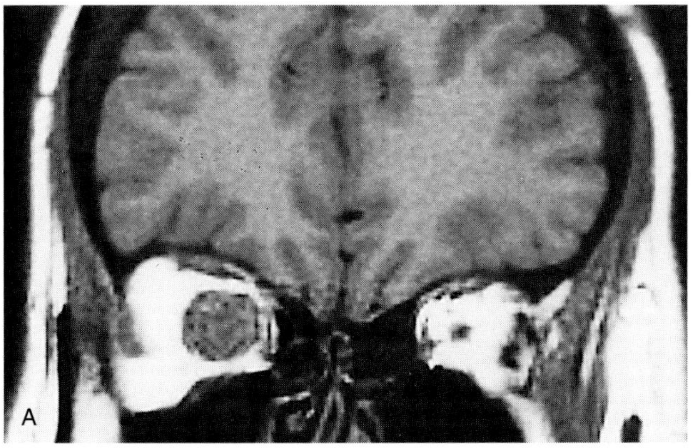

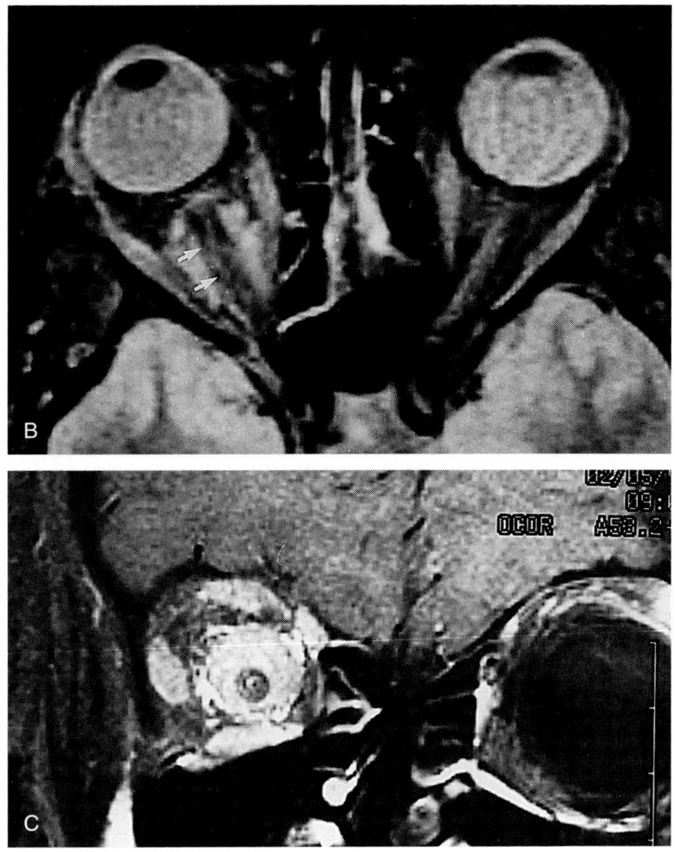

Figure 10–22. Optic nerve meningioma. **(A)** Coronal T1-weighted MRI shows a mass of the right optic nerve that is isointense to extraocular muscle. **(B)** On axial T2-weighted images the mass is hyperintense and envelops the optic nerve (arrows). **(C)** Coronal contrast-enhanced MRI with fat suppression shows marked enhancement, irregular outer margins, and sharp contrast with the centrally located optic nerve (donut sign).

Disorder of the Extraocular Muscles

Thyroid Ophthalmopathy

Synonym: Graves' ophthalmopathy.

Thyroid ophthalmopathy is the most common cause of proptosis in the adult. Some degree of orbital involvement occurs in over half of hyperthyroid patients during the course of their disease. Occasionally orbital disease may precede the clinical onset of hyperthyroidism. The major ocular abnormalities consist of lid retraction, edema and infiltration of retro-orbital fat, and most notably enlargement of the extraocular muscles, which may be severe. The condition resolves spontaneously in 90% of cases, but vision-threatening complications develop in many of the remainder.

CT Findings. CT usually demonstrates proptosis accompanied by thickening of the extraocular muscles, most commonly bilateral and roughly symmetrical. The maximum normal thickness in the belly of an extraocular muscle has been reported as 2.8 mm. The inferior recti, followed by medial recti, are most often and most severely affected. The muscle tendons are spared, with smooth tapering near the globe insertion. There may be areas of decreased attenuation within the muscle, but the muscle margins remain sharp. The retro-ocular fat may be increased in volume, even in the absence of muscle enlargement.

TABLE 10–9 | Extraocular Muscle Masses

Cause	Distinguishing Features
Thyroid ophthalmopathy	Proptosis and lid retraction Bilateral, medial and inferior recti Fusiform thickening Spares tendinous insertion
Pseudotumor	Painful orbit Unilateral and multifocal disease May involve tendinous insertion Infiltrates intraorbital fat
Metastasis	Rare, usually from breast carcinoma Focal bulbous mass, unilateral, and no preferred muscle More tendency to be bright on T2-weighted images and greater contrast enhancement

MRI Findings. MRI reveals anatomic changes similar to those of CT. The muscle is usually hypointense to retro-orbital fat on T1-weighted images. On T2-weighted images, the muscle is usually isointense with fat. However, hyperintensity of the inferior and medial recti may be observed in more severe cases.

Differential Diagnosis

See Table 10–9 and Diagram 10–3.

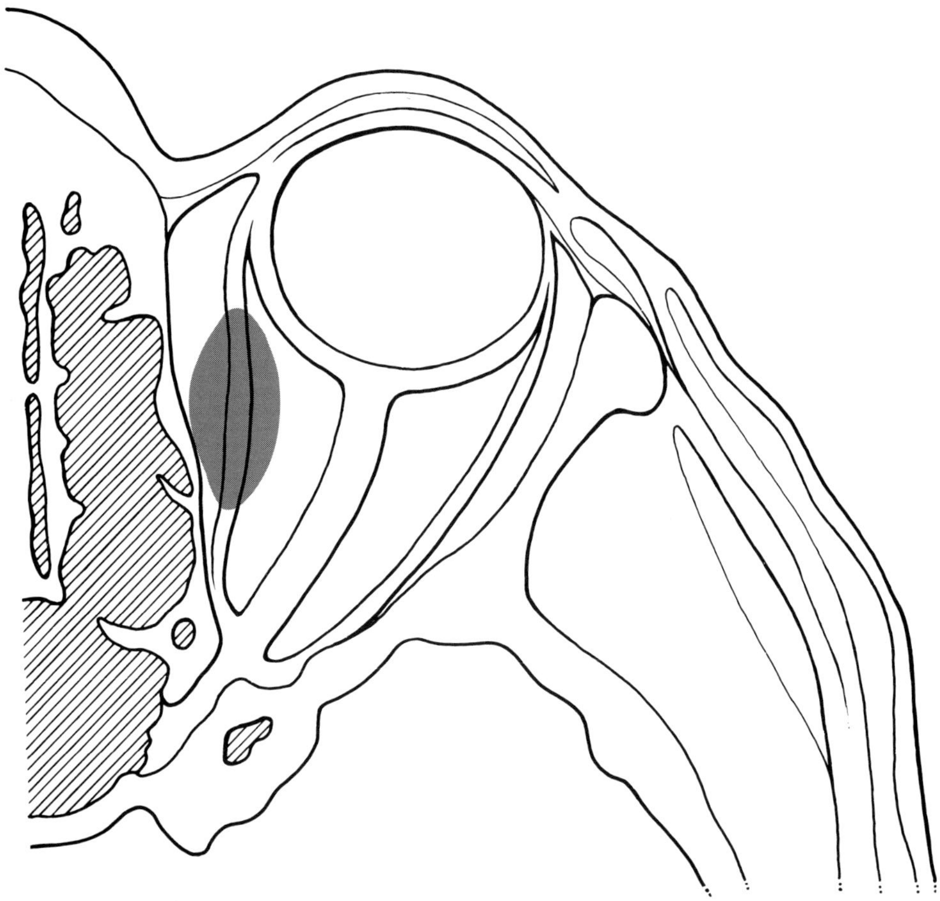

Diagram 10–3. Extraocular muscle mass. Various disorders result in focal or diffuse enlargement of one or more extraocular muscles.

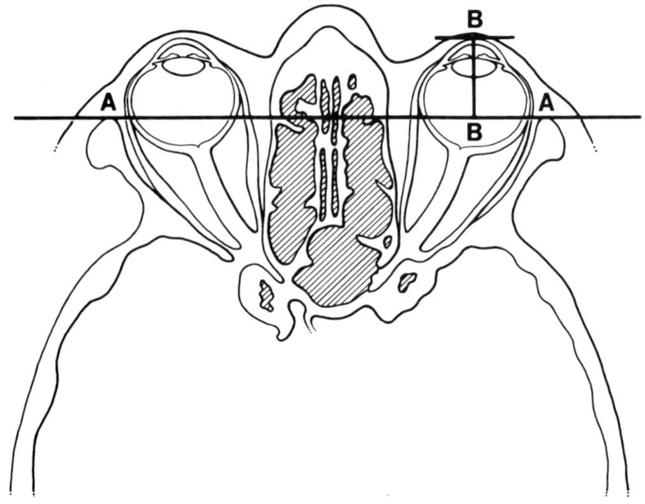

Figure 10–23. Diagnosis of proptosis. Proptosis is present when the cornea is more than 21 mm (B-B) anterior to a line connecting the lateral orbital rims (A-A).

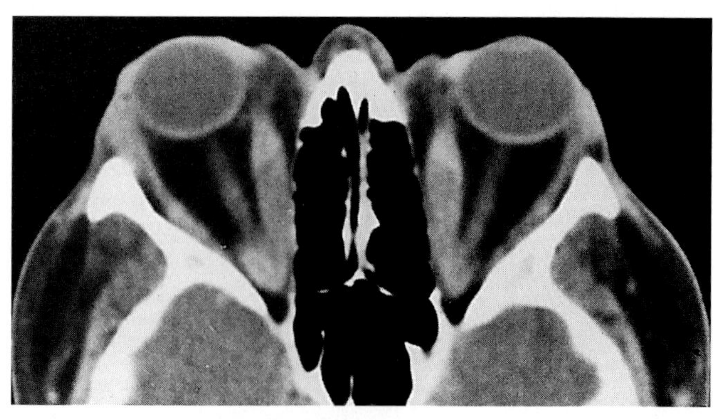

Figure 10–24. Thyroid ophthalmopathy. CT shows proptosis and bilateral symmetrical thickening of the medial recti with sparing of the tendinous scleral insertion.

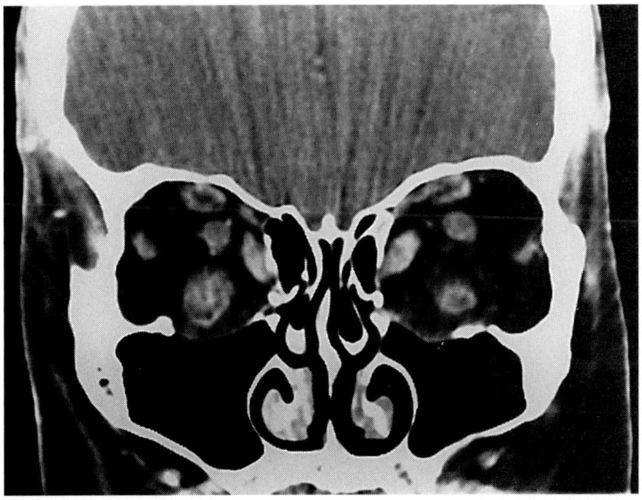

Figure 10–25. Thyroid ophthalmopathy. Coronal CT shows marked thickening of the right inferior rectus and mild thickening of the medial recti and left inferior rectus. Coronal imaging is required for adequate assessment of superior and inferior recti.

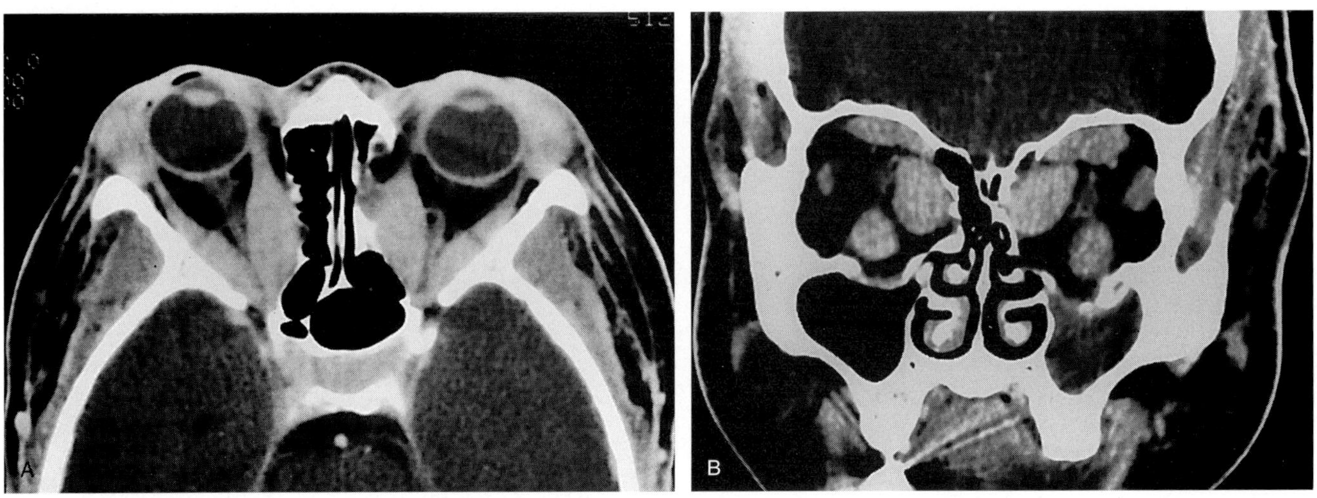

Figure 10–26. Thyroid opththalmopathy. **(A)** Axial CT shows severe thickening of the medial and lateral recti bilaterally. There is also marked lacrimal enlargement, which may occasionally be present. **(B)** Coronal CT shows superior and inferior rectus involvement as well. With such severe muscle enlargement, symptoms of orbital apex obstruction may ensue.

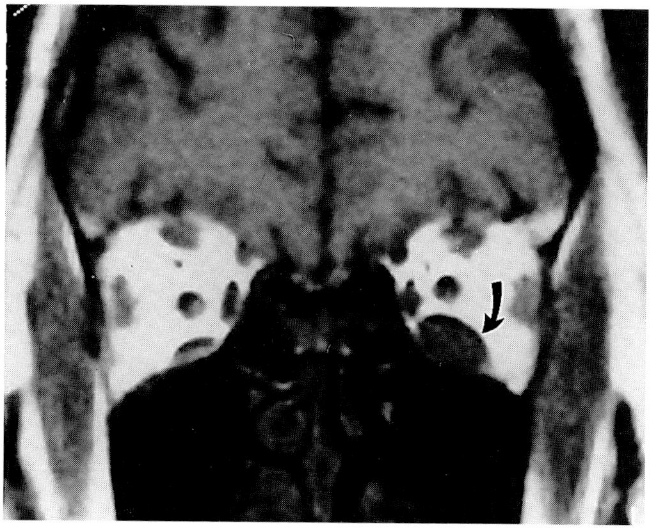

Figure 10–27. Thyroid ophthalmopathy. Coronal T1-weighted MRI shows thickening and mild hypointensity of the left inferior rectus (arrow).

Disorders of the Orbit

Orbital Varix

An orbital varix is a congenital venous malformation composed of single or multiple enlarged orbital veins. Affected individuals present with intermittent proptosis aggravated by exercise or increased venous pressure. A varix is the leading cause of spontaneous orbital hemorrhage.

CT Findings. CT shows a round or lobulated sharply marginated intraconal or extraconal mass that enhances intensely with contrast. A unique feature of an orbital varix is its ability to enlarge during the Valsalva maneuver. Proptosis may be present, which may also be enhanced by the Valsalva maneuver. Color flow Doppler ultrasound provides a useful adjunct in establishing the diagnosis.

MRI Findings. MRI demonstrates a vascular mass whose signal intensity varies depending on the pulse sequence and flow direction and velocity.

Differential Diagnosis

Hemangioma is a common cause of an intensely enhancing mass but does not change with the Valsalva maneuver or evidence flow characteristics on MRI. Secondary orbital varices may occur secondary to carotid-cavernous fistulas or arteriovenous malformations.

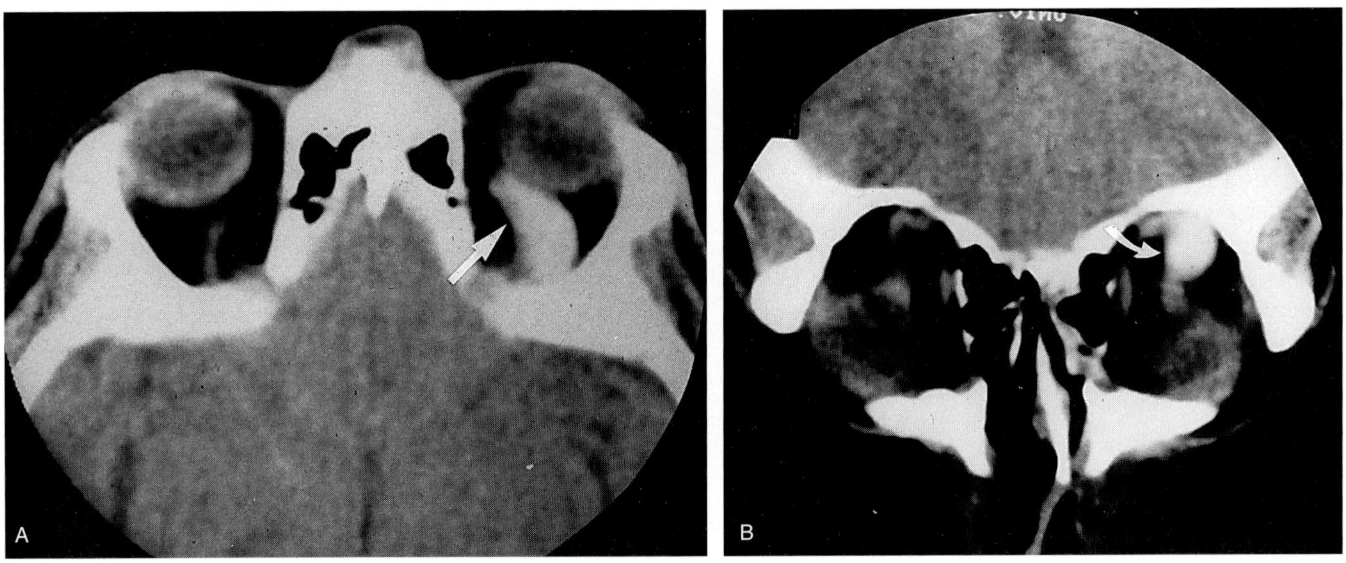

Figure 10–28. Orbital varix. **(A)** Axial and **(B)** coronal CT show an intensely enhancing mass (arrow) corresponding to an enlarged superior ophthalmic vein.

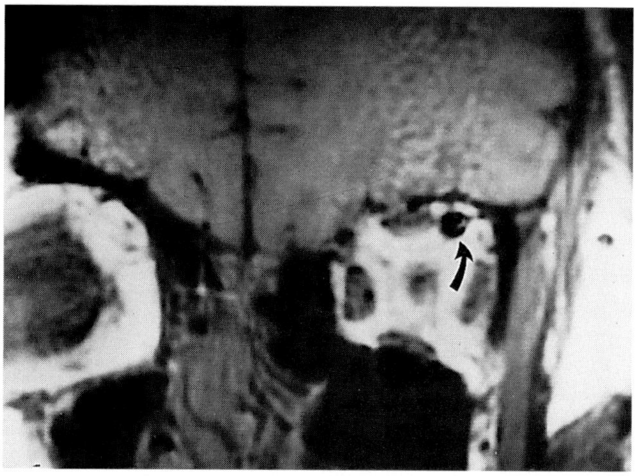

Figure 10–29. Carotid-cavernous fistula with dilated superior ophthalmic vein. Coronal T1-weighted MRI shows an enlarged left superior ophthalmic vein (arrow) with intraluminal flow void.

Pseudotumor

Orbital pseudotumor is a common inflammatory condition of unknown etiology characterized by the acute onset of pain, palpebral and conjunctival edema, proptosis, and ophthalmoplegia. Histology reveals a nonspecific inflammatory cell infiltrate. Most cases resolve following a course of systemic and sometimes intraocular corticosteroids.

CT Findings. Pseudotumor is usually unilateral (75%) and multifocal within the affected orbit. It may manifest any of the following CT findings alone or in any combination:

- Proptosis
- Thickened and enhancing sclera
- Intraorbital mass
- Infiltration of retro-orbital fat
- Thickening of extraocular muscles or optic nerve
- Enlargement of lacrimal gland

MRI Findings. MRI may manifest any of the anatomic findings described for CT. The retro-orbital masses and extraocular muscle enlargement are isointense to muscle on T1-weighted images and isointense or minimally hyperintense to fat on T2-weighted images and exhibit moderate contrast enhancement.

TABLE 10–10 **Intraconal Masses**

Cause	Distinguishing Features
Hemangioma	Adults Well-demarcated hyperdense mass with marked enhancement
Lymphangioma	Children and young adults Irregular margins, complex, and septated May be hyperintense on T1-weighted MRI.
Varix	Enlarges with Valsalva MRI signal indicates flow
Pseudotumor	Younger adults Acute onset of painful orbit Multifocal disease Scleral thickening often present
Lymphoma	Older adults Gradual onset of proptosis Homogeneous mass with irregular margins Usually anterosuperior orbit
Metastasis	Infiltrating mass with irregular margins
Nerve sheath tumor	Derived from branches of the third to seventh cranial nerves May displace optic nerve

TABLE 10–11 **Extraconal Masses**

Cause	Distinguishing Features
Cellulitis/abscess	Sinusitis or foreign body usually present
Lymphoma	Older adults Gradual onset of proptosis Homogeneous mass with irregular margins Usually anterosuperior orbit
Pseudotumor	Younger adults Acute onset of painful orbit Usually multifocal
Varix	Enlarges with Valsalva MRI signal indicates flow
Hemangioma	Adults Well-demarcated hyperdense mass with marked enhancement Usually intraconal
Lymphangioma	Children and young adults Irregular margins, complex, and septated May be hyperintense on T1-weighted MRI
Wegener's granulomatosis	Bone erosion and sinusitis Coexistent pulmonary or renal disease
Rhabdomyosarcoma	Solid homogeneous mass in children Rapidly growing and locally invasive.

Differential Diagnosis

Because of its protean manifestations, orbital pseudotumor can mimic virtually any other cause of an orbital mass lesion. Diffuse involvement may resemble cellulitis. Extraocular muscle involvement may resemble thyroid ophthalmopathy. Lacrimal involvement may resemble sarcoid or lymphoid tumors. Isolated masses must be distinguished from metastases. (See Tables 10–10 to 10–12 and Diagrams 10–4 to 10–6.)

Text continued on page 488

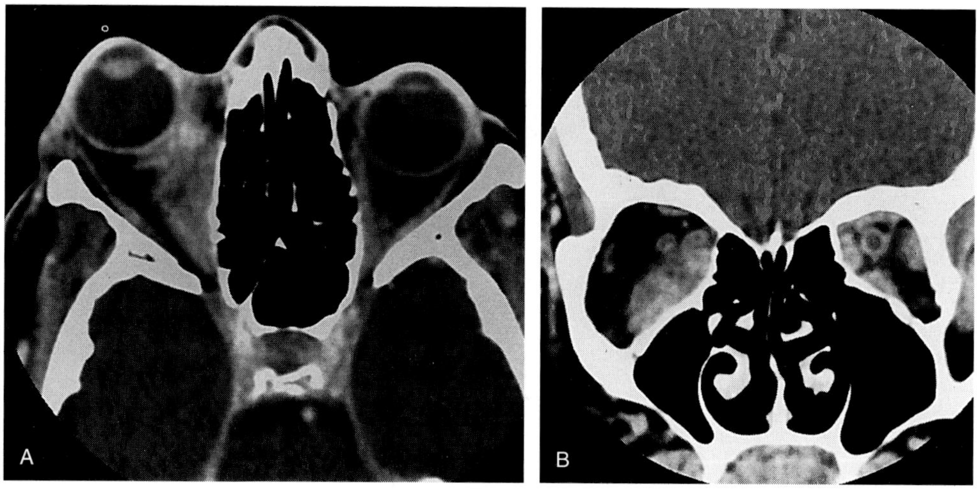

Figure 10–30. Pseudotumor. **(A)** Axial and **(B)** coronal contrast-enhanced CT show an irregular enhancing mass encompassing the right medial and inferior recti and retro-ocular fat.

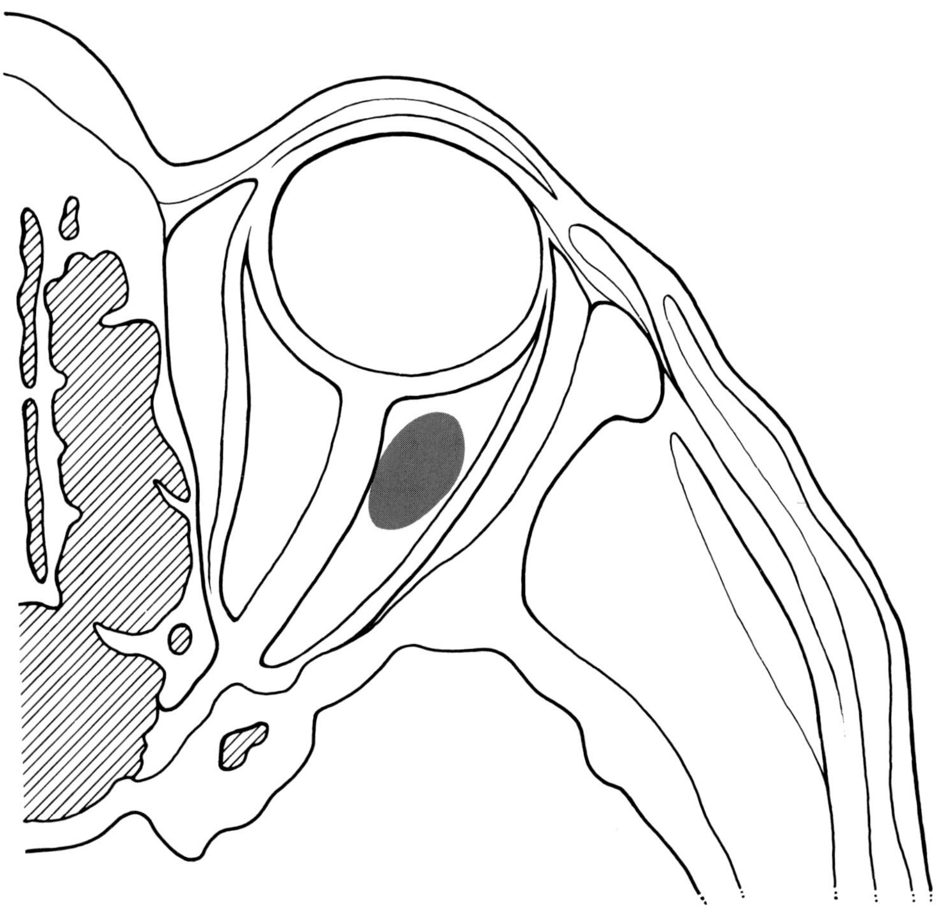

Diagram 10–4. Intraconal mass. An intraconal mass lies within a cone bordered anteriorly by the globe and around its circumference by the extraocular muscles and investing fascia.

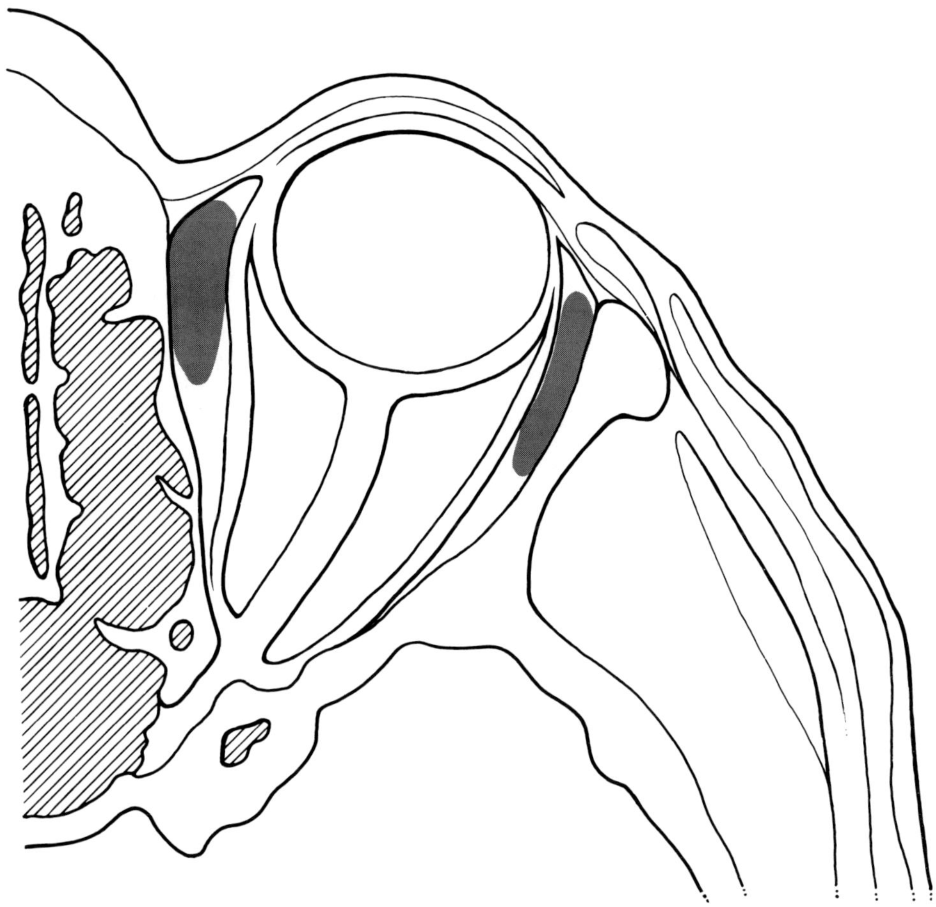

Diagram 10–5. Extraconal mass. Extraconal masses lie outside the muscle cone but within the bony orbit. Secondary bone involvement may be encountered, especially with neoplasms.

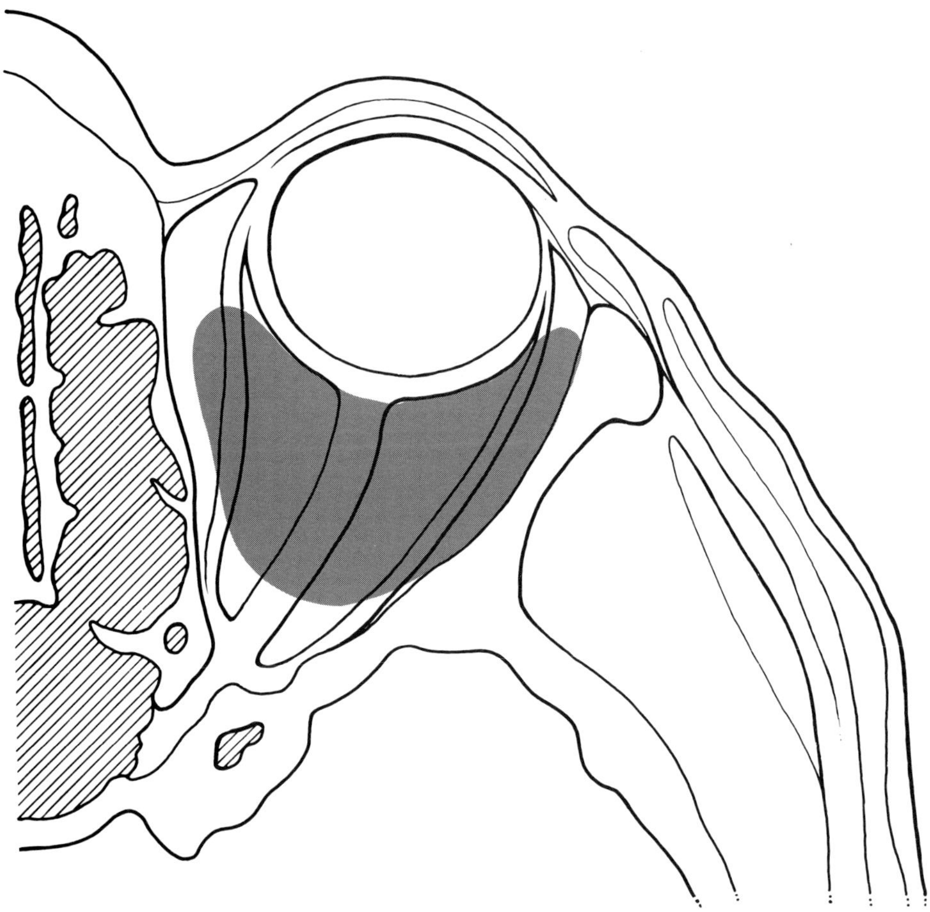

Diagram 10–6. Diffuse orbital mass. Such disorders may present with involvement of both intraconal and extraconal compartments or completely fill the orbit.

TABLE **10–12** **Diffuse Orbital Masses**

Cause	Distinguishing Features
Pseudotumor	Younger adults Acute onset of painful orbit Usually multifocal Sinuses not involved
Lymphoma	Older adults Gradual onset of proptosis Homogeneous mass with irregular margins Usually anterosuperior orbit
Wegener's granulomatosis	Sinusitis, bone erosion, and pulmonary and renal disease
Cellulitis	Sinusitis or foreign body present

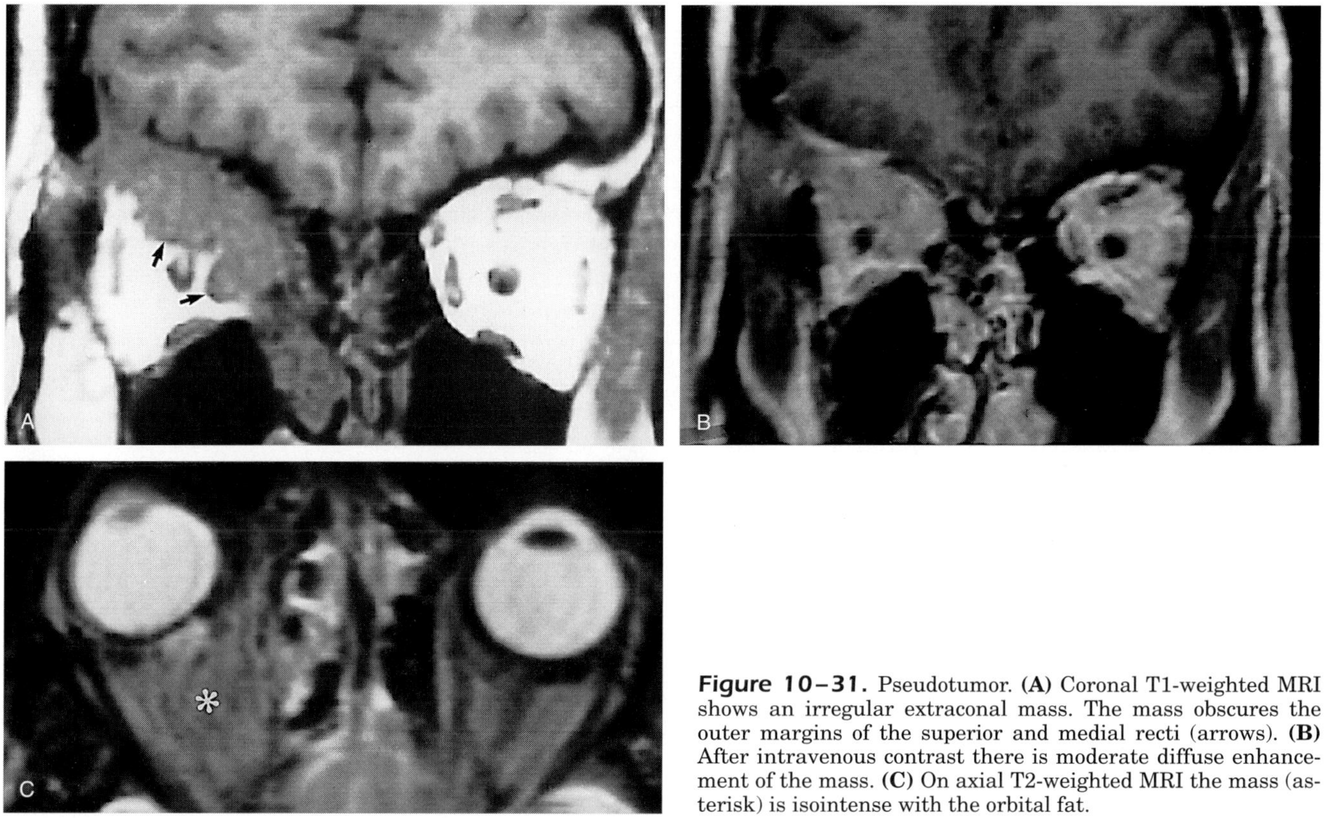

Figure 10–31. Pseudotumor. **(A)** Coronal T1-weighted MRI shows an irregular extraconal mass. The mass obscures the outer margins of the superior and medial recti (arrows). **(B)** After intravenous contrast there is moderate diffuse enhancement of the mass. **(C)** On axial T2-weighted MRI the mass (asterisk) is isointense with the orbital fat.

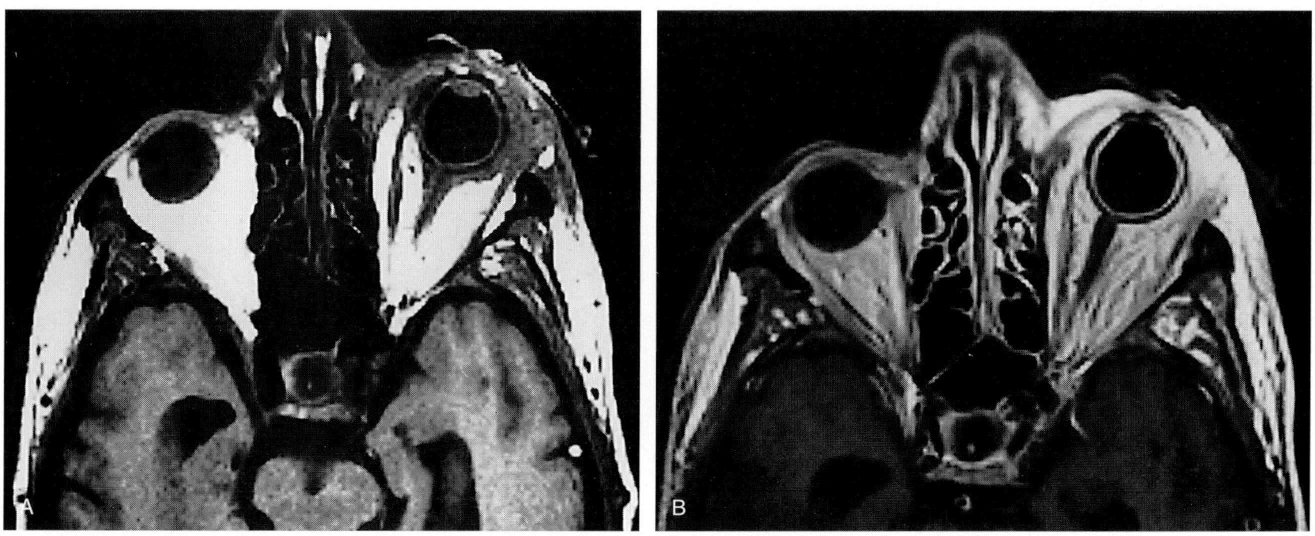

Figure 10–32. Pseudotumor with scleritis. Axial T1-weighted MRI **(A)** before and **(B)** after intravenous contrast shows irregular soft tissue thickening encompassing the left globe. The inflammatory tissue enhances intensely after contrast. There was a small associated choroidal detachment.

Cellulitis

Preseptal cellulitis is an acute pyogenic cellulitis of the eyelids and surrounding tissues. The tough fibrous orbital septum normally prevents retrograde spread of infection into the orbit.

Orbital cellulitis is a much more serious pyogenic infection of the orbit proper. It usually occurs as a complication of sinusitis, contaminated foreign body, or retrograde thrombophlebitis. Patients present with a painful red swollen eye, proptosis, and ophthalmic nerve deficits. The role of imaging is to distinguish preseptal from orbital involvement and to demonstrate abscess formation.

CT Findings. Swelling of the eyelids, proptosis, scleral thickening, subperiosteal abscesses, thickening of the extraocular muscles, and increased attenuation of the orbital fat may all be seen. Abscesses usually exhibit ring enhancement, but solid enhancement can also occur. Predisposing conditions such as sinusitis, foreign bodies, or fractures are usually evident. Complications such as epidural abscess, subdural empyema, meningitis, cerebritis, or brain abscess may be present and should be carefully searched for.

MRI Findings. Palpebral and periorbital edema manifest diminished signal on T1-weighted images and increased signal on T2-weighted images. Thrombosis of the superior ophthalmic vein may occur with the finding of increased signal rather than flow void in the lumen. Sinusitis and fractures are readily identified, but MRI is less effective than CT in the detection of foreign bodies. Complicating intracranial disease may be more readily detected with contrast-enhanced MRI.

Differential Diagnosis

Similar findings may be caused by pseudotumor, trauma and hemorrhage, or edema of other etiologies, such as superior vena cava occlusion.

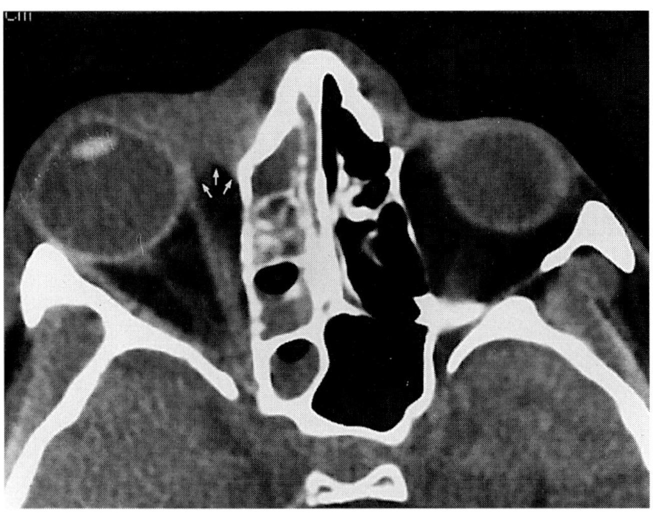

Figure 10–33. Preseptal cellulitis. Note the right-sided periorbital edema and lateral displacement of globe. The spread of infection is limited by the orbital septum (arrows).

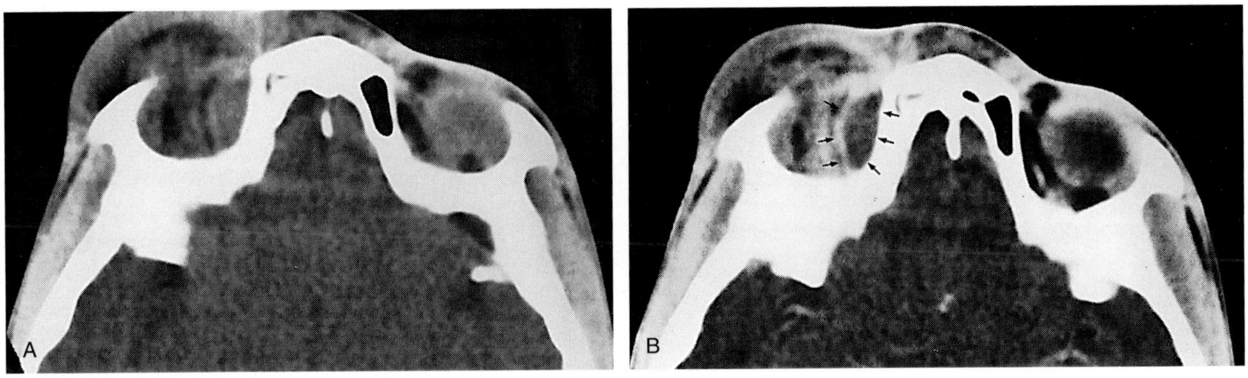

Figure 10–34. Orbital abscess. **(A)** Axial CT shows right orbital cellulitis with subperiosteal abscess. **(B)** The abscess (arrows) shows rim enhancement following intravenous contrast. (See also Fig. 3–11.)

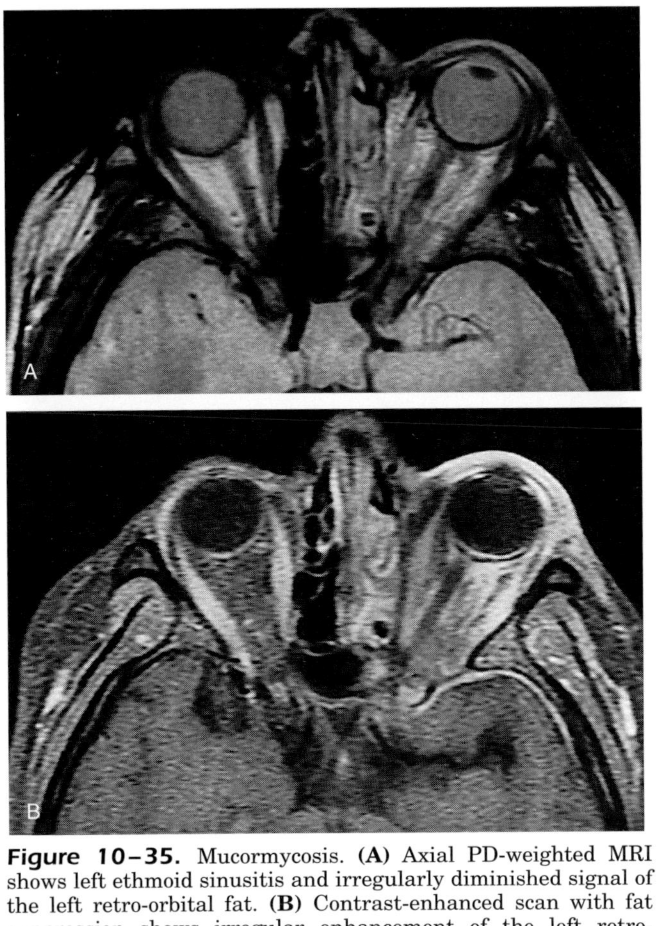

Figure 10–35. Mucormycosis. **(A)** Axial PD-weighted MRI shows left ethmoid sinusitis and irregularly diminished signal of the left retro-orbital fat. **(B)** Contrast-enhanced scan with fat suppression shows irregular enhancement of the left retro-orbital fat, highlighting the left optic nerve, which does not enhance.

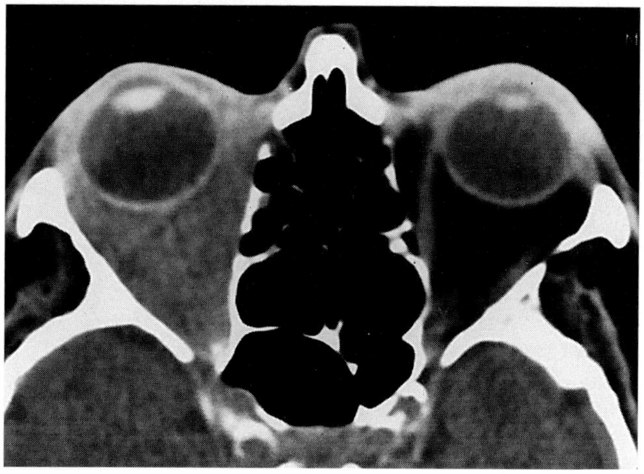

Figure 10–36. Wegener's granulomatosis. CT shows a soft tissue mass diffusely involving the right orbit.

Vascular Tumors

Cavernous hemangiomas are the most common orbital tumors in adults. They are benign slow-growing tumors, usually intraconal, and most common in middle-aged women. Proptosis is the usual presenting sign.

Capillary hemangiomas present in young infants, grow rapidly during the first year of life, and usually regress spontaneously by age 6. They may be primary to the orbit or primarily cutaneous with secondary orbital extension.

Lymphangiomas are hamartomatous collections of blood vessels, lymphatic channels, and smooth muscle that present with proptosis in children and young adults. They form irregular multicystic septate masses with a strong propensity to spontaneous and recurrent hemorrhage.

CT Findings. A hemangioma appears as a well-demarcated, rounded, and usually intraconal mass, typically hyperdense and with diffuse intense contrast enhancement. It occurs most commonly in the superior and lateral quadrants of the cone. Calcifications (phleboliths) are infrequent but when present are nearly specific.

Lymphangiomas form poorly defined inhomogeneous masses with irregular borders and a tendency to cross anatomic boundaries. Variable heterogeneous enhancement occurs after intravenous contrast. Cystlike areas may be present due to resolving hemorrhage.

MRI Findings. Hemangiomas are isointense to muscle on T1-weighted images and markedly hyperintense on T2-weighted images. Spontaneous thrombosis may occur, resulting in a more heterogeneous appearance. Marked enhancement occurs with intravenous contrast. Lymphangiomas may be suspected by the recognition of resolving hemorrhage.

Differential Diagnosis

See Tables 10–10 and 10–11 and Diagrams 10–4 and 10–5.

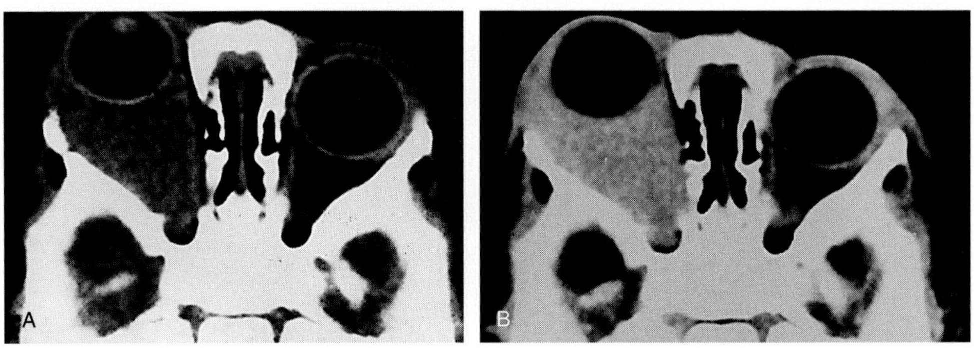

Figure 10–37. Capillary hemangioma. CT **(A)** before and **(B)** after contrast show a diffuse mass of the right orbit with intense homogeneous enhancement.

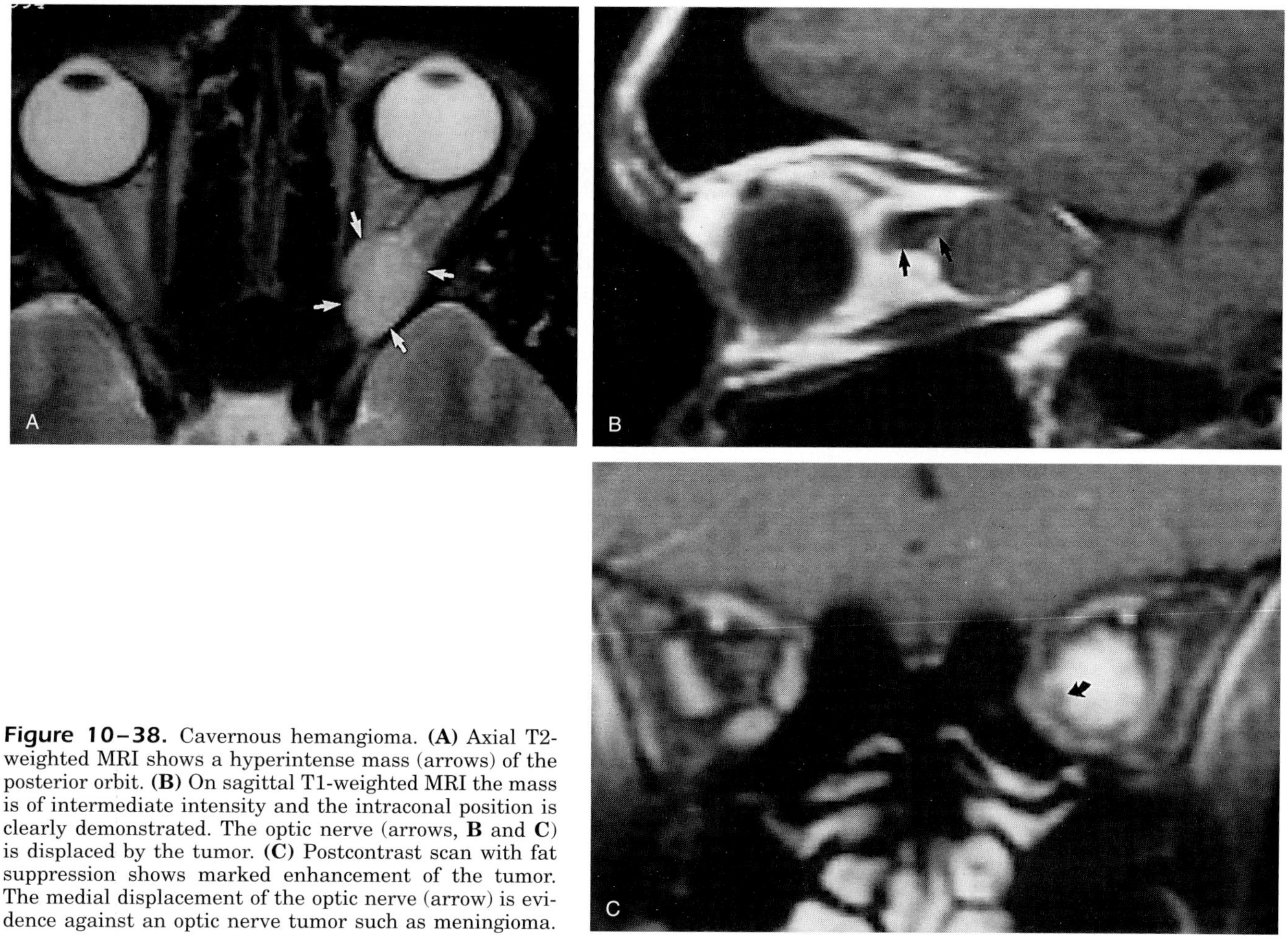

Figure 10–38. Cavernous hemangioma. **(A)** Axial T2-weighted MRI shows a hyperintense mass (arrows) of the posterior orbit. **(B)** On sagittal T1-weighted MRI the mass is of intermediate intensity and the intraconal position is clearly demonstrated. The optic nerve (arrows, **B** and **C**) is displaced by the tumor. **(C)** Postcontrast scan with fat suppression shows marked enhancement of the tumor. The medial displacement of the optic nerve (arrow) is evidence against an optic nerve tumor such as meningioma.

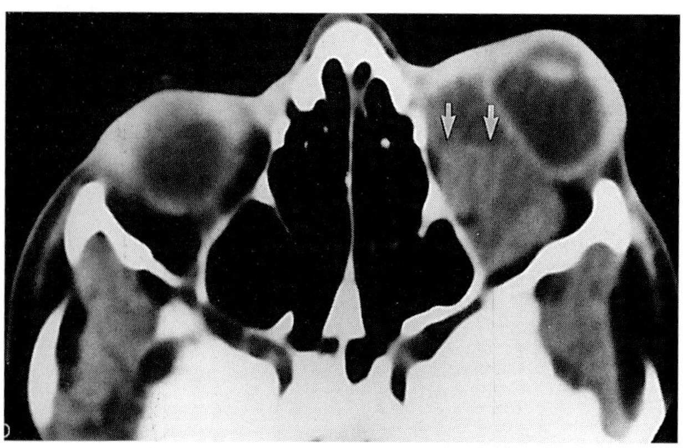

Figure 10–39. Lymphangioma. CT shows a mass of the medial left orbit causing severe proptosis. The fluid-fluid level (arrows) due to hemorrhage is characteristic of lymphangioma. (Courtesy of Dr. Taher El Gammal, Birmingham, AL.)

Lymphoma

Primary lymphoma of the orbit is usually composed of a monoclonal proliferation of B cells. It is a condition of older adult patients who present with a slowly progressive proptosis. A related entity is benign lymphoid hyperplasia, or pseudolymphoma, which is distinguished by its polyclonal population of B cells. Lymphoma is treated by radiation, with a very good prognosis if the initial tumor is limited to the orbit.

CT Findings. CT shows a sharply defined homogeneous mass of high attenuation with mild enhancement. Its margins become more irregular at interfaces with orbital fat. Although usually arising in the anterior orbit, lymphoma may also occur in the retroocular or superior compartments. Lymphomas exhibit a strong tendency to mold to adjacent structures without causing bone erosion.

MRI Findings. The morphologic features of orbital lymphoma are as described for CT. The tumor tends to be hypointense on T1-weighted images and either isointense or hyperintense on T2-weighted images.

Differential Diagnosis

See Table 10–12 and Diagram 10–6. The differential diagnosis depends on the location of the mass. Because it often involves the anterior orbit, the differential diagnosis for lacrimal gland lesions (Table 10–13) often applies. Pseudotumor, orbital cellulitis, and metastases are other common conditions that may exhibit similar imaging findings.

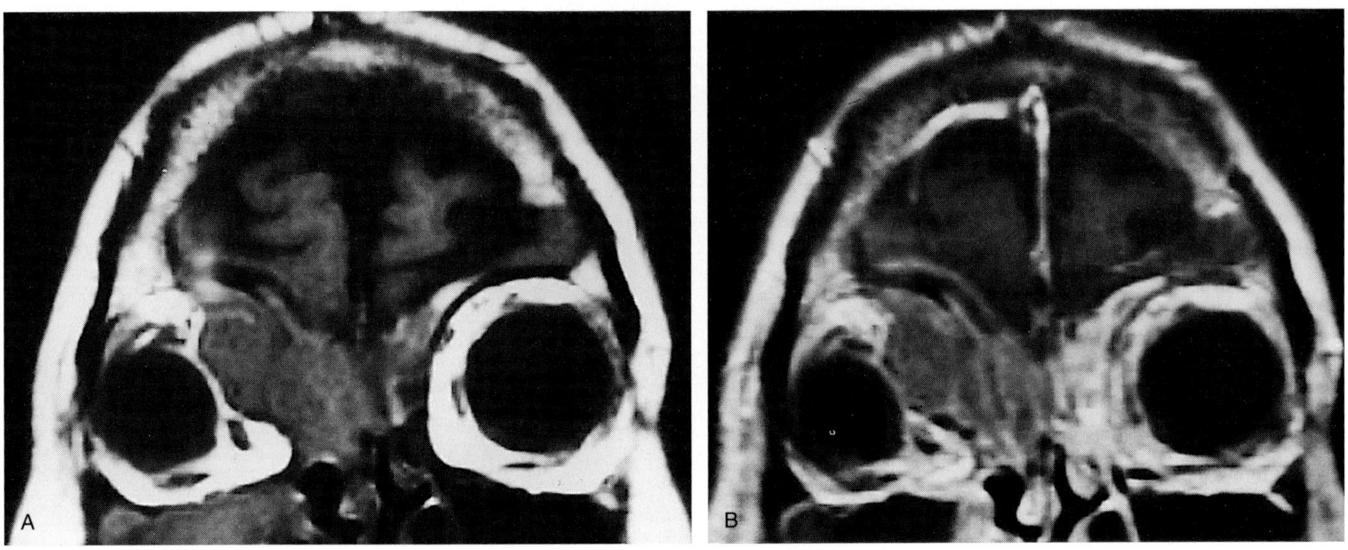

Figure 10–40. Orbital lymphoma. Coronal T1-weighted MRI shows a mass with **(A)** intermediate signal intensity involving the right medial orbit and adjoining ethmoid sinus and **(B)** mild contrast enhancement.

Rhabdomyosarcoma

Rhabdomyosarcoma is the most common primary malignant tumor of the orbit (excluding the globe) in children. It is one tenth as common as retinoblastoma. About 90% occur before age 16. Rhabdomyosarcoma arises from mesenchymal precursors of striated muscle, and patients present with rapidly progressive proptosis. The mortality rate has historically been high. Combined radiation and chemotherapy now promises a 5-year survival of up to 90%.

CT Findings. CT shows a soft tissue mass commonly associated with bone destruction and extraorbital extension.

MRI Findings. MRI shows a solid homogeneous mass that is hypointense on T1-weighted images and hyperintense on T2-weighted images. Diffuse enhancement occurs with intravenous contrast.

Differential Diagnosis

In this young age group, the main differential consideration is capillary hemangioma, which appears much more vascular on imaging studies.

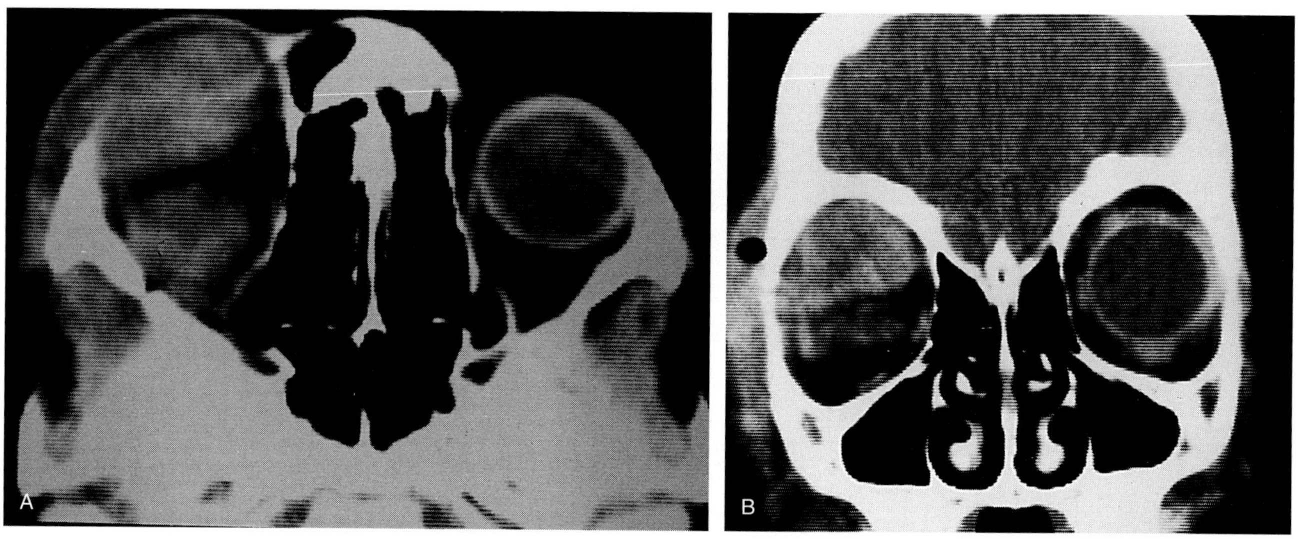

Figure 10–41. Rhabdomyosarcoma. **(A)** Axial and **(B)** coronal CT show a bulky mass of the superior right orbit. (See also Fig. 8–50.)

Lacrimal Tumors

The lacrimal gland gives rise to an assortment of inflammatory, benign, and malignant mass lesions that may be difficult or impossible to differentiate by imaging criteria alone. Inflammatory pseudotumors and benign mixed tumors are the most common lacrimal masses. The most common malignant tumor is adenoid cystic carcinoma.

CT Findings. CT shows a mass in the superolateral portion of the orbit (lacrimal fossa) with contrast enhancement in 50%. The mass usually envelops the lateral rectus muscle. The presence of fat is nearly specific for dermoid. Otherwise, no CT features reliably distinguish the various entities found in this region. Bilateral lacrimal masses are usually due to sarcoidosis or lymphoma. Tumors may be differentiated from inflammation by the presence of bone changes (remodeling, sclerosis, or destruction) and more discrete mass effect, usually sparing the palpebral lobe. Inflammation tends to cause diffuse enlargement of a gland.

MRI Findings. Signal intensities of lacrimal masses vary considerably. Experience thus far indicates that MRI is no more specific than CT in suggesting the pathologic diagnosis.

Differential Diagnosis

See Table 10–13 and Diagram 10–7.

TABLE 10–13 | **Lacrimal Masses**

Cause	Distinguishing Features
Pseudotumor	Common Multifocal Painful orbit
Lacrimal adenitis	Diffuse swelling of gland with marked enhancement
Dermoid	Fat within the mass is specific but not always present
Lymphoma	Diffusely involves gland and may be bilateral Tends to be bulkier than adenitis
Sarcoidosis	Bilateral lacrimal involvement Systemic manifestations
Adenoma	Pleomorphic adenoma or benign mixed tumor About 50% of epithelial lacrimal tumors Bone remodeling usually present Palpebral lobe usually not involved
Adenoid cystic carcinoma	About 30% of epithelial lacrimal tumors Bone remodeling or destruction present Margins tend to be more irregular than with benign tumors

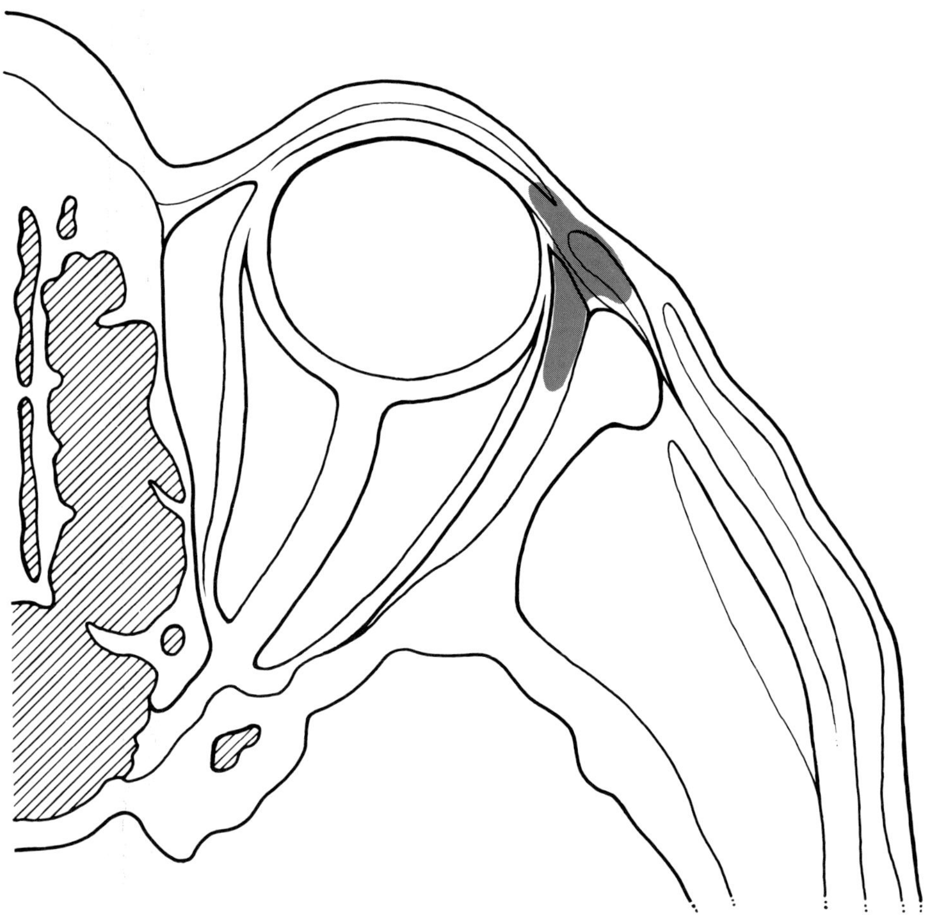

Diagram 10–7. Lacrimal mass. The lacrimal gland lies anteriorly in the superolateral quadrant of the extraconal space. It has two lobes, the palpebral that lies anterior to the globe and the deep that is lateral to the globe.

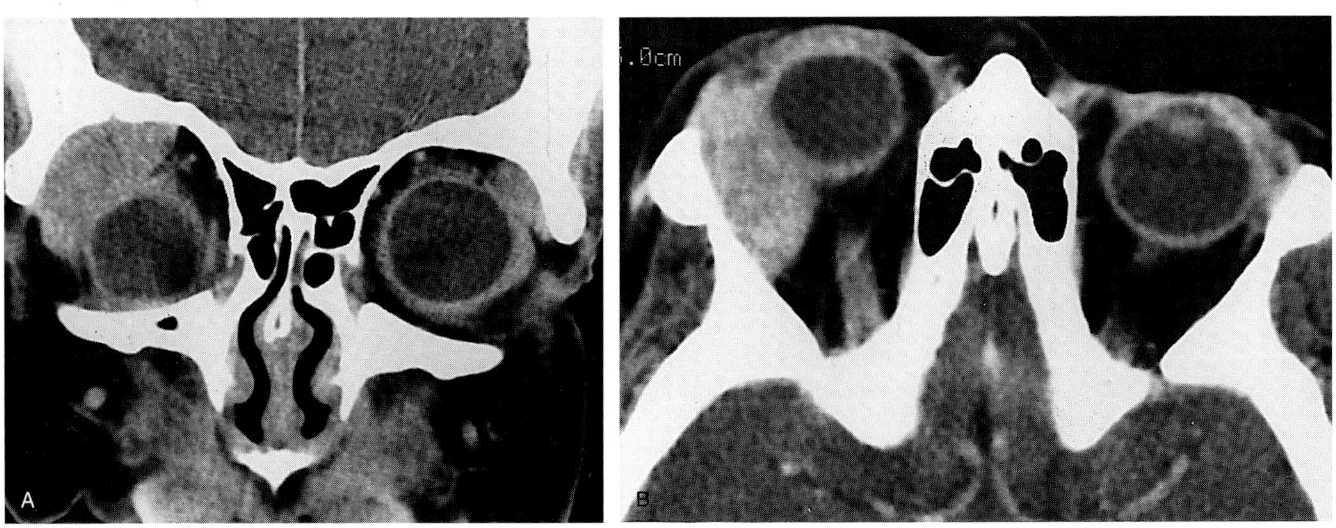

Figure 10–42. Lacrimal inflammation (pseudotumor). **(A)** Coronal and **(B)** axial CT show a homogeneous enhancing mass of the right lacrimal gland. Although inflammatory in origin, there was relative sparing of the palpebral lobe.

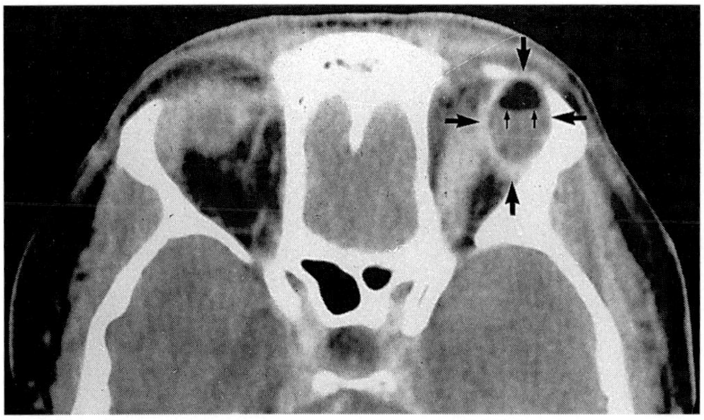

Figure 10–43. Dermoid. Axial CT shows a mass (large arrows) of the left lacrimal gland with a fat-fluid level (small arrows). The presence of fat is specific for dermoid.

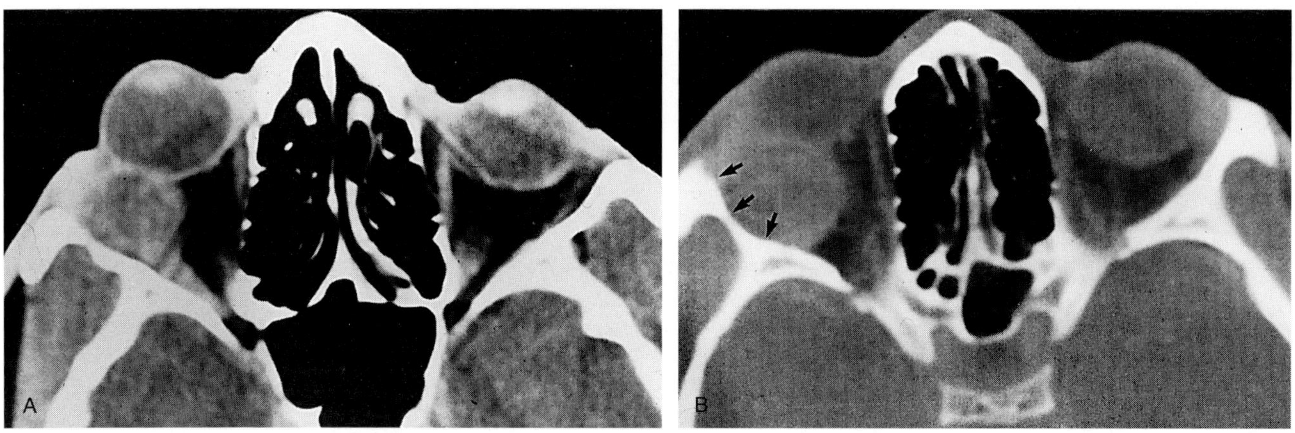

Figure 10–44. Carcinoma. **(A)** Axial CT shows a nonspecific mass of the right lacrimal gland. **(B)** Bone window shows remodeling of the lateral orbital wall (arrows), which favors a neoplasm over inflammation.

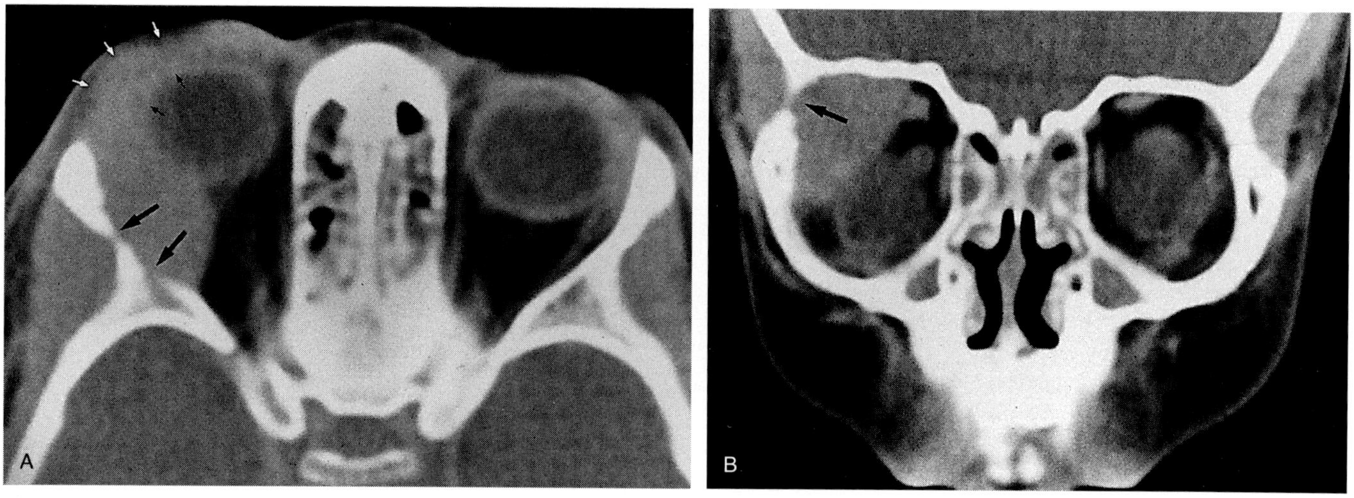

Figure 10–45. Lymphoma. **(A)** Axial contrast-enhanced CT shows a homogeneous mass of the right lacrimal gland also involving the palpebral lobe (small arrows). Both axial and **(B)** coronal scans show erosion of the lateral orbital wall (large arrows).

SUGGESTED READINGS

General

Atlas,SW. Magnetic Resonance Imaging of the Orbit: Current Status. *Magn Reson Q* 5:39-96, 1989.

Hopper,KD, Sherman,JL, Boal,DK, Eggli,KD. CT and MR Imaging of the Pediatric Orbit. *Radiographics* 12:485–503, 1992.

Wells,RG, Sty,JR, Gonnering,RS. Imaging of the Pediatric Eye and Orbit. *Radiographics* 9:1023–1044, 1989.

Coloboma

Bilaniuk,LT, Farber,M. Imaging of Developmental Anomalies of the Eye and the Orbit. *AJNR* 13:793–803, 1992.

Gardner,TW, Zaparackas,ZG, Naidich,TP. Congenital Optic Nerve Colobomas: CT Demonstration. *J Comput Assist Tomogr* 8:95–102, 1984.

Mafee,MF, Jampol,LM, Langer,BG, Tso,M. Computed Tomography of Optic Nerve Colobomas, Morning Glory Anomaly, and Colobomatous Cyst. *Radiol Clin North Am* 25:693–699, 1987.

Drusen

Ramirez,H, Blatt,ES, Hibri,NS. Computed Tomographic Identification of Calcified Optic Nerve Drusen. *Radiology* 148: 137–139, 1983.

Phthisis Bulbi

Osborne,DR, Foulks,GN. Computed Tomographic Analysis of Deformity and Dimensional Changes in the Eyeball. *Radiology* 153:669–674, 1984.

Retinal Detachment

Mafee,MF, Linder,B, Peyman,GA, et al. Choroidal Hematoma and Effusion: Evaluation with MR Imaging. *Radiology* 168:781–786, 1988.

Mafee,MF, Peyman,GA. Retinal and Choroidal Detachments: Role of Magnetic Resonance Imaging and Computed Tomography. *Radiol Clin North Am* 25:487–507, 1987.

Retinoblastoma

Mafee,MF, Goldberg,MF, Greenwald, MJ, Schulman,J, Malmed,A, Flanders,AE. Retinoblastoma and Simulating Lesions: Role of CT and MR Imaging. *Radiol Clin North Am* 25:667–682, 1987.

Provenzale,JM, Weber,AL, Klintworth,GK, McLendon,RE. Bilateral Retinoblastoma with Coexistent Pinealoblatoma (Trilateral Retinoblastoma). *AJNR* 16:157–165, 1995.

Smirniotopoulos,JG, Bargallo,N, Mafee,MF, et al. Differential Diagnosis of Leukokoria: Radiologic-Pathologic Correlation. *RadioGraphics* 14:1059–1079, 1994.

Melanoma

Lorigan,JG, Wallace,S, Mavligit,GM. The Prevalence and Location of Metastases from Ocular Melanoma: Imaging Study in 110 Patients. *AJR* 157:1279–1281, 1991.

Mafee,MF, Peyman,GA, McKusick,MA. Malignant Uveal Melanoma and Similar Lesions Studied by Computed Tomography. *Radiology* 156:403–408, 1985.

Mihara,F, Gupta,KL, Murayama,S, Lee,N, Bond,JB, Haik,BG. MR Imaging of Malignant Uveal Melanoma: Role of Pulse Sequence and Contrast Agent. *AJNR* 12:991–996, 1991. *AJR* 157:1087–1092, 1991.

Peyman,GA, Mafee, MF. Uveal Melanoma and Similar Lesions: The Role of Magnetic Resonance Imaging and Computed Tomography. *Radiol Clin North Am* 25:471–486, 1987.

Tong,KA, Osborn,AG, Mamalis,N, Harrie,RP, Call,NB. Radiologic-Pathologic Correlation: Ocular Melanoma. *AJNR* 14: 1359–1366, 1993.

Metastasis

Atlas, SW, Grossman,RI, Savino,PJ, et al. Surface-Coil MR of Orbital Pseudotumor. *AJNR* 8:141–146, 1987.

Peyster,RG, Shapiro,MD, Haik,BG. Orbital Metastasis: Role of Magnetic Resonance Imaging and Computed Tomography. *Radiol Clin North Am* 25:647–662, 1987.

Optic Neuritis

Hudgins,PA, Newman,NJ, Dillon,WP, Hoffman,JC. Radiation-Induced Optic Neuropathy: Characteristic Appearances on Gadolinium-enhanced MR. *AJNR* 13:235–238, 1992.

Merandi,SF, Kudryk,BT, Murtagh,FR, Arrington,JA. Contrast-Enhanced MR Imaging of Optic Nerve Lesions in Patients with Acute Optic Neuritis. *AJNR* 12:923–926, 1991.

Optic Nerve Glioma

Azar-Kia,B, Naheedy,MH, Elias,DA, Mafee,MF, Fine,M. Optic Nerve Tumors: Role of Magnetic Resonance Imaging and Computed Tomography. *Radiol Clin North Am* 25:561–581, 1987.

Optic Nerve Meningioma

Hendrix,LE, Kneeland,JB, Haughton,VM, et al. MR Imaging of Optic Nerve Lesions: Value of Gadopentate Dimeglumine and Fat-Suppression Technique. *AJR* 155:849–854, 1990.

Peyster,RG, Hoover,ED, Hershey,BL, Haskin,ME. High Resolution CT of Lesions of the Optic Nerve. *AJR* 140:869–874, 1983.

Thyroid Ophthalmopathy

Barrett,L, Glatt,HJ, Burde,RM, Gado,MH. Optic Nerve Dysfunction in Thyroid Eye Disease: CT. *Radiology* 167:503–507, 1988.

Hosten,N, Sander,B, Cordes,M, Schubert,CJ, Schorner,W, Felix,R. Graves Ophthalmopathy: MR Imaging of the Orbits. *Radiology* 172:759–762, 1989.

Nugent,RA, Belkin,RI, Neigel,JM, et al. Graves' Orbitopathy: Correlation of CT and Clinical Findings. *Radiology* 177:675–682, 1990.

Ohnishi,T, Noguchi,S, Murakami,N, et al. Extraocular Muscles in Graves Ophthalmopathy: Usefulness of T2 Relaxation Time Measurements. *Radiology* 190:857–862, 1994.

Orbital Varix

Shnier,R, Parker,GD, Hillinan,JM, Pollei,SR, Smoker,WRK. Orbital Varices: A New Technique for Noninvasive Diagnosis. *AJNR* 12:717–718, 1991.

Wildenhain,PM, Lehar,SC, Dastur,KJ, Dodd,GD. Orbital Varix: Color Flow Imaging Correlated with CT and MR Studies. *J Comput Assist Tomogr* 15:171–173, 1991.

Pseudotumor

Atlas,SW, Grossman,RI, Savino,PJ, et al. Surface-Coil MR of Orbital Pseudotumor. *AJNR* 8:141–146, 1987.

Curtin,HD. Pseudotumor. *Radiol Clin North Am* 25:583–599, 1987.

Harr,DL, Quencer,RM, Abrams,GW. Computed Tomography and Ultrasound in the Evaluation of Orbital Infection and Pseudotumor. *Radiology* 142:395–401, 1982.

Cellulitis

Atlas,SW, Bilaniuk,LT, Zimmerman,RA, Hackney,DB, Goldberg,HI, Grosman,RI. Orbit: Initial Experience with Surface Coil Spin Echo MR Imaging at 1.5T. *Radiology* 164: 501–509, 1987.

Weber,AL, Mikulis,DK. Inflammatory Disorders of the Paraorbital Sinuses and Their Complications. *Radiol Clin North Am* 25:615–630, 1987.

Zimmerman,RA, Bilaniuk,LT. CT of Orbital Infection and Its Cerebral Complications. *AJR* 134:45–50, 1980.

Vascular Tumors

Atlas,SW, Grossman,RI, Hackney,DB, Goldberg,HI, Bilaniuk, LT, Zimmerman,RA. STIR MR Imaging of the Orbit. *AJR* 151:1025–1030, 1988. *AJNR* 9:969–974, 1988.

Graeb,DA, Rootman,J, Robertson,WD, Lapointe,JS, Nugent,RA, Hay,EJ. Orbital Lymphangiomas: Clinical, Radiologic, and Pathologic Characteristics. *Radiology* 175:417–421, 1990.

Savoiardo,M, Strada,L, Passerini,A. Cavernous Hemangiomas of the Orbit: Value of CT, Angiography, and Phlebography. *AJNR* 4:741–744, 1983.

Willing,SJ, Faye-Peterson,O, Aronin,P, Faith,S. Radiologic-Pathologic Correlation: Capillary Hemangioma of the Meninges. *AJNR* 14:529–536, 1993.

Lymphoma

Erickson,BA, Harris,GJ, Enke,CA, et al. Periocular Lymphoproliferative Diseases: Natural History, Prognostic Factors, and Treatment. *Radiology* 185:63–70, 1992.

Flanders, AE, Espinosa,GA, Markiewicz,DA, Howell,DD. Orbital Lymphoma: Role of CT and MRI. *Radiol Clin North Am* 25:601–613, 1987.

Rhabdomyosarcoma

Hopper,KD, Sherman,JL, Boal,DK, Eggli,KD. CT and MR Imaging of the Pediatric Orbit. *Radiographics* 12:485–503, 1992.

Sagerman,RH. Orbital Rhabdomyosarcoma: A Paradigm for Irradiation. *Radiology* 187:605–607, 1993.

Vade,A, Armstrong,D. Orbital Rhabdomyosarcoma in Childhood. *Radiol Clin North Am* 25:701–714, 1987.

Lacrimal Tumors

Forbes,GS, Sheedy,PF, Waller,RR. Orbital Tumors Evaluated by Computed Tomography. *Radiology* 136:101–111, 1980.

Mafee,MF, Haik,BG. Lacrimal Gland and Fossa Lesions: Role of Computed Tomography. *Radiol Clin North Am* 25:767–779, 1987.

Nugent,RA, Lapointe,JS, Rootman,J, Robertson,WD, Graeb,DA. Orbital Dermoids: Features on CT. *Radiology* 165:475–478, 1987.

CHAPTER
ELEVEN

Congenital Diseases of the Spine

The term spinal dysraphism applies to a spectrum of disorders resulting from the faulty or incomplete fusion of midline spinal structures—mesenchymal, bony, and osseous (see Tables 11–1 and 11–2). If there is exposed neural tissue or a meningeal sac, the malformation is further classified as spina bifida aperta. The occult spinal dysraphisms are covered by skin with no exposed neural tissue or obvious cystic mass. Most isolated spinal malformations of clinical significance represent some form of dysraphism.

Another category of congenital malformations of the spine results from systemic genetic disorders. This includes the dwarfisms (represented by achondroplasia), the mucopolysaccharidoses, and neurofibromatosis. The cranial findings of neurofibromatosis were presented in Chapter 2. The spinal changes will be presented here.

The format herein is the same as in Chapter 2. When dealing with congenital malformations, one is primarily concerned with the identification of anatomic alterations that are not modality specific. For each condition, the essential findings that permit the diagnosis are given, followed by ancillary findings that are more variably present.

TABLE 11–2 | **Key Abnormalities Associated with the Major Congenital Spinal Disorders**

	Dorsal Sac	Cutaneous Defect	Myelodysplasia	Dorsal Bony Defect	Sacral Agencies	Split Cord	Lipoma	Tethered Cord	Syrinx	Tonsillar Herniation
Meningocele	+	+	•	•			•			
Meningomyelocele	+	+	+	+		•	•	•	•	+
Myelocele		+	+	+			•	•	•	
Lipomeningomyelocele		•	+	+			+	•		
Caudal regression	•		•	+	+	•	•			
Diastematomyelia						+	•	+	•	
Lipoma				•			+	•		
Tethered cord				•			•	+		
Syringohydromyelia									+	•

\+ = Always or nearly always present.
• = Sometimes present.

Spina Bifida Aperta

Meningocele

The meningocele is a posterior midline protrusion of the dura and arachnoid forming a CSF-filled sac. The incidence is approximately 1 in 10,000 births. Most occur in the lumbosacral area, and they are commonly but not invariably associated with the Chiari II malformation. Meningoceles are generally diagnosed clinically and corrected at birth. Diagnostic imaging is not routinely required.

TABLE 11–1 | **Classification of Spinal Dysraphism**

Spina bifida cystica (spina bifida aperta)
- Meningocele
- Meningomyelocele
- Lipomeningomyelocele

Occult spinal dysraphism
- Diastematomyelia
- Hydromyelia and syringomyelia
- Spinal lipoma
- Lipomeningomyelocele
- Tethered cord
- Caudal regression syndrome
- Dorsal dermal sinus
- Neurenteric cyst
- Split notochord and dorsal enteric fistula

Primary Abnormalities

- Spinal bony defect (usually but not always posterior)
- Dorsal sac filled with CSF and communicating with spinal subarachnoid space through bony defect
- May contain nerve roots but no cord elements in dorsal sac

Ancillary Findings

- The posterior bony defect is usually limited in severity and extent
- The following abnormalities have been described in association with meningocele:
  —Lipomas
  —Glial and smooth muscle heterotopias
  —Myelodysplasia (defective development of the spinal cord)

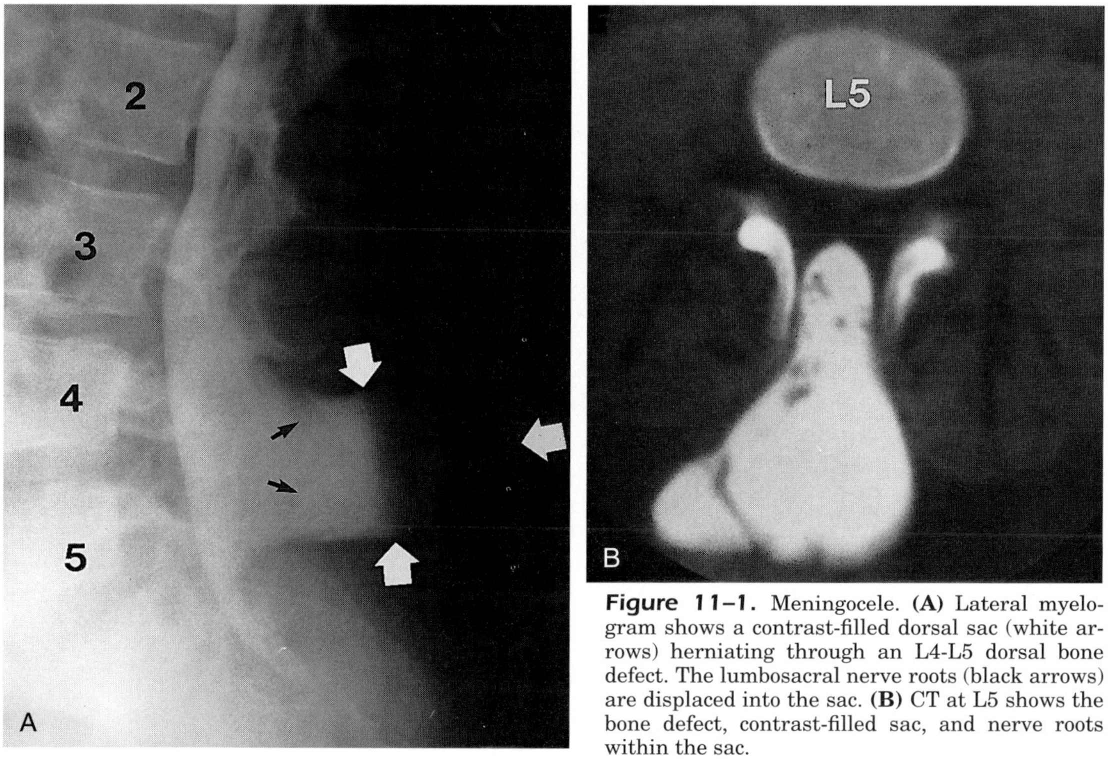

Figure 11–1. Meningocele. **(A)** Lateral myelogram shows a contrast-filled dorsal sac (white arrows) herniating through an L4-L5 dorsal bone defect. The lumbosacral nerve roots (black arrows) are displaced into the sac. **(B)** CT at L5 shows the bone defect, contrast-filled sac, and nerve roots within the sac.

Myelocele and Meningomyelocele

The myelocele is a more complex anomaly in which there is externalization of a deformed distal spinal cord due to failure of midline closure. The meningomyelocele is a myelocele associated with a ventral enlargement of the subarachnoid space producing a sac. In both, the terminal cord is split dorsally and its dorsal halves laterally rotated, forming the so-called neural placode. As a result, both ventral and dorsal roots originate from the anterior cord surface. The dorsal groove is continuous with the central canal of the spinal cord. A Chiari II malformation is almost invariably present.

Imaging is seldom required of unoperated meningoceles and myelomeningoceles, as operative repair is usually attempted immediately after birth. Postoperatively, imaging plays a necessary role in the detection of other anomalies, such as syringohydromyelia, and complications, such as late onset tethering.

Primary Abnormalities

- Defect in dorsal elements of spine, usually more severe than with simple meningocele
- Overexpansion of ventral subarachnoid space with posterior displacement of dysplastic terminal spinal cord
- Cutaneous defect overlying malformation with externalization of neural tissue

Ancillary Findings

- Dysplasia of involved spinal cord, which is split open posteriorly and becomes flattened rather than tubular (neural placode)
- Nerve roots arise from ventral surface of neural placode
- Tethered cord
- Abnormally horizontal course of nerve roots
- Chiari II malformation almost invariably present
- Other bony anomalies: kyphosis, scoliosis, hemivertebrae
- Enlarged spinal canal at level of malformation

Associated Conditions

- Lipoma
- Thickened filum terminale
- Diastematomyelia in 30–45%
- Syringohydromyelia in 30–75%

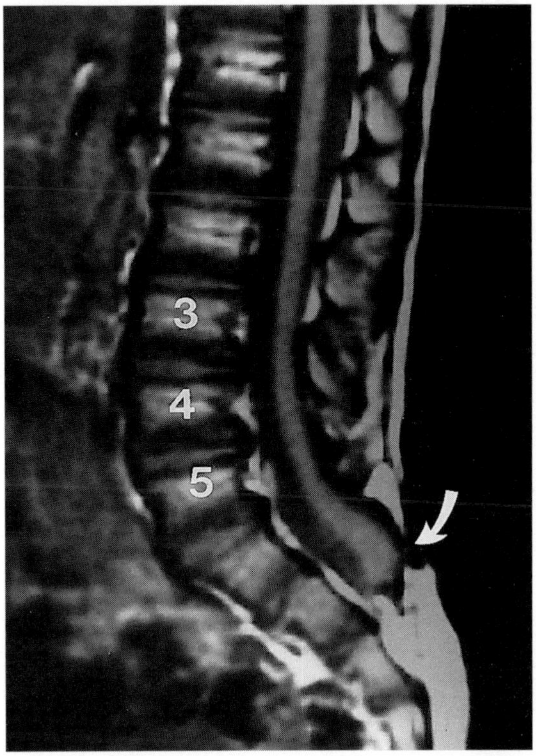

Figure 11–2. Repaired meningomyelocele. Sagittal MRI shows a tethered cord with dysplastic terminal segment, the neural placode. The placode is adherent to the dorsal soft tissues at the site of repair (arrow).

Occult Spinal Dysraphism

Lipomyelomeningocele and Lipomyelocele

The lipomyelomeningocele is characterized by a fibrofatty mass adherent to the dorsal surface of a dysplastic terminal cord. The lipoma herniates through a posterior spinal defect and is continuous posteriorly with subcutaneous fat. As with the meningomyelocele, the distal cord is split dorsally, forming a neural placode, and the spinal roots exit from the ventral surface of the placode. This dysraphism may be open or occult, depending on whether there is a sac (lipomeningomyelocele) or not (lipomyelocele).

Primary Abnormalities

- Wide dorsal defect in vertebrae and dura
- Dysplasia of the affected cord producing the so-called neural placode (see meningomyelocele)
- Fat extending from subcutaneous tissue through bony defect to dorsal surface of neural placode
- Intact overlying skin
- Expansion of ventral subarachnoid space with dorsal displacement of neural elements

Ancillary Findings

- Enlarged spinal canal at level of malformation
- Malformation usually lumbosacral in location
- Tethered cord
- Indentation of posterior cord surface by the lipoma
- Nerve roots arise from ventral surface of neural placode
- Lipoma may lie off midline with lateral rotation of neural placode and nerve roots

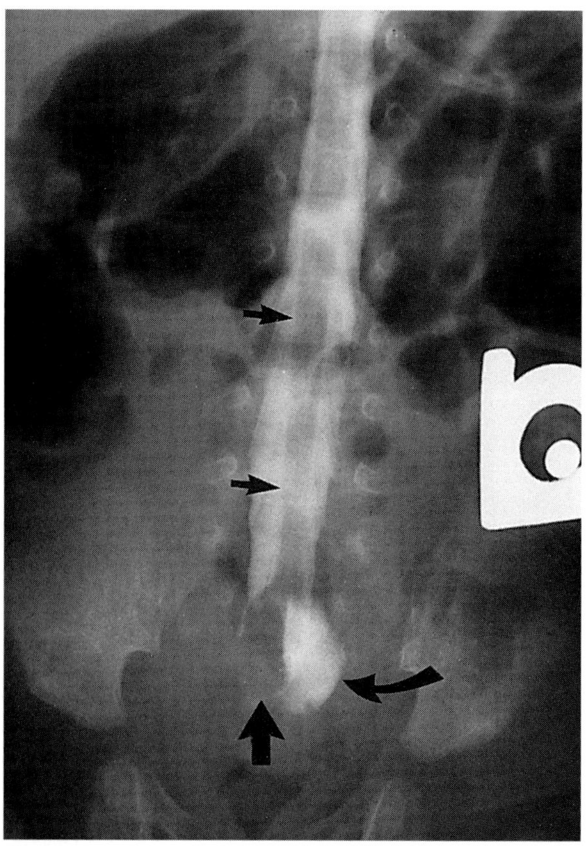

Figure 11–3. Lipomeningomyelocele. AP myelogram shows a tethered cord (thin arrows), small dorsal sac (curved arrow), and filling defect due to the lipoma (thick arrow).

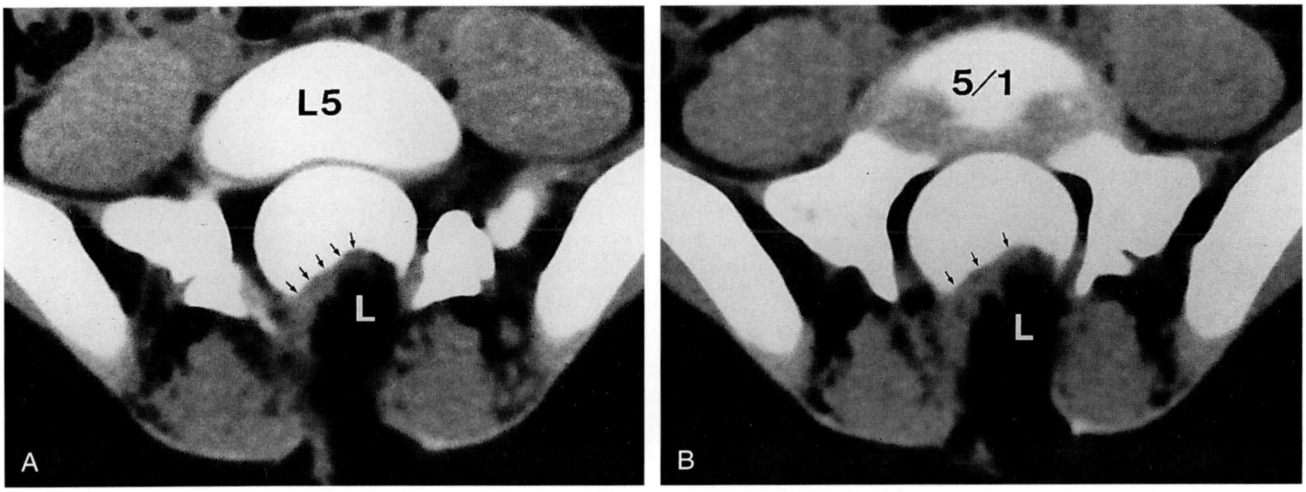

Figure 11–4. Lipomeningomyelocele. **(A,B)** Axial CT myelogram shows a wide dorsal bony defect, expansion of the ventral subarachnoid space, lipoma (L), and neural placode (arrows).

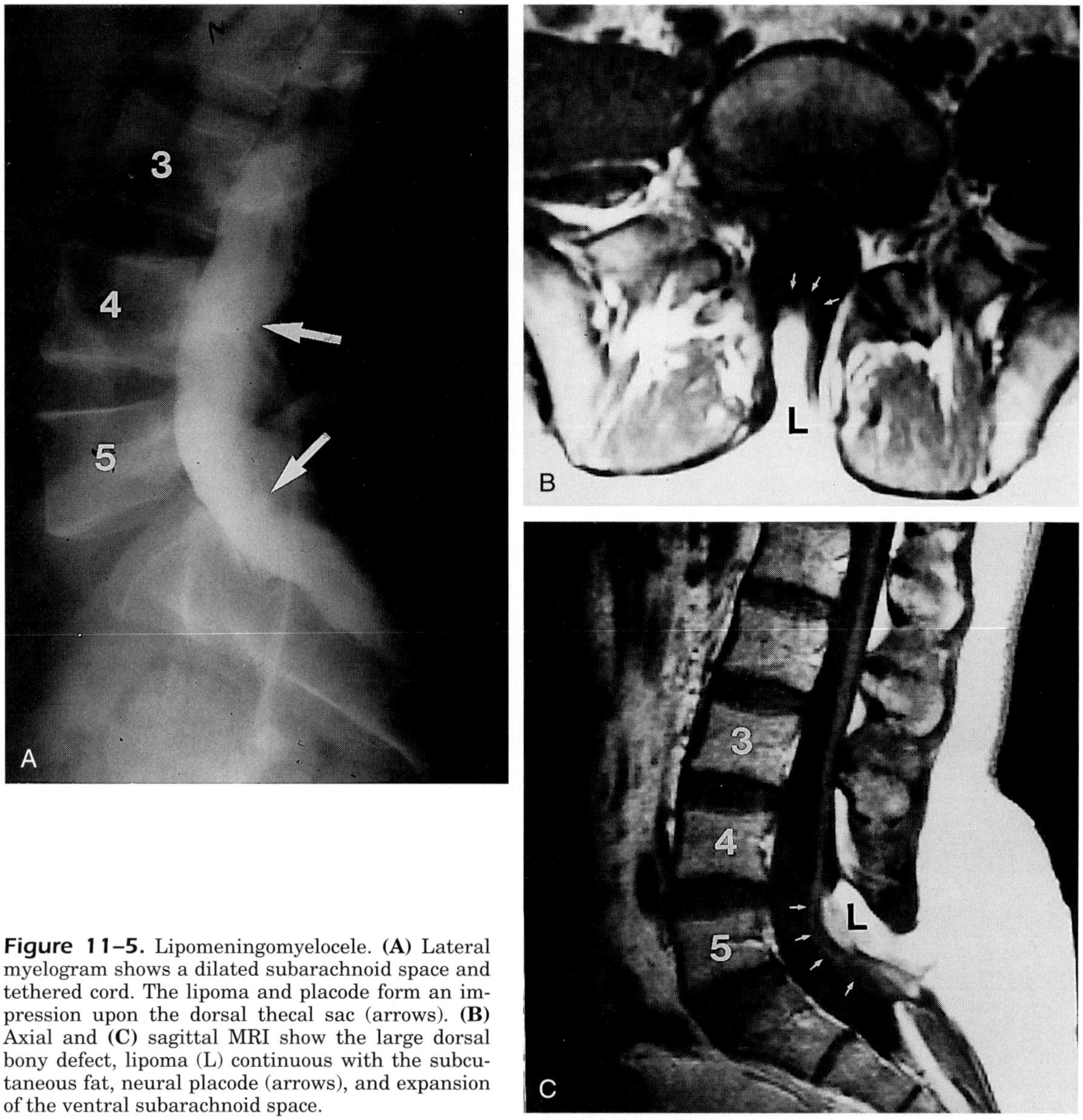

Figure 11–5. Lipomeningomyelocele. **(A)** Lateral myelogram shows a dilated subarachnoid space and tethered cord. The lipoma and placode form an impression upon the dorsal thecal sac (arrows). **(B)** Axial and **(C)** sagittal MRI show the large dorsal bony defect, lipoma (L) continuous with the subcutaneous fat, neural placode (arrows), and expansion of the ventral subarachnoid space.

Diastematomyelia

Diastematomyelia is a condition in which the spinal cord is split sagittally into two hemicords for a variable distance, with each hemicord possessing its own ventral and dorsal root. It is presumed to originate from a splitting of the notochord or its cellular precursors during fetal development. There are two types of diastematomyelia. About 50% of patients have a split cord with a normal undivided arachnoid-dural sleeve and no septum (type 1). The other 50% manifest a split cord with two separate dural sleeves and a fibrous, cartilaginous, or bony septum (type 2).

Primary Abnormality

- Sagittal, longitudinal splitting of the spinal cord into right and left halves

Ancillary Findings

- Usually occurs between T9 and S1
- Often asymmetrical, with unequally sized cord segments
- Spinal anomalies may result in anteroposterior orientation (rather than side by side) of the divided cord and dural sleeve
- Septum (if present) usually between L1 and L4
- Fibrous bands between cord and dura (meningocele manqué) that may tether the cord, which may be very subtle or indistinguishable on imaging studies
- Vertebral anomalies: fusion defects, butterfly vertebrae, hemivertebrae, vertebral fusions, diminished disc height, scoliosis, kyphosis

Associated Conditions

- Tethered cord in over 75% and thickened filum terminale
- Meningomyelocele
- Dermal sinus
- Lipoma
- Myelodysplasia
- Syringohydromyelia in approximately 50%

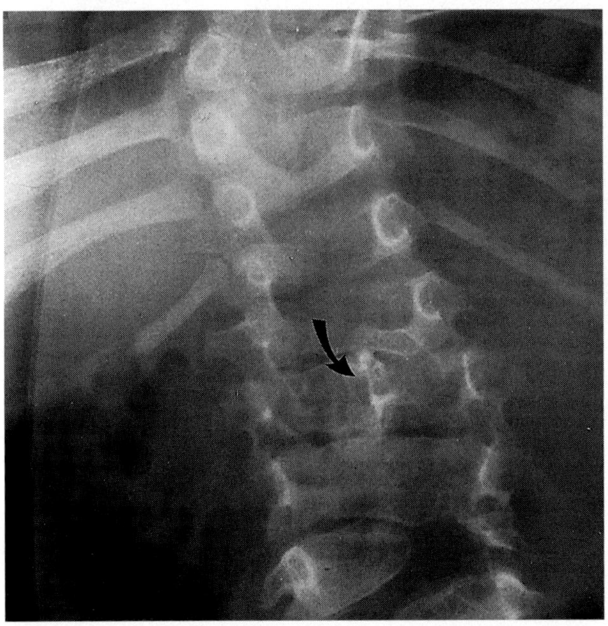

Figure 11–6. Diastematomyelia (type 2). AP radiograph shows a midline bony spur (arrow) at L2 indicating type 2 diastematomyelia. Patient exhibits scoliosis and fusion defects of other vertebrae.

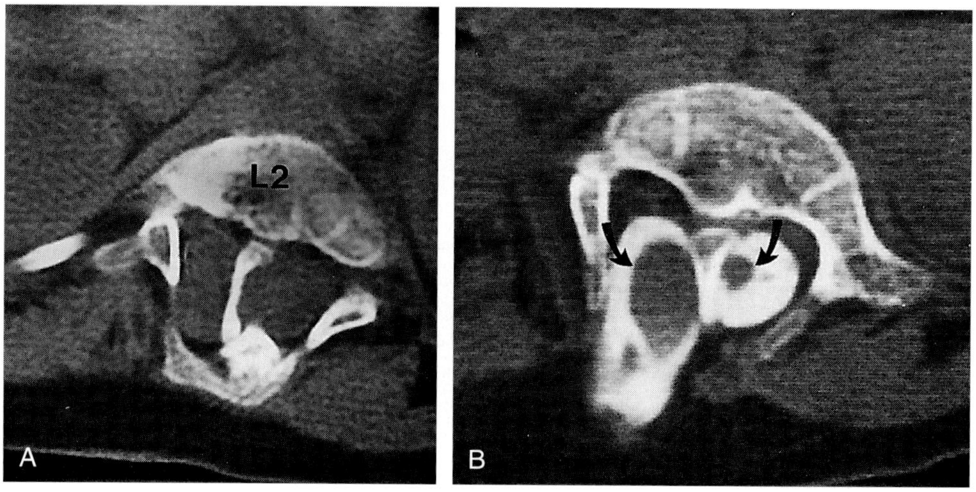

Figure 11–7. Diastematomyelia (type 2). **(A)** CT at L2 shows a thick midline bony spur dividing the spinal canal and dysplasia of the posterior bony elements. **(B)** CT myelogram shows each hemicord (arrows) in its separate sleeve and surrounded by contrast. The right hemicord is expanded by syringohydromyelia.

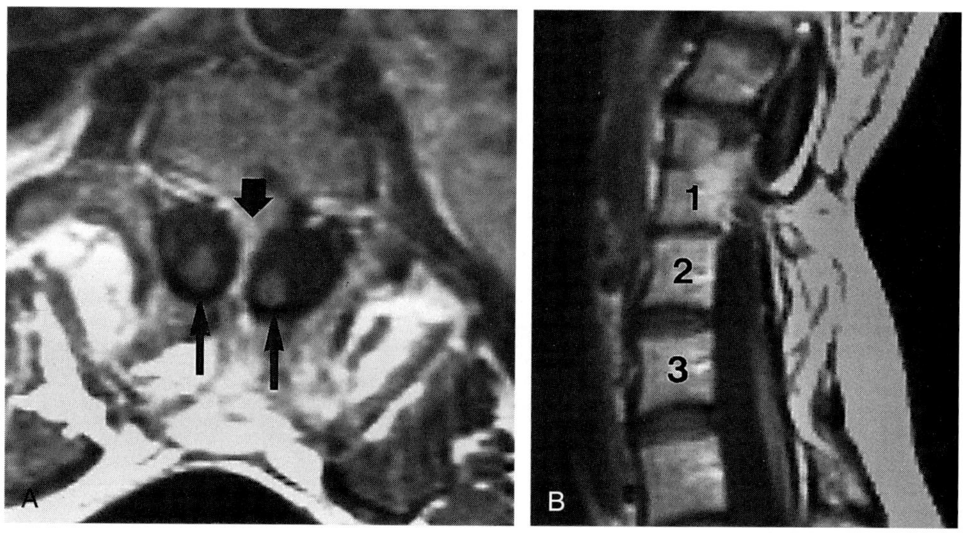

Figure 11–8. Diastematomyelia (type 2). **(A)** Axial MRI at T12-L1 shows two hemicords (thin arrows) and a midline bony septum (thick arrow). **(B)** Sagittal MRI shows the midline septum with hypoplasia and fusion of T12 and L1.

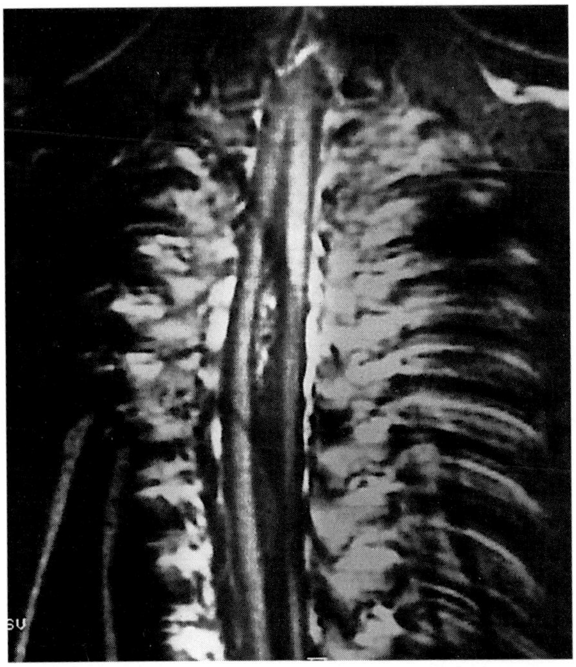

Figure 11–9. Diastematomyelia (type 2). Coronal MRI shows a midline bony septum and splitting of the cord throughout the thoracic region.

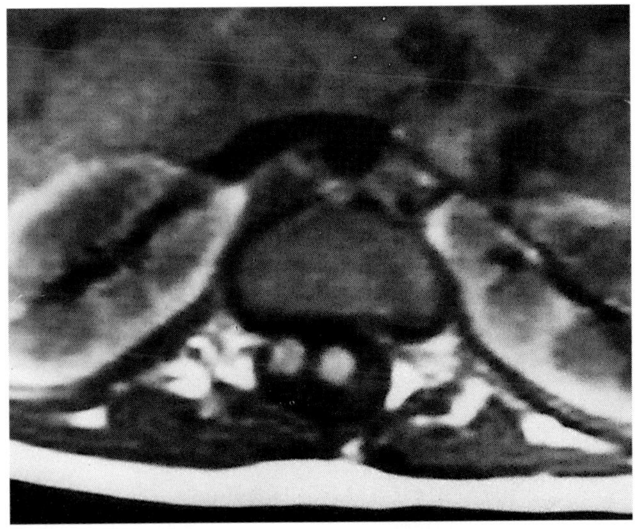

Figure 11–10. Diastematomyelia (type 1). Axial MRI at L1-L2 shows two hemicords within a single dural sleeve.

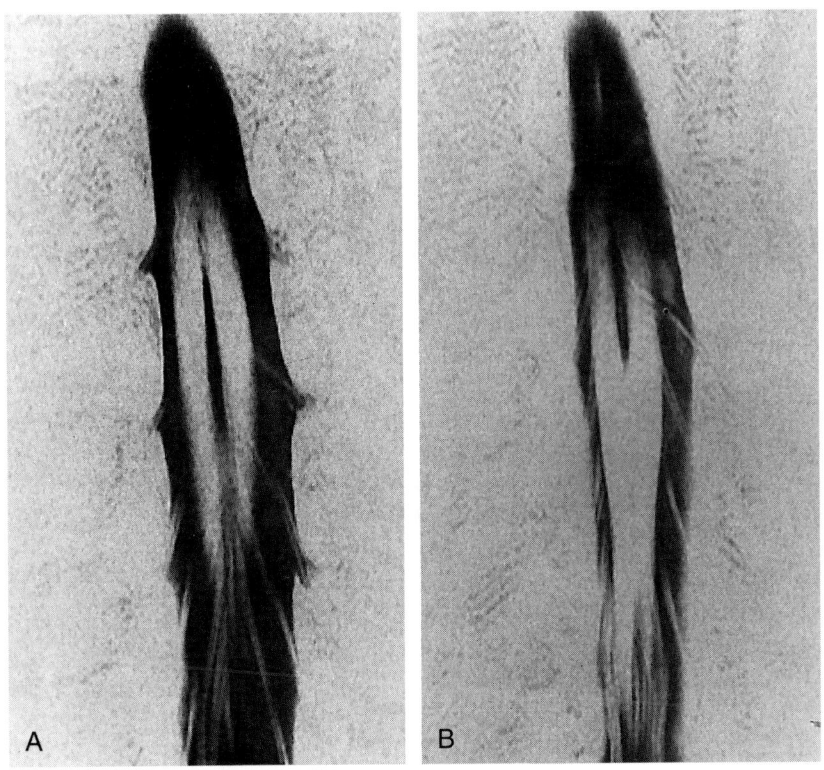

Figure 11–11. Diastematomyelia (type 1). **(A,B)** MR myelogram shows two hemicords within a single expanded dural sleeve, each hemicord giving rise to its own set of nerve roots. (Courtesy of Dr. Taher El Gammal, Birmingham, AL.)

Neurenteric Cyst

The embryonic notochord develops in the third week of gestation. The notochord and accompanying mesoderm separate the yolk sac and amniotic cavity, except for a transient small communication called the neurenteric canal. Incomplete regression of this canal may result in ectoendodermal adhesions or a neurenteric cyst and interfere with future notochordal development, leading to spinal defects or diastematomyelia. In addition to the spine, neurenteric cysts may appear in the posterior fossa or posterior mediastinum. Patients present anytime from infancy through the fifth decade, usually with symptoms of radicular pain or spastic paraparesis or quadriparesis.

Primary Abnormality

- Cystic mass in the spinal canal with or without intramedullary component and ventral to the spinal cord, or cyst in posterior mediastinum

Ancillary Findings

- Cyst often multilobulated
- Most commonly lower cervical and upper thoracic spine
- Rarely in lumbar spine or cerebellopontine angle
- Expansion of spinal canal
- Vertebral segmentation anomalies
- Kyphosis
- Spina bifida
- Ventral spinal defects rare but highly suggestive of the diagnosis

Associated Conditions

- Diastematomyelia
- Klippel-Feil anomaly

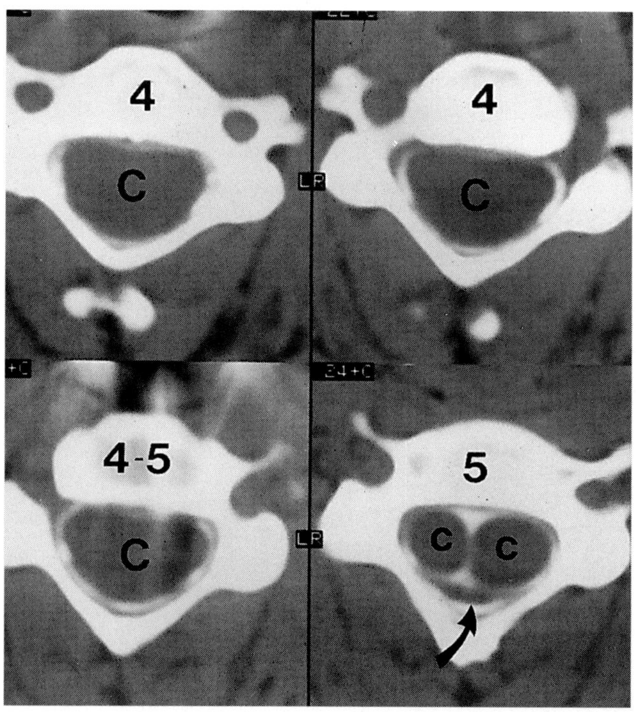

Figure 11–12. Neurenteric cyst. CT myelogram shows a mass with both intramedullary and extramedullary components. At C4 there is marked expansion of the spinal cord by the cyst (C). At C5 the cord (arrow) is posteriorly displaced and severely atrophic. A bilobulated exophytic component of the cyst lies in the ventral intradural compartment.

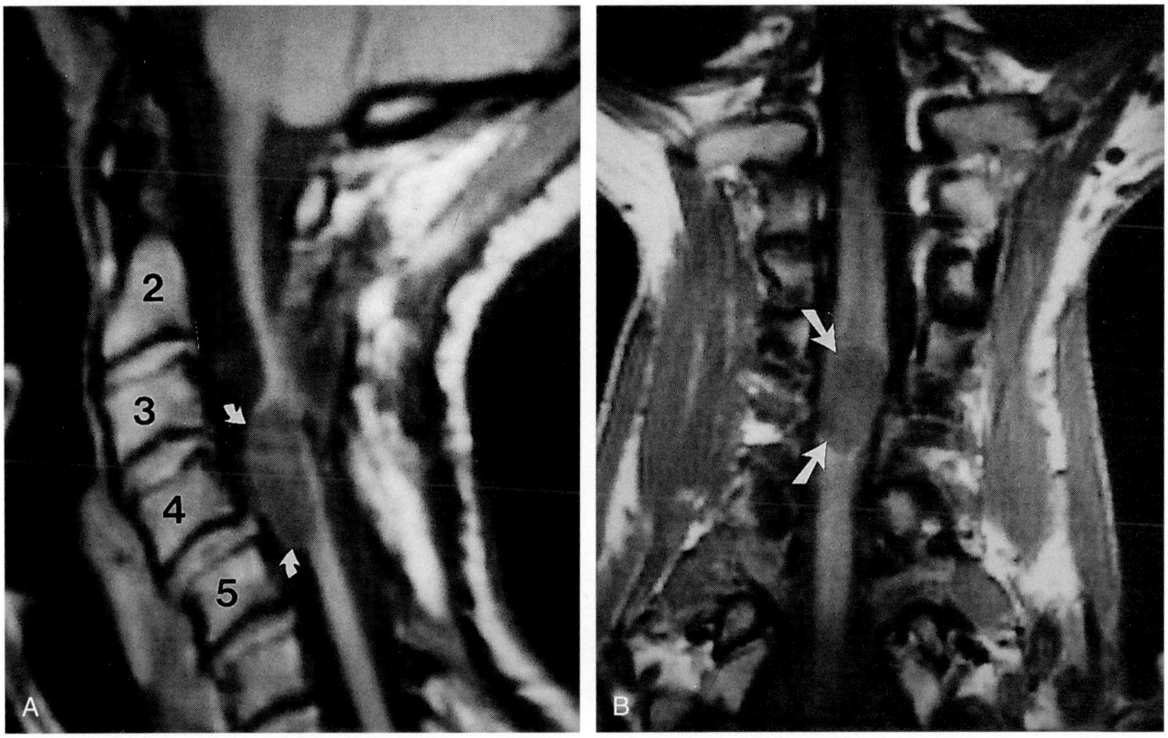

Figure 11–13. Neurenteric cyst. **(A)** Sagittal T1-weighted MRI shows a laminectomy defect from C2 to C6. A cystic mass (arrows) ventral to the cord at C4-C5 is of higher signal intensity than CSF but lower than cord parenchyma. **(B)** Coronal T1-weighted image shows the midline position of the cyst. (Reprinted with permission from Brooks,BS, Duvall,ER, El Gammal,T, et al. Neuroimaging Features of Neuroenteric Cysts: Analysis of Nine Cases and Review of the Literature. AJNR 14:735–746, 1993, © by American Society of Neuroradiology.)

Hydromyelia and Syringomyelia

Hydromyelia is a cystic dilatation of the central spinal canal and is lined by ependyma. Syringomyelia (syrinx) is defined as a spinal cord cyst separate from the central canal and lined by neuroglial tissue. The two are clinically and radiologically indistinguishable, and it is common practice to use the terms interchangeably or combine them (syringohydromyelia). Most cases are congenital; a minority are caused by trauma or tumors (see Table 11–3). The symptoms and clinical course are highly variable. It is generally recommended that every de novo case of syringohydromyelia have at least one contrast-enhanced MRI to exclude an underlying tumor. Once this has been done, noncontrast MRI is sufficient for routine follow-up.

TABLE 11–3 | Causes of Syringomyelia (Hydromyelia)

Congenital malformation of craniocervical junction (Chiari I and II)
Posterior fossa cyst
Posterior fossa neoplasm
Basal arachnoiditis
Spinal arachnoiditis
Trauma
Intramedullary neoplasm
Cord infarction

Primary Abnormality

- Longitudinally oriented, CSF-filled cavity in the spinal cord

Ancillary Findings

- Chiari I or II malformation usually present with related anomalies of the craniocervical junction
- Hyperintensity of adjacent cord parenchyma on T2-weighted images sometimes present
- Partial transverse septations commonly present
- May not be perfectly isointense with CSF due to flow, protein, past hemorrhage, or other factors
- Delayed CT scanning after intrathecal contrast will show filling of the central cavity; this procedure has been rendered unnecessary by MRI

Simple syrinx versus tumor-associated cyst:

- Simple syrinx exhibits sharp interface with cord parenchyma.
- The contents of a simple syrinx should be isointense with CSF on all sequences.
- No cord enhancement occurs with a simple syrinx.

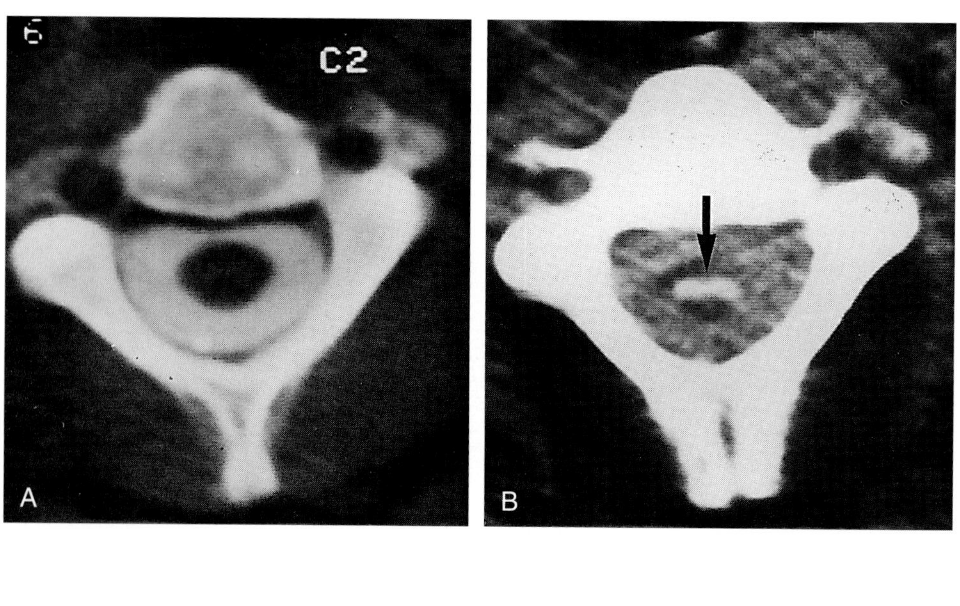

Figure 11–14. Syrinx. **(A)** CT myelogram shows a normal-sized cord at the C2 level. **(B)** Twenty-four-hour delayed scan shows dense accumulation of contrast (arrow) within the cord.

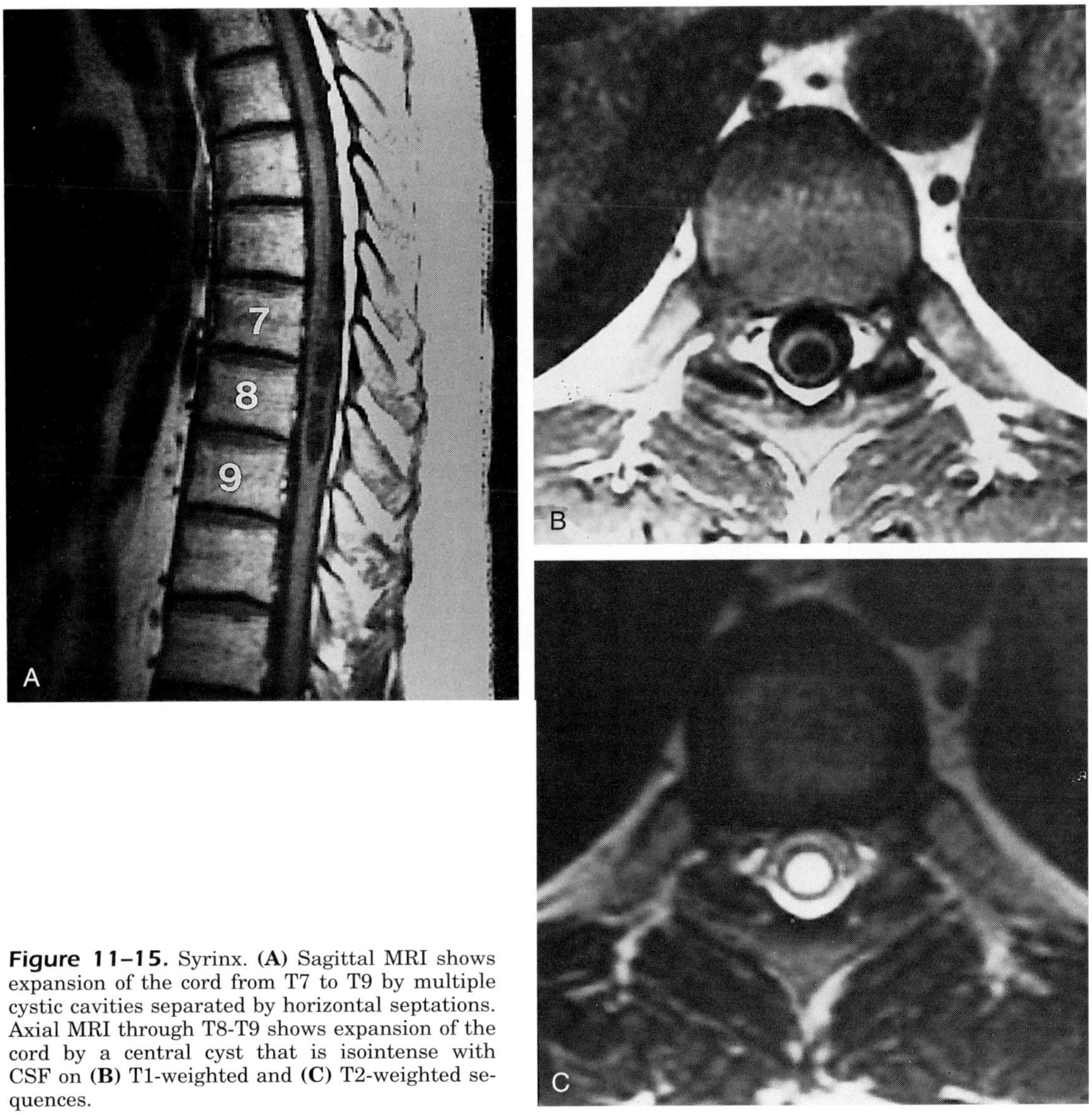

Figure 11–15. Syrinx. **(A)** Sagittal MRI shows expansion of the cord from T7 to T9 by multiple cystic cavities separated by horizontal septations. Axial MRI through T8-T9 shows expansion of the cord by a central cyst that is isointense with CSF on **(B)** T1-weighted and **(C)** T2-weighted sequences.

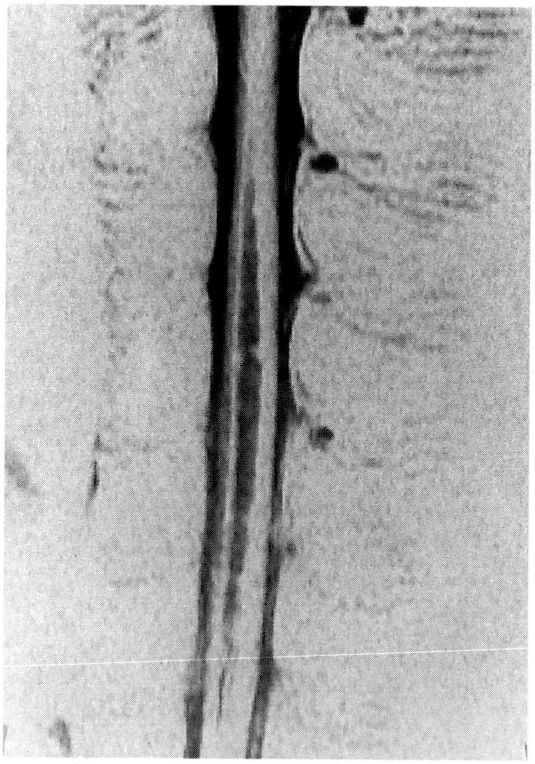

Figure 11–16. Syrinx. MR myelogram shows expansion of the spinal cord with a central cystic cavity extending from T3 to T7. (Courtesy of Dr. Taher El Gammal, Birmingham, AL.)

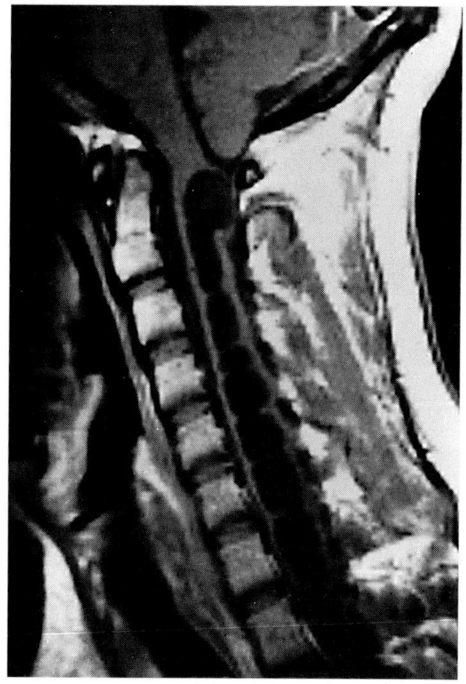

Figure 11–17. Syrinx and Chiari I. Sagittal MRI shows cystic expansion of the cervical cord and tonsillar herniation. Note the stack of coins appearance of the cord (horizontal septations) in this patient.

Spinal Lipoma

Most lipomas (84%) occur as part of the lipomyelomeningocele complex. Fibrolipomas of the filum terminale constitute at least 12% and probably much more, as they are now a common incidental finding on lumbar MRI. Isolated intradural lipomas constitute the remaining 4%. It is believed that lipomas are induced when embryonic mesenchyme becomes exposed to the ependyma, which forms the central canal. This impedes dorsal closure of the neural folds, resulting in an open neural placode (see lipomeningomyelocele). Thus even the intradural lipomas are actually subpial-juxtamedullary lesions that lie in the groove of a dorsally divided spinal cord.

Primary Abnormality

- Fatty mass in extradural, intradural, or combined extradural-intradural locations

Ancillary Findings

- Linear streaks of soft tissue coursing through the lipoma, which may represent fibrous bands, vessels, meninges, or neural tissue
- Usually posterior to cord and lie within midline dorsal cord defect
- May be cervical, thoracic, or lumbar
- Dorsal defect in dura sometimes presents with transdural extension of lipoma
- Small localized spina bifida may be present
- Widening of the spinal canal, erosion of pedicles, and thinning of the posterior elements due to mass effect
- Mass effect may occur from either extradural or intradural components
- Tethered cord

Associated Condition

- Dorsal dermal sinus

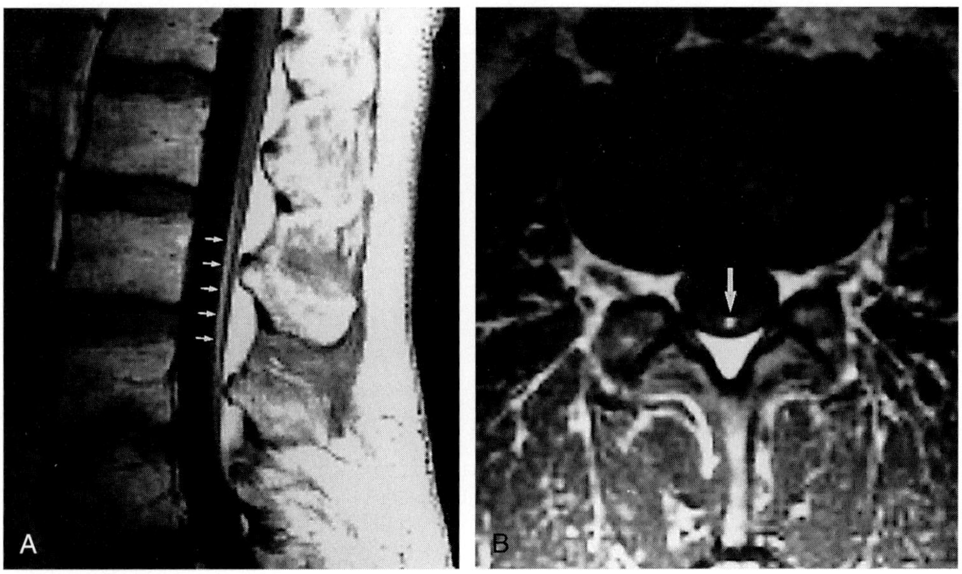

Figure 11–18. Fibrolipoma of filum terminale. **(A)** Sagittal and **(B)** axial MRI show a small hyperintense mass (arrows) extending along several centimeters of the filum. As in most cases, the cord is not tethered.

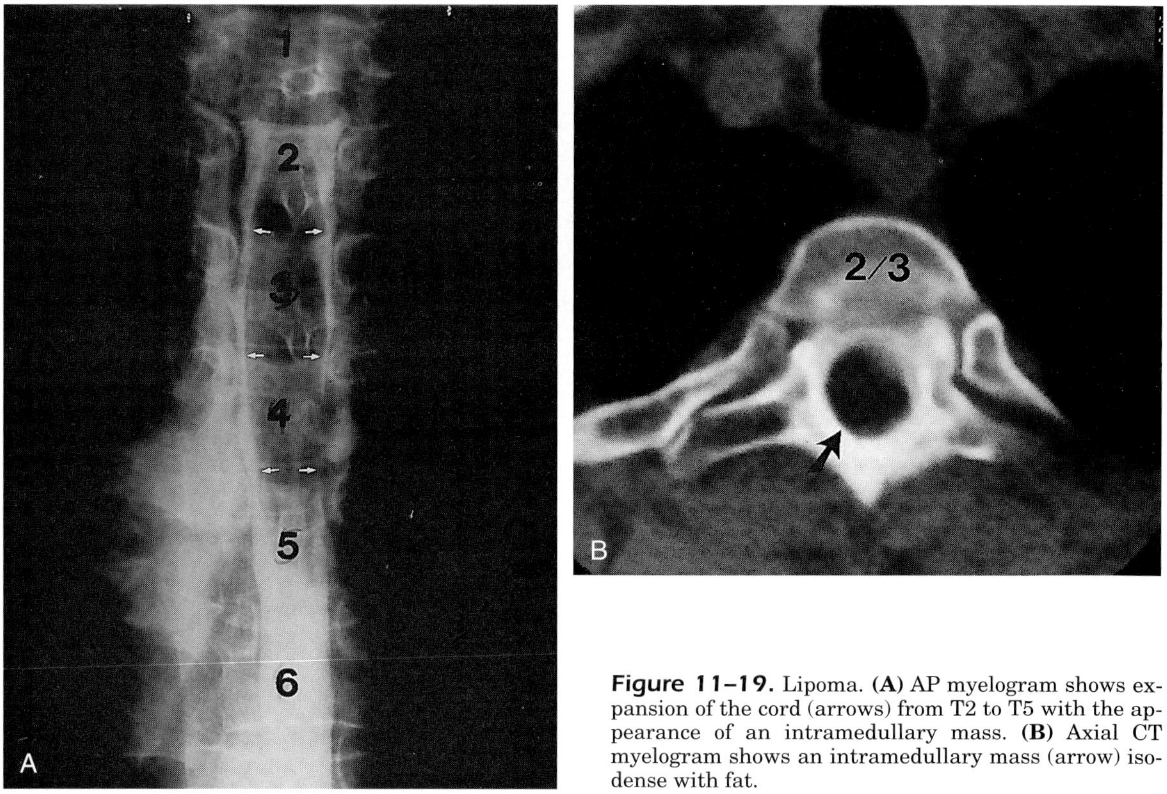

Figure 11–19. Lipoma. **(A)** AP myelogram shows expansion of the cord (arrows) from T2 to T5 with the appearance of an intramedullary mass. **(B)** Axial CT myelogram shows an intramedullary mass (arrow) isodense with fat.

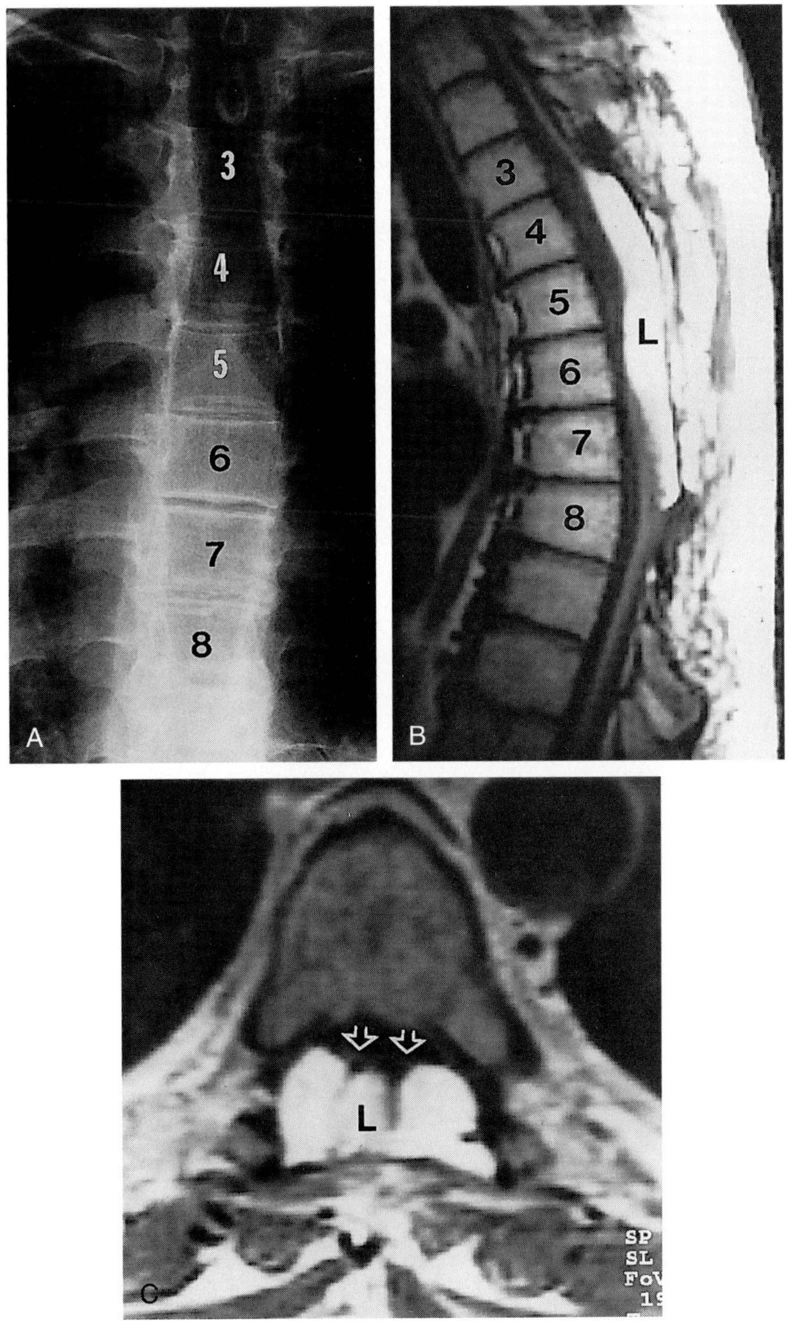

Figure 11–20. Lipoma. **(A)** AP radiograph shows absence of the posterior elements from T3 to T7, widening of the spinal canal, and hypoplasia of the pedicles. **(B)** Sagittal and **(C)** axial MRI show a lipoma (L) from T3 to T8. The cord (arrows) is dysplastic.

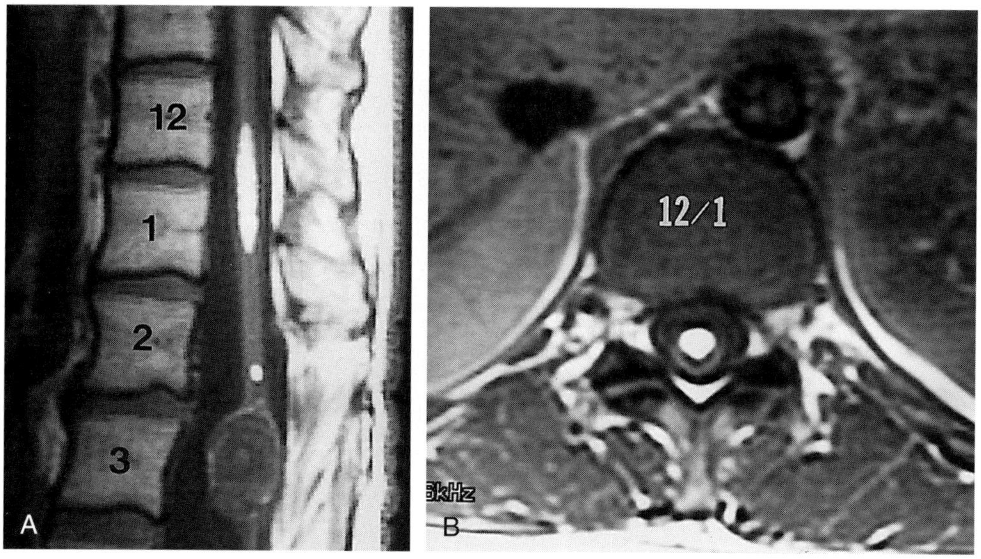

Figure 11–21. Lipoma and epidermoid. In this unusual case, **(A)** sagittal and **(B)** axial T1-weighted MRI show a purely intramedullary lipoma at T12-L1 and intact dorsal elements. A second small lipoma is present at lower L2. The mass in the conus at L3 is an epidermoid.

Tethered Cord

In the neonate, the spinal cord terminates at L3. More rapid growth of the spinal column relative to the cord results in a terminal cord level of about L1 L2 by age 12. Conditions that prevent this relative ascent of the cord may result in gait disturbance and lower cord dysfunction. Tethering of the cord is associated to some degree with nearly all of the dysraphisms. Isolated spinal cord tethering is usually associated with a thickened filum terminale. Although most patients present in late adolescence, the disorder can first present clinically well into late adulthood.

Primary Abnormality

- Abnormally low conus medullaris

Criteria for abnormally low conus medullaris:
Less than 6 years old: Below L3 vertebral body
More than 12 years old: Below L2-L3 disc space

Ancillary Findings

- May occur as primary disorder or in combination with other dysraphic conditions (spinal bifida occulta present in 33–100% of cases)
- Posterior displacement of distal spinal cord
- Widening of subarachnoid space
- Abnormally horizontal orientation of nerve roots
- Long tapering of conus or thickened filum terminale (normal filum measures <2 mm thick)
- Fibrolipomas of the filum in 23%
- Conus best visualized on axial images but may be hard to distinguish from the cauda equina on sagittal images
- Scoliosis present in 25%

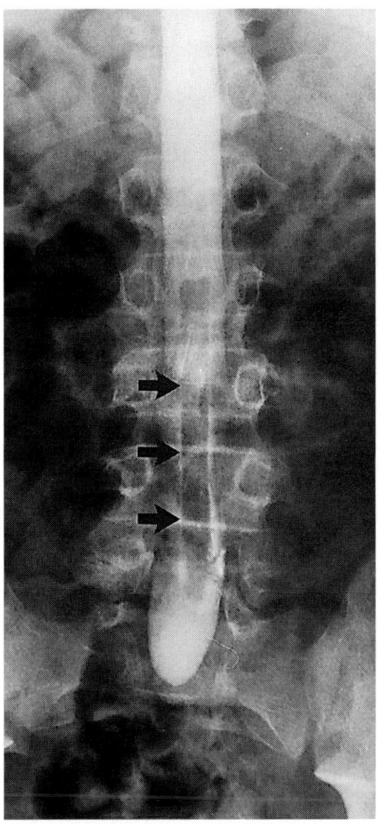

Figure 11–22. Tethered cord. AP myelogram shows a dilated terminal sac with tethering of the cord (arrows) to L5-S1.

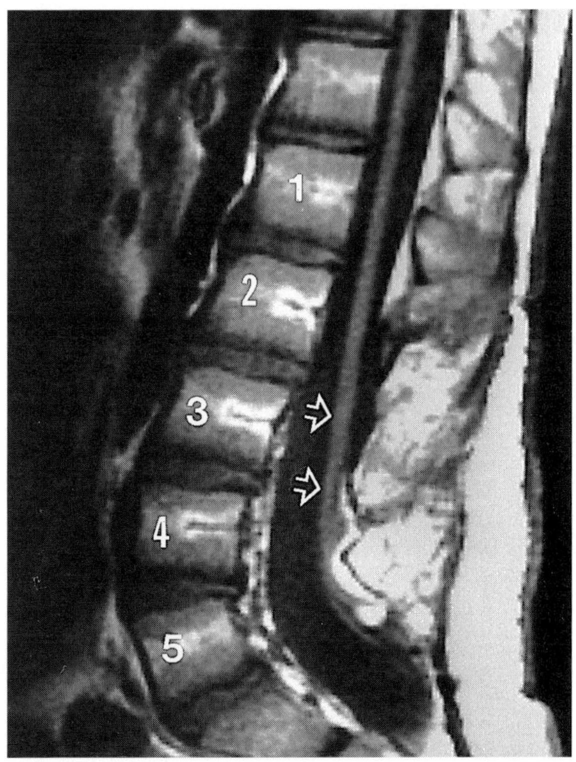

Figure 11–23. Tethered cord/lipomyelomeningocele. Sagittal MRI shows a tethered cord with the conus (arrows) dorsally adherent to a lipoma at L4-L5. There is enlargement of the ventral subarachnoid space and absence of posterior elements from L2 to S1.

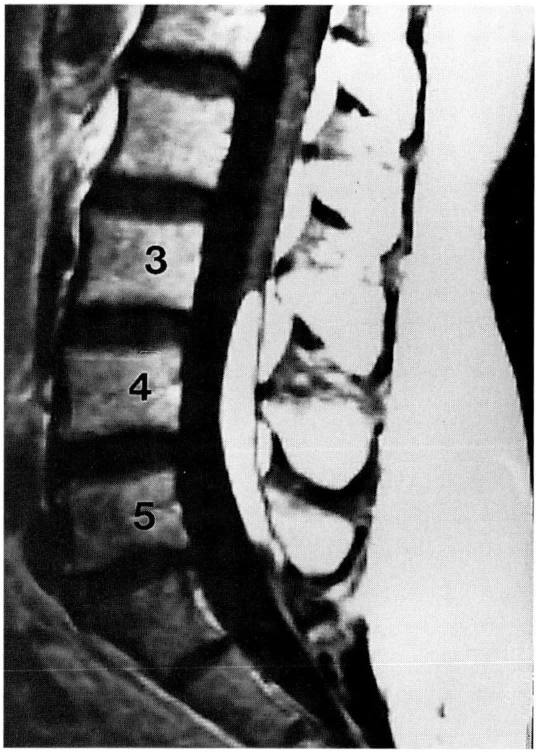

Figure 11–24. Tethered cord and filum lipoma. A large lipoma of the filum is present from L3 to S1 with tethering of the spinal cord. The posterior elements remain intact.

Caudal Regression Syndrome

The caudal regression syndrome is a condition of failure of caudal development ranging from complete fusion of the lower extremities, to atresia of the lower spine, to mere anal atresia. In most cases, the sacrum is absent, with partial agenesis of the lumbar spine. The level of atresia is usually below L1 and often limited to the sacrum. The distal cord is dysplastic and usually terminates caudally at the level of agenesis.

Primary Abnormality

- Congenital hypoplasia or atresia of caudal spinal elements
- May include coccyx, sacrum, lumbar spine, or lower thoracic spine

Ancillary Findings

- In complete absence of the sacrum, the ilia may articulate with each other
- Subarachnoid space may terminate at the top of the malformation or continue downward to normal position
- May be unilateral, with partial or complete sacral agenesis limited to one side
- Tethered cord, meningocele, or subcutaneous lipoma may be seen in those cases with fully formed dural sac
- Wedge-shaped appearance of terminal spinal cord

Associated Conditions

- Diastematomyelia
- Lipomeningomyelocele
- Intradural lipoma
- Dermoid cyst
- Dermal sinus

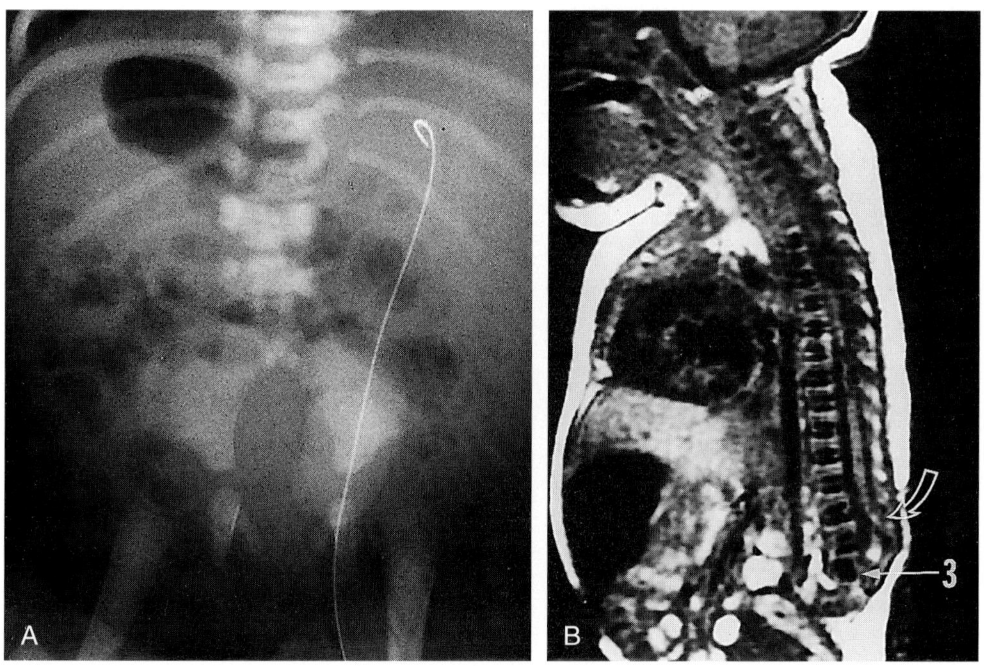

Figure 11–25. Caudal regression syndrome. **(A)** AP radiograph shows absence of the sacrum and lower two lumbar segments. Rudiments of L3 articulate with the iliac wings. **(B)** Sagittal MRI shows termination of the spinal column at L3 and the cord at L2 (open arrow).

Systemic Genetic Disorder

Neurofibromatosis

The clinical features and cranial manifestations of neurofibromatosis types 1 and 2 were discussed in Chapter 2. Both types share the same wide spectrum of spinal anomalies. However, there is a greater tendency to hypoplastic bone anomalies in type 1 and a greater tendency to nerve root and cord tumors in type 2.

Spinal Dysplasia

Hypoplastic Bone Changes

- More common in type 1 neurofibromatosis
- Hypoplasia or aplasia of pedicles, which may result in enlargement of foramina
- Hypoplasia of ribs or transverse processes
- Hypoplasia of vertebral bodies
- Posterior (sometimes anterior) scalloping of vertebral bodies

Secondary Effects of Osseous Hypoplasia

- Scoliosis (usually mild)
- Lateral meningocele

Hyperplastic Bone Changes

- Focal overgrowth of pedicle or vertebral arch
- Increased height of vertebral bodies

Effects of Dural Dysplasia

- Posterior scalloping of vertebral bodies
- Lateral thoracic and anterior sacral meningoceles

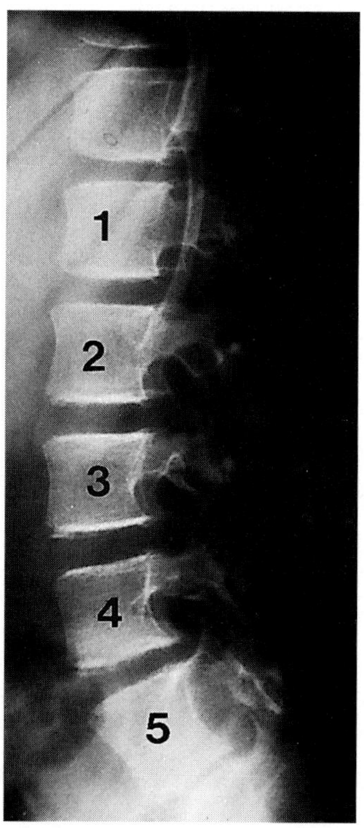

Figure 11–26. Neurofibromatosis I (vertebral scalloping). Lateral radiograph shows marked posterior scalloping of vertebral bodies L1 through L5. This is almost always due to dural ectasia and not tumor.

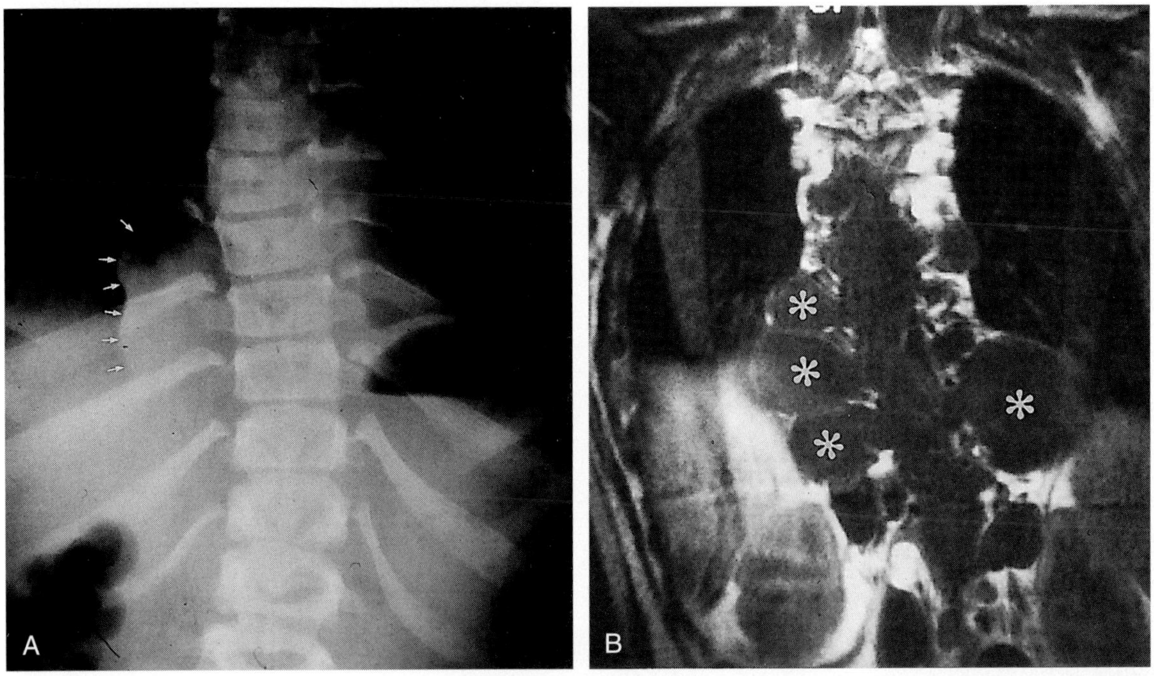

Figure 11–27. Neurofibromatosis 1 (lateral meningoceles). **(A)** AP radiograph shows scoliosis, widening of the spinal canal, hypoplasia or thinning of the pedicles, and right paraspinal soft tissue masses (arrows). **(B)** Coronal T1-weighted MRI shows multiple paraspinal masses isointense with CSF and communicating with the subarachnoid space through enlarged root sleeves. The larger meningoceles are indicated with asterisks. (Courtesy of Dr. Yoginder Vaid, Birmingham, AL.)

Nerve Sheath Tumors

Primary Findings

- Schwannomas, neurofibromas, or meningiomas
- Malignant degeneration in 5–10% of patients
- Nearly equal incidence in cervical, thoracic, and lumbar spine
- Soft tissue mass that may be intradural (70%), dumbbell (15%), or extradural (15%)
- Calcifications are infrequent
- More common in type 2 neurofibromatosis

The imaging features and diagnosis of nerve sheath tumors are addressed in Chapter 12.

Secondary Bone Changes

- Erosion of pedicles and enlargement of foramina
- Vertebral body erosion or destruction

Nerve sheath tumors in neurofibromatosis:

1. All central lesions (intracranial) are schwannomas.
2. Nearly all peripheral lesions (subcutaneous, peripheral nerves) are neurofibromas.
3. Spinal nerve sheath tumors are usually neurofibromas in type 1.
4. Spinal nerve sheath tumors are usually schwannomas in type 2.

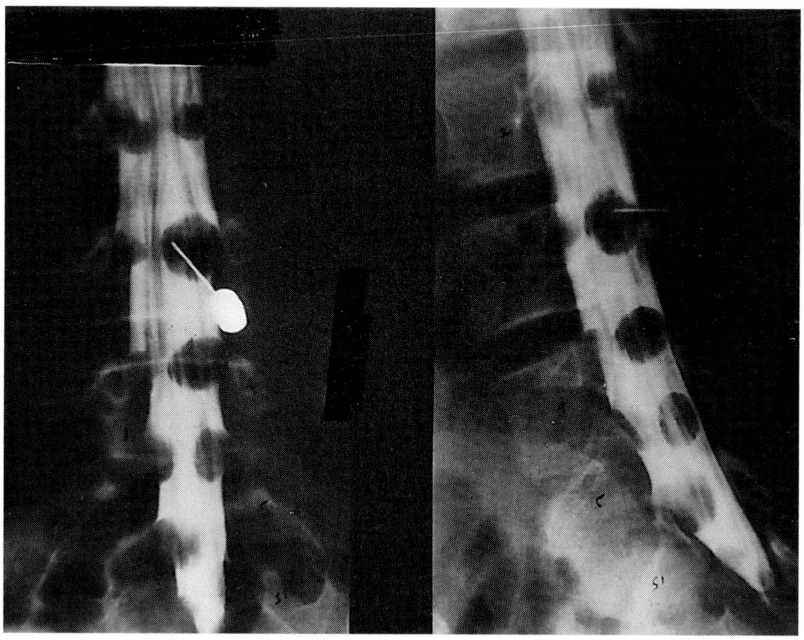

Figure 11–28. Neurofibromatosis 2 (nerve sheath tumors). AP and oblique myelogram show bilateral filling defects at every lumbar level.

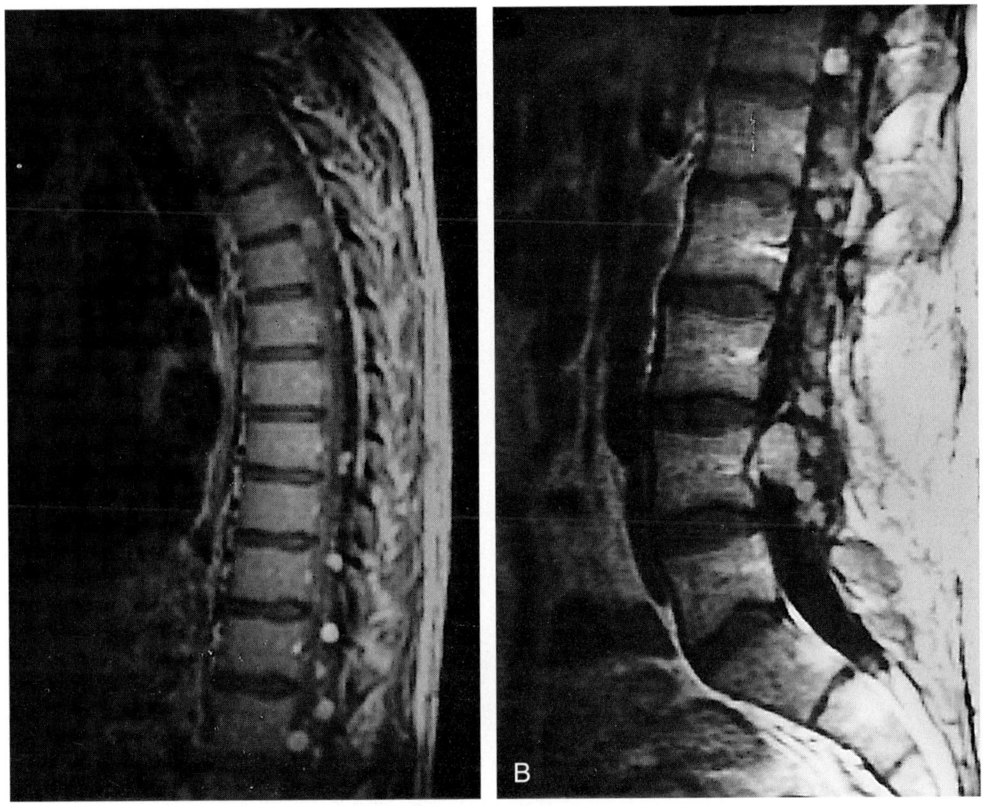

Figure 11–29. Neurofibromatosis II (nerve sheath tumors). Sagittal contrast-enhanced MRI of **(A)** thoracic and **(B)** lumbar spine show numerous discrete enhancing nodules of varying size in this individual with neurofibromatosis.

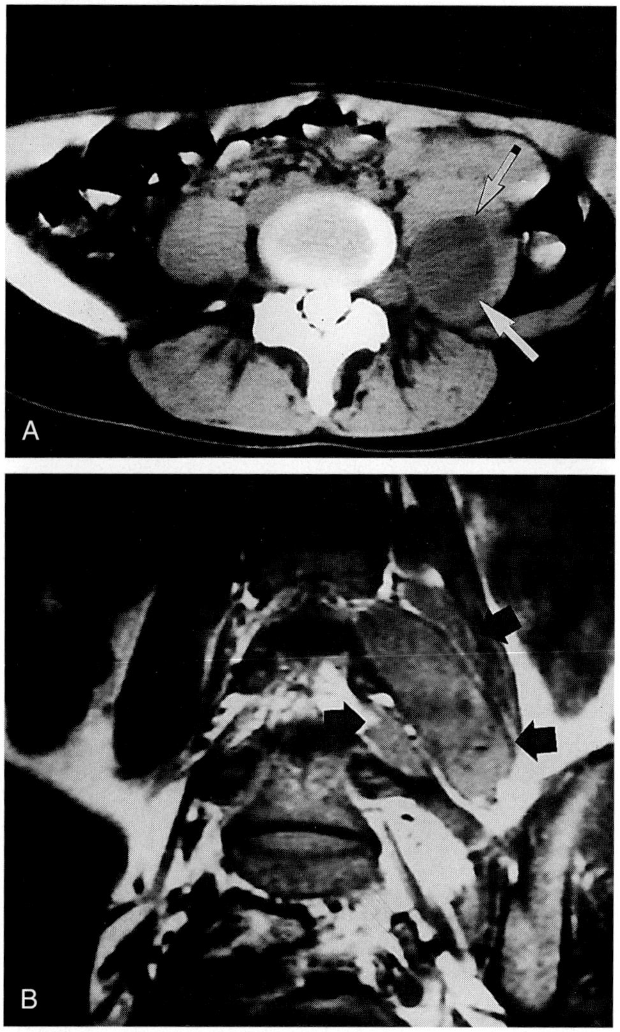

Figure 11–30. Neurofibromatosis II (plexiform neurofibroma). **(A)** Axial CT shows a large mass (arrows) of the left lumbar plexus. The mass is hypodense relative to the psoas muscle. There is contrast in the subarachnoid space. Total axis myelography was negative. **(B)** Coronal T1-weighted MRI shows marked enlargement of multiple lumbar nerve roots forming a conglomerate mass (arrows).

Spinal Cord Tumors

- Ependymomas (most frequent)
- Astrocytomas
- More common in type 2 neurofibromatosis

The imaging findings and diagnosis of spinal cord tumors are addressed in Chapter 12.

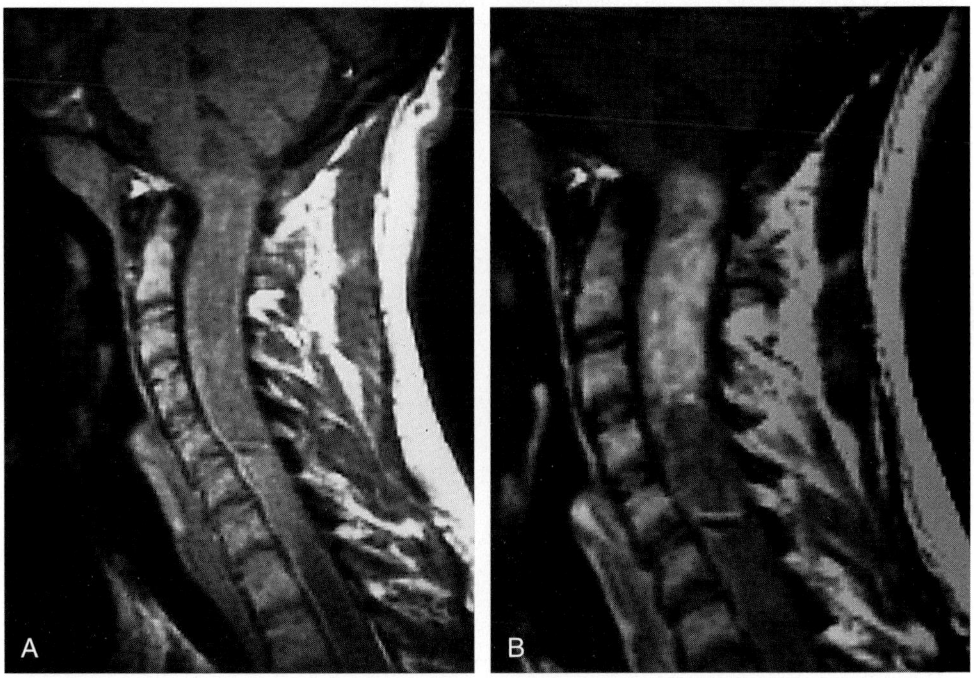

Figure 11–31. Neurofibromatosis II (spinal cord neoplasm, probable ependymoma). **(A)** Sagittal T1-weighted MRI shows a mass involving the medulla and complete cervical cord. There is enlargement of the spinal canal. **(B)** Dense enhancement of the central component is observed after intravenous contrast.

RECOMMENDED READINGS

Spinal Dysraphism

Barkovich,AJ, Naidich,TP. Congenital Anomalies of the Spine. In Barkovich,AJ: *Pediatric Neuroimaging*. New York: Raven Press, 1990, pp 227–271.

Brunberg,JA, Latchaw,RE, Kanal,E, Burk,L, Albright,L. Magnetic Resonance Imaging of Spinal Dysraphism. *Radiol Clin North Am* 26:181–205, 1988.

Davis,PC, Hoffman,JC, Ball,TI, et al. Spinal Abnormalities in Pediatric Patients: MR Imaging Findings Compared with Clinical, Myelographic, and Surgical Findings. *Radiology* 166:679–685, 1988.

DeLaPaz,RL. Congenital Anomalies of the Lumbosacral Spine. *Neuroimaging Clin North Am* 3:425–442, 1993.

Korsvik,HE, Keller,MS. Sonography of Occult Dysraphism in Neonates and Infants with MR Imaging Correlation. *Radiographics* 12:297–306, 1992.

Nievelstein,RAJ, Valk,J, Smit,LME, Vermeij-Keers,C. MR of the Caudal Regression Syndrome: Embryologic Implications. *AJNR* 15:1021–1029, 1994.

Scatliff,JH, Kendall,BE, Kingsley,DPE, Britton,J, Grant,DN, Hayward,RD. Closed Spinal Dysraphism: Analysis of Clinical, Radiological, and Surgical Findings in 104 Consecutive Patients. *AJNR* 10:269–277, 1989.

Syringohydromyelia

Batnitzky,S, Price,HI, Gaughan,MJ, Hall, PV, Rosenthal,SJ. The Radiology of Syringohydromyelia. *Radiographics* 3: 585–611, 1983.

Slasky,BS, Bydder,GM, Niendorf,HP, Young,IR. MR Imaging with Gadolinium-DTPA in the Differentiation of Tumor, Syrinx, and Cyst of the Spinal Cord. *JCAT* 11:845–850, 1987.

Williams,AL, Haughton,VM, Pojunas,KW, Daniels,DL, Kilgore, DP. Differentiation of Intramedullary Neoplasms and Cysts by MR. *AJR* 149:159–164, 1987.

Neurofibromatosis

Braffman,B, Naidich,TP. The Phakomatoses: Part I. Neurofibromatosis and Tuberous Sclerosis. *Neuroimaging Clin N Am* 4:299–324, 1994.

Burk,DL, Brunberg,JA, Kanal,E, Latchaw,RE, Wolf,GL. Spinal and Paraspinal Neurofibromatosis: Surface Coil MR Imaging at 1.5T. *Radiology* 162:797–801, 1987.

Egelhoff,JC, Bates,DJ, Ross,JS, Rothner,AD, Cohen,BH. Spinal MR Findings in Neurofibromatosis Types 1 and 2. *AJNR* 13:1071–1077, 1992.

Yaghmai,I. Spine Changes in Neurofibromatosis. *Radiographics* 6:261–285, 1986.

CHAPTER
TWELVE

Inflammatory and Neoplastic Diseases of the Spine

This chapter encompasses a broad spectrum of disorders, both neoplastic and non-neoplastic in nature. Only the more common entities are presented. Syringohydromyelia was discussed in Chapter 11. For most of these conditions, MRI has become the imaging procedure of choice. However, CT and even myelography continue to serve a useful adjunctive role and occasionally become necessary when contraindications to MRI exist.

As in the cranium, correct localization of a mass is a necessary preliminary to arriving at an accurate diagnosis. This subject is explored at the beginning of this chapter.

LOCALIZATION OF SPINAL MASSES

Spinal masses are traditionally divided into three categories based on the anatomic compartment of origin:

- Intramedullary: Mass arising within the spinal cord
- Intradural/extramedullary: Mass arising within the dura but outside the spinal cord, including tumors of the intradural nerve roots
- Extradural: Mass arising outside the dural sleeve, including all primary skeletal lesions

The imaging features used in localizing spinal mass lesions are outlined in Table 12–1 and the accompanying figures. The general differential diagnoses are provided in Table 12–2.

TABLE 12–2 Differential Diagnosis of Spinal Masses by Location

Differential Diagnosis
Intramedullary
Ependymoma
Astrocytoma
Hemangioblastoma
Syrinx
Multiple sclerosis
Transverse myelitis
Contusion
Hematoma
Metastasis
Arteriovenous malformation
Cavernous hemangioma
Infarction
Intradural/extramedullary
Meningioma
Schwannoma and neurofibroma
Metastasis
Arteriovenous malformation
Dural fistula
Subarachnoid and arachnoid cyst
Disc fragment
Subdural hematoma
Extradural
Herniated disc
Metastasis
Osteomyelitis and epidural abscess
Hemangioma
Synovial cyst
Schwannoma and neurofibroma
Chordoma
Primary bone tumors
Epidural hematoma

TABLE 12–1 Localization of Spinal Masses

	Intramedullary	Intradural/Extramedullary	Extradural
Spinal cord	Enlarged in coronal and sagittal planes and in cross-sectional diameter	Displaced or compressed in cross section	Displaced or compressed in cross section and at least one longitudinal plane
Subarachnoid space	Reduced at level of mass with smooth tapering above and below Edges are pushed toward the bony canal	May be enlarged in one longitudinal plane but reduced in the other Reduced at level of mass with focal enlargement or cap above and below	Reduced at level of mass with smooth tapering above and below Outer edges displaced from cortical margin of adjacent bony canal
Bony changes	Absent or smooth expansion of spinal canal	Absent or smooth compressive changes May see foraminal enlargement with dumbbell tumors	Bony destruction or vertebral collapse often present

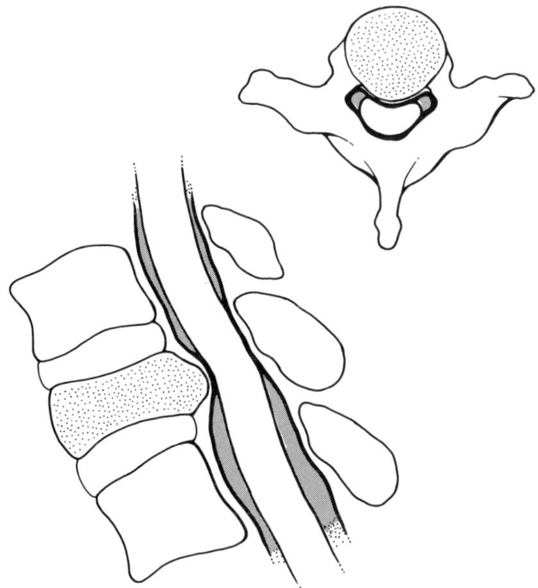

Figure 12–1. Features of an extradural mass. This graphic illustrates the features of an extradural mass using vertebral body metastasis as the prototype. The axial image illustrates effacement of the subarachnoid space and deformity of the ventral cord. On the sagittal view the cord is posteriorly displaced and ventrally deformed. The subarachnoid space as seen on myelography or MRI tapers smoothly to an acute angle above and below the mass. The dura is displaced toward the center of the spinal canal. Pathology outside the dural sleeve, such as disc degeneration or vertebral body abnormalities, is typically present.

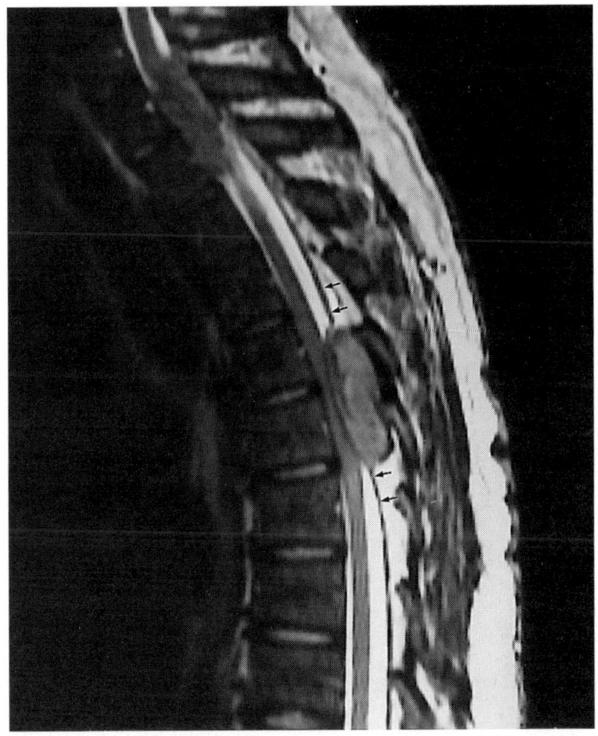

Figure 12–2. Extradural mass (lymphoma). Sagittal T2-weighted MRI shows anterior displacement of the spinal cord and dura (arrows) by a soft tissue mass in the posterior extradural space. The subarachnoid space tapers to a point above and below the tumor.

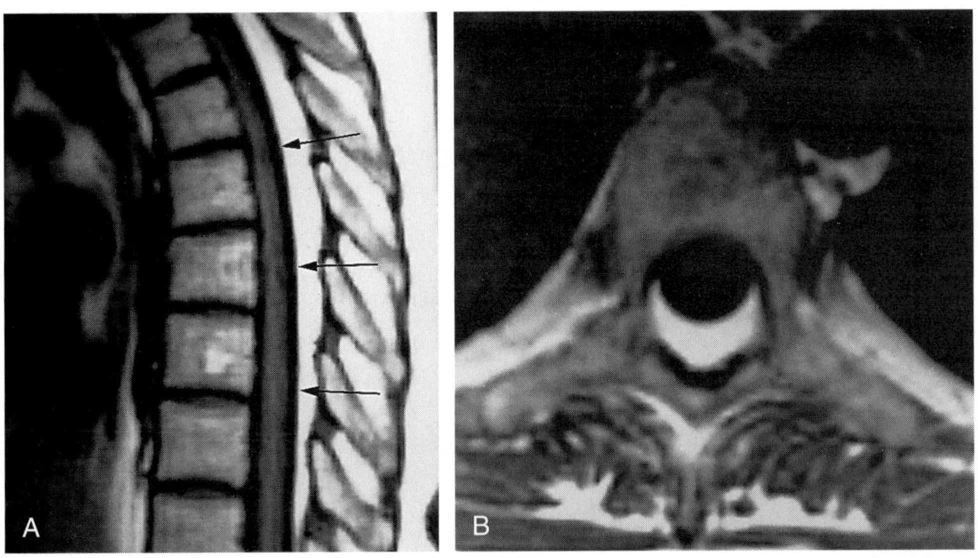

Figure 12–3. Extradural mass (epidural lipomatosis). **(A)** Sagittal and **(B)** axial T1-weighted MRI shows extensive accumulation of fat in the posterior epidural space with a thickness of 6-9 mm (normal is 3-6 mm). The dura is displaced anteriorly (arrows). This condition may be incidental and asymptomatic. Symptomatic cases are usually caused by exogenous corticosteroids.

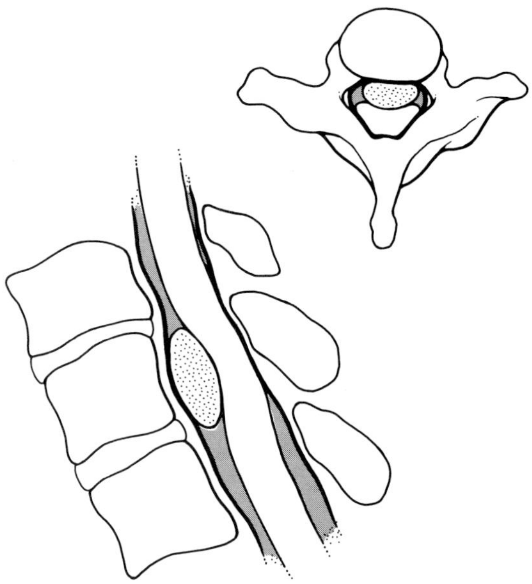

Figure 12–4. Features of an intradural extramedullary mass. This graphic illustrates the features of an intradural mass such as meningioma. On axial and sagittal images the spinal cord is displaced by the mass and deformed where it is in contact with the mass. The subarachnoid space opposite the mass tapers smoothly to an acute angle, but the ipsilateral subarachnoid space is expanded above and below forming a cap over both ends of the mass. The vertebrae and discs are usually normal except in the case of intraforaminal tumors.

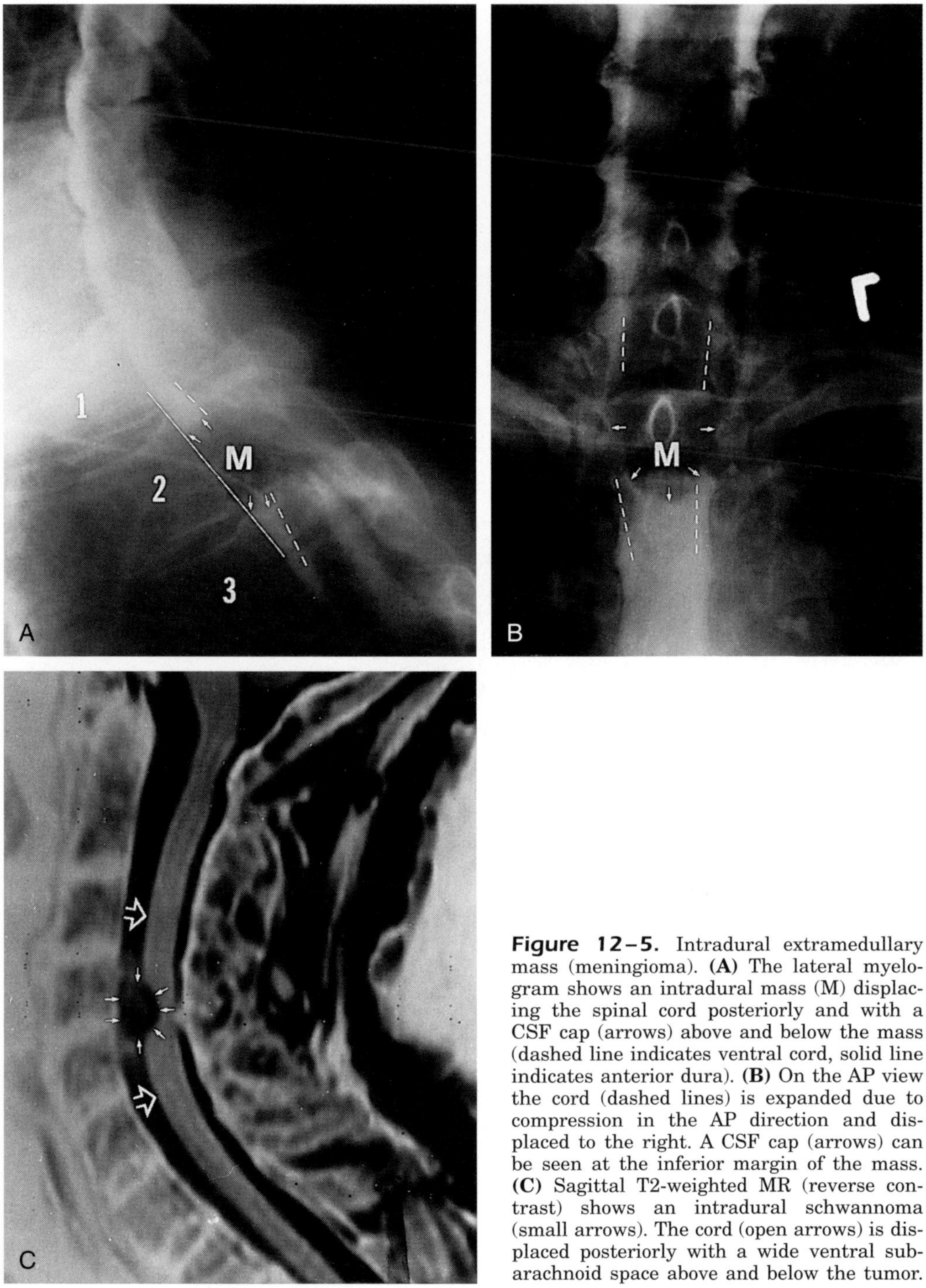

Figure 12–5. Intradural extramedullary mass (meningioma). **(A)** The lateral myelogram shows an intradural mass (M) displacing the spinal cord posteriorly and with a CSF cap (arrows) above and below the mass (dashed line indicates ventral cord, solid line indicates anterior dura). **(B)** On the AP view the cord (dashed lines) is expanded due to compression in the AP direction and displaced to the right. A CSF cap (arrows) can be seen at the inferior margin of the mass. **(C)** Sagittal T2-weighted MR (reverse contrast) shows an intradural schwannoma (small arrows). The cord (open arrows) is displaced posteriorly with a wide ventral subarachnoid space above and below the tumor.

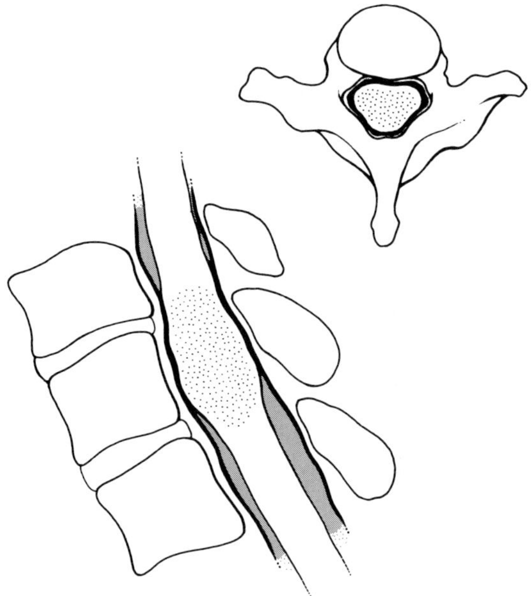

Figure 12–6. Features of an intramedullary mass. This graphic illustrates the features of an intramedullary mass such as astrocytoma. The dura is in its normal position, and the nearby discs and vertebrae are normal or thinned. The spinal canal is normal in size or even expanded. There is expansion of the spinal cord, a finding that must be confirmed in two planes or in cross section. Expansion of the cord in one plane is frequently seen with extramedullary tumors, in which case compression will be seen in an orthogonal plane (see Figure 12–32**C**). The subarachnoid space tapers smoothly above and below the mass.

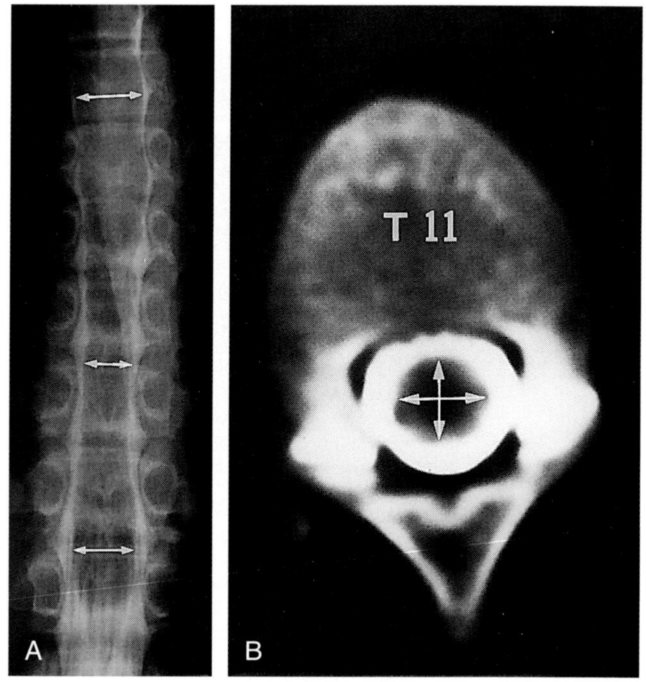

Figure 12–7. Intramedullary mass (astrocytoma). **(A)** AP myelogram shows expansion of the entire thoracic cord (arrows). This is almost always due to astrocytoma. **(B)** Axial CT myelogram shows expansion of the cord in both diameters with a normal outer margin of the dural sleeve.

Inflammatory Conditions

Arachnoiditis

Arachnoiditis is a condition of chronic inflammation of the spinal meninges resulting in fibrous adhesions of the spinal cord, nerve roots, and subarachnoid space. Affected patients usually present with pain radiating to the extremities. Spinal surgery is the most common precipitating factor. Infectious meningitis, trauma, subarachnoid hemorrhage, intrathecal anesthetics or steroids, and myelographic contrast agents (especially Pantopaque) represent other important causes. Arachnoiditis may in turn cause spinal subarachnoid cysts or syringomyelia (see Chapter 11).

Myelographic and CT Findings. Myelography remains the best technique for diagnosing arachnoiditis in the cervical and thoracic spine and is equivalent to MRI in the lumbar spine. Myelography may reveal the featureless sac, in which there is partial or complete amputation of the root sleeves and nonvisualization of nerve roots within the sac, which have become adherent to the walls of the sac. In other cases, clumping of nerve roots produces discrete large filling defects in the contrast-filled sac or adhesions produce a somewhat amorphous-looking subarachnoid space filled by interconnected irregular clumps of contrast or myelographic block (usually low lumbar).

CT myelography shows somewhat better the nerve roots, which may be adherent to the dural sleeve or clumped together within the subarachnoid space.

MRI Findings. MRI detection of arachnoiditis is mostly restricted to the lower lumbar spine, using axial T1- and T2-weighted sections. Three patterns of abnormality have been characterized on MRI:

- Central clumping of nerve roots within the thecal sac
- Adherence of nerve roots to the walls of the thecal sac
- Soft tissue mass filling the thecal sac

Following intravenous contrast, mild enhancement of the nerve roots occurs in about 50% of cases. The degree of enhancement is much less than that seen with most primary or metastatic tumors.

Differential Diagnosis

Intrathecal tumor seeding may produce similar imaging findings. It may be identified by the usual strong enhancement on contrast-enhanced MRI.

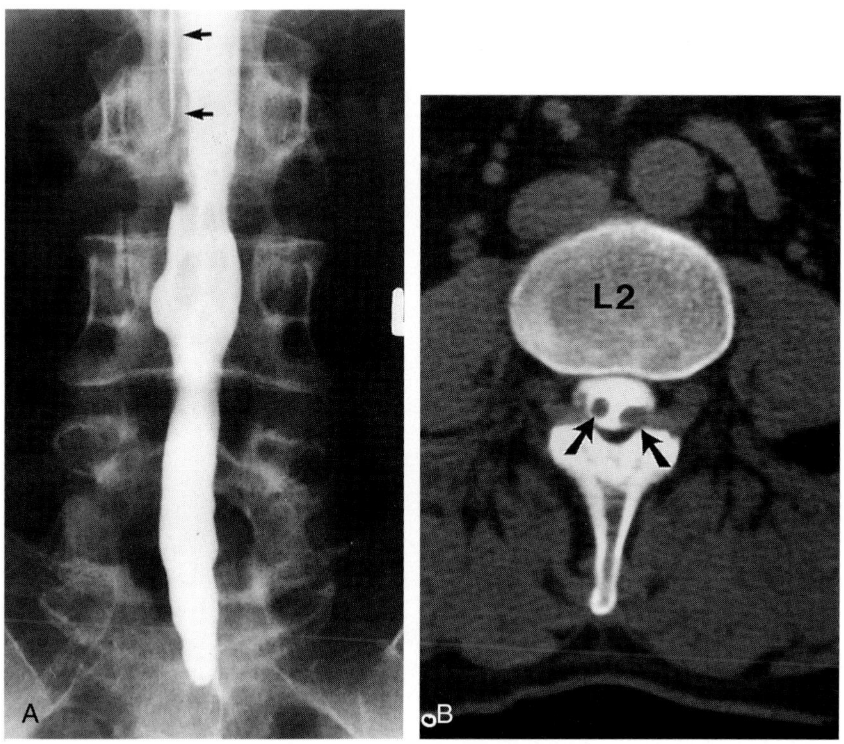

Figure 12–8. Arachnoiditis (same patient as Figure 12–10). **(A)** AP myelogram shows an amorphous, irregular thecal sac and nonvisualization of nerve roots below L3 (the empty sac sign). Clumping of nerve roots is present at L3 (arrows). **(B)** Axial CT shows clumping of the nerve roots (arrows).

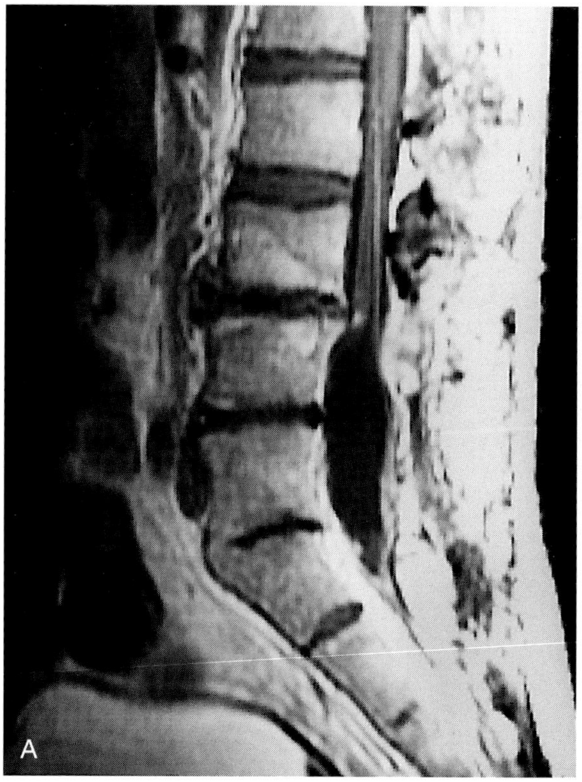

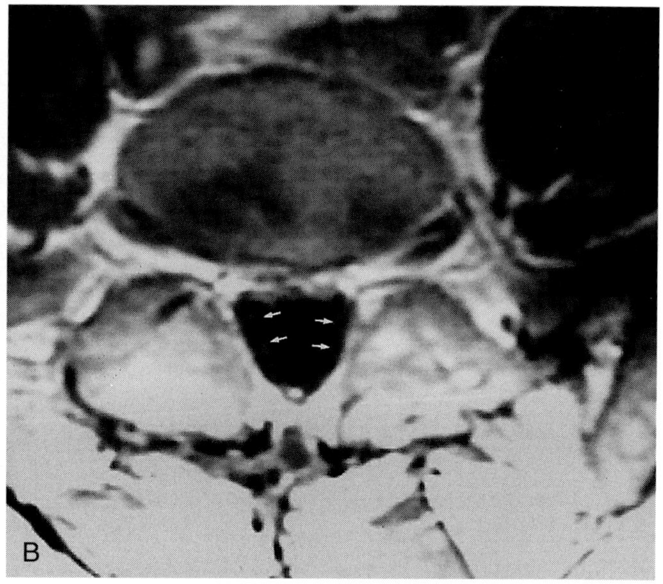

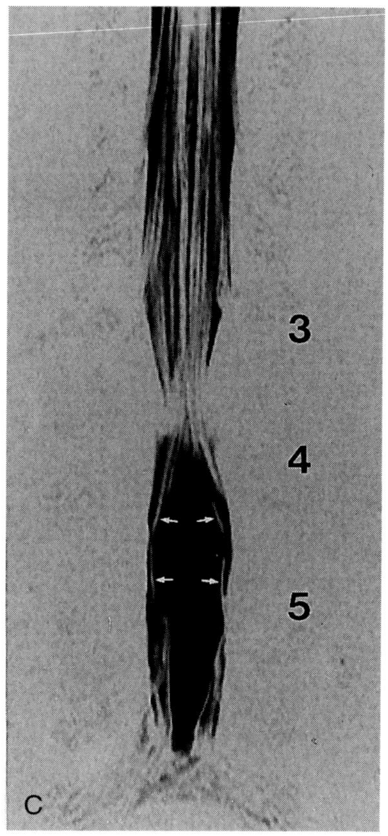

Figure 12–9. Arachnoiditis. **(A)** Sagittal contrast-enhanced MRI shows enhancement of the cauda equina and an empty sac at L4-L5. **(B)** Axial MRI at L4-L5 shows clumping of nerve roots (arrows) to the lateral walls of the thecal sac. **(C)** AP MR myelogram shows the empty sac at L4-L5 and adherence of roots (arrows) to the lateral walls of the thecal sac. There is severe stenosis at L3-L4. (**C** courtesy of Dr. Taher El Gammal, Birmingham, AL.)

Subarachnoid Cyst

Subarachnoid cysts develop when granulation tissue and adhesions in the subarachnoid space lead to CSF-containing pseudocysts that may exert pressure effects upon the spinal cord and nerve roots. They most often occur in the thoracic spine, followed by cervical and lumbar. There is usually a history of trauma, epidural anesthesia, or spinal surgery with subsequent development of arachnoiditis. Affected patients usually present with progressive pain and paraparesis.

Myelographic and CT Findings. Myelography may be nonspecific, showing only the presence of an extramedullary intradural mass or complete block. In many instances, the cysts accumulate contrast that may remain concentrated and hyperdense relative to the remaining CSF and does not shift with a change in position. CT may show a loculated hyperdense collection of contrast with a thin or indistinguishable wall and displacement of the cord. Bony erosion is occasionally encountered with larger lesions. Findings of arachnoiditis are typically present.

MRI Findings. The signal intensity of the cyst should equal CSF on all sequences. In cases of loculation or reduced flow, however, it may be somewhat brighter, and with turbulent flow it may become darker. The presence of a mass can sometimes only be inferred from displacement or deformity of the spinal cord. Septations are visible in about half of cases. No enhancement should occur after intravenous contrast.

Differential Diagnosis

True arachnoid cysts occur without arachnoiditis or a history of antecedent trauma. Cord atrophy with enlargement of the subarachnoid space and intramedullary cysts (syrinx or myelomalacia) may imitate the MRI appearance of subarachnoid cysts.

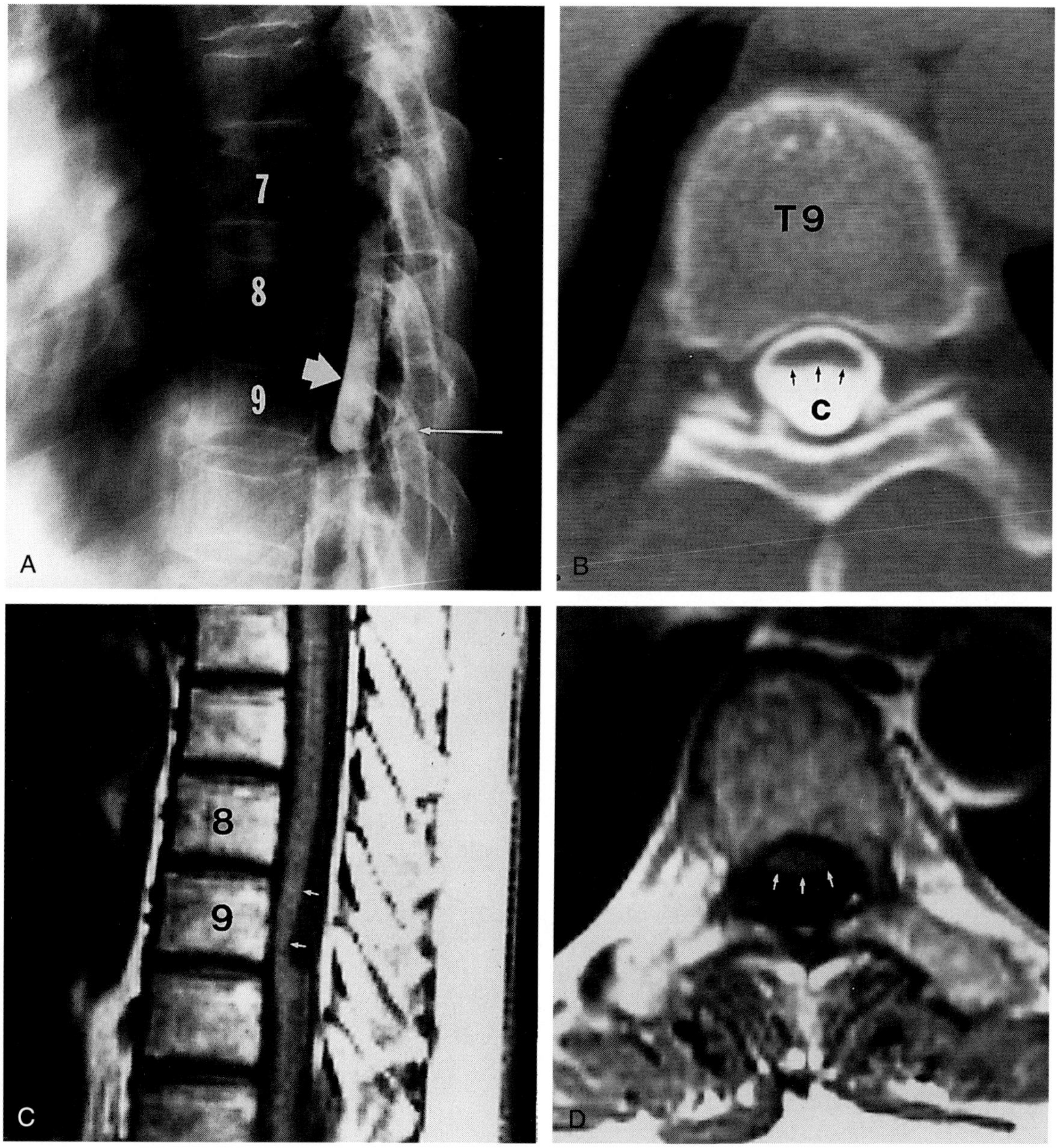

Figure 12–10. Subarachnoid cyst and arachnoiditis (same patient as Figure 12–8). **(A)** Lateral myelogram shows accumulation of contrast material within a cyst (large arrow) dorsal to the cord. Small arrow indicates plane of section in **B**. **(B)** CT through the cyst (c) shows ventral displacement and flattening of the cord (arrows). Contrast within the cyst is isodense with the opacified CSF. **(C)** Sagittal and **(D)** axial T1-weighted MRI show deformity of the cord (arrows) by a posterior mass isointense with CSF.

Multiple Sclerosis

Multiple sclerosis (MS) is discussed in detail in Chapter 5. In a substantial percentage of cases, only the spinal cord is involved on initial presentation. Changes of MS may be seen anywhere within the spinal cord. Typical presenting symptoms consist of pain, numbness, or motor deficits.

Myelographic and CT Findings. Occasionally focal cord enlargement or atrophy may be seen. Both CT and myelography are usually normal and insensitive for the detection of demyelination in the cord.

MRI Findings. MRI may reveal multiple areas of hyperintensity in the cord on proton-density and T2-weighted images. The margins are indistinct, and the lesions tend to be multiple and extend over several vertebral levels. Either solid or ring enhancement may be seen in the acute phase. The cord is usually normal in size but may be either enlarged in the acute phase or atrophic in advanced chronic disease. Intracranial lesions are seen in about 70% of cases, but a significant proportion present with spinal lesions and no evidence of intracranial disease.

TABLE 12–3 | Differential Diagnosis of Localized Signal Abnormality in Cord

Multiple sclerosis
Transverse myelitis
Myelomalacia
Syringohydromyelia
Astrocytoma
Ependymoma
Hemangioblastoma
Arteriovenous malformation
Infarction
Contusion

Differential Diagnosis

See Table 12–3. The finding of typical white matter hyperintensities in the brain is the most useful clue to MS. The diagnosis is confirmed by a set of established clinical criteria.

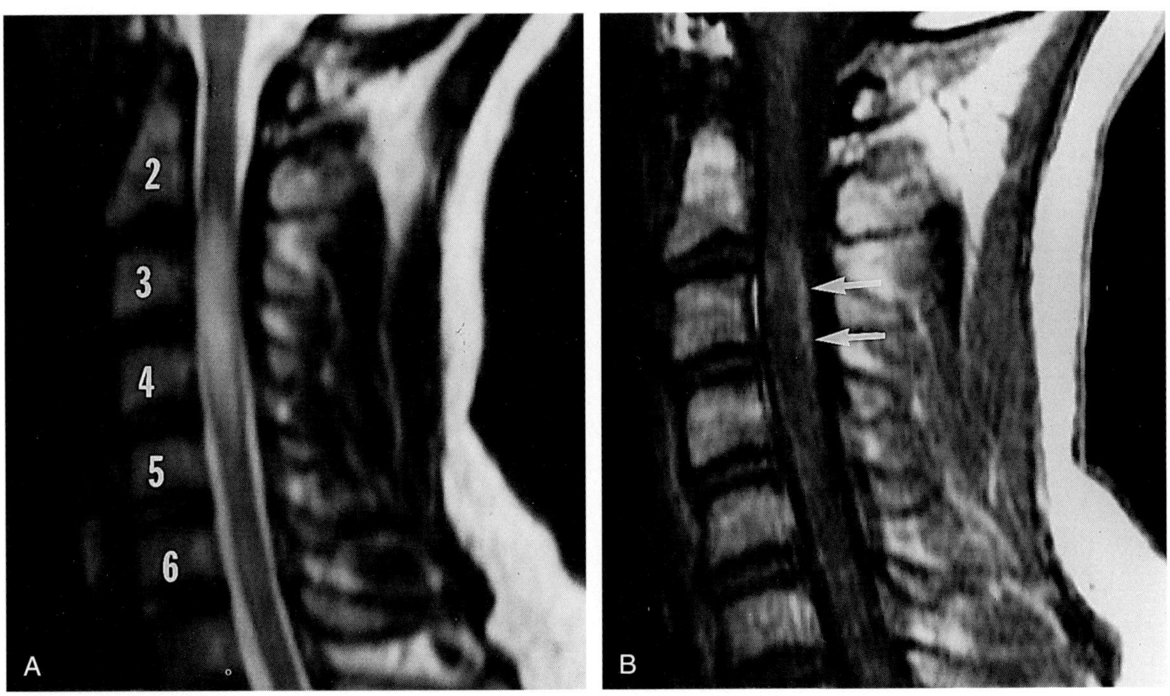

Figure 12–11. Acute MS. **(A)** Sagittal T2-weighted MRI shows a flame-shaped hyperintensity within the cord from lower C2 to the top of C5. **(B)** Mild peripheral enhancement (arrows) occurs after intravenous contrast.

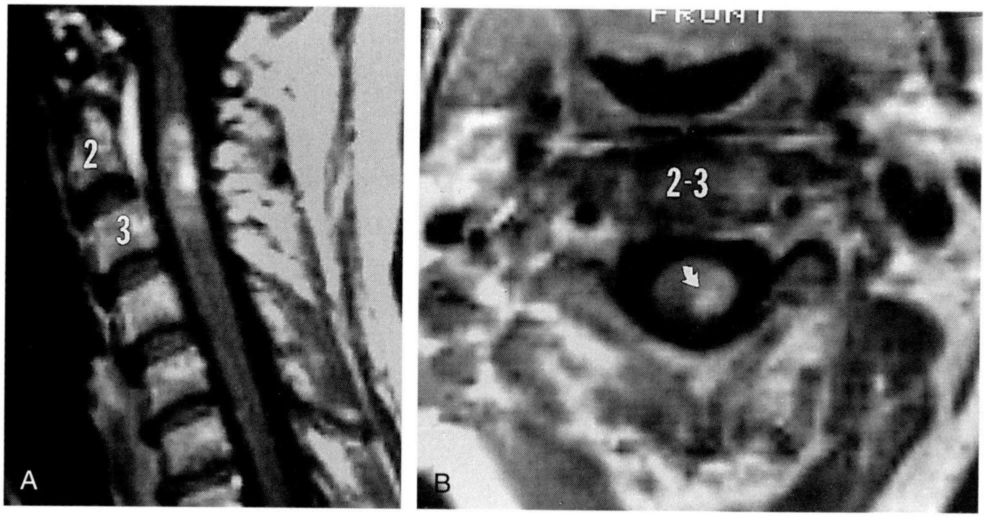

Figure 12–12. Acute MS. **(A)** Sagittal and **(B)** axial contrast-enhanced MRI show intense homogeneous enhancement (arrow in **B**) within the cord at C2–C3.

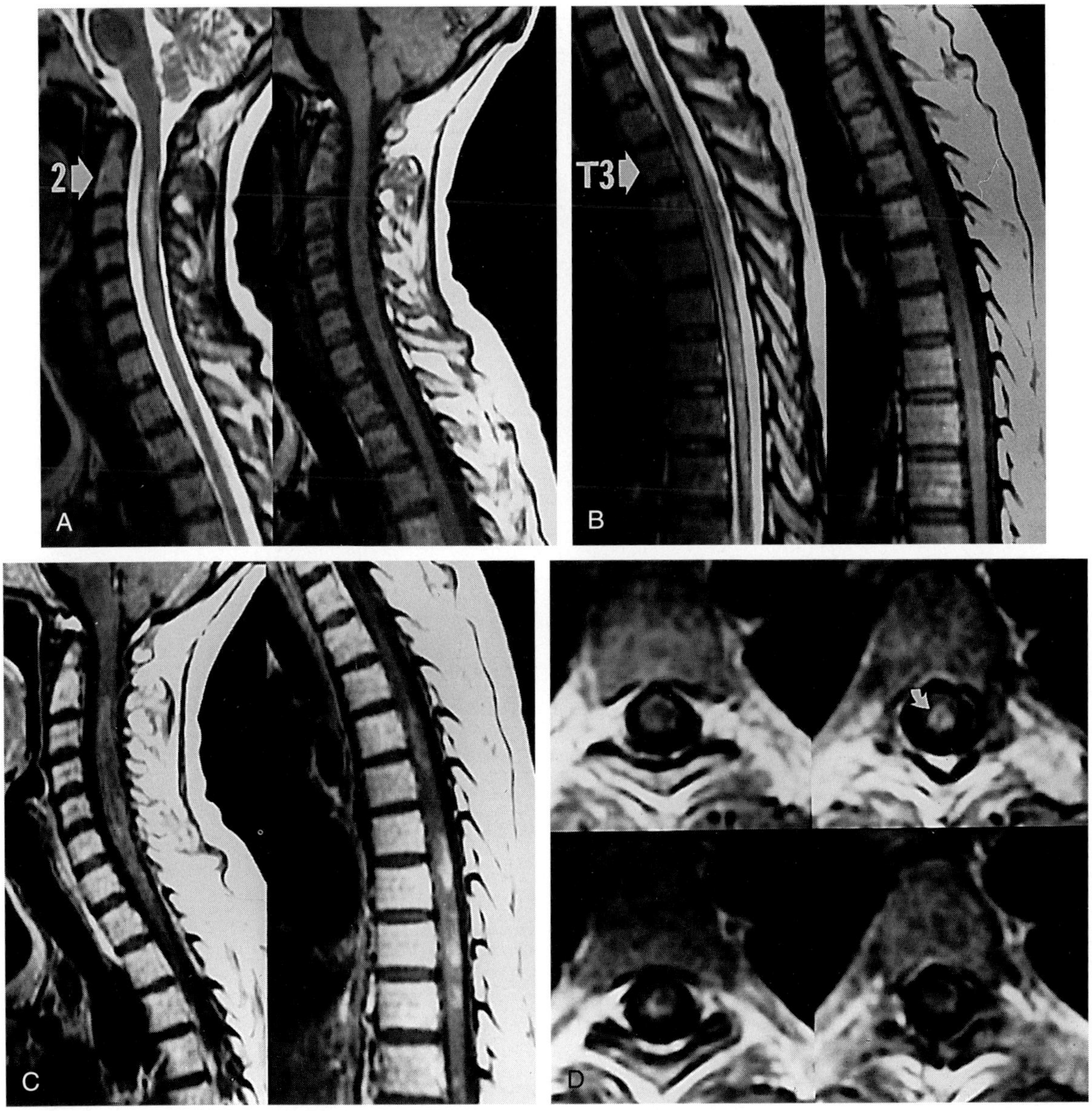

Figure 12–13. Acute MS. **(A,B)** Sagittal T2-weighted (left) and T1-weighted (right) images of the spine show edema and demyelination involving most of the spinal cord. The cord is enlarged from C2 to C6 and T3 to T9. Postcontrast **(C)** sagittal and **(D)** axial images show extensive patchy enhancement (arrow in **D**) in the cord, which is most severe posteriorly.

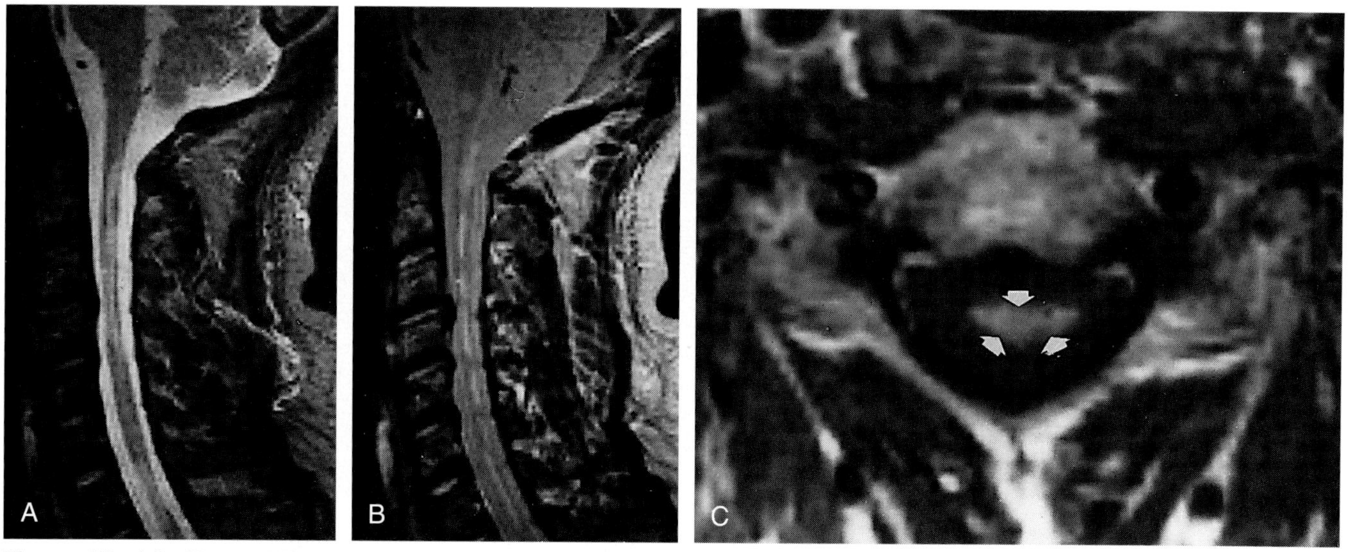

Figure 12–14. Chronic MS. Sagittal **(A)** T2-weighted and **(B)** PD-weighted MRI show atrophy and hyperintensity throughout the cervical spinal cord. **(C)** Axial T1-weighted image shows marked cord atrophy (arrows). Common causes of cord atrophy include MS, trauma, collapsed syrinx, and chronic compression.

Discitis and Osteomyelitis

Bacterial seeding of the spine may occur by way of surgery, trauma, hematogenous spread, or direct spread from a contiguous infection. Hematogenous spread from genitourinary, cutaneous, or pulmonary infections appears to be most common. *Staphylococcus aureus* is the offending organism in 60% of cases, and *Enterobacter* species cause about 30%. Less common pathogens include *Mycobacterium tuberculosis, Salmonella, Candida,* and other gram-negative rods. The infection usually originates in the anterior vertebral body and spreads into the disc space, subligamentous spaces, and adjoining vertebrae. The advancing infection may completely bypass the disc, especially in tuberculous and fungal infections. Osteomyelitis most often involves the lumbar spine, followed by the thoracic and then cervical spine. Tuberculous spondylitis is most common at L1. Most cases respond to systemic antibiotics. Abscesses, especially epidural ones, may require surgical drainage.

Radiographic and CT Findings. Plain radiographs may show end plate destruction, loss of disc space, and vertebral collapse late in the course of the illness. CT is more sensitive for bone destruction earlier in the course and may also show soft tissue changes ranging from paraspinal soft tissue swelling to extensive paraspinal abscess formation. Extensive paraspinal calcification may develop in tuberculous abscesses. Myelography should be performed only in those who cannot undergo MRI but may reveal an extradural mass or complete block.

MRI Findings. In about 65% of cases of pyogenic origin, MRI shows decreased signal intensity on T1-weighted images and increased signal intensity on T2-weighted images in the intervertebral disc and the marrow of both adjoining vertebral bodies. In 25% of cases, additional levels are involved. Loss of the intranuclear cleft, a low signal area in the center of the disc usually seen on T2 sequences by age 30, is another clue to an infected disc. The disc space may be narrowed, and as bone destruction progresses the dark cortical line of the end plate begins to disappear. Both the vertebral bodies and the disc enhance after intravenous contrast.

Soft tissue changes may range from mild swelling adjacent to the disc to extensive abscess formation. These changes are hypointense on T1-weighted images and hyperintense on T2-weighted images, and usually exhibit heterogeneous contrast enhancement.

An epidural abscess produces a mass that is hypointense on T1-weighted images and hyperintense on T2-weighted images. The diagnosis is facilitated with intravenous contrast, after which solid or heterogeneous enhancement occurs in most cases. An abscess commonly extends over two to four vertebral levels.

TABLE 12–4 | Differential Diagnosis of Osteomyelitis

Degenerative disc disease	May show similar signal changes in vertebral bodies Disc shows diminished rather than increased signal on T2-weighted images Disc enhancement is rare
Lymphoma	May involve contiguous vertebrae but spares disc space
Myeloma	Elevated serum immunoglobulins Usually multifocal and extensive Paravertebral soft tissue swelling focal or absent Discs spared
Chordoma	Unifocal mass May cross disc space Calcifications frequent Much more rare than osteomyelitis
Postoperative discectomy	May normally see enhancement of disc space and posterior annulus Enhancement of vertebral marrow is infrequent

Differential Diagnosis

See Table 12–4.

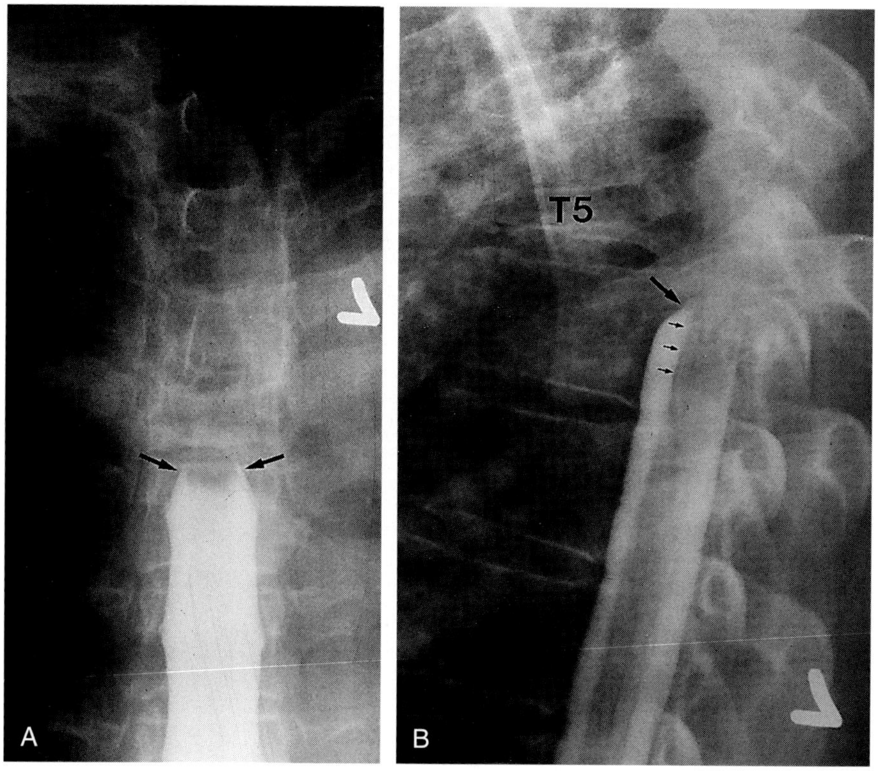

Figure 12–15. Osteomyelitis and epidural abscess. **(A)** AP and **(B)** lateral myelograms show the appearance of complete block at T5. Findings indicating the extradural nature of the process include collapse of T5, central displacement of the dural sleeve (large arrows), and tapering of the subarachnoid space to the point of the mass. The cord is posteriorly displaced (small arrows in **B**).

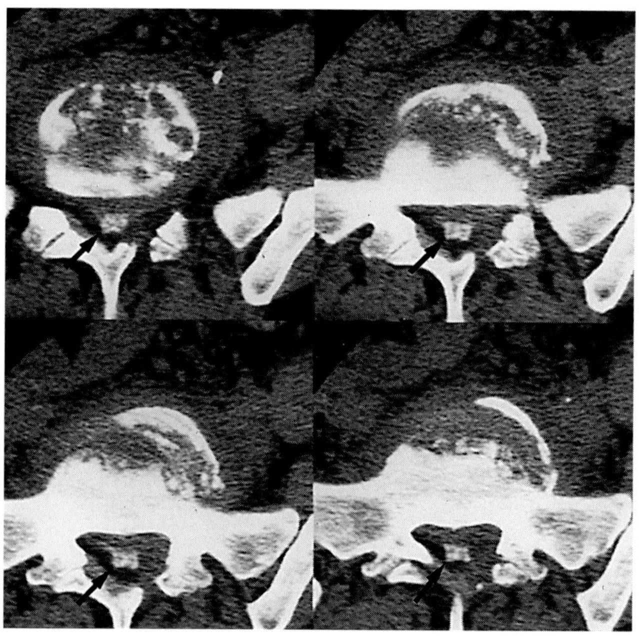

Figure 12–16. Osteomyelitis. Axial CT myelogram through L5-S1 shows extensive end plate destruction and marked paravertebral soft tissue swelling. The terminal thecal sac (arrows) is compressed.

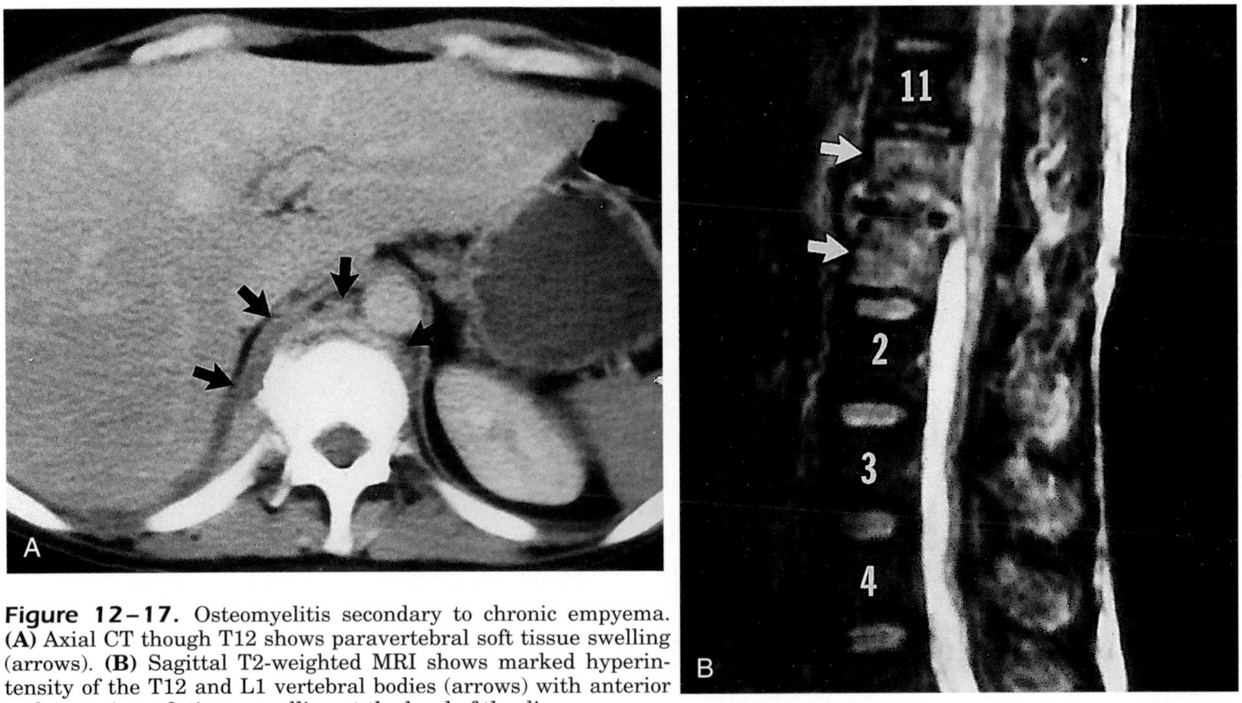

Figure 12–17. Osteomyelitis secondary to chronic empyema. **(A)** Axial CT though T12 shows paravertebral soft tissue swelling (arrows). **(B)** Sagittal T2-weighted MRI shows marked hyperintensity of the T12 and L1 vertebral bodies (arrows) with anterior and posterior soft tissue swelling at the level of the disc.

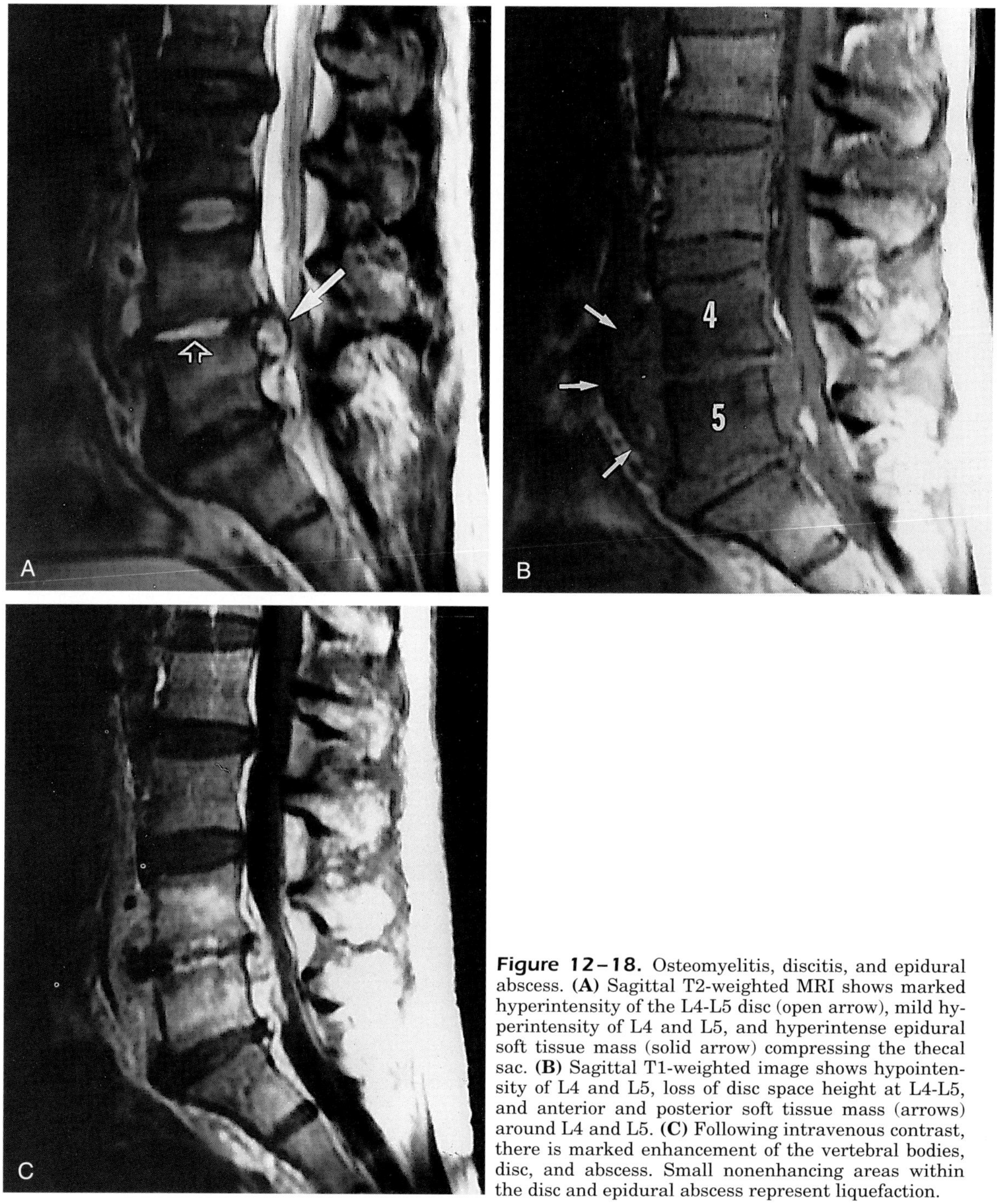

Figure 12–18. Osteomyelitis, discitis, and epidural abscess. **(A)** Sagittal T2-weighted MRI shows marked hyperintensity of the L4-L5 disc (open arrow), mild hyperintensity of L4 and L5, and hyperintense epidural soft tissue mass (solid arrow) compressing the thecal sac. **(B)** Sagittal T1-weighted image shows hypointensity of L4 and L5, loss of disc space height at L4-L5, and anterior and posterior soft tissue mass (arrows) around L4 and L5. **(C)** Following intravenous contrast, there is marked enhancement of the vertebral bodies, disc, and abscess. Small nonenhancing areas within the disc and epidural abscess represent liquefaction.

Vascular Malformations

Extramedullary Arteriovenous Malformation

Synonyms: Dural arteriovenous malformation (or fistula), radiculomeningeal vascular malformations.

Spinal dural arteriovenous fistula is a condition of middle-aged and elderly adults. Over 80% occur in males. The lesion is composed of (1) an arteriovenous shunt outside the dura but in proximity to a nerve root and (2) an enlarged, arterialized intradural vein draining the fistula. Most are seen in the lower thoracic and upper lumbar regions. Patients present with slowly progressive paraparesis, paresthesia, and bladder dysfunction due to venous hypertension and resulting ischemic myelopathy. Hemorrhage rarely, if ever, occurs.

Myelographic Findings. Myelography should include supine views of the thoracic region. The cord is usually normal. A fistula should be suspected when abnormally prominent serpiginous filling defects are identified in the subarachnoid space, especially posterior to the cord.

MRI Findings. The actual nidus or fistula site is almost never identifiable on MRI. Abnormally prominent vessels may be visible in the spinal CSF or on the surface of the cord. These may be more prominent after intravenous contrast. Mild cord swelling with enlargement of the cord contour, decreased signal on T1-weighted images, and increased signal on T2-weighted images are usually present in the lower cord and conus medullaris. Enhancement of the abnormal cord commonly occurs following intravenous contrast.

Angiographic Findings. Complete spinal angiography may be necessary to identify the precise location of the fistula, which is usually supplied by a single pedicle. Selective injection of the feeding pedicle reveals a small tangle of vessels feeding the fistula, which lies outside the dura in proximity to a nerve root. Venous drainage extends into the coronal venous plexus surrounding the spinal cord, and abnormally enlarged vessels may extend for a considerable distance. The veins may be slow to fill, and imaging should continue for at least 20 seconds following injection.

Differential Diagnosis

See Table 12–5. Multiple serpiginous filling defects are seen on myelography in the redundant lumbar nerve root syndrome. These represent tortuous stretched nerve roots, are always associated with severe lumbar stenosis, and occur above a myelographic block.

With high-quality MRI, especially using phased array coils, it is common to see normal enhancing vessels posterior to the cord. Many of these patients have undergone complete spinal angiography with negative results. This MRI appearance, with normal underlying cord parenchyma, may be referred to as "pseudo-AVM."

TABLE 12–5 | Differential Diagnosis of Spinal Vascular Malformations

	Intramedullary AVM	Dural AVF
Age/sex	Children and young adults (mean age 20)	Middle-aged and elderly men
Clinical presentation	Acute hemorrhage	Progressive myelopathy
Relative incidence	20%	80%
Location of nidus	Spinal cord	On or adjacent to dura
Feeding vessels	Anterior spinal arteries	Posterior spinal arteries
Myelography	Enlarged cord and multiple enlarged vessels	Enlarged tortuous draining veins and normal cord
MRI	AVM nidus in cord Vessels in subarachnoid space	Cord hyperintensity on T2-weighted images but no nidus Vessels in subarachnoid space
Angiography	AVM in intradural or intramedullary location Multiple large feeding arteries Aneurysms Rapid shunting Large draining veins	AVM in extradural location Normal-size single feeding artery Nidus may be subtle with delayed venous drainage Single large draining vein

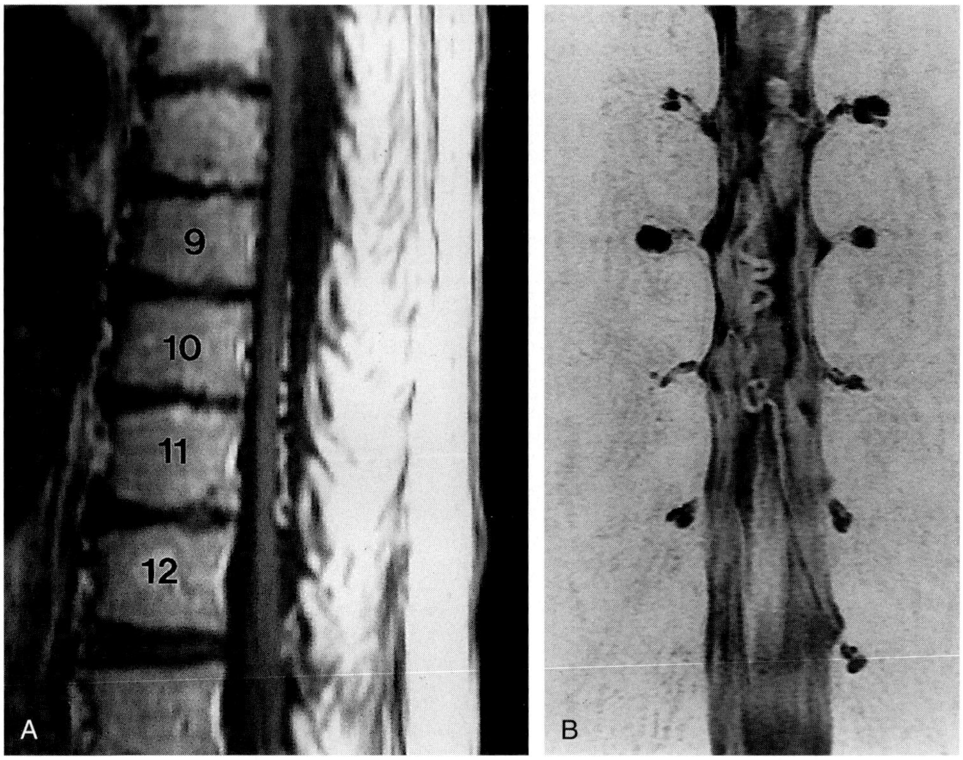

Figure 12–19. Pseudo-AVM. **(A)** Sagittal contrast-enhanced MRI shows marked enhancement of serpiginous vessels dorsal to the cord at T10-T11. **(B)** MR myelogram (AP projection) shows tortuous filling defects. Complete spinal angiography was negative. (**B** courtesy of Dr. Taher El Gammal, Birmingham, AL.)

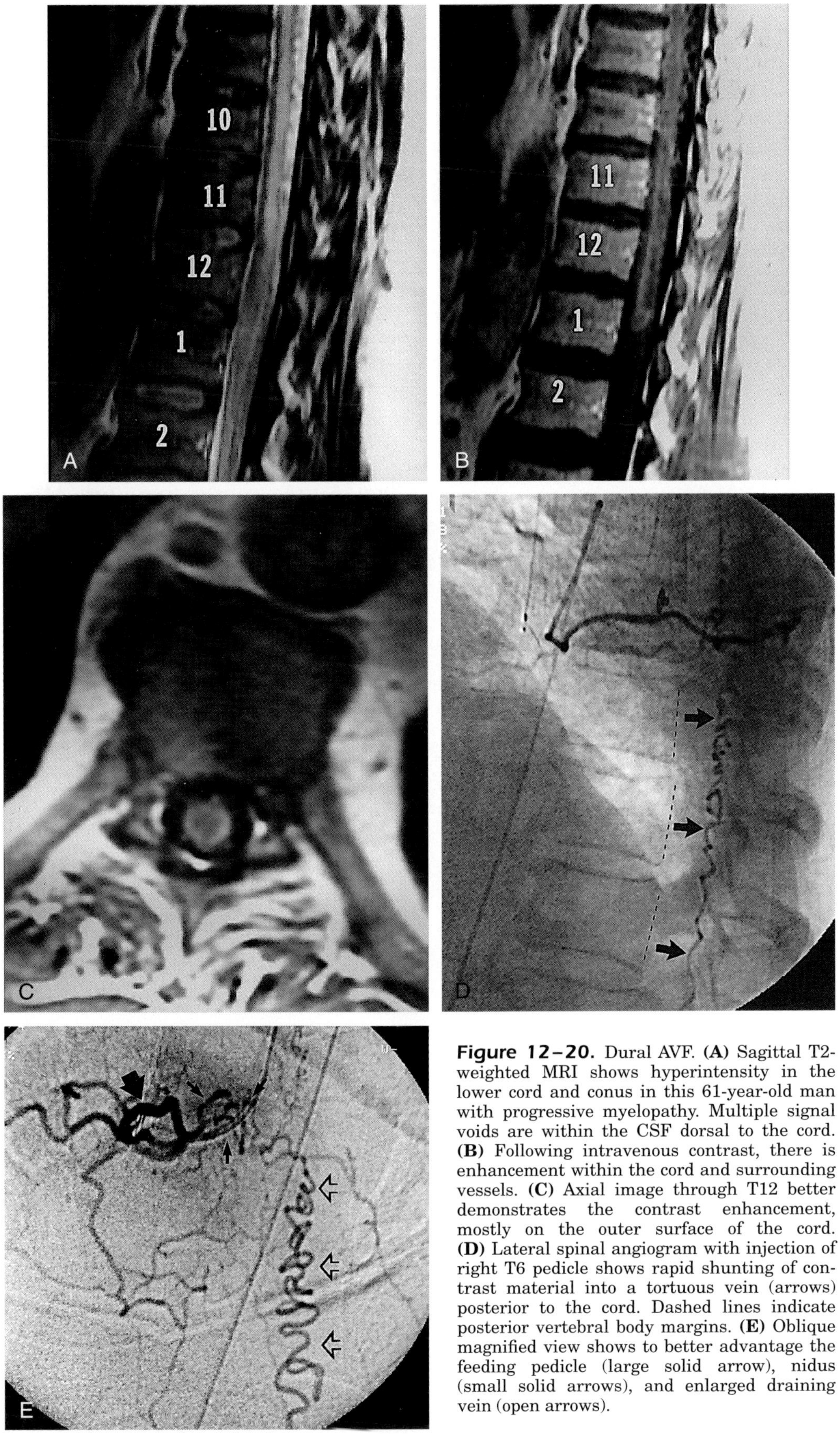

Figure 12–20. Dural AVF. **(A)** Sagittal T2-weighted MRI shows hyperintensity in the lower cord and conus in this 61-year-old man with progressive myelopathy. Multiple signal voids are within the CSF dorsal to the cord. **(B)** Following intravenous contrast, there is enhancement within the cord and surrounding vessels. **(C)** Axial image through T12 better demonstrates the contrast enhancement, mostly on the outer surface of the cord. **(D)** Lateral spinal angiogram with injection of right T6 pedicle shows rapid shunting of contrast material into a tortuous vein (arrows) posterior to the cord. Dashed lines indicate posterior vertebral body margins. **(E)** Oblique magnified view shows to better advantage the feeding pedicle (large solid arrow), nidus (small solid arrows), and enlarged draining vein (open arrows).

Intramedullary Arteriovenous Malformation

Arteriovenous malformations (AVMs) of the spinal cord usually occur with acute subarachnoid or spinal cord hemorrhage in a child or young adult. AVMs are about one fourth as common as spinal dural arteriovenous fistulae. Spinal AVMs exhibit the same features as cerebral AVMs, namely, multiple enlarged feeding arteries, a nidus of tangled arteriovenous shunts, and enlarged draining veins. They are distributed throughout the cord, with a slightly higher frequency in the thoracic levels.

Myelographic and CT Findings. Myelography will usually demonstrate an area of fusiform enlargement of the cord. The abnormal feeding and draining vessels produce multiple tortuous curvilinear filling defects in the opacified subarachnoid space, indicating the vascular nature of the process. CT with intrathecal contrast shows multiple filling defects in the subarachnoid space and an enlarged cord.

MRI Findings. The nidus of an AVM of the cord demonstrates an intramedullary or peripheral mass deforming the cord contour with signal characteristics indicative of flow (signal void or flow-related enhancement). Abnormally enlarged vessels, mostly representing draining veins, appear as curvilinear structures in the surrounding CSF. With very large lesions, enlarged intercostal or lumbar arterial feeders may be identified. Signal abnormalities in the adjacent cord may be present as a result of edema, hemorrhage, or thrombosis.

Angiographic Findings. Complete spinal angiography is required in the clinical management of these malformations to identify all vessels feeding the malformation as well as the primary supply to the spinal cord. The usual characteristics of an AVM are present, consisting of (1) enlarged arterial feeders, (2) a nidus of small complex vessels, (3) early venous filling, and (4) enlarged draining veins. Aneurysms may be present in arteries supplying the malformation or within the malformation. Intramedullary AVMs are usually supplied by the anterior spinal artery. Less often they are supplied by one of the posterior spinal arteries in addition to, or instead of, the anterior spinal artery.

Differential Diagnosis

See Table 12–5.

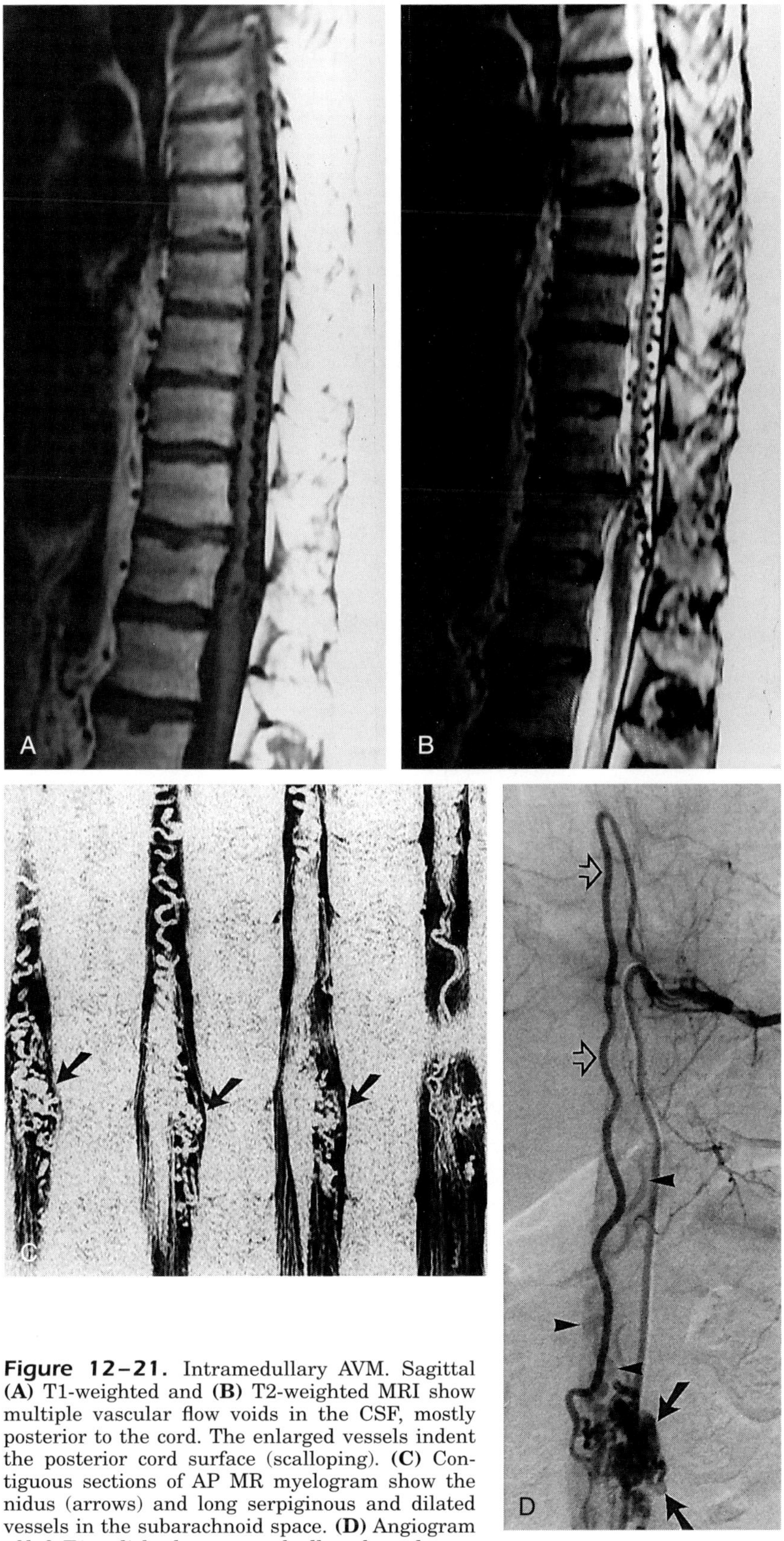

Figure 12–21. Intramedullary AVM. Sagittal **(A)** T1-weighted and **(B)** T2-weighted MRI show multiple vascular flow voids in the CSF, mostly posterior to the cord. The enlarged vessels indent the posterior cord surface (scalloping). **(C)** Contiguous sections of AP MR myelogram show the nidus (arrows) and long serpiginous and dilated vessels in the subarachnoid space. **(D)** Angiogram of left T9 pedicle shows a markedly enlarged anterior spinal artery (open arrows), nidus (large solid arrows), and early draining vein (arrowheads). (**C** courtesy of Dr. Taher El Gammal, Birmingham, AL.)

Vertebral Hemangioma

Hemangiomas are common in the vertebrae, with an incidence as high as 11% documented at autopsy. The vast majority are diagnosed incidentally and remain asymptomatic throughout life. Some behave more aggressively and may expand, leading to symptoms of back pain or even cord compression. The histology in most cases is that of cavernous hemangioma, and the most common sites are the lower thoracic and upper lumbar vertebral bodies.

Radiographic Findings. Hemangiomas of the vertebra frequently manifest a distinct, virtually pathognomonic appearance on spine radiographs. There is decreased density of the vertebral body, with accentuation of the vertical trabecula giving a striated or corduroy appearance. A honeycomb trabecular pattern may also occur.

CT Findings. Hemangiomas characteristically exhibit a polka dot pattern resulting from dense vertical trabeculae scanned in cross section, set against a background of lower attenuation. The background attenuation may be as low as fat (−70 to −90 HU). More aggressive lesions tend to exhibit a background attenuation more closely approximating soft tissue (20 to 40 HU) and may progress to posterior element involvement, bone expansion or destruction, vertebral compression, and spinal canal encroachment.

MRI Findings. Hemangiomas are a common incidental finding on MRI. The usual appearance is a mass within the vertebral body exhibiting a mottled hyperintensity on both T1- and T2-weighted images. With high resolution techniques, the coarsened trabecula appear as hypointense structures within the mass. Highly aggressive lesions contain little or no fat and are hypointense on T1-weighted images. Extraosseous extension may be present, leading to cord compression.

Differential Diagnosis

Focal fatty transformation of the marrow is also hyperintense on T1-weighted images but not on true T2-weighted images. Fat remains hyperintense on T2-weighted fast spin echo scans. The rare aggressive and hypercellular hemangiomas must be distinguished from other primary and metastatic vertebral tumors, such as plasmacytoma, giant cell tumor, and lymphoma.

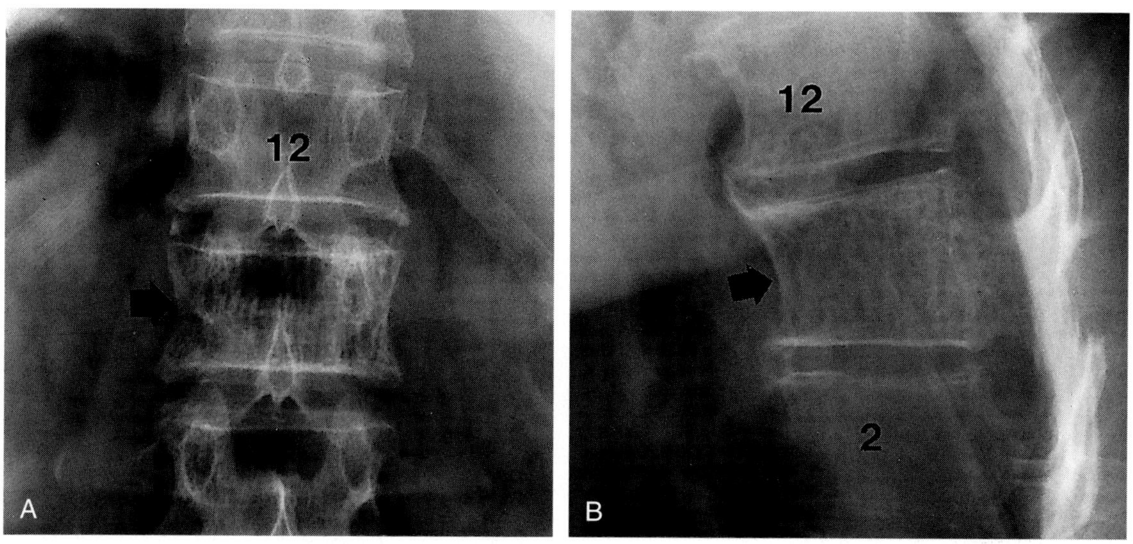

Figure 12–22. Hemangioma. **(A)** AP and **(B)** lateral radiographs show lucency of L1 (arrow) with thick and dense vertical trabeculae.

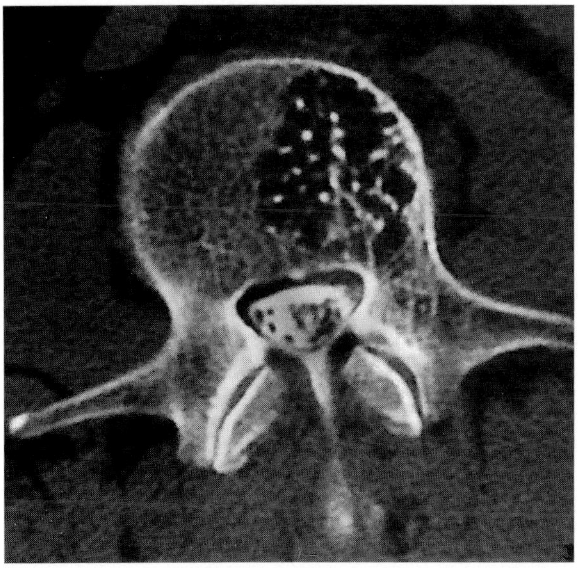

Figure 12–23. Hemangioma. CT myelogram shows a large lucency within L2 punctuated by dense sclerotic vertical trabeculae in cross section. The very low background density indicates a large fatty component. There is no effect on the thecal sac from this incidentally discovered hemangioma.

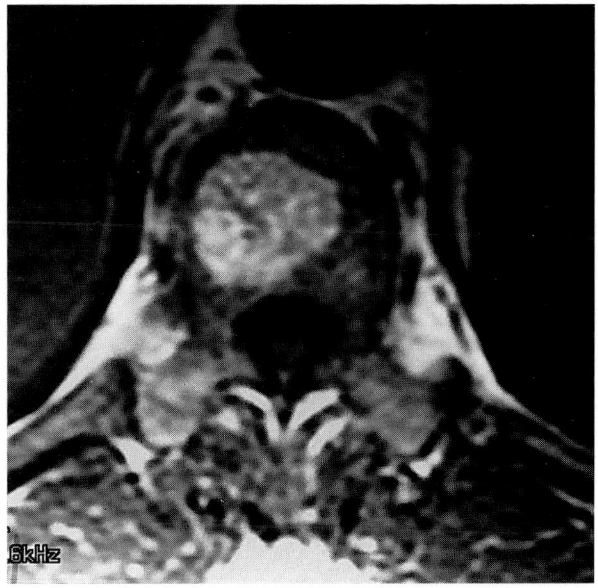

Figure 12–24. Hemangioma. Axial T1-weighted MRI shows a hyperintense mass with a large fatty component punctuated by hypointensities caused by vertical trabeculae in cross section.

Primary Neoplasms

Astrocytoma

Astrocytomas compose about 30% of all intramedullary spinal neoplasms but less than 1% of all CNS tumors. The ratio of cerebral to spinal astrocytomas is 20 to 1. They occur more commonly in males and usually present in the first three decades of life. Astrocytomas arise most commonly in the cervical cord, followed by the thoracic cord, with clinical manifestations of weakness, pain, incontinence, and sensory deficits. About 75% are low-grade tumors (fibrillary or pilocytic) with a good prognosis following resection.

Myelographic and CT Findings. Myelography reveals expansion of the spinal cord or complete block. CT with intrathecal contrast shows cord enlargement with effacement of the subarachnoid space. Pressure erosion of the bony canal is present in up to 50% and is manifested by thinning of the pedicles and laminar arch and scalloping of the posterior vertebral body.

MRI Findings. MRI reveals expansion of the spinal cord, usually with decreased signal intensity on T1-weighted images and increased signal intensity on T2-weighted images. Long segments or even the entire cord may be involved. Nearly all enhance after contrast, usually in a patchy irregular manner with areas of cystic change or necrosis. Syringohydromyelia is occasionally present and usually cervical in location. There is considerable overlap with the appearance of ependymoma, and the two cannot be reliably distinguished by imaging findings.

TABLE 12–6 | Neoplasms of the Spinal Cord

Tumor	Proportion of Cord Tumors	Comments
Ependymoma	65%	Usually conus or filum terminale May present with hemorrhage Increased incidence with type 2 neurofibromatosis
Astrocytoma	30%	More common than ependymomas within the cervicothoracic cord Younger age of presentation
Hemangioblastoma	3%	One third have von Hippel-Lindau disease with multiple tumors
Cavernous hemangioma	Rare	Resembles intracerebral cavernomas, with enhancing core and distinctive hemosiderin rim
Metastasis	Rare	Most often from lung carcinoma Discrete solid enhancing mass

Differential Diagnosis

See Table 12–6.

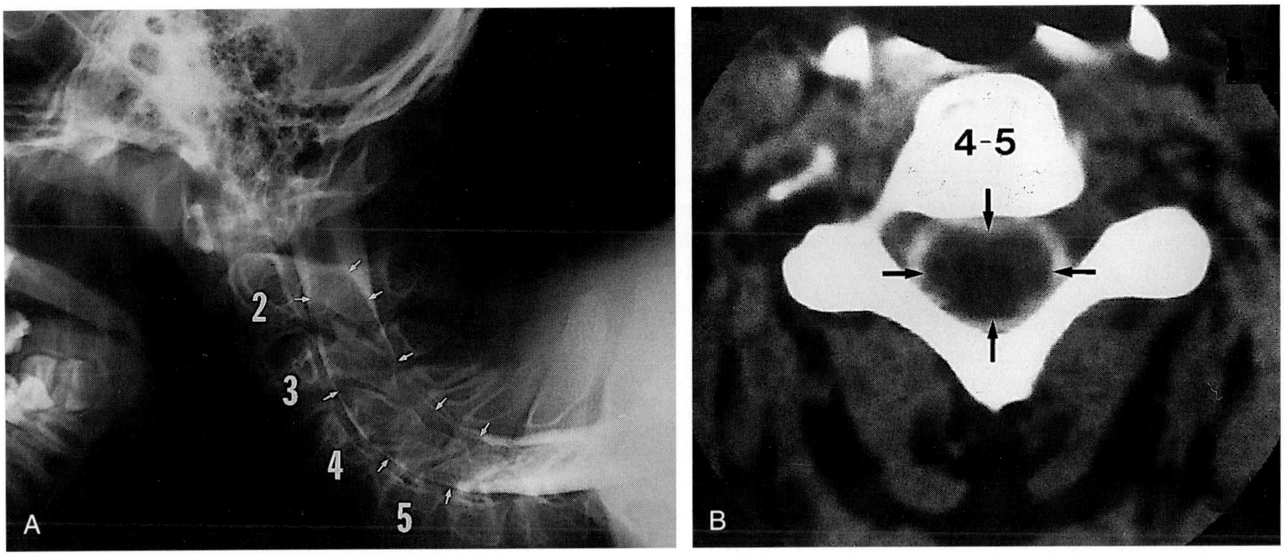

Figure 12–25. Astrocytoma. **(A)** Lateral myelogram shows fusiform expansion of the cord (arrows) from C2 to C6. **(B)** Axial CT myelogram through C4-C5 shows circumferential expansion of the cord (arrows).

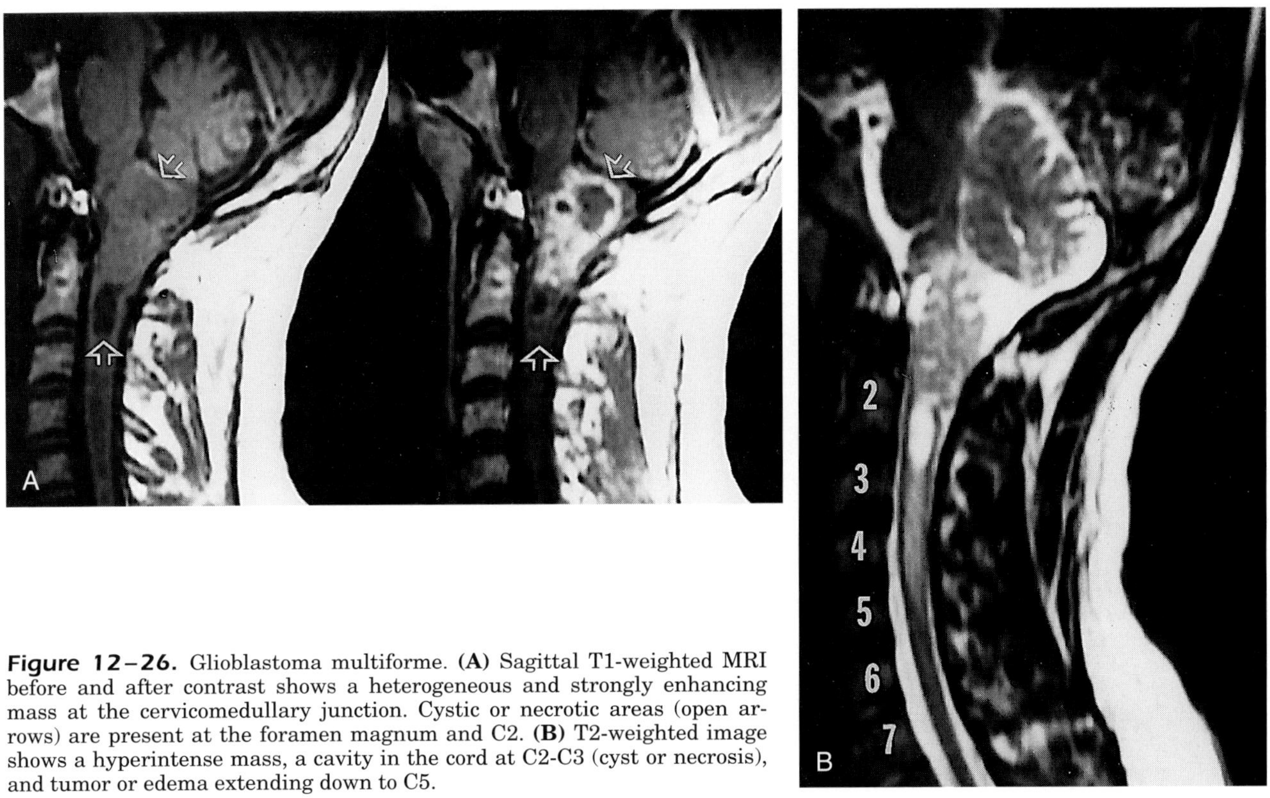

Figure 12–26. Glioblastoma multiforme. **(A)** Sagittal T1-weighted MRI before and after contrast shows a heterogeneous and strongly enhancing mass at the cervicomedullary junction. Cystic or necrotic areas (open arrows) are present at the foramen magnum and C2. **(B)** T2-weighted image shows a hyperintense mass, a cavity in the cord at C2-C3 (cyst or necrosis), and tumor or edema extending down to C5.

Ependymoma

Ependymomas compose about 65% of all intramedullary neoplasms. They are slightly more common in males and tend to occur in the third through sixth decades, peaking in the fourth. Most spinal ependymomas arise from the lower cord, particularly the conus medullaris, or the filum terminale. Patients often present with local or radicular pain. Some ependymomas are highly vascular and may become manifest with spontaneous subarachnoid hemorrhage.

Myelographic and CT Findings. Myelography reveals enlargement of the spinal cord or an intradural mass in the lumbar spinal canal. Complete block may be present. CT with intrathecal contrast shows expansion of the cord and effacement of the surrounding subarachnoid space. Enlargement of the spinal canal due to mass effect is present in 15–35%, with scalloping of the posterior vertebral body and thinning and separation of the pedicles.

MRI Findings. MRI shows enlargement of the spinal cord, especially the conus, or a mass below the cord arising from the filum terminale. The mass typically extends over one to five vertebral segments. Ependymomas tend to be isointense with the cord on T1-weighted images and hyperintense on T2-weighted images. It has been reported that prominent hypointensity on T2 images within the tumor or at the tumor margins, probably due to hemorrhage, is strongly suggestive of ependymoma. Intense, homogeneous, and sharply marginated enhancement occurs in most cases. Intratumoral cysts may be seen on enhanced studies. Syringohydromyelia is occasionally present and usually cervical in location.

Differential Diagnosis

See Table 12–6.

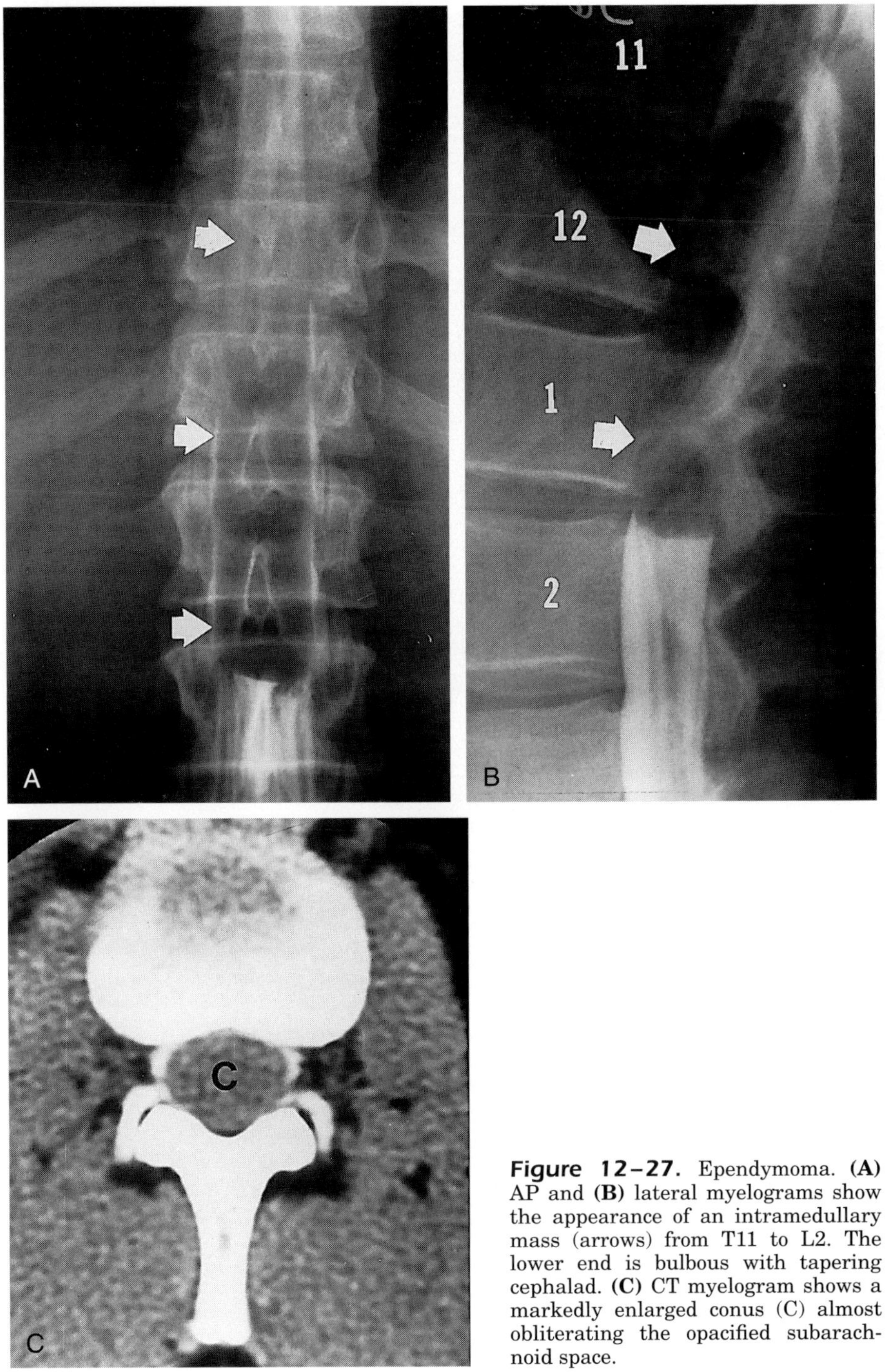

Figure 12–27. Ependymoma. **(A)** AP and **(B)** lateral myelograms show the appearance of an intramedullary mass (arrows) from T11 to L2. The lower end is bulbous with tapering cephalad. **(C)** CT myelogram shows a markedly enlarged conus (C) almost obliterating the opacified subarachnoid space.

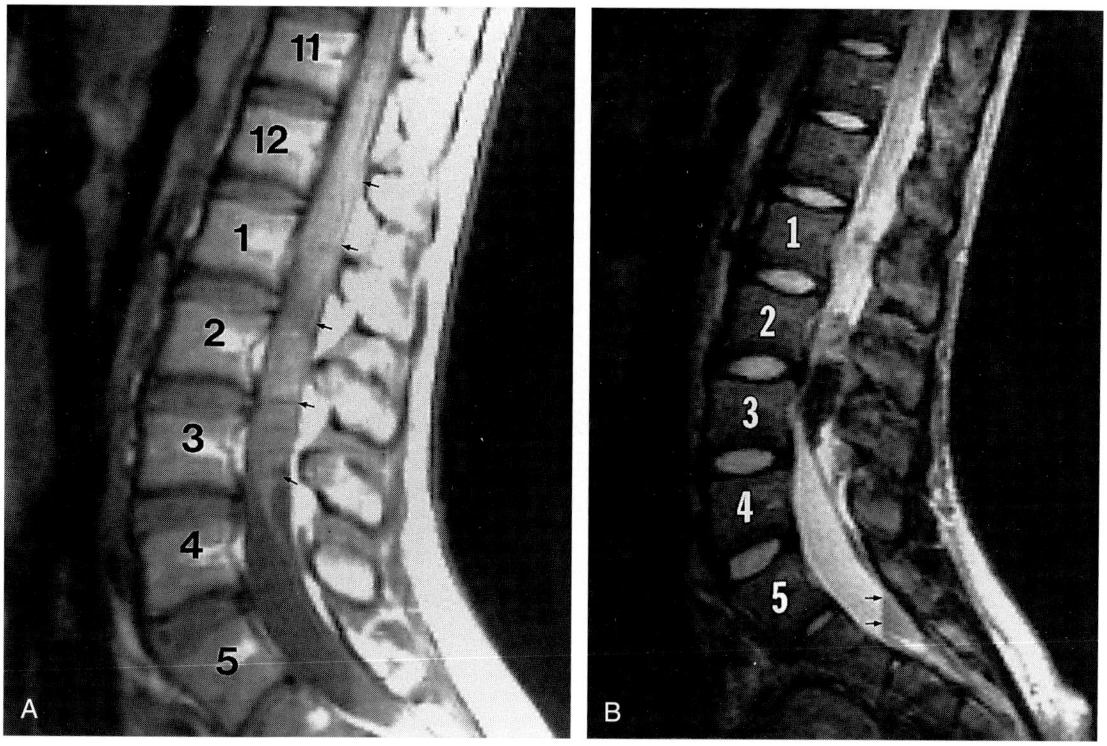

Figure 12–28. Ependymoma. **(A)** Sagittal T1-weighted MRI shows a mass (arrows) extending from L3 to at least T10. **(B)** T2-weighted MRI shows hyperintensity of the tumor, marked hypointensity at L2-L3 due to hemorrhage, and fluid-fluid level (arrows) in the subarachnoid space at S1-S2 caused by layering of blood products.

Hemangioblastoma

Hemangiomas account for approximately 3% of all intramedullary neoplasms. Like cerebral hemangioblastomas, they may be solid (40%) or cystic (60%), with enhancing mural nodules. About 60% arise in the thoracic cord, and 40% in the cervical cord. One third of spinal hemangioblastomas are associated with von Hippel-Lindau disease (Table 12–7).

Myelographic and CT Findings. Myelography and CT reveal the common features of cord tumors: cord expansion, effacement of the subarachnoid space, and possibly block. Intense enhancement of the mass has been observed on CT.

MRI Findings. MRI reveals expansion of the cord. In 60% of cases, there is a well-defined cyst or full-blown syrinx with enhancing mural nodule. The cyst may involve multiple cord segments. The remaining 40% exhibit a solid cord mass with intense enhancement. The hypervascular nature of these tumors may be reflected in the visualization of serpiginous flow voids dorsal to the cord. Hemangioblastomas are multiple in 20% of patients, usually those with von Hippel-Lindau disease.

Angiographic Findings. Spinal angiography will reveal the vascular nature of these tumors, with enlarged feeding arteries, intense staining, and early venous drainage.

TABLE 12–7 Incidence of Features of von Hippel-Landau Disease

Feature	Incidence
Single or multiple cerebral hemangioblastomas	36–60%
Single or multiple spinal hemangioblastomas	5%
Renal cell carcinoma	25–38%
Retinal angiomatosis	>50%
Pheochromocytoma	>10%
Pancreatic cysts	60–80%
Renal cysts	60–100%
Epididymal cysts (males)	50–60%

Differential Diagnosis

See Table 12–6.

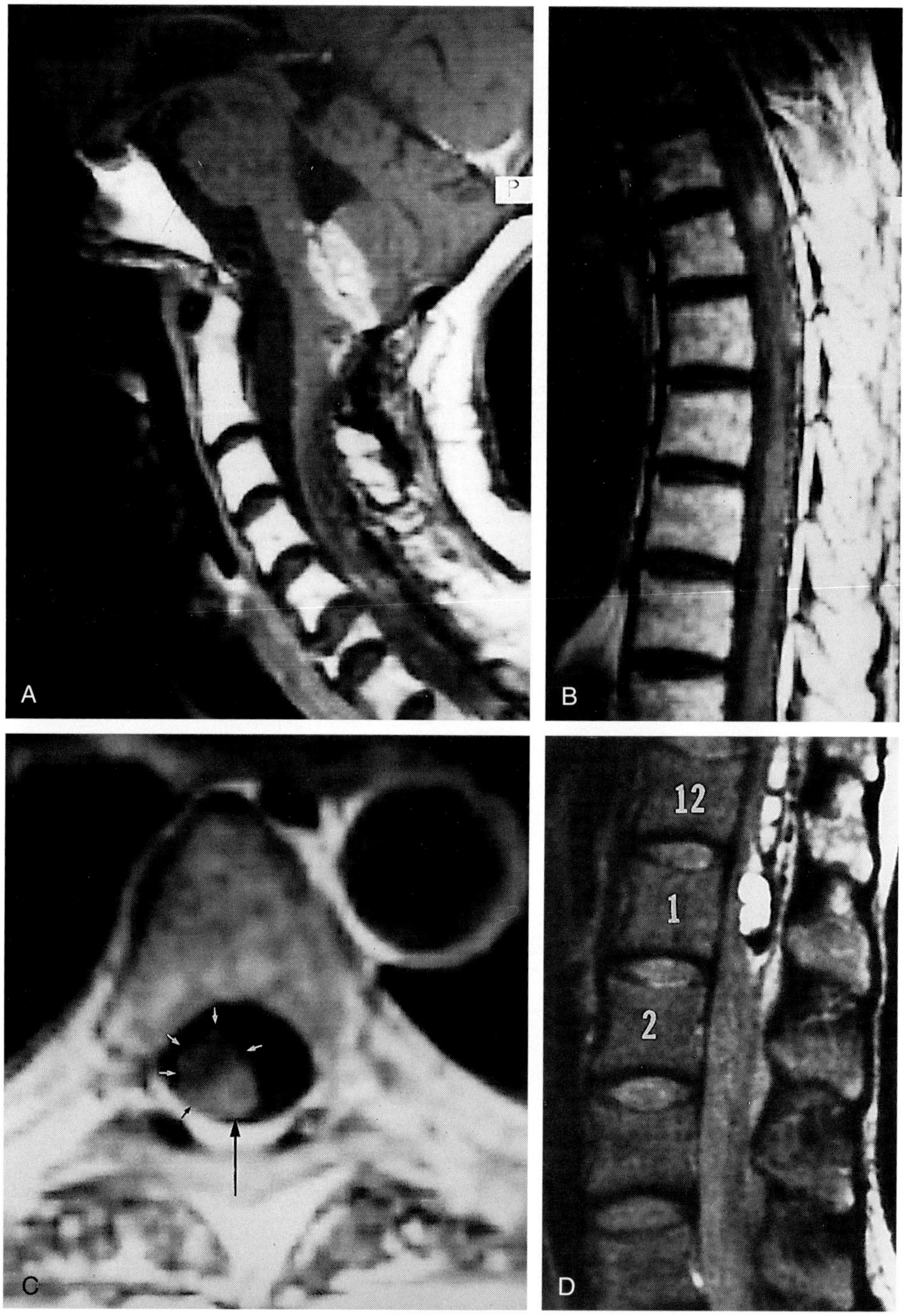

Figure 12–29. Multiple hemangioblastomas (von Hippel-Lindau syndrome). **(A,B)** Sagittal contrast-enhanced MRI shows a solid intensely enhancing mass of the inferior vermis, multiple enhancing tumors of the cord, and enlarged enhancing vessels in the spinal subarachnoid space. **(C)** Axial contrast-enhanced image establishes the intramedullary location of a tumor (long arrow) on the dorsal spinal cord (short arrows). **(D)** Sagittal T2-weighted image of the lumbar spine shows cavitation/cyst formation and hemorrhage in the lower cord and conus medullaris (T12 and L1).

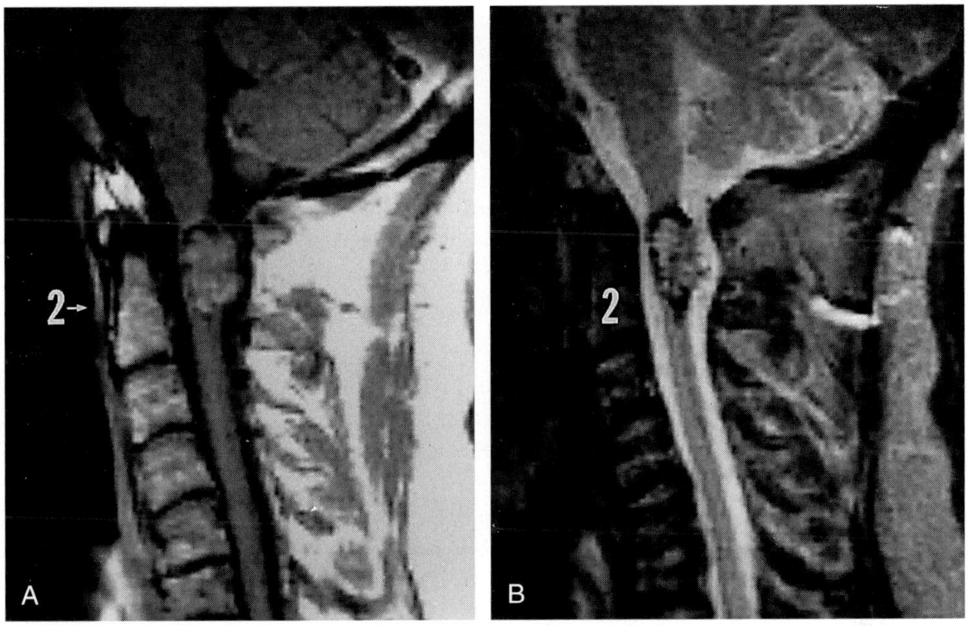

Figure 12–30. Cavernous hemangioma. **(A)** Sagittal contrast-enhanced MRI shows an intramedullary mass at C1-C2 with moderate central enhancement. **(B)** T2-weighted image shows the features of a markedly hypointense hemosiderin rim, nodular mulberrylike texture, and central hyperintensity.

Meningioma

Meningiomas compose about 25% of all spinal tumors and are the second most common spinal tumor after schwannomas. There is a strong (9 to 1) female predominance with a peak incidence in the fifth and sixth decades. About 80% originate in the thoracic spine, 15% in the cervical spine, and 5% in the lumbar spine. Most meningiomas arise posterolateral to the cord. Cervical lesions, however, tend to arise at the craniocervical junction and are usually anterior to the cord. Multiple meningiomas may be encountered in neurofibromatosis.

Myelographic and CT Findings. Myelography reveals the presence of an extramedullary intradural mass. A small percentage are purely extradural. These findings are also reflected on intrathecally enhanced CT. Without intrathecal contrast, CT may show a hyperdense mass with marked enhancement. Only about 10% manifest calcification or bony changes (hyperostosis, erosion, foraminal enlargement).

MRI Findings. The signal characteristics are variable, but most meningiomas are isointense or hypointense relative to the spinal cord on both T1- and T2-weighted images. Intense uniform enhancement typically results from intravenous contrast. A dural tail sign may be present and is a distinguishing feature of meningiomas.

Differential Diagnosis

Meningioma must be distinguished from other causes of extramedullary intradural masses, especially nerve sheath tumor (Table 12–2). Features favoring meningioma include middle age and female gender, location in the thoracic spine or foramen magnum, absence of bone changes and calcification, solid enhancement, and position ventral to the cord.

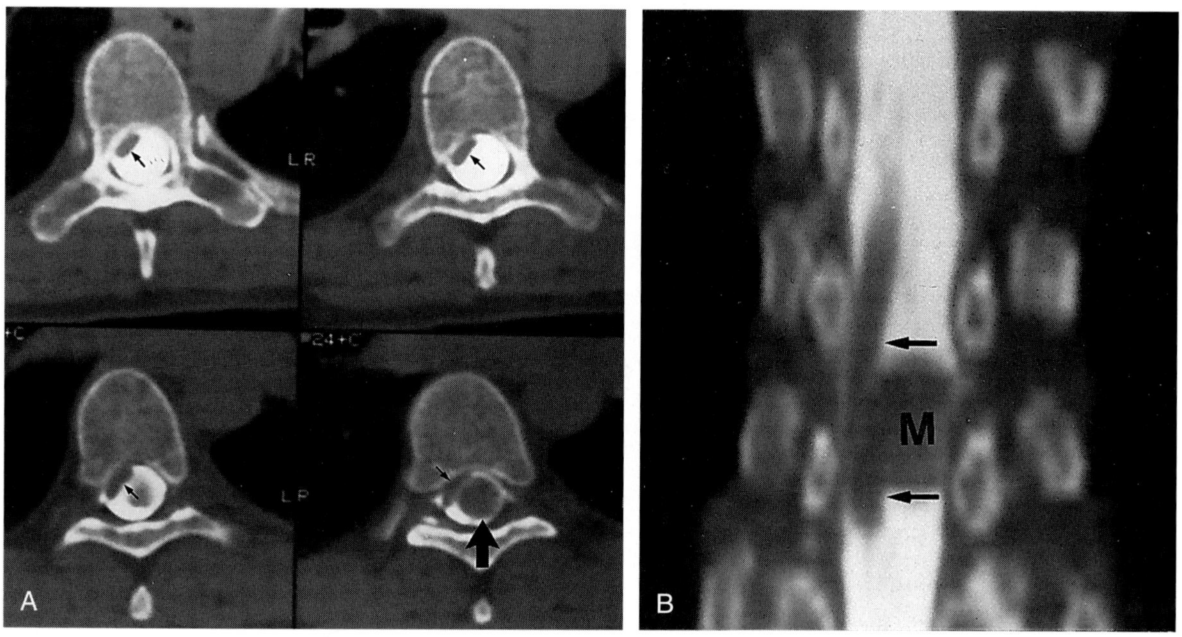

Figure 12–31. Meningioma. **(A)** Contiguous sections of a CT myelogram show anterolateral displacement of the spinal cord (small arrows) by an intradural extramedullary mass (large arrow). **(B)** Coronal reformatted image shows the classic appearance of an intradural extramedullary mass (M) displacing the cord (arrows) to the right. Note the CSF cap above and below the mass.

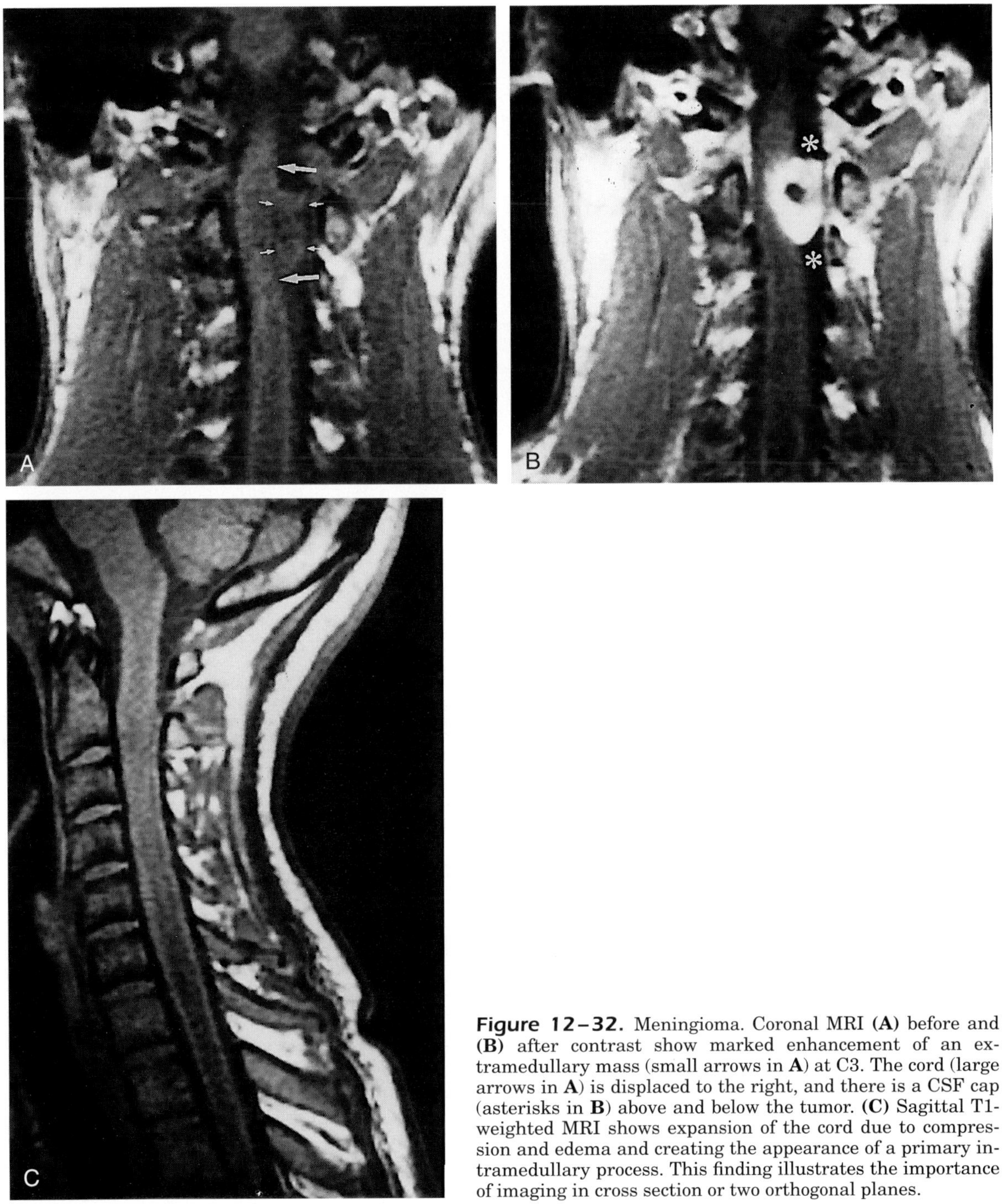

Figure 12–32. Meningioma. Coronal MRI **(A)** before and **(B)** after contrast show marked enhancement of an extramedullary mass (small arrows in **A**) at C3. The cord (large arrows in **A**) is displaced to the right, and there is a CSF cap (asterisks in **B**) above and below the tumor. **(C)** Sagittal T1-weighted MRI shows expansion of the cord due to compression and edema and creating the appearance of a primary intramedullary process. This finding illustrates the importance of imaging in cross section or two orthogonal planes.

Schwannoma and Neurofibroma

Nerve sheath tumors are the most common intraspinal neoplasm, accounting for about 30%. Almost all are schwannomas, except in patients with neurofibromatosis, in whom neurofibromas also occur. Schwannomas usually present in the fourth and fifth decades and are slightly more common in females. Their level of occurrence is evenly distributed along the spinal axis. Multiple nerve sheath tumors are common in neurofibromatosis, particularly type 2. Radicular pain is the most frequent clinical manifestation, and solitary schwannomas are amenable to surgical resection, usually with preservation of the nerve root.

Myelographic and CT Findings. Usually myelography will demonstrate the classic appearance of an ovoid extramedullary intradural mass. Approximately 15% are dumbbell tumors extending from within the dura through a neural foramen, and approximately 15% are purely extradural. CT with intrathecal contrast will show the mass displacing the cord or completely effacing the subarachnoid space at the level of the tumor. On CT, neurofibromas are hypodense relative to muscle, whereas schwannomas tend to be isodense to muscle. Smooth bony erosion of the vertebral body or margins of the neural foramen is frequently present.

MRI Findings. The appearance is variable. In most cases, however, schwannomas are hyperintense relative to the spinal cord and CSF on T2-weighted images and isointense to hypointense to the cord on T1-weighted images. After intravenous contrast, they enhance heterogeneously. A pattern of enhancement limited to the periphery (ring enhancement) is highly suggestive of the diagnosis. Neurofibromas are hyperintense on T2-weighted images but often with a central area of decreased signal intensity.

Angiographic Findings. Angiography is normally reserved only for large cervical lesions. On selective angiography, schwannomas are moderately hypervascular. They are characterized by tortuous and irregular tumor vessels, the absence of arteriovenous shunting, and "puddles" of contrast 1 to 4 mm in size extending over the late arterial to late venous phases.

Differential Diagnosis

Nerve sheath tumors must be distinguished from other causes of extramedullary intradural tumors, especially meningiomas. Factors favoring nerve sheath tumors include multiplicity, bone remodeling, extradural extension, and heterogeneous or ring enhancement.

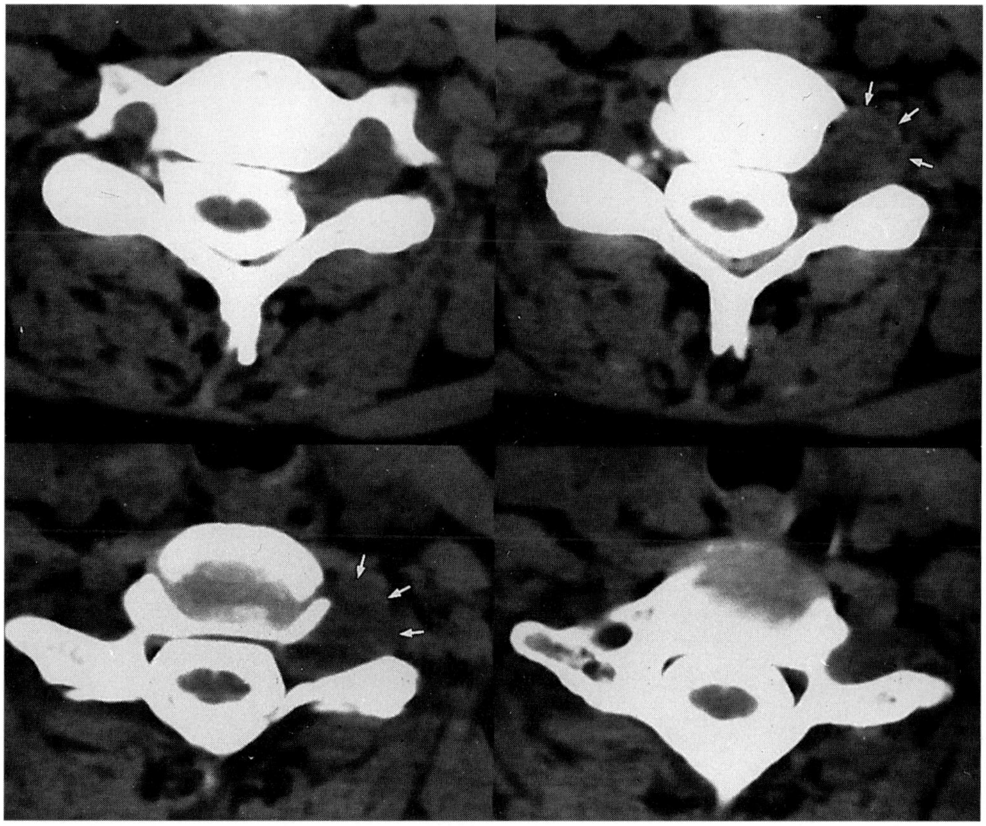

Figure 12–33. Schwannoma. (extradural). CT myelogram shows a soft tissue mass (arrows) filling and expanding the left C6-C7 neural foramen.

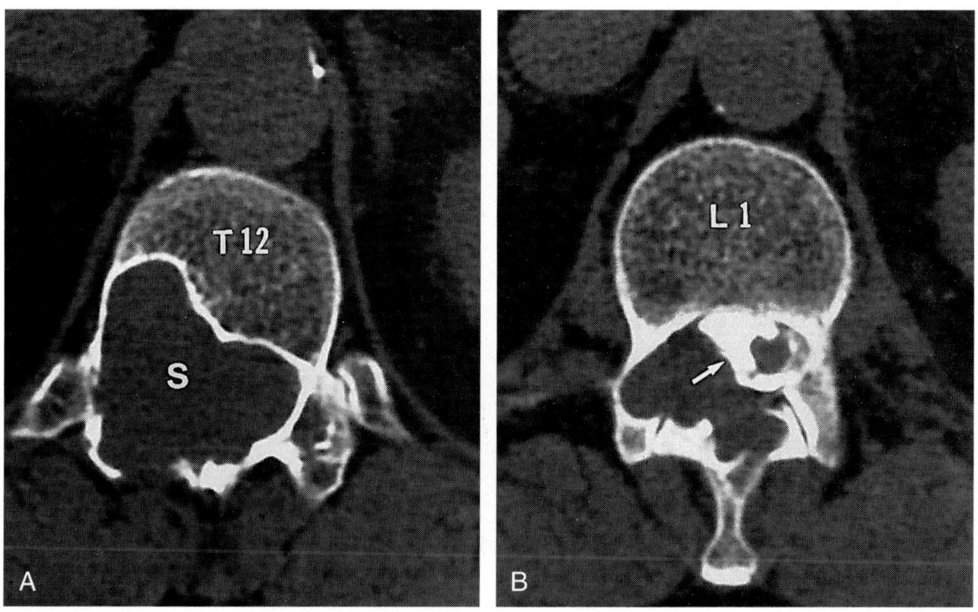

Figure 12–34. Schwannoma. CT myelogram at **(A)** T12 and **(B)** L1 shows a schwannoma (S) causing marked expansion of the spinal canal with bony remodeling rather than destruction. At L1 the thecal sac (arrow) and conus are displaced to the left. The subarachnoid space is obliterated at T12. Bone remodeling is most characteristic of nerve sheath tumors. It is also caused by dural ectasia, AVM, neurenteric cyst, intramedullary tumors, and, rarely, herniated disc.

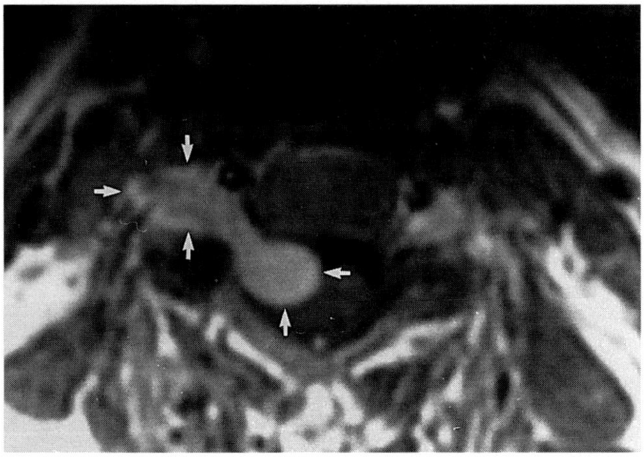

Figure 12–35. Dumbbell schwannoma. Axial contrast-enhanced MRI shows a bilobulated schwannoma with both intradural and extradural components.

Chordoma

Chordomas are rare tumors arising from notochordal remnants in the axial skeleton. They are slow growing but locally aggressive, and bone destruction is almost always present. About 50% originate in the sacrum, 35% in the clivus, and 15% in the vertebrae. Sacral chordomas usually present with localized bone pain and rectal dysfunction and are most common in the fifth through seventh decades. Systemic metastases can and often do occur.

CT Findings. CT shows a soft tissue mass with extensive bone destruction but leaving small sclerotic residual bone fragments. The soft tissue mass usually expands into the presacral space and is heterogeneous in character, with coarse calcifications and low attenuation areas caused by necrosis or myxoid material.

MRI Findings. MRI shows a mass, usually arising from the sacrum and demonstrating intraosseous marrow replacement. Chordomas are hypointense on T1-weighted images and hyperintense on T2-weighted images, with more marked hyperintensity in areas of necrosis or myxoid material. Enhancement is seen after intravenous contrast. With the rarer vertebral chordomas, epidural encroachment and cord compression are frequently present. Invasion of the intervertebral disc and adjacent vertebral body may occur, mimicking osteomyelitis.

TABLE 12–8 Differential Diagnosis of Destructive Process of Vertebrae or Sacrum

Metastasis
Myeloma
Osteomyelitis
Chordoma
Aneurysmal bone cyst
Giant cell tumor
Osteosarcoma (rare)
Chondrosarcoma (rare)
Hemangioma (rarely destructive)

Differential Diagnosis

See Table 12–8.

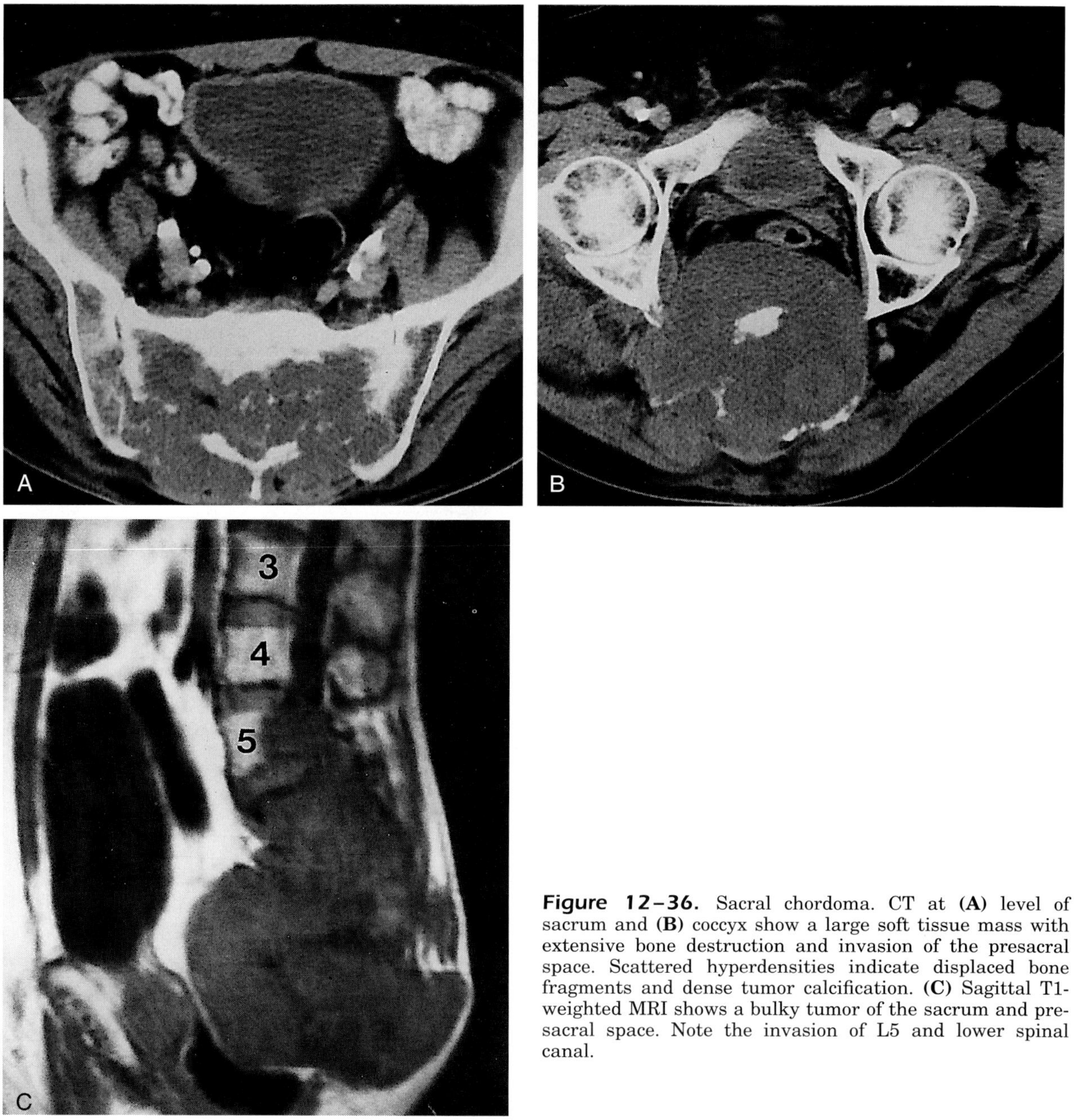

Figure 12–36. Sacral chordoma. CT at **(A)** level of sacrum and **(B)** coccyx show a large soft tissue mass with extensive bone destruction and invasion of the presacral space. Scattered hyperdensities indicate displaced bone fragments and dense tumor calcification. **(C)** Sagittal T1-weighted MRI shows a bulky tumor of the sacrum and presacral space. Note the invasion of L5 and lower spinal canal.

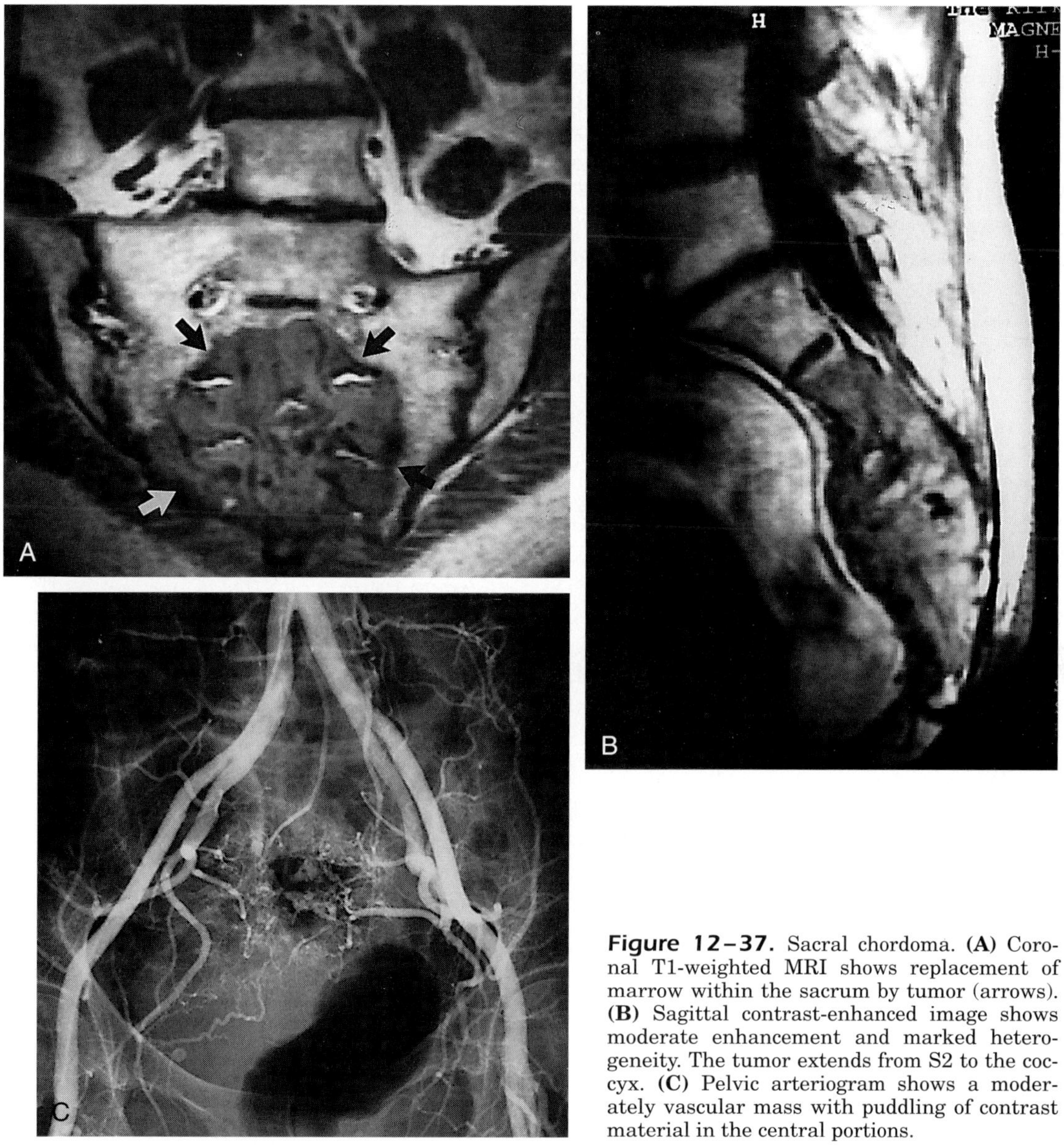

Figure 12–37. Sacral chordoma. **(A)** Coronal T1-weighted MRI shows replacement of marrow within the sacrum by tumor (arrows). **(B)** Sagittal contrast-enhanced image shows moderate enhancement and marked heterogeneity. The tumor extends from S2 to the coccyx. **(C)** Pelvic arteriogram shows a moderately vascular mass with puddling of contrast material in the central portions.

Secondary Neoplasms

Leptomeningeal Metastasis

Metastatic disease to the leptomeninges is usually an ominous event seen with advanced CNS and systemic malignancies. It may occur in up to 50% of patients with acute lymphoblastic and myelogenous leukemias. However, lymphoma, breast carcinoma, and lung carcinoma are the most common non-CNS primaries. Meningeal metastases are seen in the lumbar, thoracic, and cervical spinal canal, in decreasing order of frequency. Definitive diagnosis relies on CSF cytology. To achieve maximum sensitivity requires multiple punctures obtaining large quantities of CSF. Treatment is mostly palliative, consisting of radiotherapy or intrathecal chemotherapy.

Myelographic and CT Findings. Findings at myelography reflect tumor seeding of the subarachnoid space and meninges. This causes nodularity and irregularity of the thecal sac, nerve roots, and spinal cord. Obliteration of root sleeves or the thecal sac or complete myelographic block may also occur. Postmyelography CT may show filling defects within the CSF, effacement or obliteration of the subarachnoid space, or enlargement of the cord diameter with an irregular nodular surface.

MRI Findings. Contrast-enhanced MRI is comparable to CT myelography in sensitivity for meningeal metastatic disease and is complementary to CSF cytology in establishing the diagnosis. Unenhanced MRI may show small nodules in the CSF that are isointense to cord or diffusely increased signal intensity of the CSF on T1-weighted images. Intravenous contrast improves the sensitivity somewhat, although probably to no higher than 40%. Enhanced MRI may show small enhancing nodules, enhancement of the nerve roots, pial enhancement on the surface of the spinal cord, or homogeneous enhancement of large portions of the subarachnoid space.

TABLE 12–9 Leading Sources of Metastases to the Subarachnoid Space

CNS Primary
Medulloblastoma
Ependymoma
Pineal region tumors (pineocytomas and germ cell tumors)
Glioblastoma
Systemic Primary
Lung carcinoma
Breast carcinoma
Lymphoma
Leukemia
Melanoma
Gastrointestinal carcinoma

Differential Diagnosis

Enhancement in the subarachnoid space may be caused by normal vessels, arteriovenous malformations, nerve sheath tumors, meningiomas, sarcoidosis, or meningitis. See Table 12–9.

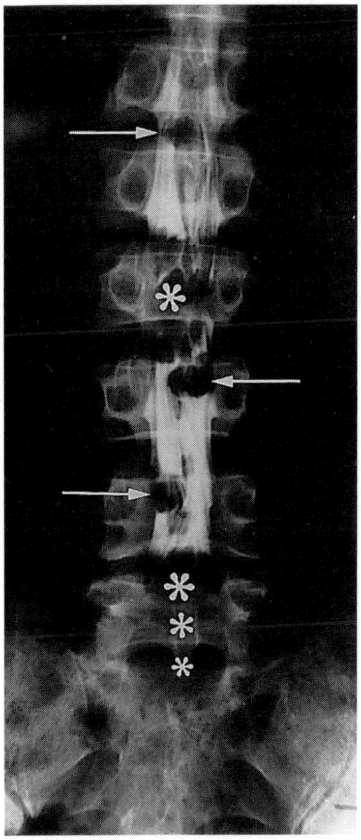

Figure 12–38. Leptomeningeal metastases (adenocarcinoma). AP myelogram shows multiple intradural masses. Smaller metastases appear as discrete filling defects (long arrows). Larger masses cause more extensive areas of nonfilling (asterisks). (Courtesy of Alan Lovell, MD, Birmingham, AL).

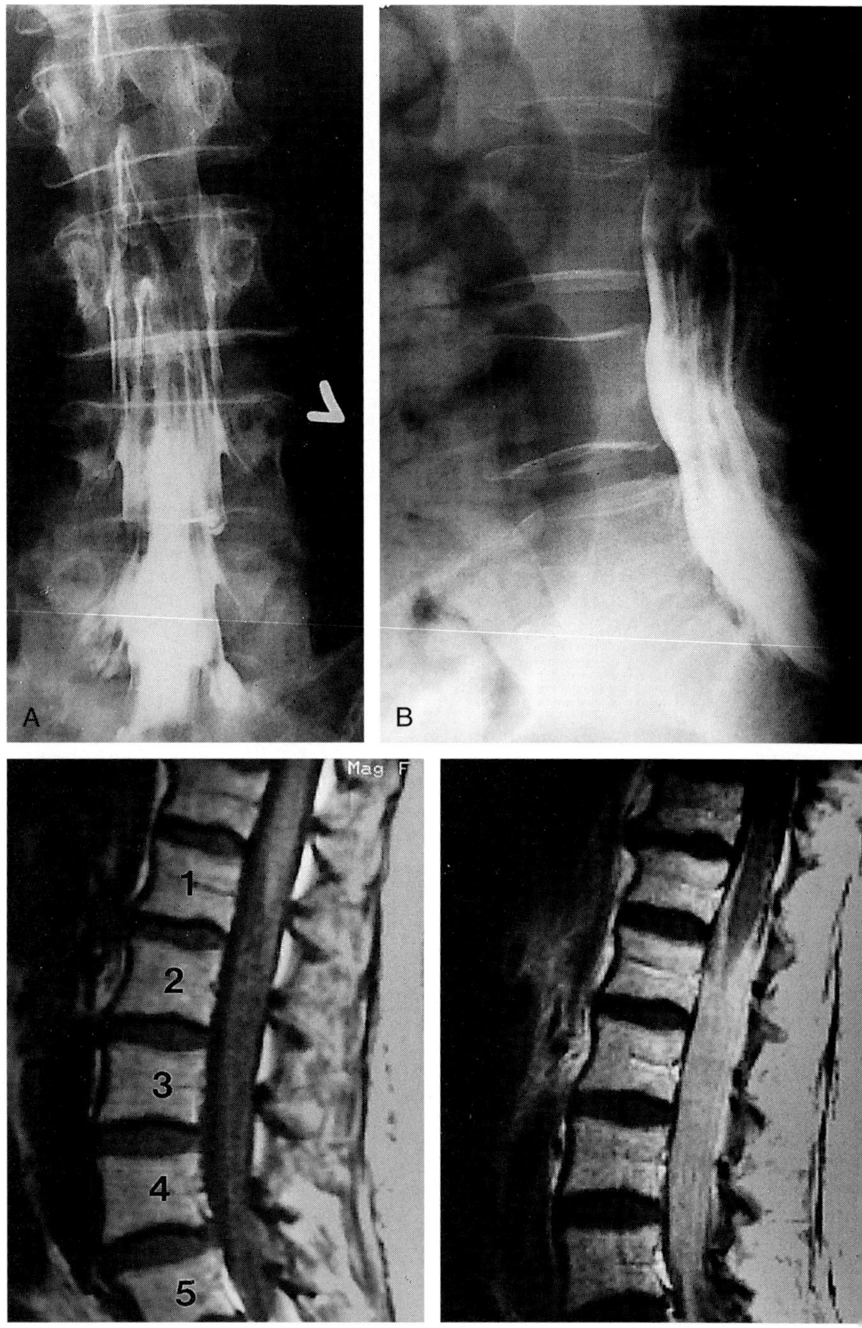

Figure 12–39. Leptomeningeal metastases (lymphoma). **(A)** AP and **(B)** lateral myelograms show marked thickening of the roots of the cauda equina. **(C)** Sagittal T1-weighted MRI shows mildly increased signal intensity from the cauda equina and lumbar CSF. The tip of the conus is at L1. **(D)** After intravenous contrast there is marked enhancement within the entire lumbar subarachnoid space highlighting the conus, which does not enhance.

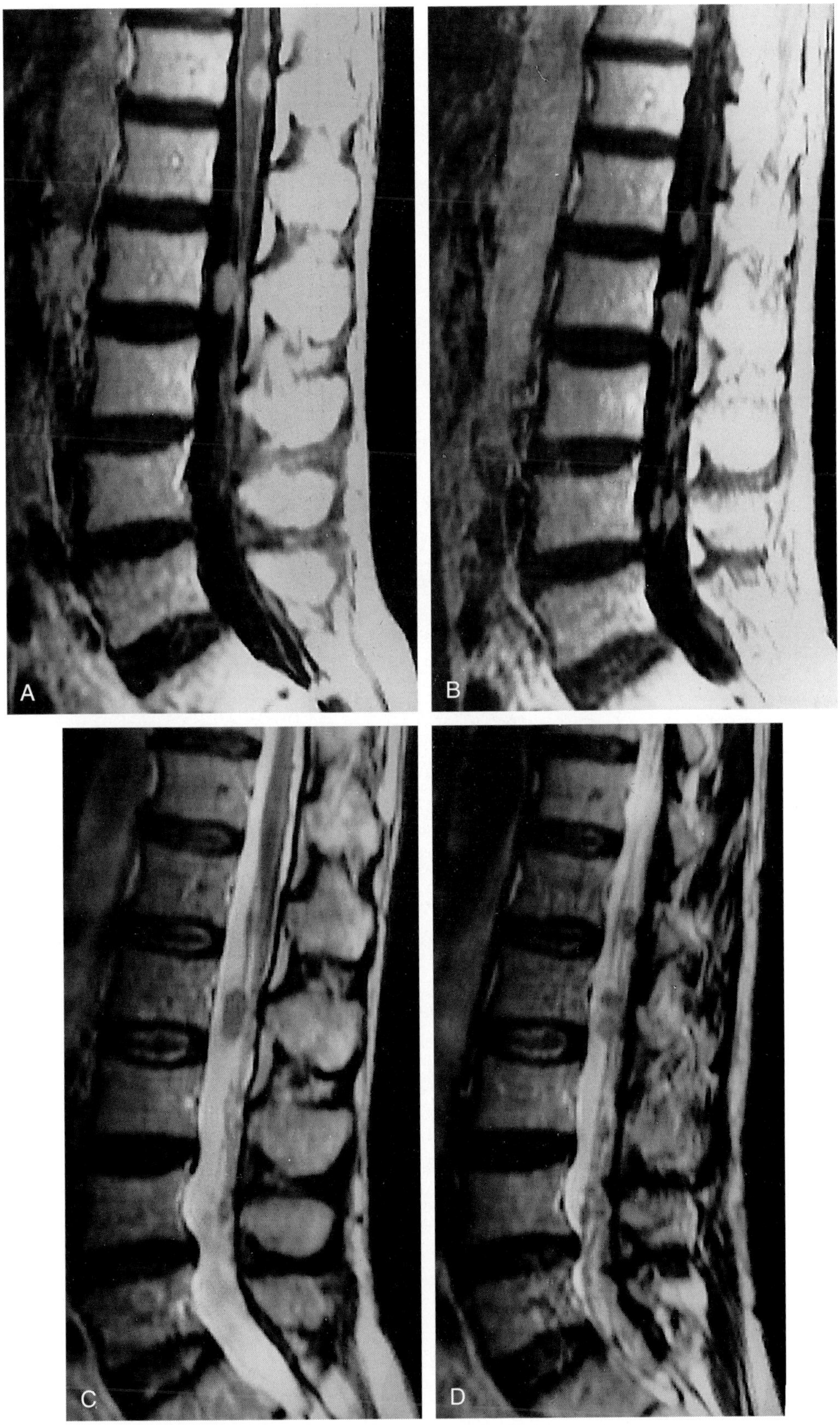

Figure 12–40. Leptomeningeal metastases **(A,B)** Sagittal contrast-enhanced MRI shows enhancement of intradural masses, pial enhancement on the surface of the conus, and enhancement of nerve roots. **(C,D)** On sagittal T2-weighted MRI the intradural masses and thickened nodular nerve roots are hypointense relative to CSF, whereas the pial involvement of the conus cannot be identified.

Spinal Metastasis and Multiple Myeloma

Spinal metastases are second in frequency to brain metastases among oncologic patients with CNS complications. In most cases, the process remains limited to the vertebra and may be asymptomatic or patients present only with bone pain. The minority who develop compression of the cord or cauda equina present with radicular pain, weakness, or sensory deficits. This is a true medical emergency, as cord compression may progress rapidly to paraplegia or quadriplegia with a poor chance of recovery. It is also noteworthy that in a sizable percentage of cases (up to 50% in some series), spinal metastases are the first indication of a malignant process. Therefore, the index of suspicion must be high, and a negative history for malignancy is irrelevant. The most common primary tumors are lymphoma and cancers of the lung, breast, prostate, and kidney. The vast majority of patients are over 50 years of age. Multiple myeloma, which is primary rather than metastatic, manifests similar clinical and imaging features.

The lumbar spine is the most frequent site of metastases diagnosed by imaging. However, the thoracic spine is the most frequent site of metastases causing cord compression. Multiple vertebrae are involved in up to 90% of patients.

Myelographic and CT Findings. Myelography may reveal extradural compression of the subarachnoid space or complete block. With early lesions, CT shows lysis of trabecular bone in the vertebral body, with subsequent destruction of cortical bone. The posterior vertebral body is most often involved, followed by the anterior body and then pedicles. Sclerotic metastases may be encountered both de novo, as commonly seen with prostatic carcinoma, or secondarily, as with treated metastatic breast carcinoma.

MRI Findings. The usual MRI appearance is the identification within the vertebral marrow of multiple well-defined round or oval areas of hypointensity on T1-weighted images and hyperintensity on T2-weighted images. Other patterns of signal intensity are uncommonly encountered. Solitary lesions are uncommon but not rare. Progressive growth leads to bone destruction and expansion of tumor into the epidural space with cord compression. Other patterns of metastatic involvement include (1) diffuse replacement of marrow (hypointense on T1-weighted images, hyperintense on T2-weighted images), especially encountered with multiple myeloma, (2) patchy or variegated marrow replacement (similar signal characteristics as the prior pattern), and (3) sclerotic metastases (hypointense on T1- and T2-weighted images).

Intravenous contrast agents should be used selectively. After intravenous contrast, the enhancement of metastases and myeloma exceeds the enhancement of normal marrow. If the normal marrow is cellular (hypointense on T1-weighted images), intravenous contrast aids in the detection of tumors. In the more typical situation of fatty adult marrow (hyperintense on T1 sequences), enhanced tumor may be isointense with, and therefore indistinguishable from, normal marrow. The finding of increased marrow enhancement may be helpful to differentiate the diffuse pattern of multiple myeloma from normal cellular marrow.

TABLE 12–10 | Differential Diagnosis of Vertebral Marrow Signal Patterns on MRI

	Hypointense on T1-Weighted Images	Hyperintense on T1-Weighted Images
Hypointense on T2-weighted images	Myelofibrosis Osteopetrosis Sclerotic metastases	Acute hemorrhage
Intermediate signal intensity on T2-weighted images	Leukemias Hodgkin's disease Normal cellular marrow of early childhood	Focal fatty marrow Radiation therapy Aplastic anemia Type 2 degenerative change
Hyperintense on T2-weighted images	Hemangioma Osteomyelitis Metastasis* Multiple myeloma Type 1 degenerative change Acute compression fracture* Use of fast spin echo technique without fat suppression	Hemangioma Subacute hemorrhage

*See Table 12–11.

TABLE 12–11 Differentiation of Benign Versus Malignant Compression Fractures

Acute Benign Compression Fracture	Pathologic Compression Fracture
Normal signal intensity of uninvolved vertebrae	Metastases frequently seen in other vertebrae
Sharply angulated anterior or posterior margins in sagittal plane	Smooth convex anterior and posterior margins
Heterogeneous (and usually focal) signal alteration in marrow	Homogeneous (and usually diffuse) signal alteration of marrow

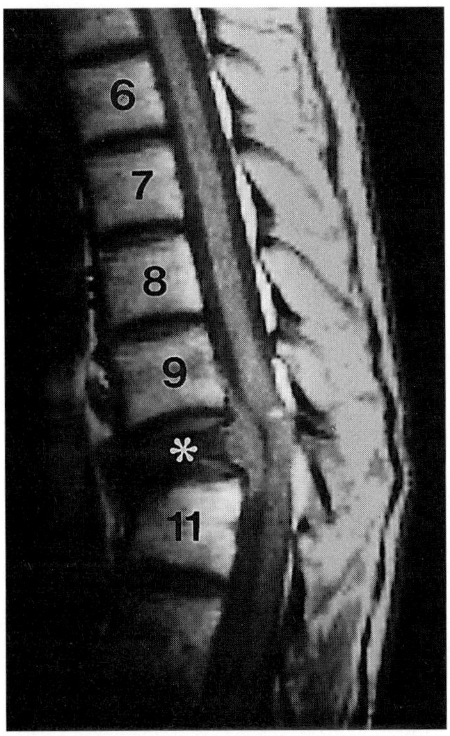

Figure 12–41. Vertebral metastasis with cord compression (hepatoma). Sagittal T1-weighted MRI shows collapse of T10 (asterisk) with a large anterior epidural soft tissue mass obliterating the subarachnoid space and compressing the spinal cord.

Differential Diagnosis

Metastases and multiple myeloma must be distinguished from numerous conditions that may cause signal alteration within the vertebral marrow (Table 12–10). Most often metastases are multiple, of variable size, and easily distinguished from fatty marrow on T1-weighted images. The diagnosis becomes more problematic when the normal marrow is cellular or in the presence of acute vertebral body compression (Table 12–11).

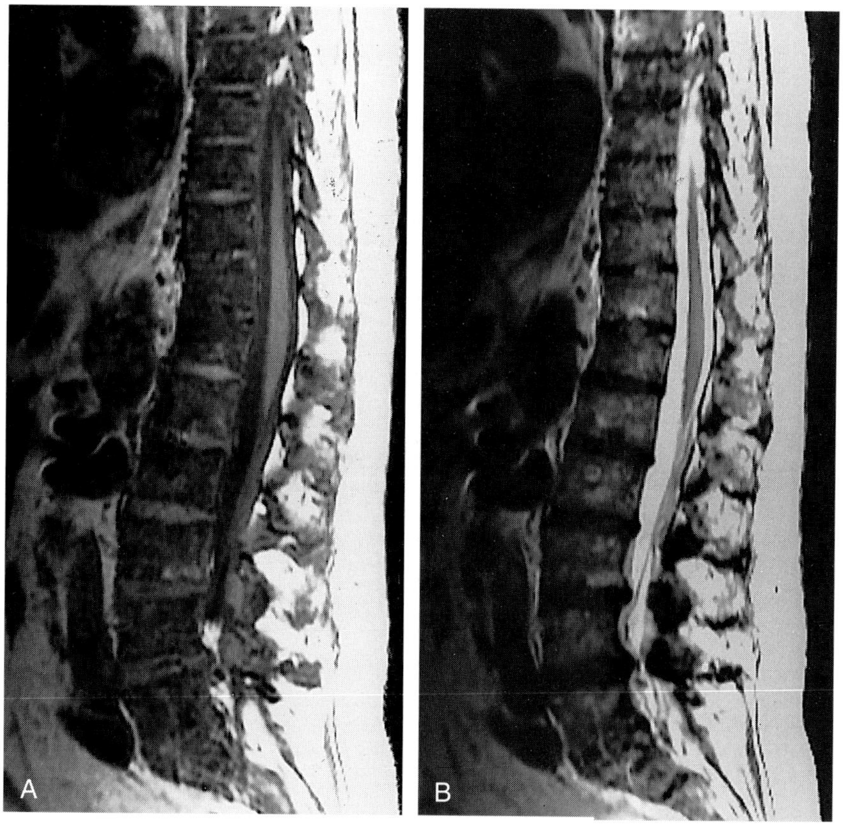

Figure 12–42. Vertebral metastases (prostatic carcinoma). Sagittal **(A)** T1-weighted and **(B)** T2-weighted MRI show diffuse hypointensity of the vertebral marrow, which is most striking in **A**. This is due to diffuse blastic metastatic disease.

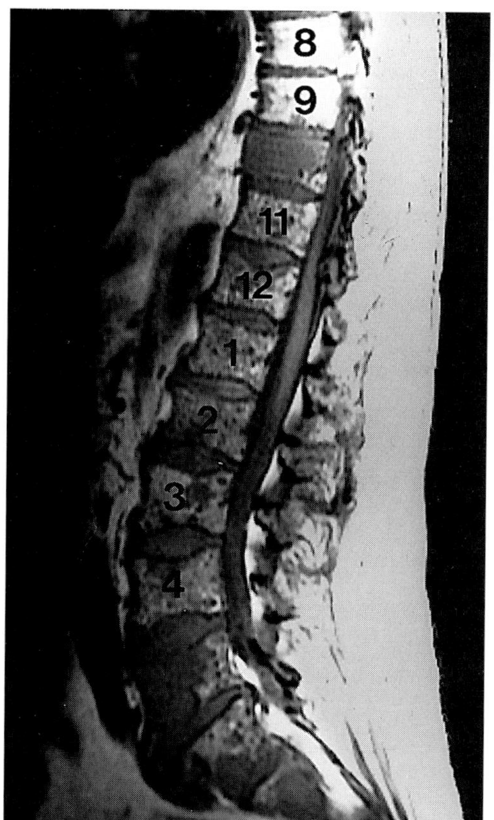

Figure 12–43. Multiple myeloma. Sagittal T1-weighted MRI shows multiple, variably sized foci of soft tissue against a background of hyperintense fatty marrow. There is almost complete marrow replacement in T10 and L5. The marked hyperintensity within T8 and T9 indicates complete fatty transformation secondary to radiotherapy.

RECOMMENDED READINGS

Arachnoiditis

Bangert,BA, Ross,JS. Arachnoiditis Affecting the Lumbosacral Spine. *Neuroimaging Clin North Am* 3:517–524, 1993.

Johnson,CE, Sze,G. Benign Lumbar Arachnoiditis: MR Imaging with Gadopentetate Dimeglumine. *AJNR* 11:763–770, 1990. *AJR* 155:873–880, 1990.

Ross,JS, Masaryk,TJ, Modic,MT. MR Imaging of Lumbar Arachnoiditis. *AJR* 149:1025–1032, 1987.

Subarachnoid Cyst

Bangert,BA, Ross,JS. Arachnoiditis Affecting the Lumbosacral Spine. *Neuroimaging Clin North Am* 3:517–524, 1993.

Sklar,E, Quencer,RM, Green,BA, Montalvo,BM, Post,MJD. Acquired Spinal Subarachnoid Cysts: Evaluation with MR, CT Myelography, and Intraoperative Sonography. *AJNR* 10: 1097–1104, 1989. *AJR* 153:1057–1064, 1989.

Multiple Sclerosis

Maravilla,KR, Weinreb,JC, Suss,R, Nunnally,RL. Magnetic Resonance Demonstration of Multiple Sclerosis Plaques in the Cervical Cord. *AJR* 144:381–385, 1985.

Wallace,CJ, Seland,TP, Fong,TC. Multiple Sclerosis: The Impact of MR Imaging. *AJR* 158:849–857, 1992.

Discitis and Osteomyelitis

Boden,SD, Davis,DO, Dina,TS, Sunner,JL, Wiesel,SW. Postoperative Diskitis: Distinguishing Early MR Imaging Findings from Normal Postoperative Disk Space Changes. *Radiology* 184:765–771, 1992.

Sandhu,FS, Dillon,WP. Spinal Epidural Abscess: Evaluation with Contrast-Enhanced MR Imaging. *AJNR* 12: 1087–1093, 1991, *AJR* 158:405–411, 1992.

Shanley, DJ. Tuberculosis of the Spine: Imaging Features. *AJR* 164:659–664, 1995.

Sharif,HS. Role of MR Imaging in the Management of Spinal Infections. *AJR* 158:1333–1345, 1992.

Sklar,EML, Post,MJD, Lebwohl,NH. Imaging of Infection of the Lumbosacral Spine. *Neuroimaging Clin North Am* 3: 577–590, 1993.

Van Lom,KJ, Kellerhouse,LE, Pathria,MN, et al. Infection versus Tumor in the Spine: Criteria for Distinction with CT. *Radiology* 166:851–855, 1988.

Extramedullary Arteriovenous Malformation

Choi,IS. Spinal Dural Arteriovenous Fistula: The Role of PVA Embolization. *AJNR* 13:941–942, 1992.

Larson,EM, Desai,P, Hardin,CW, Story,J, Jinkins,JR. Venous Infarction of the Spinal Cord Resulting from Dural Arteriovenous Fistula: MR Imaging Findings. *AJNR* 12:739–743, 1991.

Mascalchi,M, Bianchi,MC, Quilici,N, et al. MR Angiography of Spinal Vascular Malformations. *AJNR* 16:289–297, 1995.

Terwey,B, Becker,H, Thron,AK, Vahldiek,G. Gadolinium-DTPA Enhanced MR Imaging of Spinal Dural Arteriovenous Fistulas. *J Comput Assist Tomogr* 13:30–37, 1989.

Willinsky,R, Lasjaunias,P, Terbrugge,K, Hurth,M. Angiography in the Investigation of Spinal Dural Arteriovenous Fistula. *Neuroradiology* 32:114–116, 1990.

Intramedullary Arteriovenous Malformation

Biondi,A, Merland,JJ, Hodes,JE, Pruvo,JP, Reizine,D. Aneurysms of Spinal Arteries Associated with Intramedullary Arteriovenous Malformations. I. Angiographic and Clinical Aspects. *AJNR* 13:913–922, 1992.

Choi,IS, Berenstein,A. Surgical Neuroangiography of the Spine and Spinal Cord. *Radiol Clin North Am* 26(5):1131–1141, 1988.

Minami,S, Sagoh,T, Nishimura,K, et al. Spinal Arteriovenous Malformation: MR Imaging. *Radiology* 169:109–115, 1988.

Vertebral Hemangioma

Laredo,JD, Assouline,E, Gelbert,F, Wybier,M, Merland,JJ, Tubiana,JM. Vertebral Hemangiomas: Fat Content as a Sign of Aggressiveness. *Radiology* 177:467–472, 1990.

Laredo,JD, Reizine,D, Bard,M, Merland,JJ. Vertebral Hemangiomas: Radiologic Evaluation. *Radiology* 161:183–189, 1986.

Ross,JS, Masaryk,TJ, Modic,MT, Carter,JR, Mapstone,T, Dengel,FH. Vertebral Hemangiomas: MR Imaging. *Radiology* 165:165–169, 1987.

Astrocytoma

Bazan,C. Imaging of Lumbosacral Spine Neoplasms. *Neuroimaging Clin North Am* 3:591–608, 1993.

Parizel,PM, Belériaux,D, Rodesch,G, et al. Gd-DTPA-Enhanced MR Imaging of Spinal Tumors. *AJR* 152:1087–1096, 1989. *AJNR* 10:249–258, 1989.

Zimmerman,RA, Bilaniuk,LT. Imaging of Tumors of the Spinal Canal and Cord. *Radiol Clin North Am* 26:965–1007, 1988.

Ependymoma

Nemotto,Y, Inoue,Y, Tashiro,T, et al. Intramedullary Spinal Cord Tumors: Significance of Associated Hemorrhage at MR Imaging. *Radiology* 182:793–796, 1992.

Parizel,PM, Balériaux,D, Rodesch,G, et al. Gd-DTPA-Enhanced MR Imaging of Spinal Tumors. *AJR* 152:1087–1096, 1989. *AJNR* 10:249–258, 1989.

Hemangioblastoma

Choyke,PL, Glenn,GM, Walther,MM, Patronas,NJ, Linehan,WM, Zbar,B. von Hippel-Lindau Disease: Genetic, Clinical, and Imaging Features. *Radiology* 194:629–642, 1995.

Kaffenberger,DA, Shah,CP,Murtagh,FR, Wilson,C, Silberger,ML. MR Imaging of Spinal Cord Hemangioblastoma Associated with Syringomyelia. *J Comput Assist Tomogr* 12:495–498, 1988.

Nelson,DR, Yuh,WTC, Waziri,MH, et al. MR Imaging of Hippel-Lindau Disease: Value of Gadopentetate Dimeglumine. *J Magn Reson Imaging* 1:469–476, 1991.

Sato,Y, Waziri,M, Smith,W, et al. Hippel-Lindau Disease: MR Imaging. *Radiology* 166:241–246, 1988.

Meningioma

Bazan,C. Imaging of Lumbosacral Spine Neoplasms. *Neuroimaging Clin North Am* 3:591–608, 1993.

Zimmerman,RA, Bilaniuk,LT. Imaging of Tumors of the Spinal Canal and Cord. *Radiol Clin North Am* 26:965–1007, 1988.

Schwannoma and Neurofibroma

Abramowitz,J, Dion,JE, Jensen,ME, et al. Angiographic Diagnosis and Management of Head and Neck Schwannomas. *AJNR* 12:977–984, 1991. *AJR* 157:1309–1316, 1991.

Burk,DL, Brunberg,JA, Kanal,E, Latchaw,RE, Wolf,GL. Spinal and Paraspinal Neurofibromatosis: Surface Coil MR Imaging at 1.5T. *Radiology* 162:797–801, 1987.

Friedman,DP, Tartaglino,LM, Flanders,AE. Intradural Schwannomas of the Spine: MR Findings with Emphasis on Contrast-Enhancement Characteristics. *AJR* 158:1347–1350, 1992.

Chordoma

Meyer,JE, Lepke,RA, Lindfors,KK, et al. Chordomas: Their CT Appearance in the Cervical, Thoracic, and Lumbar Spine. *Radiology* 153:693–696, 1984.

Rosenthal,DI, Scott,JA, Mankin,HJ, Wismer,GL, Brady,TJ. Sacrococcygeal Chordoma: Magnetic Resonance Imaging and Computed Tomography. *AJR* 145:143–147, 1985.

Sze,G, Uichano,LS, Brant-Zawadski,MN, et al. Chordomas: MR Imaging. *Radiology* 166:187–191, 1988.

Leptomeningeal Metastasis

Lim,V, Sobel,DF, Zyroff,J. Spinal Cord Pial Metastases: MR Imaging with Gadopentetate Dimeglumine. *AJNR* 11: 975–982, 1990. *AJR* 155:1077–1084, 1990.

Stanley,P, Senac,MO, Segall,HD. Intraspinal Seeding from Intracranial Tumors in Children. *AJR* 144:157–161, 1985.

Yousem,DM, Patrone,PM, Grossman,RI. Leptomeningeal Metastases: MR Evaluation. *J Comput Assist Tomogr* 14:255–261, 1990.

Spinal Metastasis and Multiple Myeloma

Algra,PR, Bloem,JL, Tissing,H, Falke,THM, Arndt,JW, Verboom,LJ. Detection of Vertebral Metastases: Comparison Between MR Imaging and Bone Scintigraphy. *Radiographics* 11:219–232, 1991.

Algra,PR, Heimans,JJ, Valk,J, Nauta,JJ, Lachniet,M, Van Kooten,B. Do Metastases in Vertebra Begin in the Body or the Pedicles? Imaging Study in 45 Patients. *AJR* 158: 1275–1279, 1992.

Baker,LL, Goodman,SB, Perkash,I, Lane,B, Enzmann,DR. Benign versus Pathologic Compression Fractures of Vertebral Bodies: Assessment with Conventional Spin-Echo, Chemical Shift, and STIR MR Imaging. *Radiology* 174:497–502, 1990.

Carmody,RF, Yang,PJ, Seeley,GW, Seeger,JF, Unger,EC, Johnson,JE. Spinal Cord Compression Due to Metastatic Disease: Diagnosis with MR Imaging versus Myelography. *Radiology* 173:225–229, 1989.

Laredo,JD, Lakhdari,K, Bellaiche,L, Hamze,B, Janklewicz,P, Tubiana,JM. Acute Vertebral Collapse: CT Findings in Benign and Malignant Nontraumatic Cases. *Radiology* 194: 41–48, 1995.

Mehta,RC, Marks,MP, Hinks,RS, Glover,GH, Enzmann,DR. MR Evaluation of Vertebral Metastases: T1-weighted, Short-Inversion-Time Inversion Recovery, Fast Spin-Echo, and Inversion-Recovery Fast Spin-Echo Sequences. *AJNR* 16:281–288, 1995.

Moulopoulos,LA, Dimopoulos,MA, Alexanian,R, Leeds,NE, Libshitz,HI. Multiple Myeloma: MR Patterns of Response to Treatment. *Radiology* 193:441–446, 1994.

Moulopoulos,LA, Varma,DGK, Dimpouplos,MA, et al. Multiple Myeloma: Spinal MR Imaging in Patients with Untreated Newly Diagnosed Disease. *Radiology* 185:833–840, 1992.

MRI of Bone Marrow

Dooms,GC, Fisher,MR, Hricak,H, Richardson,M, Crooks,LE, Genant,HK. Bone Marrow Imaging: Magnetic Resonance Studies Related to Age and Sex. *Radiology* 155:429–432, 1985.

Modic,MT, Steinberg,PM, Ross,JS, Masaryk,TJ, Carter,JR. Degenerative Disk Disease: Assessment of Changes in Vertebral Body Marrow with MR Imaging. *Radiology* 166: 193–199, 1988.

Ramsey,RG, Zacharias,CE. MR Imaging of the Spine after Radiation Therapy: Easily Recognizable Effects. *AJR* 144: 1131–1135, 1985.

Smith,SR, Williams,CE, Davies,JM, Edwards,RHT. Bone Marrow Disorders: Characterization with Quantitative MR Imaging. *Radiology* 172:805–810, 1989.

CHAPTER THIRTEEN

Degenerative Diseases and Trauma of the Spine

Degenerative diseases of the spine are among the most universal medical afflictions. Surveys performed in recent years indicate that spinal MRI composes nearly 50% of an average MRI practice, most of which is for the work-up of back pain, myelopathy, or radiculopathy.

Degenerative spinal diseases include a number of pathologic entities that may occur individually or in almost any combination, converging on the vulnerable cord and nerve roots to cause compression and dysfunction. It is difficult to treat the subject justly in the confines of this chapter, but the format and process of selection used throughout this atlas are continued here.

The traumatic conditions discussed here directly involve the CNS proper: cord injuries, nerve root avulsions, and spinal hemorrhage. Spinal fractures are omitted for reasons of space and because fractures are primarily a musculoskeletal condition.

Primary Diseases

Conditions of Ligamentous Ossification

Ossification of the posterior longitudinal ligament (OPLL) is most common among the Japanese, with a peak incidence of up to 2.4%. It is notably less common in other races. Extensive ligamentous thickening and ossification may develop in the ventral spinal canal, leading to severe spinal stenosis. The etiology is unknown. Cervical levels 4, 5, and 6 are most often affected. Patients with this condition most often present in the sixth decade. Only a small number of patients develop symptoms, including neck pain, radiculopathy, and myelopathy. The condition is very slowly progressive, with surgery generally reserved for those with secondary myelopathy.

Ossification of the ligamentum flavum (OLF) is also most common among the Japanese and often coexists with OPLL. OLF is usually seen in the lower thoracic region and may cause radiculopathy or myelopathy. It is one of the most common causes of thoracic cord compression in the Far East.

CT Findings. OPLL forms a calcified mass posterior to the vertebral body extending over an average of three cervical segments. In axial section, the calcification may be rounded and convex, rectangular, or mushroomlike. The spinal canal may become severely narrowed.

OLF produces a calcified mass in the ligamentum flavum in the posterolateral thoracic or lumbar spinal canal, just anteromedial to the lamina. As it progresses, it may cause progressive foraminal or central stenosis.

MRI Findings. On sagittal and axial MRI, OPLL appears as a hypointense mass between the posterior vertebral body and CSF. PD-weighted images provide the clearest separation between the ossified ligament, vertebrae, and CSF. The ossified ligament can appear hyperintense on T1-weighted images due to fatty marrow.

OLF appears as a triangular or rounded extradural mass posterolateral to the thecal sac and hypointense on T1- and T2-weighted images. It may also show central bright signal due to fat or bone marrow formation. Other findings may include cord compression and enhancement in the cord after intravenous contrast.

In both conditions, the spinal cord may exhibit hyperintensity on T2-weighted images due to myelomalacia. This is probably the only finding for which MRI is demonstrably superior to CT.

Differential Diagnosis

Other causes of a calcified intraspinal mass include calcified disc, osteochondroma, and meningioma. These are usually limited to a single vertebral level. A low signal mass on MRI may arise from acute epidural hematoma or AVM.

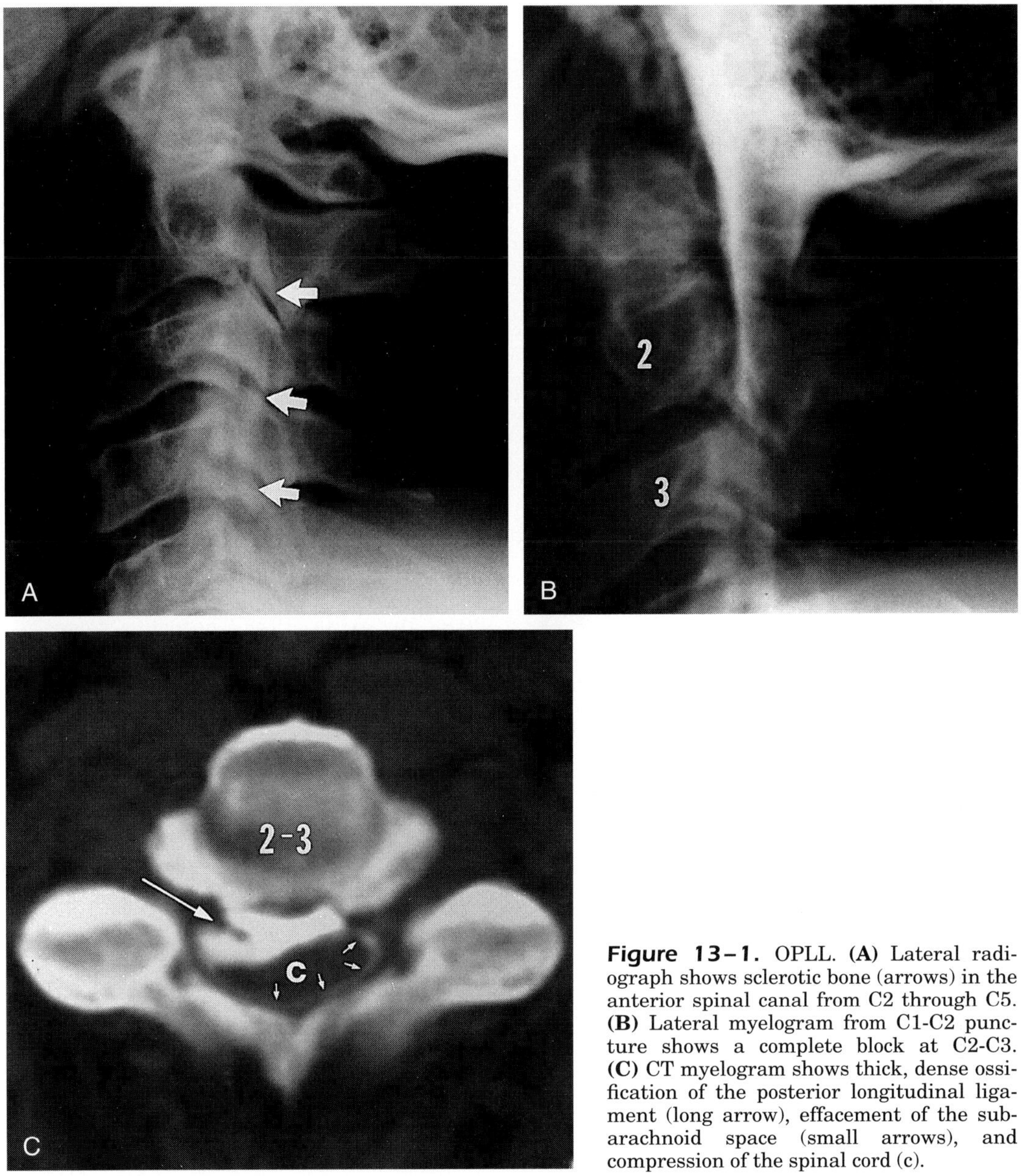

Figure 13–1. OPLL. **(A)** Lateral radiograph shows sclerotic bone (arrows) in the anterior spinal canal from C2 through C5. **(B)** Lateral myelogram from C1-C2 puncture shows a complete block at C2-C3. **(C)** CT myelogram shows thick, dense ossification of the posterior longitudinal ligament (long arrow), effacement of the subarachnoid space (small arrows), and compression of the spinal cord (c).

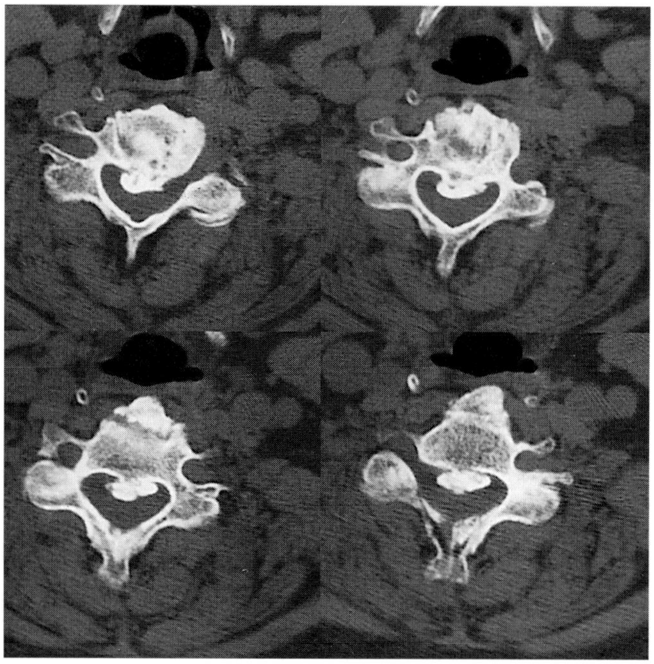

Figure 13–2. OPLL. Sequential CT sections show mushroom-like growth of ossified posterior longitudinal ligament into the spinal canal.

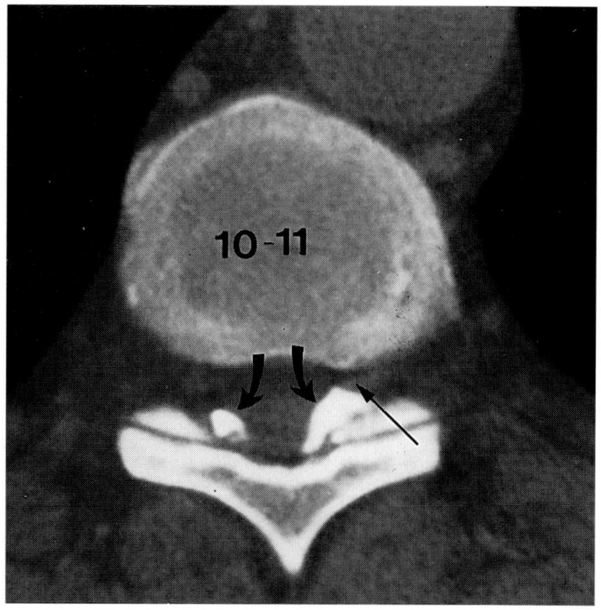

Figure 13–3. Ossification of ligamentum flavum. CT shows bilateral ossification of the ligamentum flavum (arrows) causing left foraminal stenosis (long arrow) in this patient presenting with a left T10 radiculopathy.

Rheumatoid Arthritis

Rheumatoid arthritis is a systemic disease of the synovial joints. Its pathologic features include pannus formation, erosion of cartilage and subchondral bone, fibrosis, and new bone formation. It has been reported to cause marked thickening of the dura within the spinal canal (pachymeningitis). Rheumatoid arthritis is a common disorder that most often appears in the fourth and fifth decades and is two to three times more common in females. Clinically evident extra-articular disease appears in a small minority of cases and may include vasculitis, rheumatoid nodules of the heart and lungs, pleural effusions, and pulmonary fibrosis.

Myelographic and CT Findings. Myelography and CT may show atlantoaxial subluxation with spinal stenosis and compression of the medulla. The normal distance between the anterior arch of C1 and the odontoid should not exceed 3 mm. The subluxation decreases with extension and increases with flexion. Erosion of the odontoid is common. Compared with myelography, CT may better distinguish residual bone from pannus. Vertical subluxation (craniovertebral settling, pseudobasilar invagination) is also common. This condition is present when the top of the odontoid is at or above the plane of the foramen magnum.

MRI Findings. Pannus tends to be of intermediate signal intensity on T1-weighted sequences and hyperintense on T2-weighted sequences. It is usually seen around the odontoid and may contribute to compression of the cervical cord and medulla. Sagittal MRI allows precise assessment of the canal diameter, medullary and cervical cord compression, and vertebral subluxation. In severe cases, hyperintensity may be present within the cord, indicating myelomalacia.

Differential Diagnosis

The diagnosis is usually established by serology and radiography of affected joints. Most patients are already diagnosed by the time cervical spine imaging becomes necessary. Metastasis and osteomyelitis may rarely affect C1 or C2 and produce bone erosion and a soft tissue mass. Traumatic subluxation is differentiated by history and the identification of fractures on radiography or CT.

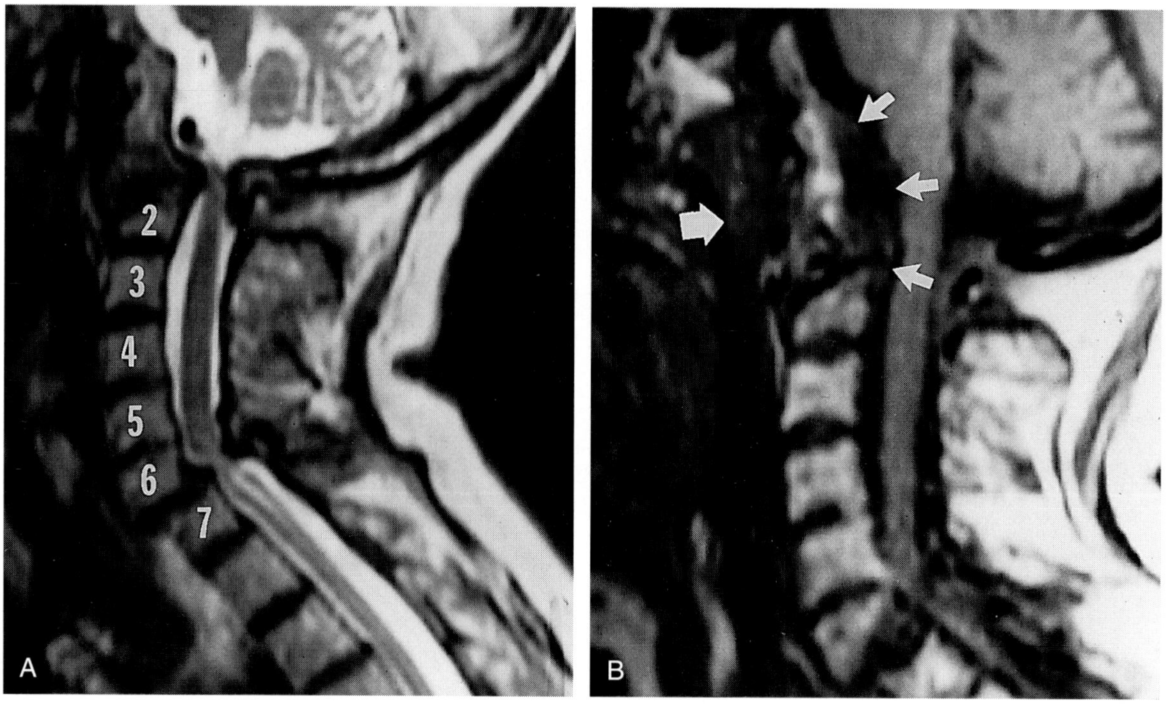

Figure 13–4. Rheumatoid arthritis. **(A)** Sagittal T2-weighted MRI shows severe stenosis due to subluxation at C1-C2 and C6-C7. The cord is severely compressed with myelomalacia at C7. **(B)** T1-weighted sagittal MRI shows pannus (arrows) with erosion of C1, odontoid process of C2, and inferior clivus.

Degenerative Conditions

Lumbar Intervertebral Disc Disease

Synonym: Intervertebral osteochondrosis.

Low back pain is a universal human affliction experienced by 80% of all adults at some time during their life. It is the second leading cause of absenteeism and the leading cause of workers' compensation claims. About 200,000 discectomies are performed annually in the United States, with billions of dollars spent in both treatment and compensation.

Among the various causes of low back pain, degenerative disease of the lumbar discs and vertebrae leads the list. It is an inevitable result of aging for the vast majority of individuals and asymptomatic in most cases. Stress and trauma are aggravating factors. Pathologically the discs become dehydrated, proteoglycans are replaced by collagen, and annular cracks and tears develop in the nucleus and annulus. Weakening of the annulus leads to bulging of the disc. Marginal osteophytes develop from the strain imposed by the outer annular fibers (Sharpey's fibers) on the vertebral end plate. Radial tears in the annulus form a conduit for migrating central disc material. When disc material extrudes beyond the outer annulus, herniation has occurred. A herniated fragment that is completely disconnected from the disc of origin is called a free fragment or sequestered disc. The term protruded disc and extruded disc are more descriptive than pathologic and have been applied inconsistently in the radiologic literature. Extruded disc usually describes herniation beyond the annulus. Protruded disc applies to a focal or diffuse bulge or subannular herniation.

Clinically most patients with symptomatic disc herniations present between the ages of 20 and 50 with back pain or radiculopathy. About 90% of herniations are equally distributed between L4-L5 and L5-S1, about 7% occur at L3-L4, and less than 3% occur at L1-L2 and L2-L3. Most herniations occur in a posterolateral (posterior paramedian) direction where the annulus is thinner and unsupported by the posterior longitudinal ligament. Herniations also occur directly posterior (central herniation) and at or lateral to the neural foramen (lateral herniation). A Schmorl's node is a herniation of disc material through the vertebral end plate. Anterior herniations also occur and can cause back pain but not radiculopathy.

Myelographic Findings. A bulging disc causes a mild convex ventral extradural deformity that is bilaterally symmetrical and usually less apparent on oblique as opposed to lateral projections. The nerve roots should not be enlarged. The deformity caused by a herniated disc is asymmetrical and more angular and laterally located and may extend above or below the disc space. The related nerve root is often widened. Both conditions may produce nonfilling (cutoff) of the related root sleeves.

About 5% of disc herniations occur lateral to the thecal sac and are undetectable by myelography. The L5-S1 level is associated with another myelographic pitfall, for here abundant epidural fat may accommodate a substantial herniated disc without any deformity of the thecal sac seen on myelography.

CT Findings. CT findings of disc degeneration include gas in the disc (vacuum phenomenon), disc calcification, Schmorl's nodes, marginal osteophytes, vertebral body sclerosis, and focal or generalized enlargement of the disc contour. The presence of epidural fat normally allows sharp definition of the posterior disc margin, separating it from the thecal sac. An enlarged disc contour, whether from herniation or bulge, leads to effacement of this epidural fat. The CT attenuation of normal and herniated disc ranges from 60 to 110 HU, higher than CSF or surrounding soft tissue. CT myelography (scanning with intrathecal iodinated contrast) came into wide use in the 1980s as the diagnostic procedure of choice for disc disease but was displaced by MRI later in the decade. With the use of intrathecal contrast, the relationships of disc and thecal sac are elegantly depicted in cross section, and the cause of dural deformity is more confidently determined.

A bulging disc manifests circumferential enlargement of the disc contour beyond the margins of the adjoining end plate and usually, but not always, with a convex posterior margin. A herniated disc forms a localized convex bulge of the disc contour. It is not always possible to distinguish a bulging disc from a herniated disc, since the key pathologic determinant (the integrity of the outer annulus) cannot always be established by imaging. Lateral herniations are lateral to the thecal sac, within or beyond the neural foramen and lateral recess. The normal fat in the neural foramen is replaced by higher density disc material.

Chronically herniated discs frequently become calcified and develop osteophytes at upper and lower margins.

MRI Findings. Signal alterations within the disc are the first MRI manifestation of the degenerative process. The loss of water results in diminished signal intensity on T2-weighted images. This may be followed by loss of disc space height, signal alterations in the marrow of the adjoining vertebrae, radial fissures in the annulus, and Schmorl's nodes. The adjoining vertebral marrow may exhibit increased or diminished signal intensity on both T1- and T2-weighted images. Radial fissures, at least acutely, are hyperintense on T2-weighted images. Acutely herniated discs manifest intermediate signal intensity on T1-weighted images and are usually hyperintense on T2-weighted images. Sagittal T2-weighted images may directly reveal disruption of the posterior longitudinal ligament and are most useful for the diagnosis of a free fragment, which is disconnected from the disc of origin.

The use of intravenous contrast is almost never necessary for the diagnosis of degenerative disease in the unoperated back. If used, however, abnormal contrast enhancement may be observed within degenerated discs and the adjoining vertebrae, adjacent to Schmorl's nodes, in lumbosacral nerve roots, and surrounding acute disc herniations.

Chronically herniated discs tend to become hypointense on T2-weighted images and often develop marginal osteophytes. They may show solid enhancement as the disk is replaced by fibrovascular connective tissue.

Comparison of Modalities. From the extent to which MRI has replaced CT and myelography in the diagnosis of disc disease, one might conclude that MRI is the superior examination, but this is not the case. CT and CT myelography possess a sensitivity of 80–95% for the diagnosis of herniated nucleus pulposus and a specificity of 68–88%. The sensitivity of MRI is 90–95%, with a specificity somewhat lower than CT myelography.

Several series have been reported comparing the accuracy of CT with MRI in the diagnosis of HNP with sometimes conflicting data. It would be fair to summarize that current MRI is roughly equivalent to CT myelography and only slightly superior to plain CT. However, even the best designed comparison of the modalities would be nearly obsolete by the time of its publication because of ongoing technological improvements. MRI is much more expensive than CT and comparable in cost to CT myelography. The greater advantage of MRI lies in its noninvasive nature and avoidance of ionizing radiation.

The issue of imaging in disc disease is further clouded by the high incidence of mild abnormalities in asymptomatic patients and the knowledge that even large disc herniations can improve dramatically without surgery.

TABLE 13–1 | Differential Diagnosis of Disc Herniation

Herniated disc	Extradural mass in ventral spinal canal Hyperdense on CT and hyperintense on T2-weighted MRI Degenerative changes in adjacent intervertebral disc
Perineural cyst	Conforms to anatomic course of nerve root Similar density on CT and signal on MRI to that of CSF Opacifies with contrast on myelography
Tumor	Bone erosion or remodeling and solid enhancement are strongly suggestive
Synovial cyst	Posterior location in proximity to degenerated facet joint Hypointense rim on T2-weighted MRI
Abscess	Nearly always associated with discitis and osteomyelitis of adjoining vertebrae
Hematoma	Signal intensity on MRI is complex and determined by the age of the clot
Arachnoiditis	Usually past history of trauma, subarachnoid hemorrhage, surgery, or pantopaque myelography Nearly always extends over several vertebral levels
Stenosis	MRI and CT both reveal multifocal degenerative changes involving discs, facet joints, and vertebrae

Differential Diagnosis

See Table 13–1.

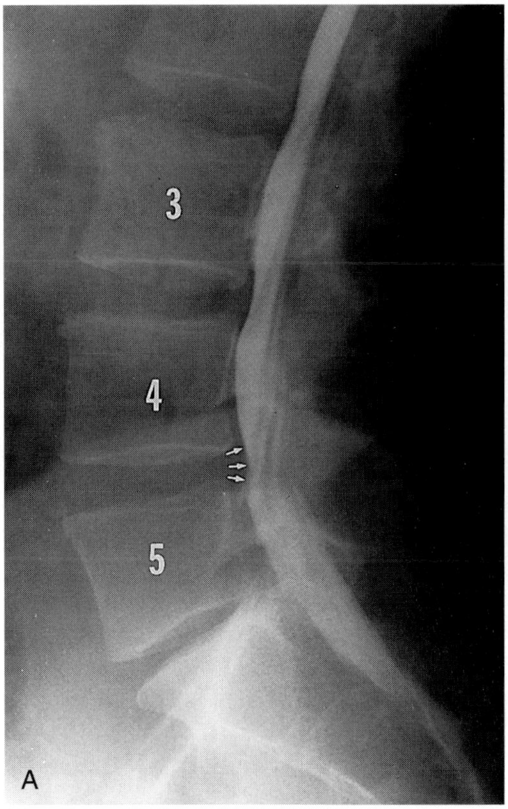

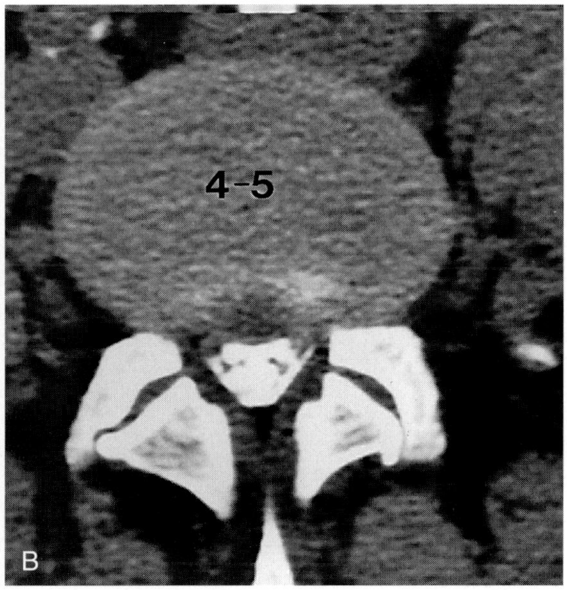

Figure 13–5. Bulging intervertebral disc. **(A)** Lateral myelogram shows a mild ventral deformity (arrows) of the thecal sac at L4-L5. **(B)** CT myelogram shows a symmetrical circumferential enlargement of the intervertebral disc margin and a smoothly convex posterior margin. The thecal sac is mildly compressed.

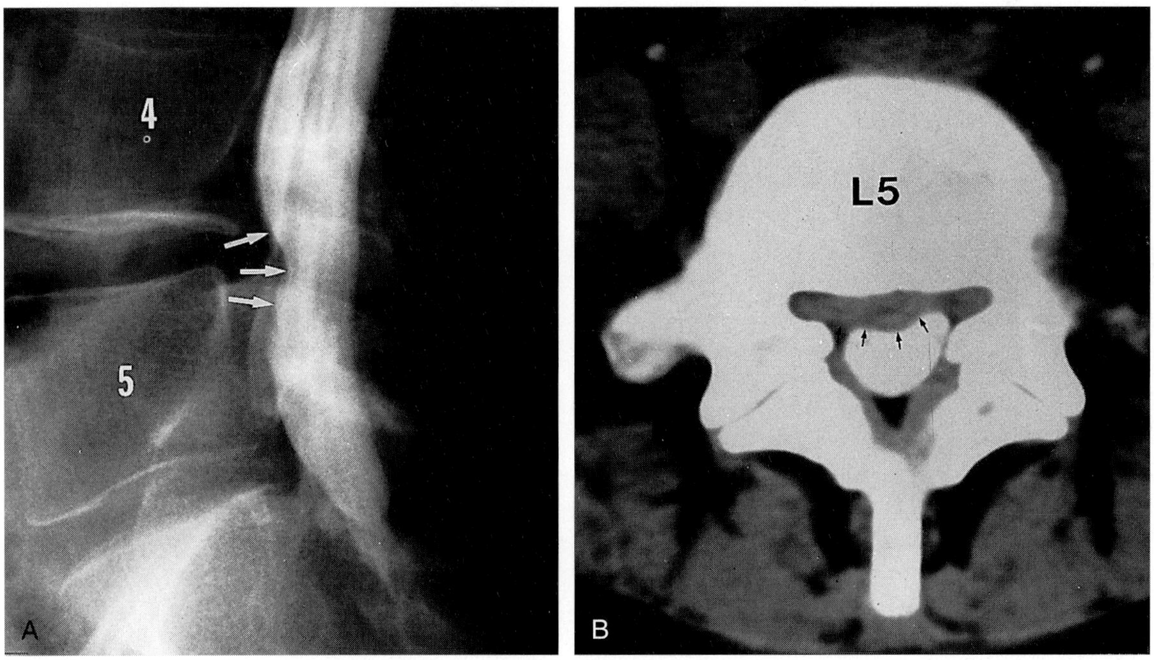

Figure 13–6. Herniated nucleus pulposus. **(A)** Lateral myelogram shows a prominent ventral extradural defect (arrows) at L4-L5 with the defect extending below the disc margin to mid L5. **(B)** CT myelogram shows disc material (arrows) posterior to L5 in the midline and right ventral epidural space (right posterior paramedian herniation).

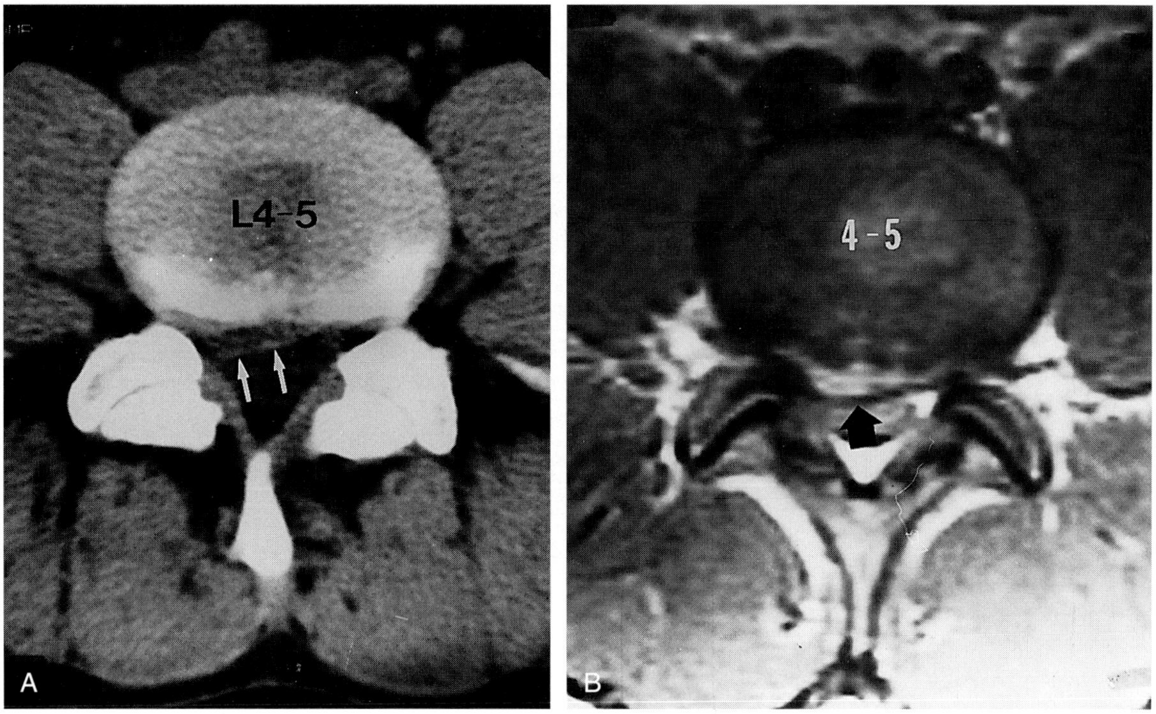

Figure 13-7. Herniated nucleus pulposus. **(A)** CT shows a right posterior paramedian disc herniation (arrows). Note the high attenuation of disc material relative to the thecal sac and surrounding fat. **(B)** On axial PD-weighted MRI the acutely herniated disc (arrow) is hyperintense relative to the parent disc.

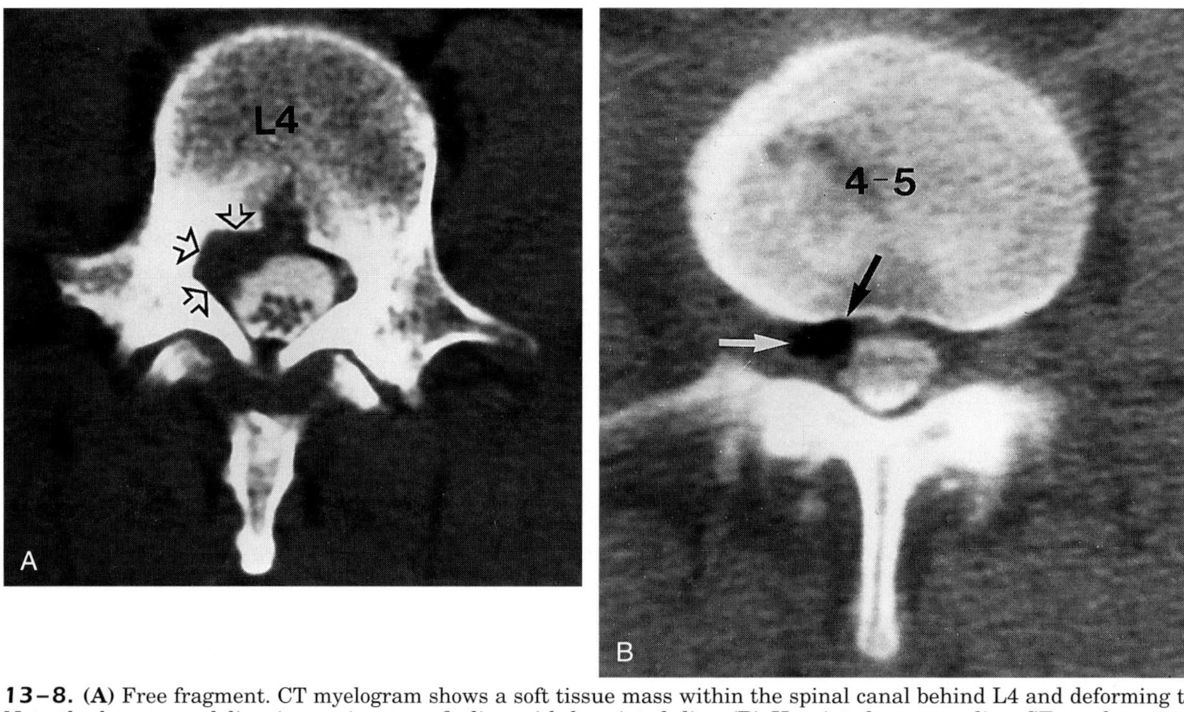

Figure 13-8. **(A)** Free fragment. CT myelogram shows a soft tissue mass within the spinal canal behind L4 and deforming the thecal sac. Note the bone remodeling (arrows), a rare finding with herniated disc. **(B)** Herniated vacuum disc. CT myelogram at L4-5 shows mild deformity of the thecal sac by a mass of air density. Other causes of epidural air include synovial cyst, epidural pneumatosis, gas-forming infection, fistula, and penetrating trauma.

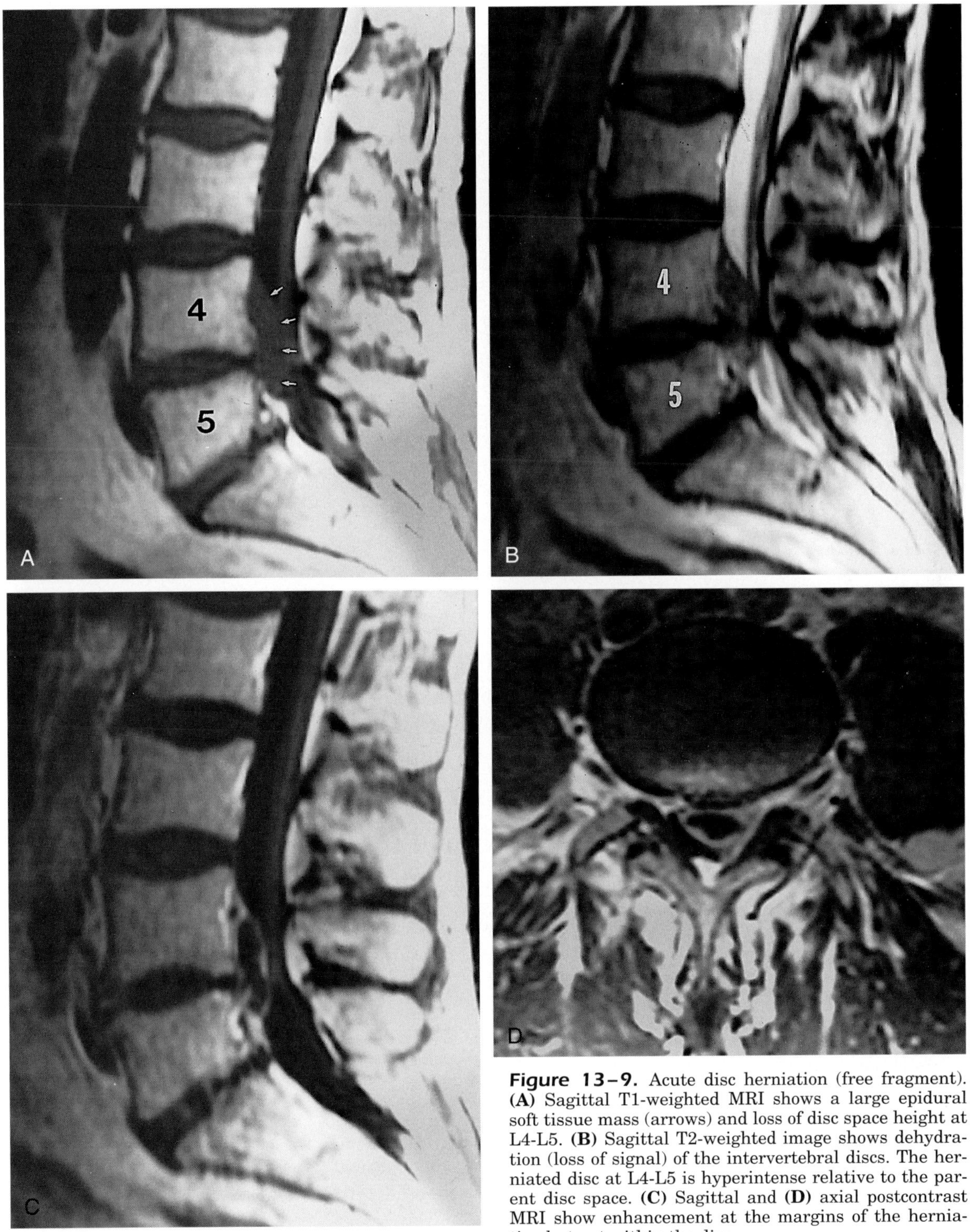

Figure 13–9. Acute disc herniation (free fragment). **(A)** Sagittal T1-weighted MRI shows a large epidural soft tissue mass (arrows) and loss of disc space height at L4-L5. **(B)** Sagittal T2-weighted image shows dehydration (loss of signal) of the intervertebral discs. The herniated disc at L4-L5 is hyperintense relative to the parent disc space. **(C)** Sagittal and **(D)** axial postcontrast MRI show enhancement at the margins of the herniation but not within the disc.

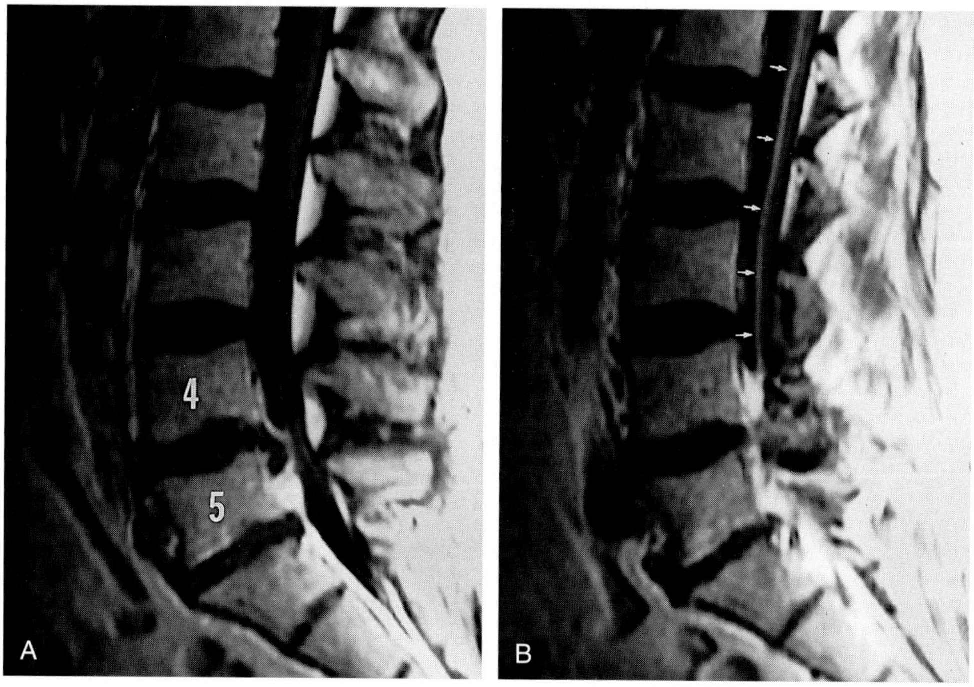

Figure 13–10. Nerve root enhancement (herniated nucleus pulposus). **(A)** Midline sagittal contrast-enhanced MRI shows enhancement at the margins of an L4-L5 herniated disc. **(B)** Paramedian sagittal image shows enhancement of a long segment of lumbar nerve root (arrows).

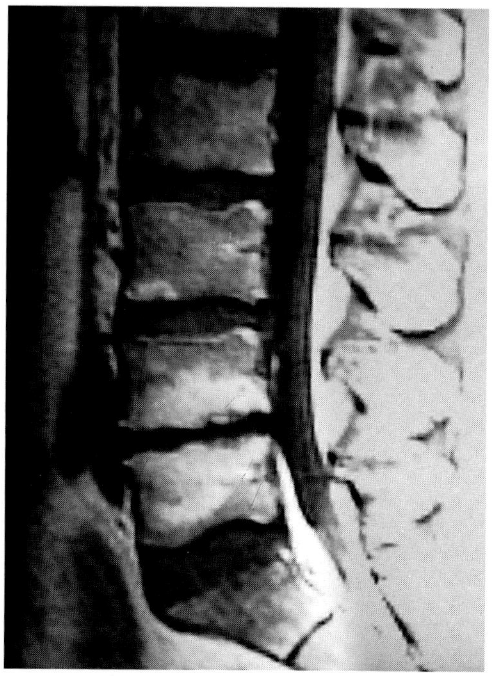

Figure 13–11. Discogenic marrow alterations. Sagittal T1-weighted MRI shows marked hyperintensity of the L4 and L5 marrow adjoining the degenerated L4-L5 disc. Degenerative change may also induce hypointensity in adjoining vertebrae on T1 sequences.

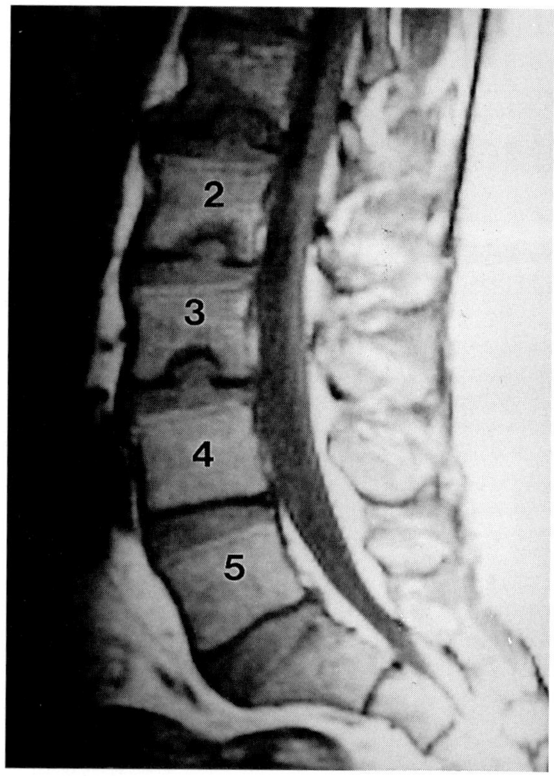

Figure 13–12. Schmorl's nodes. Sagittal T1-weighted scan shows Schmorl's nodes in the inferior end plates of L1, L2, and L3. This represents intrabody herniation of disc material. Note the hypointense rim of sclerosis in L2 and L3 and marked hypointensity in L1.

Cervical Intervertebral Disc Disease

With regard to both pathology and imaging, cervical disc disease is very similar to lumbar disc disease. To avoid redundancy, this brief discussion will emphasize only the differences.

Acute cervical disc herniation is much less common than lumbar herniation but still a common disorder. The peak incidence is in the third and fourth decades. Patients present with cervical radiculopathy, neck pain, or myelopathy. The cervical levels most often affected by both herniations and spondylosis are C6-C7 (60–75%) and C5-C6 (20–30%). There is a greater tendency in the cervical spine to form osteophytes at the posterior disc margin and uncovertebral joints, so that the differentiation of disc from osteophyte assumes greater importance.

Myelographic Findings. Plain radiographs remain an excellent technique for the diagnosis of foraminal stenosis and osteophyte but are insensitive for uncalcified (soft) disc herniations. Cervical myelography may be performed from either C1-C2 or lumbar puncture and shows a rounded or angular extradural defect at or slightly above a disc space. Posterolateral herniations usually cause amputation of the root sleeve. The pitfalls of myelography include insensitivity for far lateral herniations, difficulty in imaging through the shoulders in obese or short-necked patients, and sometimes poor opacification when the lumbar approach is used.

CT Findings. Unenhanced CT may show a hyperdense extradural mass adjoining the disc space but is limited by the absence of epidural fat in this region and beam-hardening artifacts through the shoulders. The inherent contrast between the disc and surrounding soft tissues can be increased somewhat by the use of intravenous contrast. In the 1980s, CT myelography became the gold standard for imaging the degenerated cervical spine. With the use of thin slices, this technique is highly sensitive for disc herniations, central and foraminal stenosis, and the differentiation of disc from osteophyte. With acute disc herniation, CT myelography shows displacement of the thecal sac by an anterior or anterolateral flat or convex soft tissue mass. The finding of calcification usually indicates chronic disc degeneration or osteophyte. The opacified thecal sac may be narrowed or obliterated, and the spinal cord displaced or compressed.

MRI Findings. An acutely herniated disc is of intermediate intensity (brighter than CSF) on T1-weighted images and hyperintense on T2-weighted SE and T2*-weighted GRE images (i.e., gradient-recalled echo). On axial GRE images, the hyperintense herniated disc is separated from the hyperintense CSF by a hypointense band of displaced posterior longitudinal ligament and dura. Because of its insensitivity to calcification, however, MRI is less able to diagnose osteophytes or to distinguish them from discs, ligaments, and CSF. T2-weighted images may reveal hyperintensity in the cord due to edema or myelomalacia. Intravenous contrast-enhanced MRI may improve the contrast between a herniated disc and surrounding tissue due to enhancement of the epidural venous plexus and reactive fibrovascular granulation tissue.

Differential Diagnosis

The differential diagnosis is essentially the same as that for lumbar disc herniation given in Table 13–1. The most important task is usually to differentiate soft disc herniation from chronic degeneration and osteophyte. Cervical spine radiography and CT are both highly accurate by directly demonstrating calcification within the abnormality.

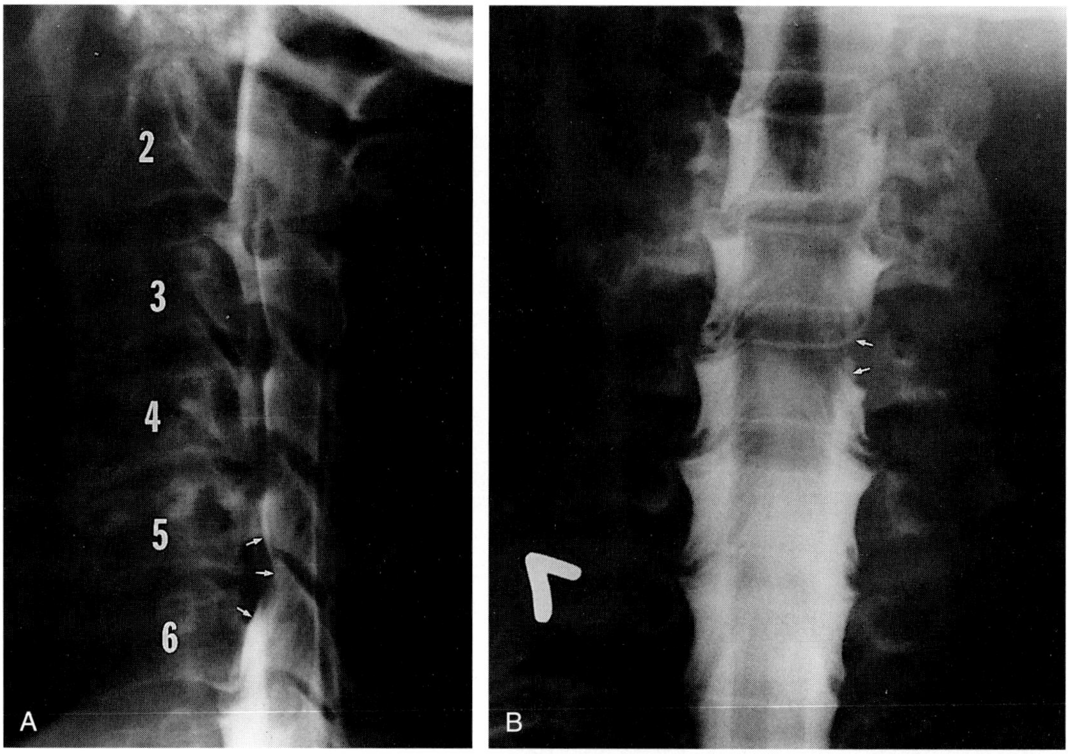

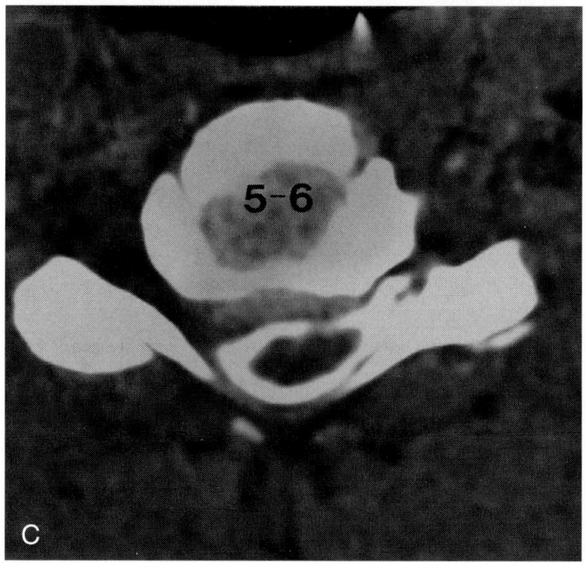

Figure 13–13. Cervical disc herniation. **(A)** Lateral and **(B)** AP myelograms show narrowing at C3-C4, C4-C5, and C5-C6 with a large ventral deformity (arrows in **A**) and right-sided root sleeve defect (arrows in **B**) at C5-C6. **(C)** CT myelogram shows a large uncalcified right paramedian disc herniation displacing the thecal sac and cord.

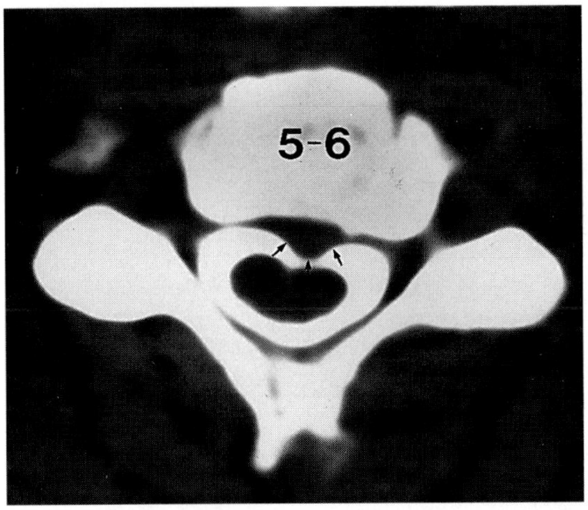

Figure 13–14. Cervical disc herniation. CT myelogram shows a markedly convex impression (arrows) upon the thecal sac caused by a nearly midline disc herniation. The cord is not affected.

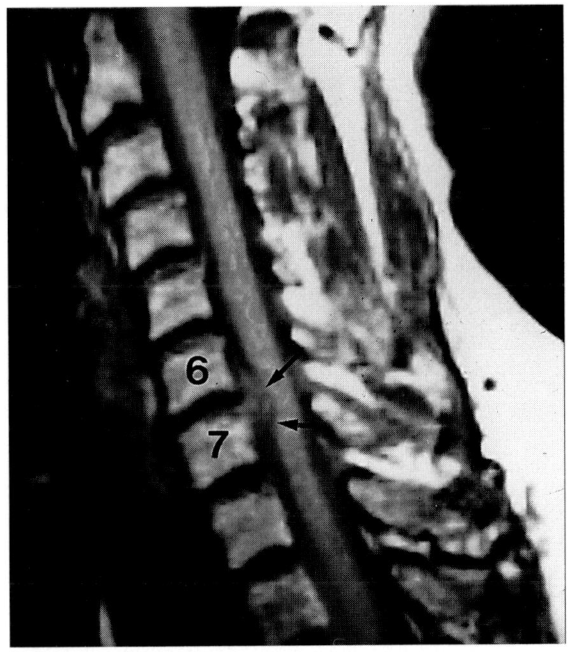

Figure 13–15. Cervical disc herniation. Sagittal T1-weighted MRI shows a large herniated disc at C6-C7 narrowing the canal and compressing the spinal cord.

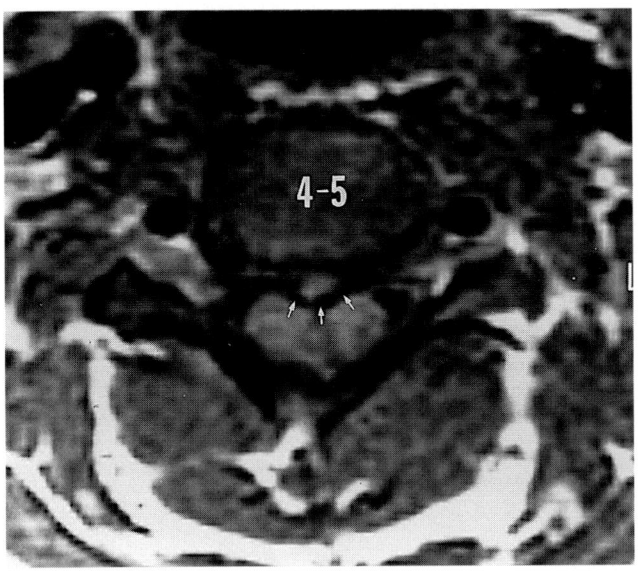

Figure 13–16. Cervical disc herniation. Axial T1-weighted scan through C4-C5 shows a herniated disc separated from the cord by a hypointense band (arrows) of dura and posterior longitudinal ligament. There is concave deformity of the ventral spinal cord.

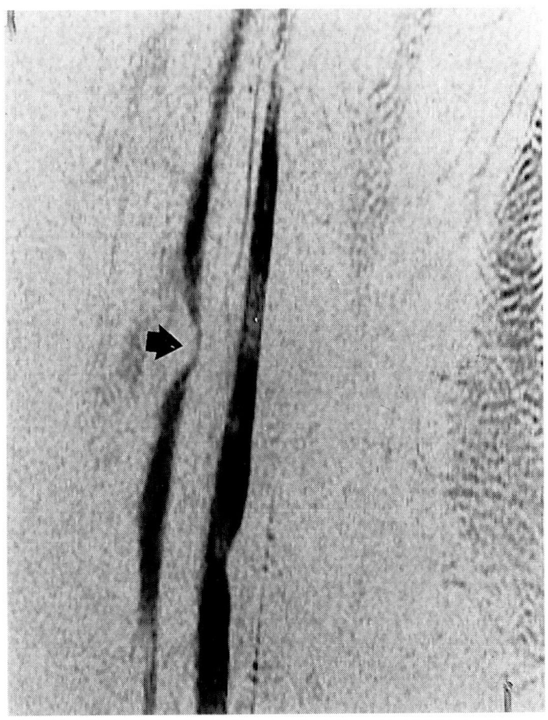

Figure 13–17. Cervical disc herniation. Oblique projection of MR myelogram shows deformity of the thecal sac (arrow) due to herniated disc at C5-C6. By itself this technique cannot distinguish disc from osteophyte. (Courtesy of Dr. Taher El Gammal, Birmingham, AL).

Cervical Spondylosis

Synonym: Spondylosis deformans.

Cervical spondylosis is a condition of the spine resulting from chronic disc degeneration, leading to marginal osteophytes of the disc space and hypertrophic osteophytes of the uncovertebral joints. This condition is extraordinarily common but usually asymptomatic. Up to 80% of adults over age 50 manifest vertebral osteophytes. Degenerative disease of the facet joints is more correctly referred to as osteoarthritis and often coexists.

Spondylosis becomes clinically important when osteophytes produce compression of the cervical roots (radiculopathy) or cord (myelopathy). Myelopathy is most likely to develop in individuals with a congenitally narrow cervical canal. Congenital or acquired stenosis both make the cervical cord much more susceptible to damage from minor trauma.

Myelographic Findings. The normal sagittal diameter of the bony cervical spinal canal measured from the posterior vertebral body to the interlaminar line should be greater than 13 mm. Anything less than 12 mm indicates stenosis. Another method is to divide the anteroposterior diameter of the spinal canal by the anteroposterior diameter of the midvertebral body at that level. A ratio of less than 0.8 indicates stenosis, whereas the mean value in normal patients is 1.0.

Routine myelography may show defects of the root sleeves, narrowing of the subarachnoid space, ventral and dorsal extradural defects due respectively to osteophytes and buckling of the ligamentum flavum, cord compression or atrophy, or myelographic block.

CT Findings. In decreasing order of incidence, CT myelographic findings may include narrowing of the subarachnoid space, marginal osteophytes, cord flattening, foraminal stenosis, root sleeve defects, cord displacement, and disc herniations. The anteroposterior diameter of the opacified subarachnoid space should be greater than 9 mm. CT is best able to distinguish acute disc herniations, which are of soft tissue density, from osteophytes, which are more or less isodense with bone. CT is ideal for showing stenosis of the neural foramina, usually caused by osteophytosis of the uncovertebral joints (joints of Luschka).

TABLE 13–2 | Differential Diagnosis of Spinal Stenosis

Common
Degenerative disease
Lymphoma
Myeloma
Metastasis
Abscess
Arachnoiditis
Postoperative fibrosis
Spondylolisthesis
Compression fracture
Uncommon
Epidural lipomatosis
Extramedullary hematopoiesis
Physiologic constriction (Valsalva maneuver)
Paget's disease
Ligamentous ossification
Synovial cysts
Achondroplasia
Hypochondroplasia
Morquio's syndrome

MRI Findings. Sagittal and axial T2-weighted images show narrowing or obliteration of the CSF surrounding the spinal cord at the level of the stenosis. Ventral deformity of the spinal cord occurs with ventral osteophytes and cord compression and is best seen on T1-weighted images. The cortical bone of osteophytes is hypointense on all sequences, whereas internally the presence of bone marrow may result in variable signal intensities.

T2-weighted images may show hyperintensity in the cord at levels of stenosis. This is believed to represent demyelination, gliosis, and myelomalacia and correlates with more severe myelopathy and a worse postoperative prognosis. CT remains better suited for the evaluation of bony changes and neural foramina, whereas MRI is superior in the noninvasive diagnosis of acute disc herniations and cord alterations. Various factors with MRI tend to cause overestimation of foraminal stenosis.

Differential Diagnosis

See Table 13–2.

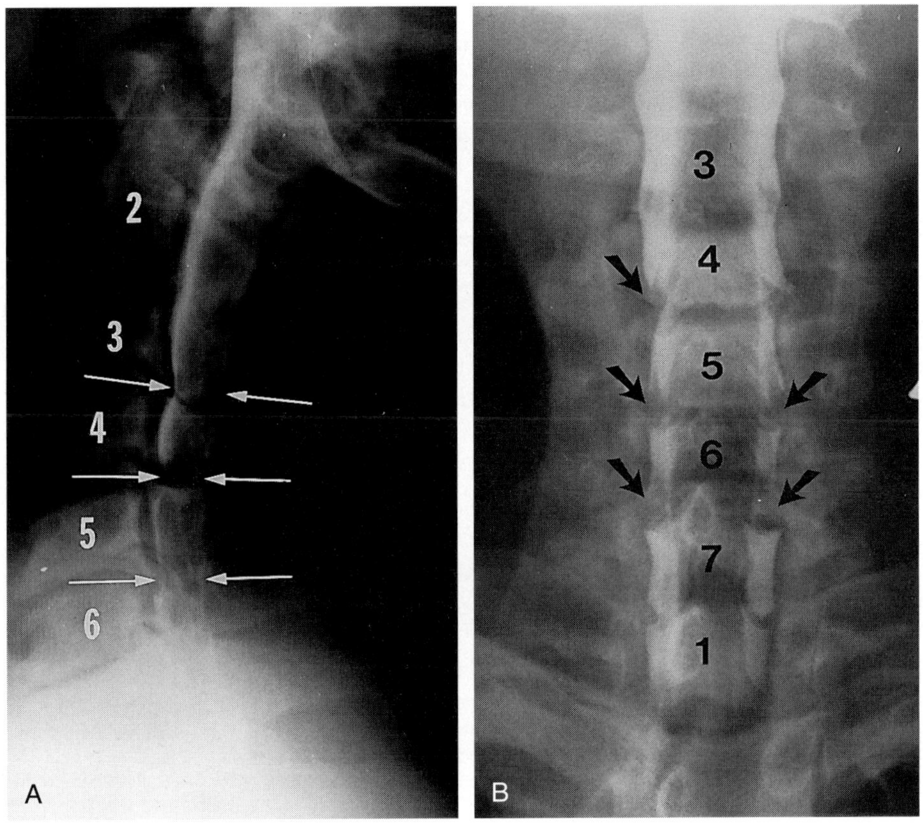

Figure 13–18. Cervical spondylosis. **(A)** Lateral myelogram shows severe stenosis (arrows) of the spinal canal from C3 to T1 with ventral defects due to spurs at C3-C4, C4-C5, and C5-C6. **(B)** AP myelogram shows nerve root sleeve defects (arrows) on the right at C3-C4, C4-C5, and C5-C6 and on the left at C5-C6 and C6-C7.

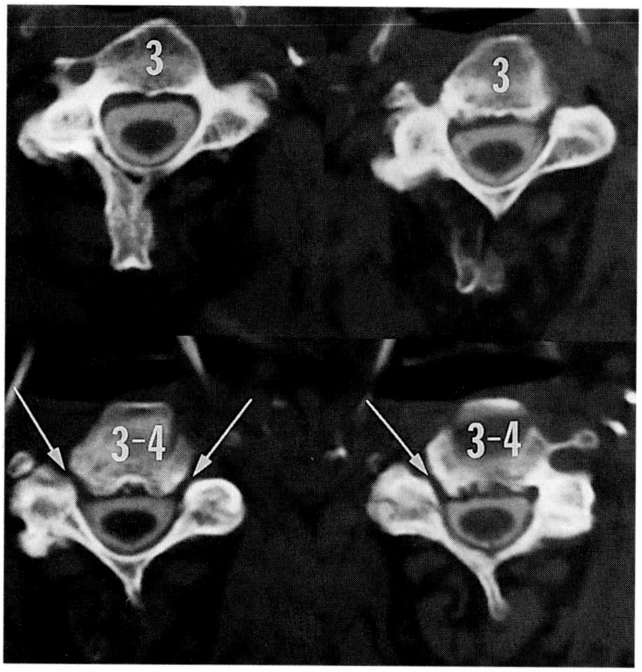

Figure 13–19. Cervical spondylosis with foraminal stenosis. CT myelogram through the C3-C4 level shows severe bilateral foraminal stenosis (arrows) due to hypertrophy of superior facets and uncinate processes. There is mild spurring along the posterior disc margin at C3-C4.

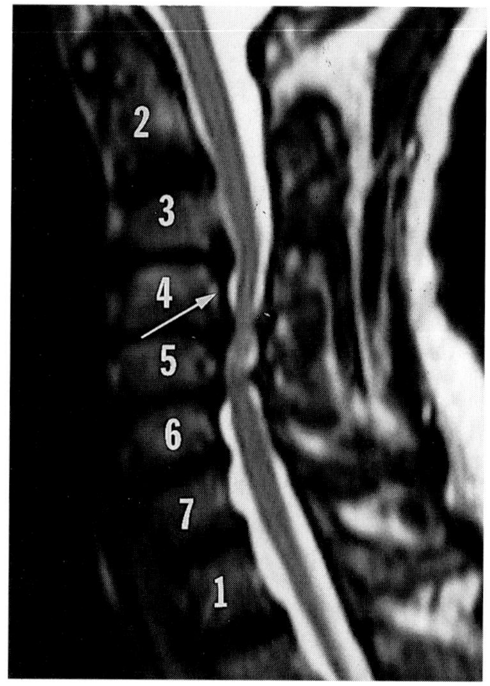

Figure 13–20. Cervical spondylosis and OPLL. Sagittal T2-weighted MRI shows large hypointense posterior osteophytes at C3-C4, C4-C5, C5-C6, and C6-C7 with degeneration of the disc spaces, severe stenosis, and myelomalacia. Note also the elevation and thickening of the posterior longitudinal ligament posterior to C4 (long arrow), an appearance compatible with OPLL (unconfirmed).

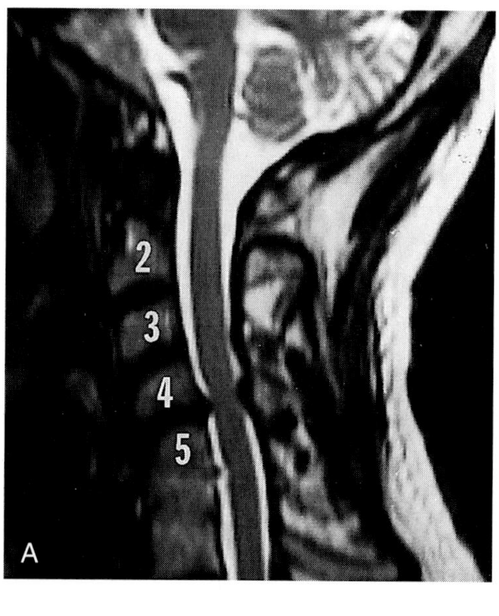

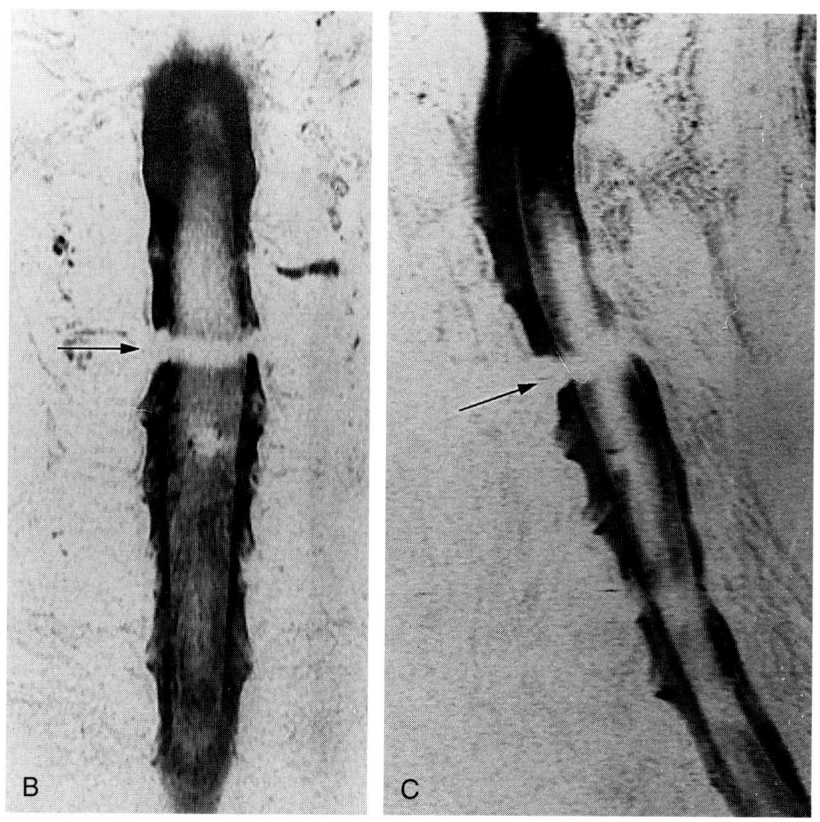

Figure 13–21. Cervical spondylosis. **(A).** Sagittal T2-weighted MRI shows narrowing of the subarachnoid space at C4-C5 because of ventral osteophyte and posterior ligamentous thickening. C5 through C7 are surgically fused. AP **(B)** and oblique **(C)** MR myelograms show obliteration of CSF at C4-C5 and severe bilateral extradural deformity (arrows).

Lumbar Stenosis

The complex structure of the lumbar spine coupled with the weight bearing and stress placed upon it render all of its individual components vulnerable to progressive degenerative change with advancing age. Isolated osteoarthritis of the facet joints may result in local pain. Commonly, however, symptoms of radicular pain and lower extremity weakness develop due to hypertrophic degenerative processes causing compression of the cauda equina and nerve roots.

Lumbar spinal stenosis may consist of narrowing of the central spinal canal, stenosis of the lateral recess, or stenosis of the neural foramina, individually or in combination. Concurrent disc degeneration is commonly present. It is a matter of debate whether primary degeneration of the disc places stress on the facet joints, promoting their secondary degeneration, or vice versa.

Stenosis of the central canal results from disc bulge or herniation, osteophytosis of the end plate, superior facet hypertrophy, spondylolisthesis with intact pars, and thickening of the ligamentum flavum. The latter is probably due more to laxity and buckling than actual hypertrophy. A congenitally narrow canal due to short pedicles or a narrow interpediculate diameter is an important predisposing factor. Both lateral recess stenosis and foraminal stenosis result from bulging of the disc, superior facet hypertrophy, vertical subluxation of the superior facet, or some combination of these. Because the nerve root exists in the upper part of the foramen just beneath the pedicle, narrowing of the inferior foramen does not cause root compression.

Myelographic Findings. Myelography demonstrates a narrow canal, compression of the dural sleeve, or complete block. The narrowing is usually both ventral and dorsal and most severe at the level of the disc space. Marked tortuosity of the cauda equina may be observed above a block. This has been dubbed the redundant lumbar nerve root syndrome and is attributed to traction and repeated stretching.

CT Findings. Plain CT and CT myelography are highly effective for the diagnosis and preoperative assessment of lumbar stenosis. CT findings include disc bulge or herniation, thickening of the ligamenta flava, and degeneration and osteophytosis of the facet joints. With advanced central canal stenosis, both anterior and posterior epidural fat is obliterated, and the dural sleeve itself may be virtually obliterated. In the case of spondylolisthesis, a scan through the plane of the disc demonstrates a double image of two overlapping end plates with the olisthetic vertebra anterior to the stationary vertebra.

Lateral recess stenosis occurs when osteophytes of the superior facet approach within 5 mm of the posterior vertebral body. Stenosis of the neural foramina may best be appreciated with parasagittal reformatted images. A good rule of thumb is that the lumbar foramina should be easily visualized in at least two contiguous sections of 4 to 5 mm.

TABLE 13–3 Useful Measurements Pertaining to the Lumbar Spine

Normal sagittal diameter of spinal canal	≥12 mm
Normal transverse diameter of spinal canal (facet joint)	≥10 mm
Normal transverse diameter of spinal canal (pedicles)	≥16 mm
Normal cross-sectional area of spinal canal	≥1.45 cm^2
Normal thickness of ligamentum flavum	<6 mm
Normal thickness of facet joint/hyaline cartilage	2–4 mm
Normal sagittal diameter of neural foramina:	
Craniocaudal	9 mm
Anteroposterior	4 mm

MRI Findings. A complete MRI examination should include sagittal T1- and T2-weighted images and axial T1- or PD-weighted images. The sagittal T2-weighted scan shows the size and contour of the thecal sac and the early stages of disc degeneration. The sagittal T1-weighted sequence is best for assessing the posterior disc margins and diameter of the neural foramina, which should normally be filled with hyperintense fat with nerve roots and ganglia readily recognizable in the upper half. Various patterns of signal abnormality occur in the vertebral marrow in association with disc degeneration (see Table 12–10). The axial images aid in distinguishing disc bulge from herniation, enable measurement of the ligamentum flavum, and show sclerosis, cartilaginous degeneration, and osteophytosis of the facet joints, although in the latter case not as accurately as CT.

Differential Diagnosis

See Table 13–2.

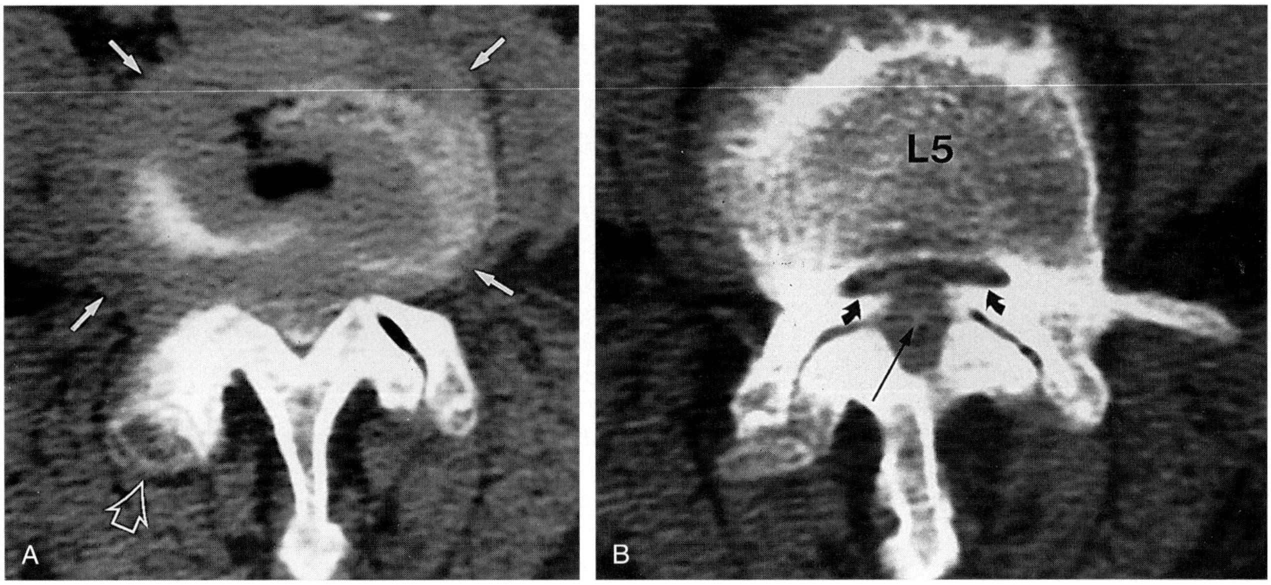

Figure 13–22. Central and lateral recess stenosis. **(A)** CT myelogram through the L4-L5 disc shows circumferential disc bulge (solid arrows), vacuum phenomenon in the disc and left facet joint, advanced hypertrophy and degeneration of the right facet joint (open arrow), and severe compression of the thecal sac. **(B)** Slightly lower section through the top of L5 shows almost total obliteration of the subarachnoid space (long arrow). Short pedicles and hypertrophy of the superior facets contribute to severe lateral recess stenosis (curved arrows) bilaterally. Other changes include thinning and sclerosis of the facet joints and obliteration of the epidural fat.

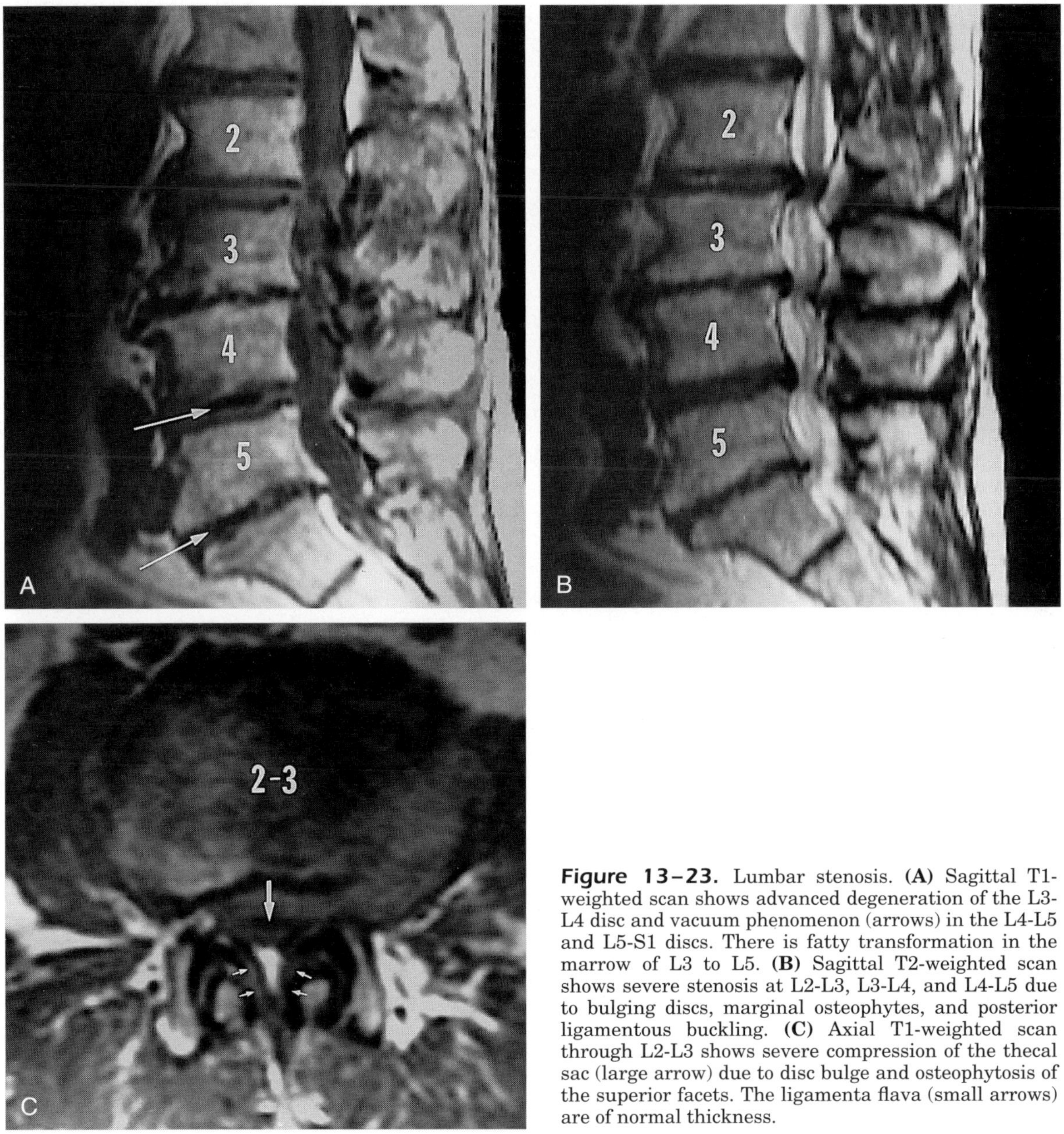

Figure 13–23. Lumbar stenosis. **(A)** Sagittal T1-weighted scan shows advanced degeneration of the L3-L4 disc and vacuum phenomenon (arrows) in the L4-L5 and L5-S1 discs. There is fatty transformation in the marrow of L3 to L5. **(B)** Sagittal T2-weighted scan shows severe stenosis at L2-L3, L3-L4, and L4-L5 due to bulging discs, marginal osteophytes, and posterior ligamentous buckling. **(C)** Axial T1-weighted scan through L2-L3 shows severe compression of the thecal sac (large arrow) due to disc bulge and osteophytosis of the superior facets. The ligamenta flava (small arrows) are of normal thickness.

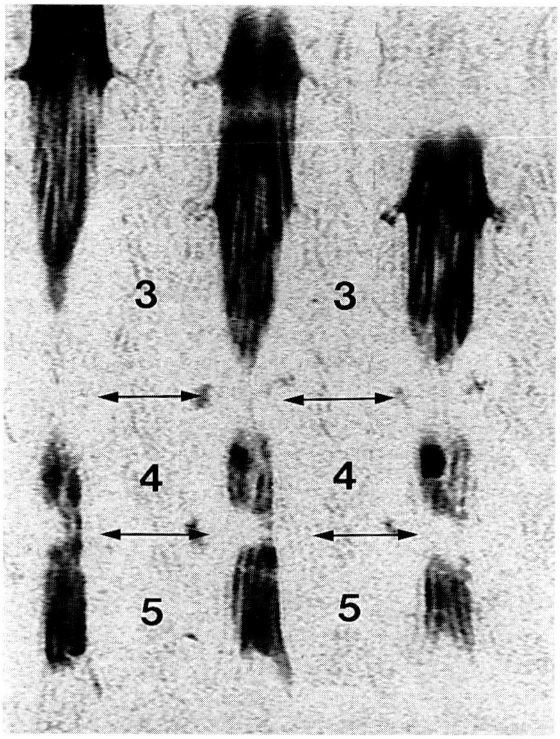

Figure 13–24. Lumbar stenosis. AP projection of MR myelogram shows obliteration of the subarachnoid space at L3-L4 and severe stenosis at L4-L5. The hyperintense structure at mid L4 is a synovial cyst (unproven). (Courtesy of Dr. Taher El Gammal, Birmingham, AL).

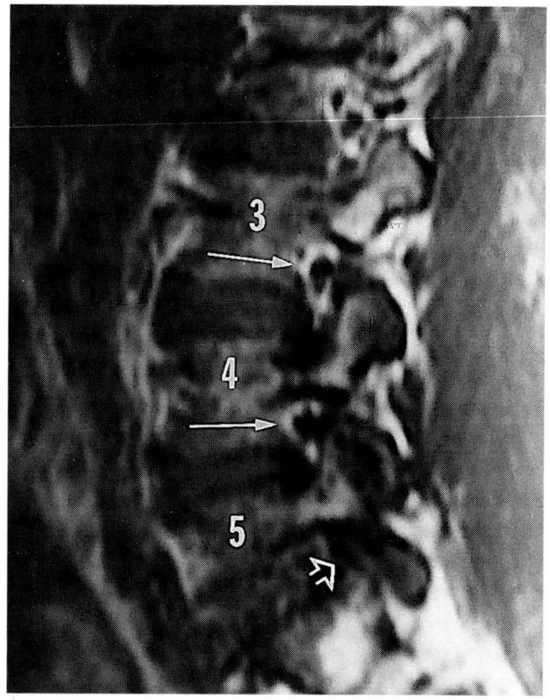

Figure 13–25. Foraminal stenosis. Sagittal T1-weighted MRI shows normal L3-L4 and L4-L5 foramina (long arrows) and severe stenosis of the L5-S1 foramen (open arrow). The dorsal root ganglia are easily identified in the upper half of the L3-L4 and L4-L5 foramina.

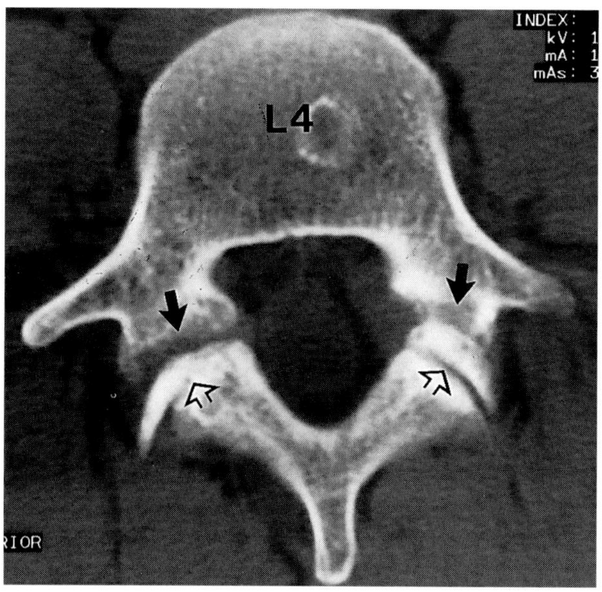

Figure 13–26. Spondylolysis. CT through L4 shows bilateral pars defects (solid arrows). The facet joints (open arrows) are more posterior and obliquely oriented; spondylolysis is usually parallel with the coronal plane. There is narrowing and sclerosis of both facet joints and a posterior osteophyte of the right superior facet.

Synovial Cyst

Synovial cysts arise from degenerated facet joints of the lumbar spine. Most occur between L3 and S1, with 75% at the L4-L5 level. Ganglion cysts are not lined by synovium and do not communicate with the joint. They otherwise behave clinically like synovial cysts. On imaging, ganglion cysts may only be differentiated by facet joint arthrography, which in the case of synovial cysts shows communication with the joint capsule. Both cysts form epidural masses in the posterior lumbar canal that may compress nerve roots and cause back pain and radiculopathy.

Myelographic and CT Findings. Myelography and CT show a posterior rounded epidural mass of 5 to 10 mm usually adjoining a facet joint in the lower lumbar spine. The attenuation is variable, and peripheral calcifications may be present. Gas (vacuum phenomenon) may be present within the facet joint and if also present within the mass is pathognomonic for synovial cyst.

MRI Findings. Synovial cysts are typically hyperintense to CSF on T2-weighted images with a hypointense rim. The signal characteristics may be highly variable, especially in the presence of hemorrhage. Subacute hemorrhage may result in marked hyperintensity on T1-weighted images. Marked peripheral enhancement occurs following intravenous contrast.

Differential Diagnosis

Epidural or cystic masses may be caused by disc fragments, perineural cysts, or nerve sheath tumors. The key findings to distinguish a synovial cyst are its proximity to the facet joint and its location deep (dorsal) to the ligamentum flavum.

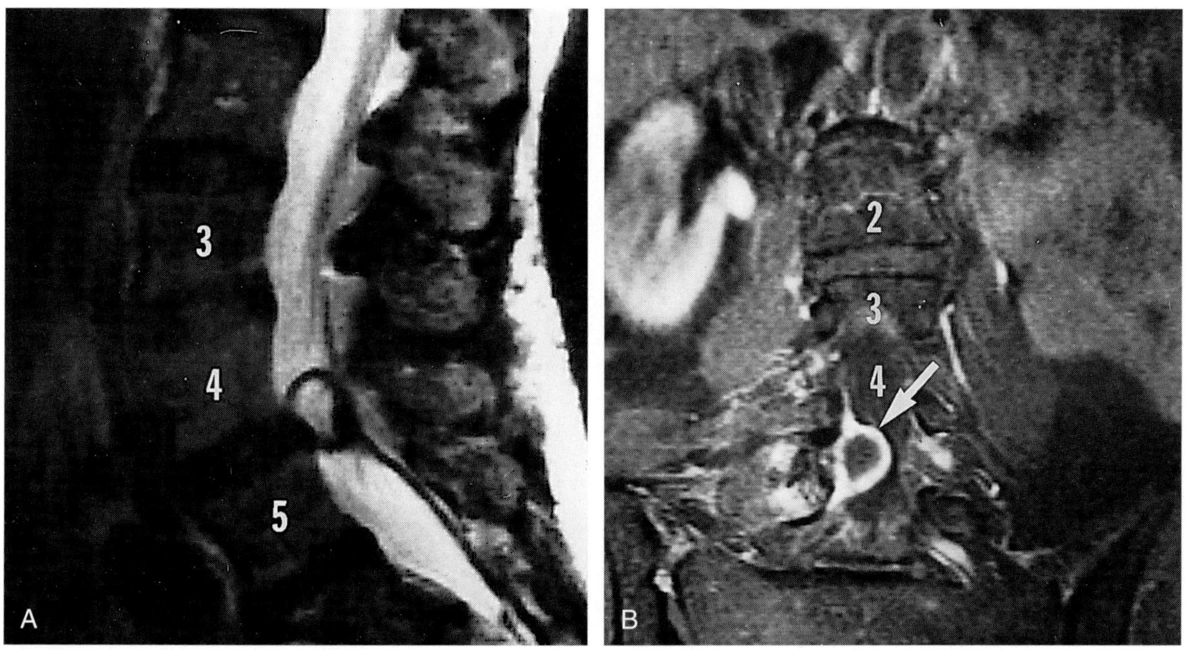

Figure 13–27. Synovial cyst. **(A)** Sagittal T2-weighted MRI shows a hyperintense cyst at L4-L5 with markedly hypointense rim. **(B)** Coronal contrast-enhanced MRI shows marked peripheral enhancement of the cyst (arrow).

Postoperative Spine

In up to 40% of patients with back pain, surgery fails to provide relief of pain or functional disability. Although the true incidence is probably closer to 15%, there is still a large cohort of patients with this condition currently referred to as the failed back surgery syndrome. The leading identified causes include postoperative epidural fibrosis, recurrent or residual disc herniation, arachnoiditis, and spinal stenosis. The usual clinical dilemma is the differentiation of disc from epidural fibrosis in a postoperative patient with an epidural mass. Patients with herniation may improve with additional surgery, whereas those with epidural fibrosis do not benefit.

Myelographic and CT Findings. Myelography alone is of little use in the differentiation of recurrent disc from postoperative scar. In general, however, recurrent disc herniations are associated with a larger extradural defect. Intrathecal contrast also does not improve the specificity of CT. Intravenous contrast, however, may increase the accuracy of CT to as high as 87%. Scar tissue in the anterior and lateral epidural space is notable for a leaky endothelium and large extracellular space. Generally speaking, recurrent disc does not enhance, whereas anterior and lateral recess scar shows demonstrable enhancement throughout.

MRI Findings. Unenhanced MRI has little advantage over other techniques, as both herniated disc and scar exhibit a similar range of signal intensities. The reported accuracy of contrast-enhanced MRI in the discrimination of disc from scar is as high as 96–100%. Generally speaking, if scanning is performed within 10 minutes of contrast injection, scar enhances but herniated disc does not.

Normal MRI findings during the first 6 postoperative months include enhancement of the decompressed nerve root, enhancement of the posterior annulus at the level of discectomy, enhancement of the facet joints, and soft tissue mass with peripheral or diffuse enhancement. In the early postoperative period, both herniated disc and normal postoperative change may show marginal or ring enhancement.

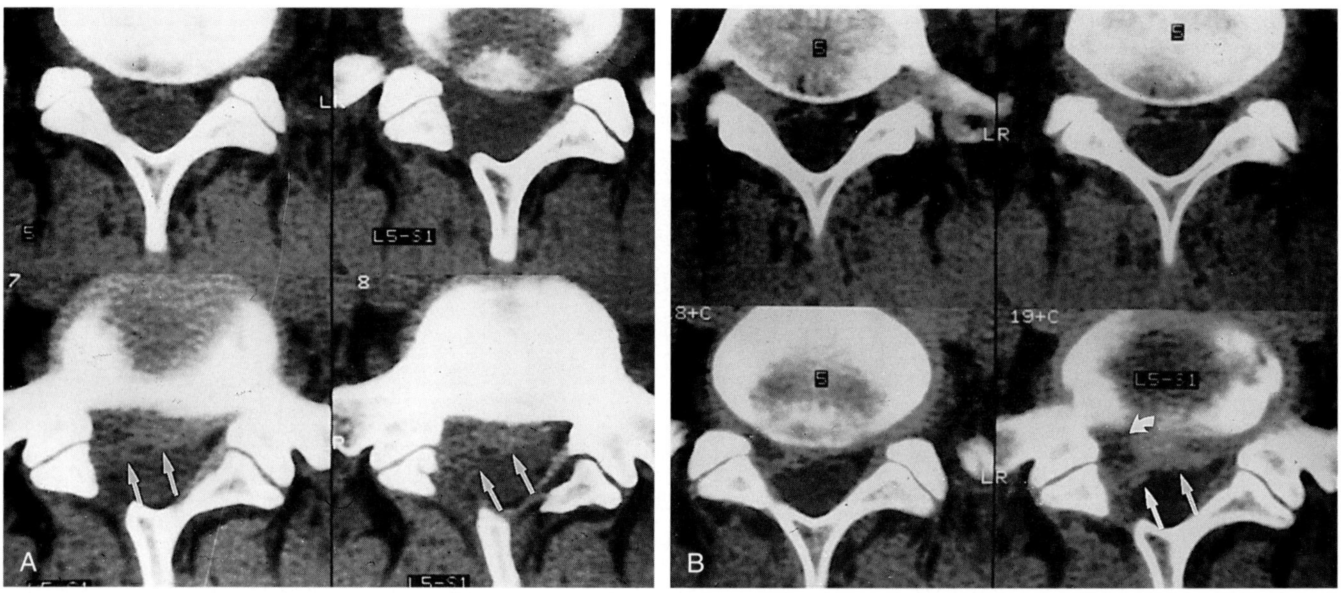

Figure 13–28. Postoperative scar and disc. **(A)** Unenhanced CT through L5-S1 shows a right laminectomy defect and soft tissue mass (arrows) obliterating the epidural fat. **(B)** Following intravenous contrast the scar enhances (straight arrows), whereas a residual disc fragment (curved arrow) does not.

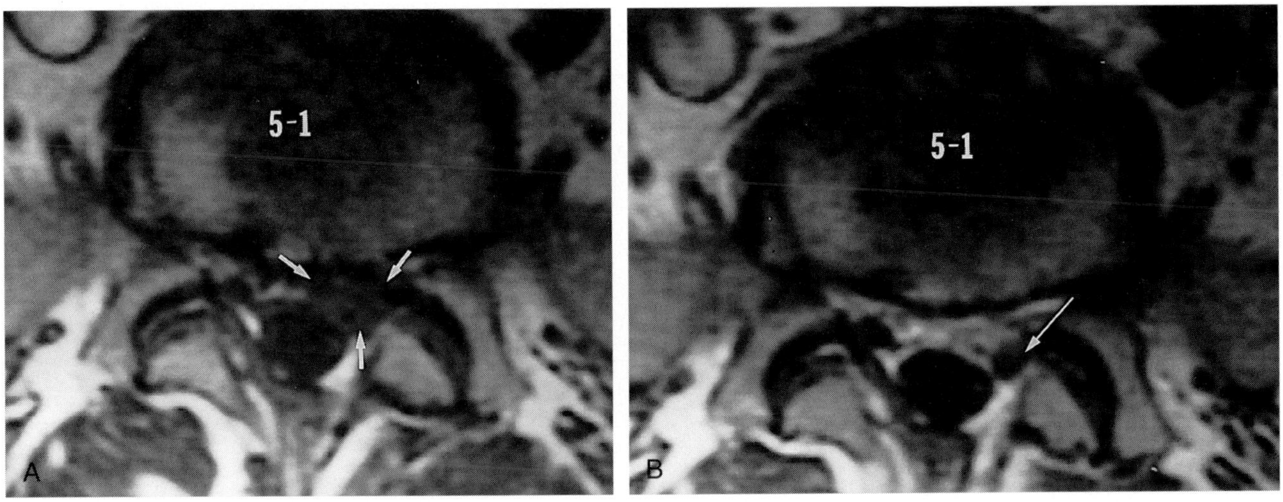

Figure 13–29. Postoperative scar. **(A)** Axial T1-weighted MRI through L5-S1 shows soft tissue mass (arrows) obliterating epidural fat and displacing the thecal sac. **(B)** Following intravenous contrast the mass enhances indicating postoperative scar. The nonenhancing posterior structure (arrow) is the normal root sleeve and should not be confused with herniated disc.

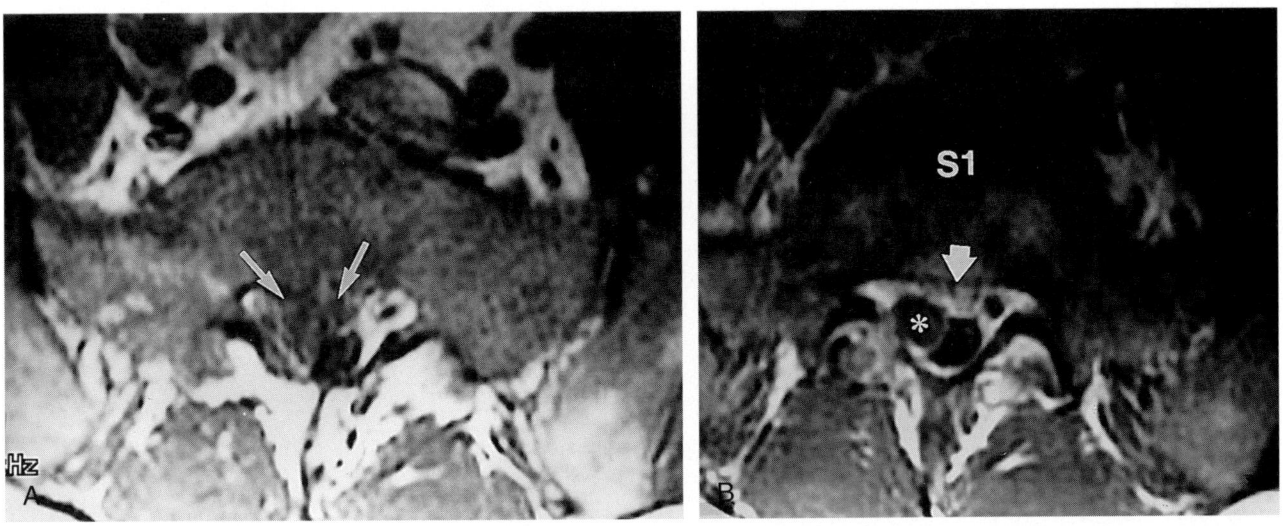

Figure 13–30. Postoperative disc. **(A)** T1-weighted MRI through S1 shows a very large epidural soft tissue mass (arrows) displacing the thecal sac and obliterating the epidural fat. **(B)** Following intravenous contrast some enhancing scar tissue is present anteriorly (arrow), and there is rim enhancement around a large recurrent disc herniation (asterisk). This finding may be normal in the immediate postoperative state.

Trauma

Nerve Root Avulsion

Direct stretch injury to the sensorimotor supply of the upper extremity can occur at the brachial plexus or the attachment of cervical spinal roots to the spinal cord. Motorcycle accidents and birth trauma are the leading causes of nerve root avulsion. Because injuries to the brachial plexus may be repaired and nerve root avulsions cannot, it is important preoperatively to exclude an avulsion by appropriate imaging.

Myelographic and CT Findings. CT myelography is highly effective at making the diagnosis of cervical root avulsion. The relevant findings consist of (1) attenuation or absence of the cervical root in its passage through the subarachnoid space, and (2) the presence of traumatic pseudomeningoceles arising at the point where a cervical root should exit. Myelography is better at visualizing the cervical roots, whereas CT is somewhat more sensitive for the pseudomeningoceles. Pseudomeningoceles represent a tear of the dura and are not synonymous with root avulsion. Although either one may be present without the other, the two injuries are associated in at least 80% of instances. Partial avulsions are less likely to be associated with a pseudomeningocele.

MRI Findings. As with myelography, MRI may directly demonstrate absence of the avulsed root. At the current state of the art, however, the avulsions are seen much less clearly than with myelography. Pseudomeningoceles appear as abnormal collections of CSF forming a well-defined homogeneous hyperintensity on T2-weighted images. Pseudomeningoceles may be exquisitely demonstrated with MR myelographic techniques.

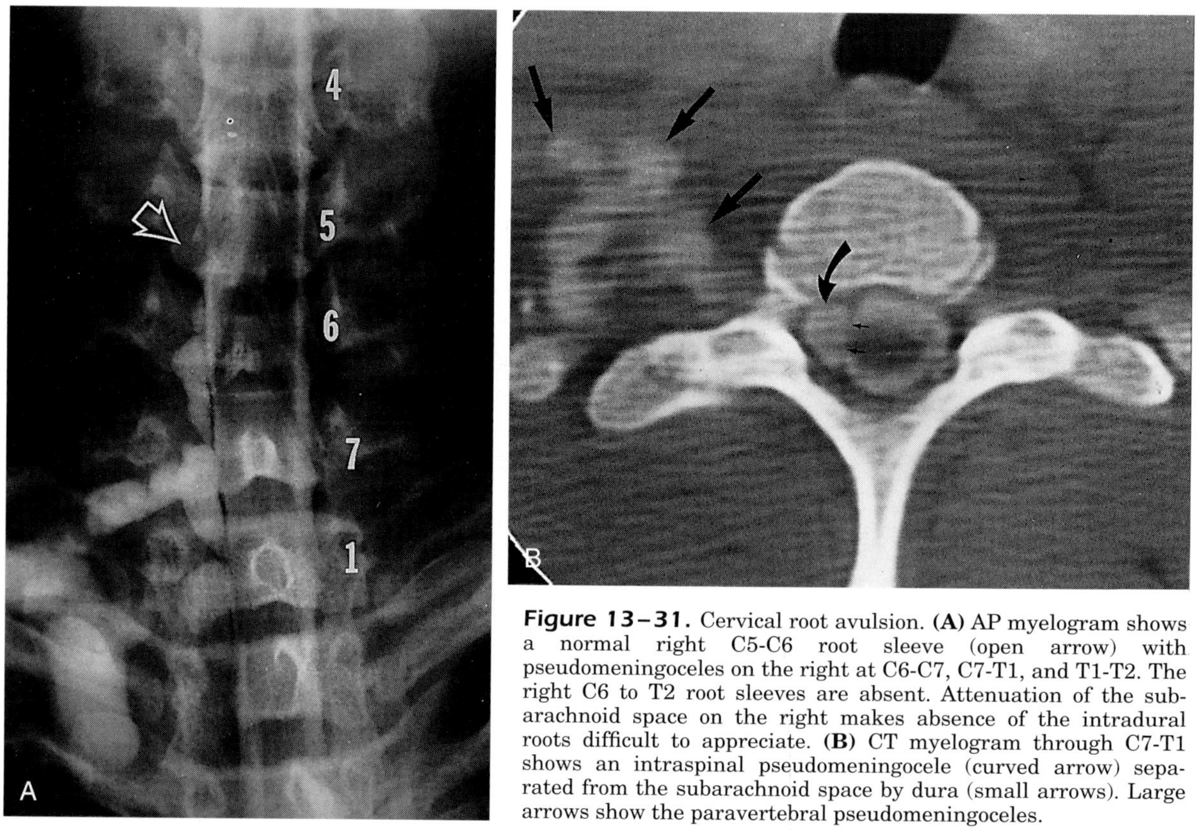

Figure 13–31. Cervical root avulsion. **(A)** AP myelogram shows a normal right C5-C6 root sleeve (open arrow) with pseudomeningoceles on the right at C6-C7, C7-T1, and T1-T2. The right C6 to T2 root sleeves are absent. Attenuation of the subarachnoid space on the right makes absence of the intradural roots difficult to appreciate. **(B)** CT myelogram through C7-T1 shows an intraspinal pseudomeningocele (curved arrow) separated from the subarachnoid space by dura (small arrows). Large arrows show the paravertebral pseudomeningoceles.

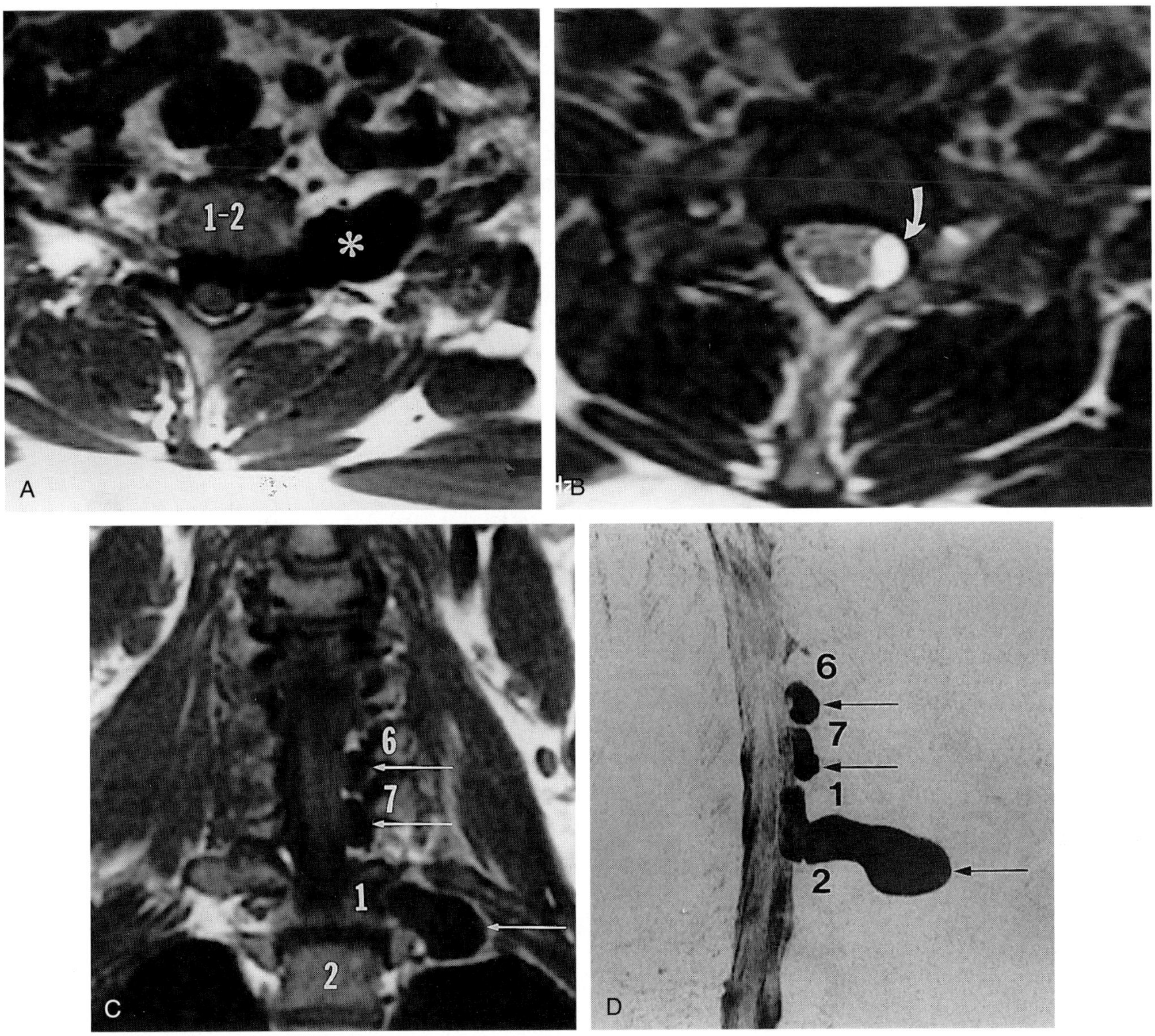

Figure 13–32. Cervical root avulsion. **(A)** Axial T1-weighted MRI shows a large paraspinal pseudomeningocele (asterisk) extending through the neural foramen. It is uniformly isointense with CSF. **(B)** On a T2-weighted image through T1, the pseudomeningocele (curved arrow) is hyperintense relative to CSF due to absence of flow. **(C)** Coronal T1-weighted MRI shows lateral pseudomeningoceles (arrows) on the left at C6-C7, C7-T1, and T1-T2. **(D)** MR myelogram (right anterior oblique projection) shows pseudomeningoceles (arrows) with absence of nerve roots. (**D** courtesy of Dr. Taher El Gammal, Birmingham, AL).

Spinal Cord Injuries

Direct blunt injuries to the spinal cord cause contusion and hemorrhage and may be seen with cervical spine fractures, ligamentous disruption, or disc herniation. The presence of cord injury is the major determinant of neurologic outcome following cervical spine trauma, and most cord injuries occur in the cervical region. Injuries to the conus are second in frequency, and blunt injury to the thoracic cord is rare. Although data are still preliminary regarding the correlation of early MRI with neurologic outcome, studies so far suggest that the prognosis of cord injury is better with nonhemorrhagic contusions and worse if hemorrhage is present (hematomyelia). Chronic sequelae of cord injury include atrophy, gliosis, myelomalacia, or syrinx.

Myelographic and CT Findings. Myelography in these patients is technically difficult due to the necessity of C1-C2 puncture and the difficulties of prone positioning. It may reveal epidural defects due to hematoma or disc herniation, enlargement of the cord due to contusion or hemorrhage, or complete myelographic block. CT enables superior delineation of most fractures but is limited in its sensitivity for cord injuries.

MRI Findings. MRI has proven valuable in the direct assessment of the spinal canal for compressive conditions and of the cord for parenchymal injury. Soft tissue injuries to the spinal ligaments and herniated discs may be apparent on MRI but undetectable on CT. Cord contusion is manifest as a localized hyperintensity on T2-weighted images often tapered at cephalic and caudal ends. Contusion is isointense or hypointense on T1-weighted images. The appearance of hemorrhage, as elsewhere, varies as a function of age but is usually distinguished from nonhemorrhagic contusion by hypointensity on T2-weighted images during the acute phase and hyperintensity on T1-weighted images in later stages.

Late after injury, MRI may demonstrate cord atrophy or syringomyelia. Signal abnormality in the cord may indicate myelomalacia or gliosis, which are hyperintense on T2-weighted images and isointense or hypointense on T1-weighted images.

Differential Diagnosis

The history of trauma and evidence of bony and soft tissue injuries readily enable differentiation of contusion from other causes of signal abnormality within the cord (see Table 12–3).

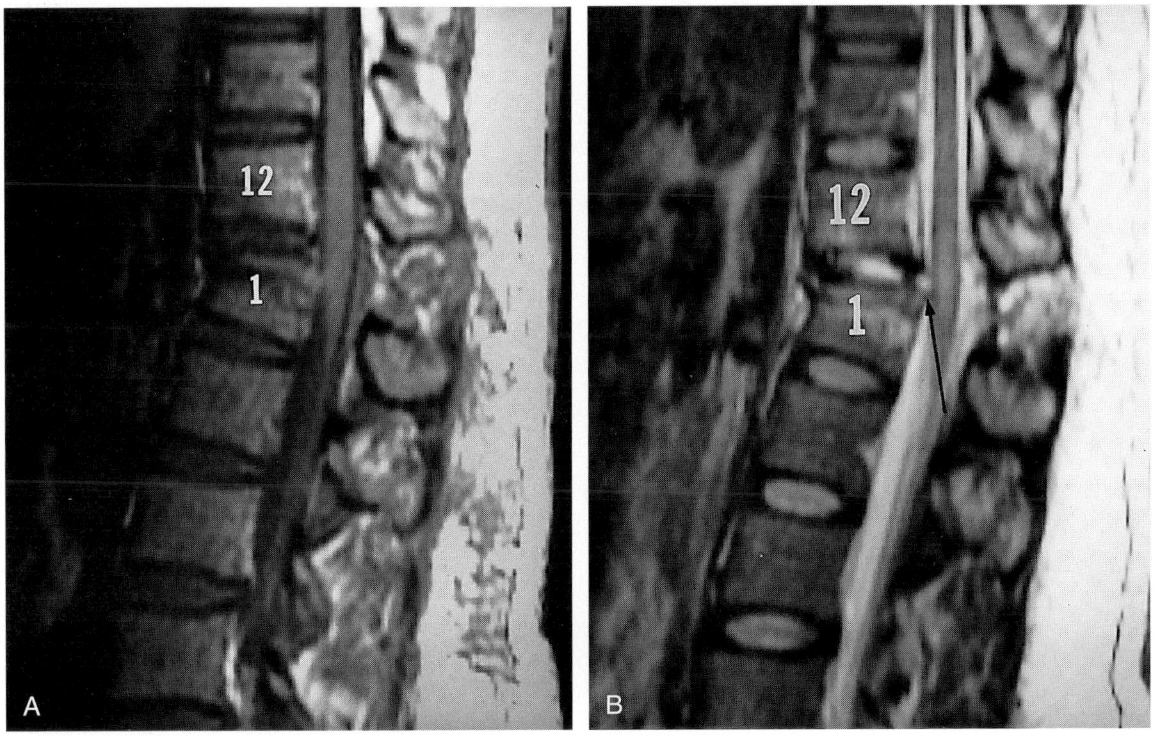

Figure 13–33. Contusion of conus. **(A)** Sagittal T1-weighted MRI shows a compression fracture of L1. The tip of the conus is at L1-L2. **(B)** T2-weighted image shows hyperintense edema in the conus and a small T12-L1 disc herniation (arrow). The signal alterations in the T12 and L1 vertebrae and T12-L1 disc space are due to hemorrhage.

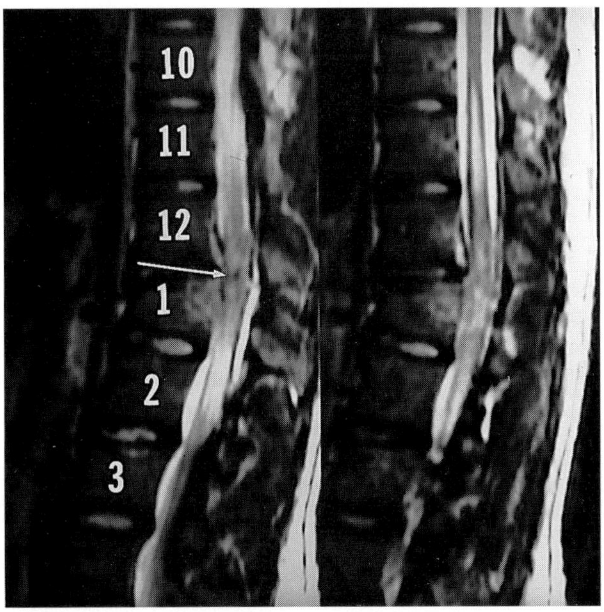

Figure 13–34. Hemorrhagic contusion of conus. Sagittal T2-weighted MRI shows anterior compression of L1, epidural hematoma posterior to T12, and severe contusion of the conus with edema extending to T10. Focal hypointensity (long arrow) at T12-L1 is a sign of cord hemorrhage.

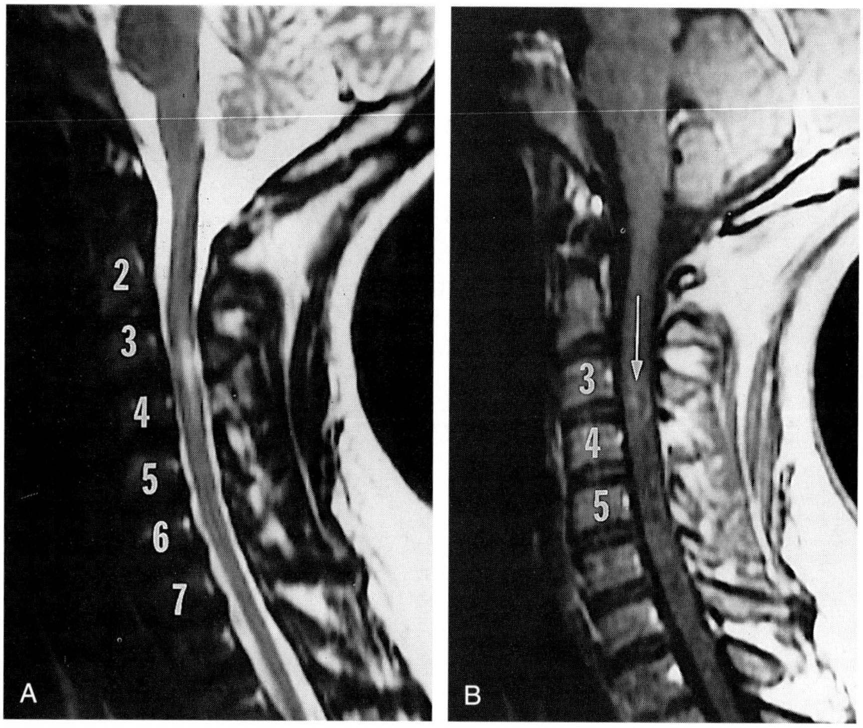

Figure 13–35. Contusion of cord. **(A)** Sagittal T2-weighted MRI shows hyperintensity in the cervical cord behind C3 and C4. **(B)** Postcontrast scan shows mild enhancement (arrow) in the cord at C3-C4. This was a hyperextension injury, and the spine is normally aligned. Fracture is not visible on these slices.

Hematoma

The patterns of hemorrhage observed in the spine parallel those in the cranium: epidural, subdural, subarachnoid, and parenchymal. Parenchymal hemorrhage (hematomyelia) may be caused by trauma, AVM, or tumors, particularly ependymoma and hemangioblastoma. Subarachnoid hemorrhage is usually a result of AVM or aneurysmal rupture in either the spine or cranium. Epidural hematoma is spontaneous in up to 50%. Other causes include vertebral fractures, epidural anesthesia, bleeding diatheses, and AVMs. Back pain is the usual presenting symptom of epidural hematoma. About 85% of spinal subdural hematomas are precipitated by lumbar puncture, especially if there is a concurrent bleeding diathesis.

CT Findings. CT may sometimes show localized or diffuse increased attenuation in the spinal canal anatomically localized to the cord, epidural compartment, or subarachnoid space. Subarachnoid hemorrhage probably cannot be differentiated from subdural hemorrhage. Lumbar epidural hematoma has an attenuation of 60 to 70 HU and may be indistinguishable from herniated nucleus pulposus.

MRI Findings. MRI may offer superior visualization of hemorrhage because of improved contrast resolution and direct sagittal imaging. The signal intensity of the hematoma is a function of its age (see Chapter 1). Subdural and subarachnoid hemorrhage may extend over a very long distance. Epidural hematoma is usually more localized, even to a single disc level, and tapered at both ends. On T2-weighted images, epidural hematoma may be separated from the CSF by a hypointense line representing the displaced dura.

Differential Diagnosis

Signal alterations in the CSF, especially hyperintensity on T1-weighted images, may result from lipoma, carcinomatosis, meningitis, or residual Pantopaque. Usually the diagnosis of hemorrhage is evident based on a clinical history of recent trauma or lumbar puncture.

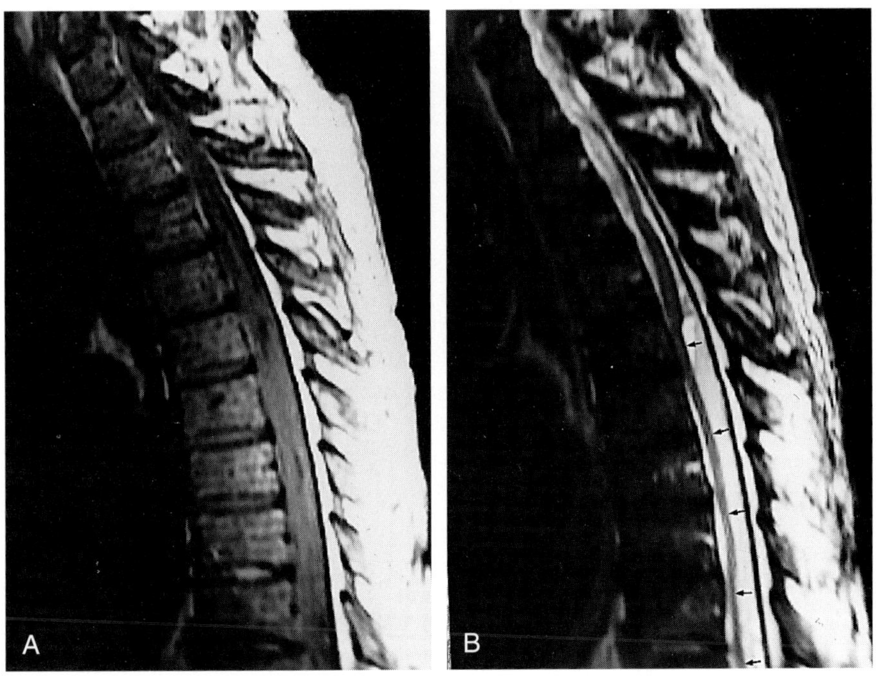

Figure 13–36. Hyperacute subdural hematoma (complication of lumbar puncture). **(A)** Sagittal T1-weighted MRI shows extensive hyperintensity of the CSF and poor delineation of the spinal cord. **(B)** On T2-weighted MRI the hematoma is of equal to or greater signal than CSF. The spinal cord (arrows) is compressed and ventrally displaced.

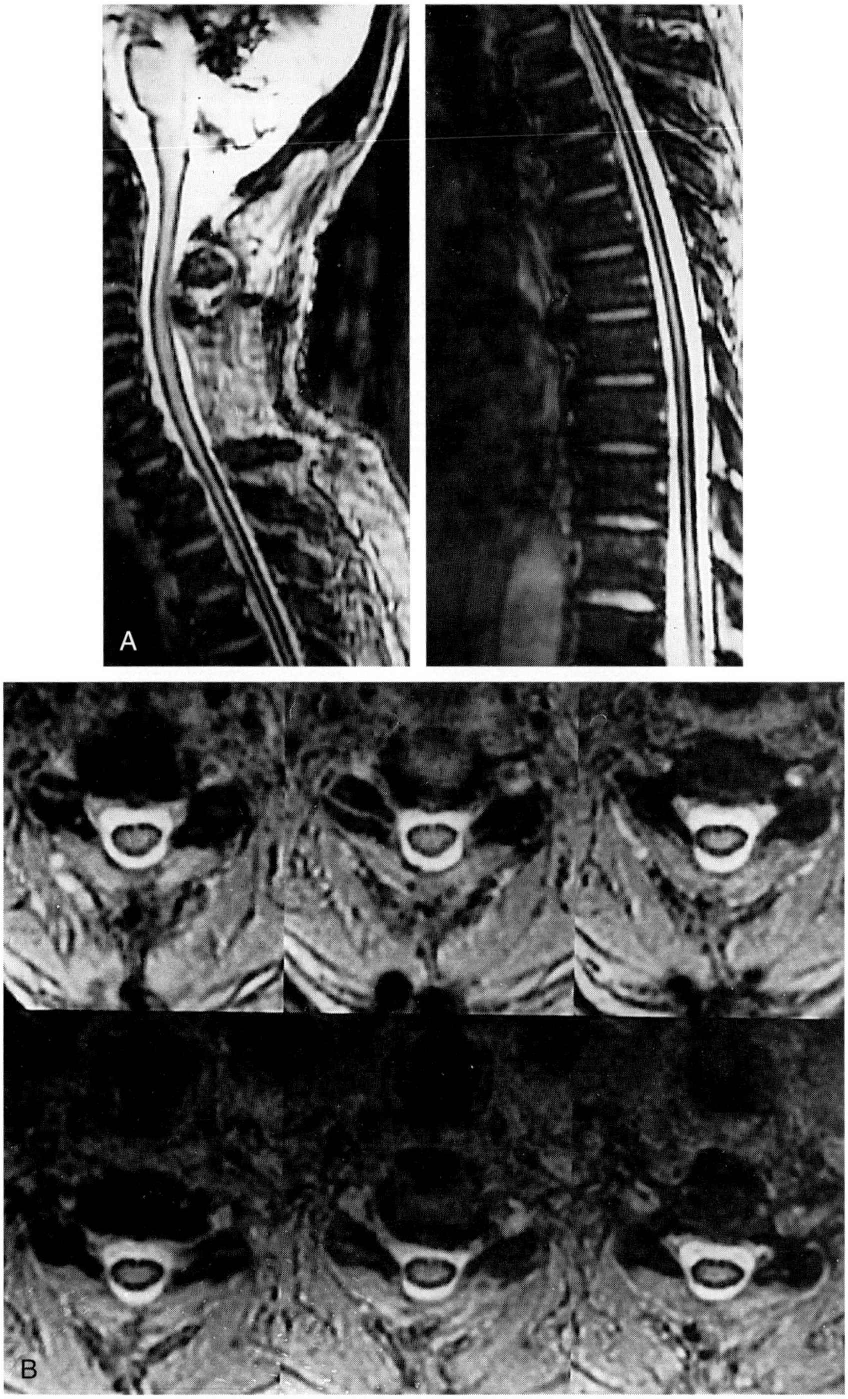

Figure 13–37. Superficial siderosis. Sagittal **(A)** and axial **(B)** T2-weighted GRE MRI shows marked hypointensity of the entire pial surface of spinal cord and brainstem. This is usually due to repeated episodes of subarachnoid hemorrhage.

RECOMMENDED READINGS

Conditions of Ligamentous Ossification

Miyasaka,K, Kaneda,K, Ito,T, et al. Ossification of Spinal Ligaments Causing Thoracic Radiculomyelopathy. *Radiology* 143:463–468, 1982.

Otake,S, Matsuo,M, Nishizawa,S, et al. Ossification of the Posterior Longitudinal Ligament: MR Evaluation. *AJNR* 13: 1059–1067, 1992.

Reinsel,TE, Andersson,GBJ. Ossification of the Posterior Longitudinal Ligament. *AJNR* 13:1068–1070, 1992.

Sugimura,H, Kakitsubata,Y, Suzuki,Y, et al. MRI of Ossification of Ligamentum Flavum. *J Comput Assist Tomogr* 16:73–76, 1992.

Rheumatoid Arthritis

Bundschuh,C, Modic,MT, Kearney,F, Morris,R, Deal,C. Rheumatoid Arthritis of the Cervical Spine: Surface-Coil MR Imaging. *AJR* 151:181–187, 1988.

Larsson,EM, Holtås,S, Zygmunt,S, Pre- and Postoperative MR Imaging of the Craniocervical Junction in Rheumatoid Arthritis. *AJR* 152:561–566, 1989.

Intervertebral Disc Disease

Brown,BM, Schwartz,RH, Frank,E, Blank,NK. Preoperative Evaluation of Cervical Radiculopathy and Myelopathy by Surface-Coil MR Imaging. *AJR* 151:1205–1212, 1988.

Czervionke,LF. Lumbar Intervertebral Disc Disease. *Neuroimaging Clin North Am* 3:465–484, 1993.

Enzman,DR. On Low Back Pain. *AJNR* 15:109–113, 1994.

Jensen,MC, Brant-Zawadski,MN, Obuchowski,N, et al. Magnetic Resonance Imaging of the Lumbar Spine in People without Back Pain. *N Engl J Med* 331:69–73, 1994.

Jinkins,JR, Whittemore,AR, Bradley,WG. The Anatomic Basis of Vertebrogenic Pain and the Autonomic Syndrome Associated with Lumbar Disk Extrusion. *AJR* 152:1277–1289, 1989.

Kieffer,SA, Sherry,RG, Wellenstein,DE, King,RB. Bulging Lumbar Intervertebral Disk: Myelographic Differentiation from Herniated Disc with Nerve Root Compression. *AJR* 138: 709–716, 1982.

Russell,EJ. Cervical Disk Disease. *Radiology* 177:313–325, 1990.

Takahashi,M, Shimomura,O, Sakae,T. Comparison of Magnetic Resonance Imaging with Myelography and Computed Tomography-Myelography in the Diagnosis of Lumbar Disc Herniation. *Neuroimaging Clin North Am* 3:487–498, 1993.

Thornbury,JR, Fryback,DG, Turski,PA, et al. Disk-caused Nerve Compression in Patients with Acute Low-Back Pain: Diagnosis with MR, CT Myelography, and Plain CT. *Radiology* 186:731–738, 1993.

Williams,AL, Haughton,VM, Daniels,DL, Grogan,JP. Differential CT Diagnosis of Extruded Nucleus Pulposus. *Radiology* 148:141–148, 1983.

Williams,AL, Haughton,VM, Meyer,GA, Ho,KC. Computed Tomographic Appearance of the Bulging Annulus. *Radiology* 142:403–408, 1982.

Cervical Spondylosis

Badami,JP, Norman,D, Barbaro,NM, et al. Metrizamide CT Myelography in Cervical Myelopathy and Radiculopathy: Correlation with Conventional Myelography and Surgical Findings. *AJR* 144:675–680, 1985.

Pavlov,H, Torg,JS, Robie,B, Jahre,C. Cervical Spinal Stenosis: Determination with Vertebral Body Ratio Method. *Radiology* 164:771–775, 1987.

Penning,L, Wilmink,JT, van Woerden,HH, Knol,E. CT Myelographic Findings in Degenerative Disorders of the Cervical Spine: Clinical Significance. *AJR* 146:793–801, 1986.

Resnick,D. Degenerative Diseases of the Vertebral Column. *Radiology* 156:3–14, 1985.

Takahashi,M, Yamashita,Y, Sakamoto,Y, Kojima,R. Chronic Cervical Cord Compression: Clinical Significance of Increased Signal Intensity on MR Images. *Radiology* 173:219–224, 1989.

Lumbar Stenosis

Grenier,N, Kressel,HY, Schiebler,ML, Grossman,RI, Dalinka, MK. Normal and Degenerative Posterior Spinal Structures: MR Imaging. *Radiology* 165:517–525, 1987.

Hacker,DA, Latchaw,RE, Yock,DH, et al. Redundant Lumbar Nerve Root Syndrome: Myelographic Features. *Radiology* 143:457–461, 1982.

Major,NM, Helms,CA. Central and Foraminal Stenosis of the Lumbar Spine. *Neuroimaging Clin North Am* 3:557–566, 1993.

McAfee,PC, Ullrich,CG, Levinsohn,EM, et al. Computed Tomography in Degenerative Lumbar Spinal Stenosis: The Value of Multiplanar Reconstruction. *Radiographics* 2:529–551, 1982.

Resnick,D. Degenerative Diseases of the Vertebral Column. *Radiology* 156:3–14, 1985.

Schellinger,D, Wener,L, Ragsdale,BD, Patronas,NJ. Facet Joint Disorders and Their Role in the Production of Back Pain and Sciatica. *Radiographics* 7:923–944, 1987.

Synovial Cyst

Jackson,DE, Atlas,SW, Mani,JR, Norman,D. Intraspinal Synovial Cysts: MR Imaging. *Radiology* 170:527–530, 1989.

Liu,SS, Williams,KD, Drayer,BP, Spetzler,RF, Sonntag,VKH. Synovial Cysts of the Lumbosacral Spine: Diagnosis by MR Imaging. *AJNR* 10:1239–1242, 1989. *AJR* 154:163–166, 1990.

Silbergleit,R, Gebarski,SS, Brunberg,JA, et al. Lumbar Synovial Cysts: Correlation of Myelographic, CT, MR, and Pathologic Findings. *AJNR* 11:777–779, 1990.

Postoperative Spine

Boden,SD, Davis,DO, Dina,TS, et al. Contrast-enhanced MR Imaging Performed after Successful Lumbar Disk Surgery: Prospective Study. *Radiology* 182:59–64, 1992.

Bundschuh,CV. Imaging of the Postoperative Lumbosacral Spine. *Neuroimaging Clin North Am* 3:499–516, 1993.

Dina,TS, Boden,SD, Davis,DO. Lumbar Spine After Surgery for Herniated Disk: Imaging Findings in the Early Postoperative Period. *AJR* 163:665–671, 1995.

Firooznia,H, Kricheff,II, Rafii,M, Golimbu,C. Lumbar Spine after Surgery: Examination with Intravenous Contrast-Enhanced CT. *Radiology* 163:221–226, 1987.

Mall,JC, Kaiser,JA. The Usual Appearance of the Postoperative Lumbar Spine. *Radiographics* 7:245–269, 1987.

Nerve Root Avulsion

Hashimoto,T, Mitomo,M, Hirabuki,N, et al. Nerve Root Avulsion of Birth Palsy: Comparison of Myelography with CT Myelography and Somatosensory Evoked Potential. *Radiology* 178: 841–845, 1991.

Volle,E, Assheuer,J, Hedde,JP, Gustor-Aeckerle,R. Radicular Avulsion Resulting from Spinal Injury: Assessment of Diagnostic Modalities. *Neuroradiology* 34:235–240, 1992.

Spinal Cord Injuries

Davis,PC, Reisner,A, Hudgins,PA, Davis,WE, O'Brien,MS. Spinal Injuries in Children: Role of MR. *AJNR* 14:607–617, 1993.

Flanders,AE, Schaefer,DM, Doan,HT, et al. Acute Cervical Spine Trauma: Correlation of MR Imaging Findings with Degree of Neurologic Deficit. *Radiology* 177:25–33, 1990.

Kulkarni,MV, Bondurant,FJ, Rose,SL, Narayana,PA. 1.5 Tesla

Magnetic Resonance Imaging of Acute Spinal Trauma. *Radiographics* 8:1059–1082, 1988.
Yamashita,Y, Takahashi,M, Matsuno,Y, et al. Chronic Injuries of the Spinal Cord: Assessment with MR Imaging. *Radiology* 175:849–854, 1990.

Hematoma

Avrahami,E, Tadmor,R, Feibel,M, Itzhak,Y. MR Demonstration of Spontaneous Acute Epidural Hematoma of the Thoracic Spine. *Neuroradiology* 31:89–92, 1989.
Friedman,DP, Flanders,AE, Tartaglino,LM. Vascular Neoplasms and Malformations, Ischemia, and Hemorrhage Affecting the Spinal Cord: MR Imaging Findings. *AJR* 162:685–692, 1994.
Gundry,CF, Heithoff,KB. Epidural Hematoma of the Lumbar Spine: 18 Surgically Confirmed Cases. *Radiology* 187: 427–431, 1993.
Laissy,JP, Milon,P, Freger,P, et al. Cervical Epidural Hematomas: CT Diagnosis in Two Cases That Resolved Spontaneously. *AJNR* 11:394–396, 1990.
Levy,JM. Spontaneous Lumbar Subdural Hematoma. *AJNR* 11:780–781, 1990.
Post,MJD, Becerra,JL, Madsen,PW, et al. Acute Spinal Subdural Hematoma: MR and CT Findings with Pathologic Correlates. *AJNR* 15:1895–1905, 1994.

Index

Note: Page numbers in *italics* refer to illustrations; page numbers followed by t refer to tables.

ISBN 0-7216-4219-5

90038

9 780721 642192